RADIOLOGY

SECRETS

RADIOLOGY

SECRETS

Second Edition

E. Scott Pretorius, MD
Associate Chairman for Education
Residency Program Training Director
Department of Radiology
Hospital of the University of Pennsylvania
Philadelphia, Pennsylvania

Jeffrey A. Solomon, MD, MBA
Assistant Professor
Interventional Radiology Section
Department of Radiology
Hospital of the University of Pennsylvania
Philadelphia, Pennsylvania

ELSEVIER
MOSBY

ELSEVIER
MOSBY

1600 John F. Kennedy Boulevard, Suite 1800
Philadelphia, PA 19103-2899

Radiology Secrets
Second Edition

ISBN: 0-323-03405-5

NOTICE

Knowledge and best practice in this field are constantly changing. As new research and experience broaden our knowledge, changes in practice, treatment and drug therapy may become necessary or appropriate. Readers are advised to check the most current information provided (i) on procedures featured or (ii) by the manufacturer of each product to be administered, to verify the recommended dose or formula, the method and duration of administration, and contraindications. It is the responsibility of the practitioner, relying on his or her own experience and knowledge of the patient, to make diagnoses, to determine dosages and the best treatment for each individual patient, and to take all appropriate safety precautions. To the fullest extent of the law, neither the Publisher nor the Editor assumes any liability for any injury and/or damage to persons or property arising out or related to any use of the material contained in this book.

Previous edition copyrighted 1998.

International Standard Book Number 0-323-03405-5

Vice President, Medical Education: Linda Belfus
Developmental Editor: Stan Ward
Senior Project Manager: Cecelia Bayruns
Marketing Manager: Kate Rubin

Printed in China.

Last digit is the print number: 9   8   7   6   5   4   3   2   1

DEDICATION

To our pets....

Zac, Brady, and Fox Pretorius
Grady, Tonka, and Gypsy Solomon

....and our parents

Jack and Ruth Solomon
Keith and Merry Pretorius

CONTENTS

XI. THORACIC RADIOLOGY

XII. ULTRASONOGRAPHY

XIII. DIAGNOSTIC RADIOLOGY AS A PROFESSION

CONTRIBUTORS

Linda J. Bagley, MD
Associate Professor, Department of Radiology, Neuroradiology Section, Hospital of the University of Pennsylvania, Philadelphia, Pennsylvania

Richard D. Bellah, MD
Associate Professor of Radiology and Pediatrics, University of Pennsylvania School of Medicine; Department of Radiology, Children's Hospital of Philadelphia, Philadelphia, Pennsylvania

Judy S. Blebea, MD
Associate Professor of Clinical Radiology, Department of Radiology, Hospital of the University of Pennsylvania, Philadelphia, Pennsylvania

William W. Boonn, MD
Resident, Department of Radiology, Hospital of the University of Pennsylvania, Philadelphia, Pennsylvania

Kerry Bron, MD
Department of Radiology, Hospital of the University of Pennsylvania, Philadelphia, Pennsylvania

Sridhar R. Charagundla, MD, PhD
Assistant Professor of Radiology, Magnetic Resonance Imaging and Cardiovascular Sections, Department of Radiology, Hospital of the University of Pennsylvania, Philadelphia, Pennsylvania

Sara C. Chen, MD
Department of Radiology, Hospital of the University of Pennsylvania, Philadelphia, Pennsylvania

Beverly G. Coleman, MD, FACR
Professor of Radiology and Associate Chair for Body Imaging; Ultrasound Section Chief, Department of Radiology, Hospital of the University of Pennsylvania, Philadelphia, Pennsylvania

Keith A. Ferguson, MD
Fellow in Body Imaging, Department of Radiology, Hospital of the University of Pennsylvania, Philadelphia, Pennsylvania

Jeffrey Scott Friedenberg, MD
Fellow in Body Imaging, Department of Radiology, Hospital of the University of Pennsylvania, Philadelphia, Pennsylvania

Gregory Goodworth, MD
Department of Radiology, Hospital of the University of Pennsylvania, Philadelphia, Pennsylvania

Andrew Gordon, MD
Department of Radiology, Hospital of the University of Pennsylvania, Philadelphia, Pennsylvania

Susan Hilton, MD
Clinical Professor of Radiology, CT Section Co-Chief, Department of Radiology, Hospital of the University of Pennsylvania, Philadelphia, Pennsylvania

Wendy C. Hsu, MD
Department of Radiology, Hospital of the University of Pennsylvania, Philadelphia, Pennsylvania

Maxim Itkin, MD
Assistant Professor of Interventional Radiology, Department of Radiology, Hospital of the University of Pennsylvania, Philadelphia, Pennsylvania

Saurabh Jha, MBBS
Department of Radiology, Hospital of the University of Pennsylvania, Philadelphia, Pennsylvania

Lisa Jones, MD, PhD
Department of Radiology, Hospital of the University of Pennsylvania, Philadelphia, Pennsylvania

Andrew J. Kapustin, MD
Fellow in Cardiovascular Imaging, Department of Radiology, Hospital of the University of Pennsylvania, Philadelphia, Pennsylvania

Woojin Kim, MD
Department of Radiology, Hospital of the University of Pennsylvania, Philadelphia, Pennsylvania

Charles T. Lau, MD
Department of Radiology, Hospital of the University of Pennsylvania, Philadelphia, Pennsylvania

Harold I. Litt, MD, PhD
Assistant Professor, Department of Radiology; Section Chief, Cardiovascular Imaging, Hospital of the University of Pennsylvania, Philadelphia, Pennsylvania

Laurie A. Loevner, MD
Professor of Radiology, Neuroradiology Section, Department of Radiology, Hospital of the University of Pennsylvania, Philadelphia, Pennsylvania

Gautham Mallampati, MD
Fellow in Magnetic Resonance Imaging, Department of Radiology, Hospital of the University of Pennsylvania, Philadelphia, Pennsylvania

Wallace T. Miller, Jr., MD
Associate Professor, Department of Radiology, Thoracic Imaging Section, Hospital of the University of Pennsylvania, Philadelphia, Pennsylvania

Jeffrey I. Mondschein, MD
Assistant Professor, Department of Radiology, Interventional Radiology Section, Hospital of the University of Pennsylvania, Philadelphia, Pennsylvania

D. Andrew Mong, MD
Assistant Professor of Pediatric Radiology, Department of Radiology, Hospital of the University of Pennsylvania, Philadelphia, Pennsylvania

Gul Moonis, MD
Assistant Professor, Department of Radiology, Neuroradiology Section, Hospital of the University of Pennsylvania, Philadelphia, Pennsylvania

Andrew Newberg, MD
Assistant Professor of Radiology, Nuclear Medicine Section, Department of Radiology, Hospital of the University of Pennsylvania, Philadelphia, Pennsylvania

Linda Kulzer Petrovich, MD
Fellow in Magnetic Resonance Imaging, Department of Radiology, Hospital of the University of Pennsylvania, Philadelphia, Pennsylvania

Avrum N. Pollock, MD, FRCPC
Director of Residency and Fellowship Programs, Department of Radiology, Division of Neuroradiology, Children's Hospital of Philadelphia, Philadelphia, Pennsylvania

E. Scott Pretorius, MD
Associate Chairman for Education, Residency Program Training Director, Department of Radiology, Hospital of the University of Pennsylvania, Philadelphia, Pennsylvania

Parvati Ramchandani, MD
Professor, Department of Radiology, Hospital of the University of Pennsylvania, Philadelphia, Pennsylvania

Neil Roach, MD
Assistant Professor, Department of Radiology, Musculoskeletal Section, Hospital of the University of Pennsylvania, Philadelphia, Pennsylvania

Mark Rosen, MD, PhD
Assistant Professor of Radiology, Magnetic Resonance Imaging and Cardiovascular Sections, Department of Radiology, Hospital of the University of Pennsylvania, Philadelphia, Pennsylvania

Susan E. Rowling, MD
Assistant Professor of Clinical Radiology, Ultrasound Section, Department of Radiology, Hospital of the University of Pennsylvania, Philadelphia, Pennsylvania

Stephen E. Rubesin, MD
Professor of Radiology, University of Pennsylvania School of Medicine; Department of Radiology, Hospital of the University of Pennsylvania, Philadelphia, Pennsylvania

Daniel Saurborn, MD
Fellow in Musculoskeletal Radiology, Department of Radiology, Hospital of the University of Pennsylvania, Philadelphia, Pennsylvania

Mary Scanlon, MD
Associate Professor of Clinical Radiology, Department of Radiology, Hospital of the University of Pennsylvania, Philadelphia, Pennsylvania

Milan Sheth, MD
Fellow in Thoracic Imaging, Department of Radiology, Hospital of the University of Pennsylvania, Philadelphia, Pennsylvania

Evan S. Siegelman, MD
Associate Professor, Department of Radiology; Section Chief, Magnetic Resonance Imaging, Hospital of the University of Pennsylvania, Philadelphia, Pennsylvania

Ross I. Silver, MD
Department of Radiology, Hospital of the University of Pennsylvania, Philadelphia, Pennsylvania

Jeffrey A. Solomon, MD, MBA
Assistant Professor, Interventional Radiology Section, Department of Radiology, Hospital of the University of Pennsylvania, Philadelphia, Pennsylvania

S. William Stavropoulos, MD
Assistant Professor, Department of Radiology, Interventional Radiology Section, Hospital of the University of Pennsylvania, Philadelphia, Pennsylvania

Drew A. Torigian, MD
Assistant Professor, Department of Radiology, Hospital of the University of Pennsylvania, Philadelphia, Pennsylvania

Susan P. Weinstein, MD
Assistant Professor, Department of Radiology, Breast Imaging Section, Hospital of the University of Pennsylvania, Philadelphia, Pennsylvania

Denise S. White, DO
Fellow in Body Imaging, Department of Radiology, Hospital of the University of Pennsylvania, Philadelphia, Pennsylvania

Courtney Woodfield, MD
Department of Radiology, Hospital of the University of Pennsylvania, Philadelphia, Pennsylvania

Christopher J. Yoo, MD
Fellow in Body Imaging, Department of Radiology, Hospital of the University of Pennsylvania, Philadelphia, Pennsylvania

Hanna M. Zafar, MD, MHS
Department of Radiology, Hospital of the University of Pennsylvania, Philadelphia, Pennsylvania

PREFACE

We both came to Penn Radiology in 1995 to be first-year residents at the University of Pennsylvania. Throughout our residencies and our preparation for our radiology board examinations, we yearned for a book that contained what we "really" needed to know, a book that neatly distilled the most important points from each subspecialty of radiology.

Sadly, we never found such a book. That, however, is exactly what we have sought to create: an eminently practical book that touches on all of the "high points" of each of radiology's subspecialties. To the extent that we have succeeded, we are indebted to our co-authors and to our many students, residents, and fellows. This book was written for you.

E. Scott Pretorius, MD
Jeffrey A. Solomon, MD, MBA

TOP 100 SECRETS

These secrets are 100 of the top board alerts. They summarize the concepts, principles, and most salient details of radiology.

1. Increasing voltage (kV) decreases contrast and increases exposure, making the film darker. Increasing milliampere-seconds (mAs) increases exposure, making the film darker.

2. A scout film should always be obtained before performing a fluoroscopy study with contrast. It allows the radiologist to determine whether an object that appears "white" on a radiograph is bone or metal versus contrast (the latter would not be on the scout film).

3. Structures in the body that are very dense (such as those that contain calcium) attenuate a large amount of the x-ray beam; thus the x-ray beam is not able to reach the film and darken it, and such structures appear white on a radiograph. Conversely, structures that are not very dense (such as air) allow the x-ray beam to penetrate and darken the film; thus such structures appear black.

4. Regions with many acoustic interfaces reflect a lot of sound back to the transducer. These are termed *echogenic* or *hyperechoic* and by convention are viewed as bright areas on ultrasound (US). Regions with few acoustic interfaces do not reflect many sound waves; they are termed *hypoechoic* and are viewed as dark areas.

5. Electron-dense structures, such as metal and bone, stop a large number of x-rays and therefore are bright on computed tomography (CT). Lower electron-density regions, such as air or fat, stop very few x-rays and are rendered as dark. Since CT images are created with x-rays, the same things that are bright and dark on plain films are bright and dark on CT.

6. T1-weighted images have a short "time to repetition" (TR) (less than 1000 ms) and a short "time to echo" (TE) (less than 20 ms). T2-weighted images have a long TR (more than 2000 ms) and a long TE (more than 40 ms).

7. To differentiate between T1- and T2-weighted images, look for simple fluid. Fluid tends to be hyperintense to virtually everything else on T2-weighted images. On T1-weighted images, fluid is of low intermediate signal. Good places to look for fluid include the urinary bladder and the cerebral spinal fluid (CSF).

8. Nuclear medicine is unique in that its strength lies in portraying the functional status of an organ rather than producing images that are predominantly anatomic in content.

9. In nuclear medicine studies, the radiologist administers a radioactive atom, either alone or coupled to a molecule, that is known to target a certain organ or organs. Its distribution is then examined to determine any pathologic condition in that particular organ.

10. PACS stands for *picture archiving and communication systems*. These are the systems used by digital radiology departments to store, network, and view imaging studies.

11. RIS stands for the *radiology information system*. The RIS manages patient scheduling and tracking, examination billing, and receipt/display of radiology reports.

12. The American College of Radiology recommends that women begin getting mammograms at age 40 and annually thereafter.

13. The BIRADS (Breast Imaging Reporting and Dictation System) lexicon was developed by the American College of Radiology to provide a clear and concise way to report mammographic results: 1 = normal, 2 = benign finding, 3 = probably benign finding (6-month follow-up mammogram recommended), 4 = suspicious finding (biopsy recommended), 5 = high likelihood of malignancy (biopsy recommended), and 6 = confirmed malignancy.

14. Breast US is useful in characterizing palpable masses or mammographically detected masses as cystic or solid. Findings in a solid lesion that are suspicious for malignancy include a hypoechoic appearance, with posterior acoustic shadowing, angular margins, spiculations, microlobulations, lesion morphology "taller" than "wide," and ductal extension of the mass.

15. Breast magnetic resonance imaging (MRI) findings suspicious for malignancy in an enhancing lesion include avid arterial phase enhancement, washout of contrast in a delayed phase, spiculated or microlobulated margins, greater enhancement peripherally than centrally, and architectural distortion.

16. Anomalous origin of the coronary arteries occurs rarely (about 1% of cardiac catheterizations). Sudden death is associated with a left main coronary artery that arises from the right sinus (particularly when the artery courses between the aorta and pulmonary artery), a right coronary artery that arises from the left sinus, and a single coronary artery. The left main coronary artery may also arise from the pulmonary trunk; this anomaly tends to present earlier, with congestive heart failure or sudden death.

17. Aortic dissections that involve the ascending aorta are surgical emergencies because the mortality rate is significantly greater in medically managed patients (approximately 90% in the first 3 months) compared with surgically treated patients. This high mortality rate is mostly due to hemopericardium, causing tamponade; acute aortic regurgitation; or involvement of coronary artery origins, causing myocardial infarction. Descending aortic dissections are usually treated medically with antihypertensive agents.

18. The most specific finding of a pulmonary embolus is a partial or complete intraluminal filling defect in a pulmonary artery. On CT angiography (CTA), the filling defect should be present on at least two contiguous sections. Abrupt cut-off of the artery also indicates a pulmonary embolus.

19. A stenosis is generally considered significant if the luminal diameter is reduced by 50% and the systolic pressure gradient is in excess of 10 mmHg across the lesion. A vessel lumen that is diminished by 50% will have a corresponding 75% reduction in a cross-sectional area, which will likely reduce flow to a clinically significant level.

20. Contraindications to barium studies of the upper gastrointestinal (GI) tract include known or suspected perforation (use water-soluble agent) and the inability of the patient to swallow (use nasogastric tube).

21. Focal hepatic lesions with T1 components that are isointense to mildly hyperintense to the surrounding liver are almost always hepatocellular in origin.

22. Almost all hepatic cysts and hemangiomas can be differentiated from malignant liver disease by the use of heavily T2-weighted (>180 msec) images.

23. On postcontrast images, the normal spleen displays alternating bands of high and low attenuation (CT) or signal (MR) in the arterial phase. The spleen appears more homogeneous in a more delayed phase.

24. Splenic laceration can be differentiated from developmental splenic cleft. Patients with laceration will have a trauma history, display a low attenuation defect with sharp edges, and have perisplenic hemoperitoneum.

25. Both MRI and CT are less specific in the characterization of splenic lesions than they are in characterization of liver, adrenal, or renal lesions.

26. The pseudocyst is the most common cystic lesion of the pancreas, accounting for about 90% of all cystic lesions in the pancreas.

27. The pancreatic neck and body are the most common portions of this organ to be injured in blunt trauma because they are compressed against the spine in blunt traumatic injuries to the abdomen.

28. The most specific CT imaging finding of acute appendicitis is an abnormal appendix that is typically dilated ≥6 mm and fluid filled. A calcified appendicolith with periappendiceal fat stranding is another highly specific CT finding.

29. If bowel ischemia is suspected on CT, one should assess the patency of the celiac artery, superior mesenteric artery, inferior mesenteric artery, portal vein, superior mesenteric vein, and inferior mesenteric vein. When the central superior mesenteric vessels are affected, the entire small bowel, along with the large bowel proximal to the distal third of the transverse colon, tend to be affected. When the central inferior mesenteric vessels are affected, the distal third of the transverse colon, the descending colon, and the sigmoid colon are generally involved.

30. A fixed filling defect in the urinary collecting system is highly suggestive of transitional cell carcinoma (TCC) and should be further evaluated with brush biopsy.

31. In a male patient with pelvic trauma, the urethra should be evaluated with a retrograde urethrogram before placement of a bladder drainage catheter.

32. An enhancing renal mass that does not contain macroscopic fat is a renal cell carcinoma until proven otherwise.

33. An enhancing renal lesion with macroscopic fat is a benign angiomyolipoma.

34. Cystic renal lesions that contain thick internal septations, thick mural calcification, or enhancing mural nodules are suggestive of cystic renal cell carcinomas and should be excised.

35. Patients with limited renal function (creatinine 1.5 and greater) generally should not receive iodinated intravenous contrast for CT. Gadolinium chelate contrast agents used for MRI are generally safe for these patients.

36. There are three ways to show that an adrenal lesion is a benign adenoma: attenuation of less than 10 HU on unenhanced CT, washout of greater than 50% on delayed CT, or signal loss of 10–15% on chemical shift MRI.

37. Most pheochromocytomas occur in the adrenal glands and enhance avidly on CT and MRI.

38. In premenopausal women, since the normal dominant follicles can range up to 3 cm (or sometimes greater), simple ovarian cysts smaller than 3 cm need no follow-up and typically resolve spontaneously.

39. MRI can generally distinguish between septate and bicornuate uteri. A septate uterus will have a smooth outer contour and a fibrous septum. A bicornuate uterus will display a depression, 1 cm or greater of the outer contour of the fundus, and a thicker, more muscular septum.

40. Most intratesticular masses are malignant. Most extratesticular masses are benign.

41. The following equipment should be present when administering conscious sedations: pharmacologic antagonists, appropriate equipment to establish airway and provide positive pressure ventilation, supplemental oxygen, and defibrillator.

42. Inferior vena cava (IVC) filters should be placed below the lowest renal vein when possible.

43. Embolization on both sides of a pseudoaneurysm, aneurysm, or arteriovenous (AV) fistula is necessary to prevent reconstitution of flow via collaterals, which causes recurrence of the lesion.

44. The two most common indication for placement of a transjugular intrahepatic portosystemic shunt (TIPS) are variceal bleeding related to portal hypertension that is refractory to endoscopic therapy or for ascites refractory to medical management. TIPS placement may act as an effective bridge to liver transplantation for patients with end-stage liver disease and the manifestations of portal hypertension.

45. There is high association between Segond fracture and anterior cruciate ligament (ACL) tear and meniscal injury.

46. When you see a fracture of the medial malleolus, do not forget to look at the proximal fibula for Maisonneuve fracture.

47. On a cervical spine radiograph, if you cannot visualize the lower cervical spine, obtain either a swimmer's view or CT. You must visualize C7–T1 to "clear" the cervical spine.

48. Osteoporosis has many secondary causes. Medical evaluation for multiple myeloma and endocrine diseases should be performed before one assumes primary osteoporosis.

49. If you see multiple lytic bone lesions in an adult, think of metastatic disease versus multiple myeloma. Primary tumors to consider in a patient with metastatic bone lesions are lung, prostate, breast, kidney, thyroid, and colorectal.

50. Patients with an osteoid osteoma classically present with pain at night relieved by aspirin.

51. Primary bone tumors that are known to occur in the epiphyseal region include giant cell tumor, chondroblastoma, and clear cell chondrosarcoma.

52. Rotator cuff tears are rare in persons younger than 40 years, except in athletes or in the setting of trauma.

53. MRI is the most sensitive modality for detection of early osteonecrosis, before femoral head cortical collapse. Early detection allows for possible joint-sparing therapies such as steroid reduction, supportive therapies such as non–weight-bearing, and core decompression.

54. A meniscal tear is diagnosed on MRI by identifying increased internal meniscal signal intensity that extends to the articular surface.

55. After the Achilles tendon, the next most likely ankle tendon to tear is the posterior tibial tendon (PTT).

56. The anterior talofibular ligament, part of the lateral ligamentous complex, is the most commonly sprained and torn ankle ligament.

57. Early plain film findings of osteomyelitis include soft tissue swelling and blurred fascial planes. After 7–10 days, bone lucencies and periosteal reaction may be seen. On MRI, bone infection generally is depicted as a region of abnormal marrow signal, which is T1 hypointense and short-tau inversion recovery (STIR) hyperintense to normal marrow.

58. Epidural hematoma is a surgical emergency. It is usually caused by an arterial injury (most commonly the middle meningeal artery), often associated with temporal bone fracture, confined by the lateral sutures, and usually lenticular in shape. Subdural hematoma is usually caused by injury to the bridging cortical veins, is not confined by the lateral sutures, and is usually crescentic in shape.

59. The differential diagnosis of an intracranial mass in a patient with HIV includes toxoplasmosis, other brain abscess, and lymphoma. Progressive multifocal leukoencephalopathy, a demyelinating disease, can sometimes appear masslike.

60. Head CT is often normal in acute stroke. The earliest sign (within 6 hours) of an acute infarct on CT is loss of the gray-white differentiation with obscuration of the lateral lentiform nucleus. Acute ischemic changes can be seen within minutes of onset of the ictus on diffusion-weighted MRI.

61. C8 is a nerve root without a body. It exits between C7 and T1. As a result, cervical nerve roots exit *above* the pedicles of the same-numbered body; thoracic and lumbar nerve roots exit *below* the pedicles of the same-numbered body.

62. One should be consistent in describing spinal degenerative disc disease. A disc bulge is a diffuse, symmetric extension of the disc beyond the end plate. A disc protrusion is a more focal extension of the disc in which the "neck" is wider than the more distal portion. A disc herniation is an extrusion of a portion of the disc in which the "neck" is the narrowest part. A disc sequestrum is a free disc fragment in the epidural space that has lost connection to the disc.

63. Inflammatory and vascular disorders of the spinal cord may mimic neoplasms.

64. Low density in a lymph node in an adult with head and neck cancer is characteristic of metastatic disease until proven otherwise.

65. The parotid glands are the only salivary glands that contain lymph nodes.

66. Neck lesions above the hyoid bone should be studied first with MRI. Pathologic findings of the neck below the hyoid bone should be primarily imaged with CT scanning.

67. CT is the imaging modality of choice for conductive hearing loss. MRI is the imaging modality of choice in adult-onset sensorineural hearing loss.

68. Tumors and other lesions within the spinal canal may be classified as *extradural* (outside the thecal sac), *intradural-extramedullary* (inside the thecal sac, but outside the cord), or *intramedullary* (inside the cord). Making this determination is the first step to selecting the correct differential diagnosis for a lesion.

69. Fluorodeoxyglucose (FDG) positron emission tomography (PET) changes the surgical management of patients in up to 40% of cases. In some cases, distant metastases or restaging indicates that the cancer is inoperable, thus preventing surgery that would have not been useful. In as many as 20% of patients, PET shows that enlarged nodes that may have prevented surgery from being considered were actually benign, so that surgery can be performed.

70. A "superscan" on bone scan implies that so much of the methylene diphosphate (MDP) is taken up by the bones that there is no significant excretion in the kidneys and bladder or uptake in the soft tissues. In a patient with cancer, a "superscan" implies widespread osseous metastases that cannot be individually distinguished but rather occupy almost the entire skeleton.

71. To classify a ventilation-perfusion (V/Q) scan as a "high probability" for pulmonary embolism (PE), the scan must have the equivalent of two or more large segmental perfusion defects (75–100% involvement of the segment) that are not matched by ventilatory abnormalities. Four or more moderately sized perfusion defects (25–75% involvement of the segment) would also represent a high probability for PE. The implication of a high probability scan suggests a greater than 80% chance of having a PE.

72. Younger male patients with "cold" thyroid nodules are more likely to have cancer than are older female patients with similar findings. Exposure of the neck to radiation is also an important risk factor for cancer in a cold nodule. Finally, US findings of mixed cystic and solid components within a cold nodule are also more suggestive of thyroid cancer. Cold nodules in the setting of a multinodular goiter are substantially less likely to be cancer than other cold nodules.

73. After renal transplantation, acute tubular necrosis (ATN) occurs almost immediately, whereas chronic rejection occurs over several days to weeks or even longer. Patients with ATN have normal or only slightly diminished perfusion of the kidney with a delayed cortical transit time (how long it takes for urine to appear in the collecting system). Rejection usually is associated with diminished flow with mildly impaired cortical function.

74. An exercise stress test should be stopped when (1) the patient cannot continue because of dyspnea, chest pain, fatigue, or musculoskeletal problems; (2) the patient has a hypertensive response; (3) the patient develops ST segment depressions of greater than 3 mm; (4) the patient has ST segment elevation, heralding a possible myocardial infarction; or (5) the patient experiences the onset of a potentially dangerous arrhythmia such as ventricular tachycardia, ventricular fibrillation, very rapid supraventricular tachycardia, or heart block.

75. A right-sided arch is associated with both tetralogy of Fallot (TOF) and truncus arteriosus (TA), but is more closely associated with TA. Since TOF is more common, however, you are more likely to see a right-sided arch with TOF.

76. Thickened aryepiglottic folds with a thickened epiglottis are indicative of epiglottitis and warrant emergent intubation.

77. If you suspect an aspirated foreign body, you should order bilateral lateral decubitus films. A normal lung will lose volume, whereas an obstructed lung will remain lucent and inflated.

78. The double-bubble sign on plain films represents an air- or fluid-filled distended stomach and duodenal bulb. It is seen in malrotation, duodenal atresia, and jejunal atresia.

79. A fleck of calcium in a normal-sized globe of a child younger than 6 years is characteristic of retinoblastoma until proven otherwise.

80. In a pediatric elbow, the medial epicondyle ossification center appears before the trochlear ossification center. If you see an ossific density in the region of the trochlea in the absence of a medial epicondylar ossification center, this is an avulsed fragment.

81. Metaphyseal corner fractures are highly sensitive and specific for child abuse.

82. The most common cause of death of an abused child is injury to the central nervous system.

83. If a pulmonary infiltrate does not resolve over time despite treatment with antimicrobial agents, be suspicious of a potential bronchoalveolar cell subtype of lung carcinoma.

84. Interstitial pulmonary edema, usually due to congestive heart failure, is the most common interstitial abnormality encountered in daily practice.

85. The majority of patients with asymptomatic mediastinal tumors have benign tumors, whereas the majority of patients with symptomatic mediastinal tumors have malignant tumors.

86. If you see a pneumothorax on chest radiography that is associated with contralateral mediastinal shift and inferior displacement of the ipsilateral hemidiaphragm, immediately notify the physician caring for the patient because a tension pneumothorax may be present. This requires emergent treatment to prevent rapid death.

87. If you see focal ovoid lucency surrounding an endotracheal tube (ETT) or a tracheostomy tube with an associated bulge in the adjacent tracheal walls, suspect overinflation of the cuff and notify the clinical staff immediately.

88. If a nasogastric, orogastric, or feeding tube is seen to extend into a distal bronchus, lung, or pleural space, notify the clinical staff immediately and suggest that tube removal be performed only after a thoracostomy tube set is at the bedside in case a significant pneumothorax develops.

89. When air embolism is suspected during line placement or use, the patient should immediately be placed in the left lateral position to keep the air trapped in the right heart chambers, supplemental oxygen should be administered, and vital signs should be monitored.

90. In a normal early pregnancy, the yolk sac should be visible sonographically by a mean gestational sac diameter of 8 mm transvaginally and 20 mm transabdominally. Similarly, an embryo should be visible sonographically by a mean gestational sac diameter of 16 mm transvaginally and 25 mm transabdominally.

91. If a pregnant patient presents with vaginal bleeding, pelvic pain, and uterine tenderness, placental abruption must be excluded.

92. The most dreaded complication of oligohydramnios is pulmonary hypoplasia.

93. Omphalocele has a worse prognosis than gastroschisis because the former is associated with an increased incidence of chromosomal abnormalities leading to other structural abnormalities.

94. Most strokes are due to emboli rather than carotid stenosis. Therefore, it is important to identify irregular atherosclerotic surfaces when examining the carotid circulation.

95. Sonographic findings in early or uncomplicated acute cholecystitis may include gallstones (which may be impacted in the gallbladder neck or cystic duct), gallbladder wall thickening, and gallbladder distention. A sonographic Murphy's sign (focal tenderness over the gallbladder when compressed by the US transducer) may also be elicited.

96. The combination of gallstones and a sonographic Murphy's sign has a positive predictive value of 92% and a negative predictive value of 95% for acute cholecystitis.

97. For a physician to be found liable for malpractice, the following four things must be demonstrated: (1) establishment of a duty of care (i.e., doctor-patient relationship); (2) breach of the duty of care, or negligence; (3) adverse outcome with injury or harm; and (4) direct causality between the negligence and outcome.

98. The three most common reasons radiologists get sued are failure of diagnosis, failure to communicate findings in an appropriate and timely manner, and failure to suggest the next appropriate procedure.

99. To become board-certified in diagnostic radiology, you must pass the written and oral examinations of the American Board of Radiology (www.theabr.org). The written examination consists of a physics portion and a clinical portion. You may take the physics portion in your second, third, or fourth year of radiology training. The clinical written portion is taken in the fall of the fourth year, and the oral examination is taken in Louisville, Ky., in June of the fourth year of residency.

100. The only thing worse than going to Louisville is going back to Louisville.

I. INTRODUCTION TO IMAGING MODALITIES

INTRODUCTION TO PLAIN FILM RADIOGRAPHY AND FLUOROSCOPY

Linda Kulzer Petrovich, MD, and E. Scott Pretorius, MD

CHAPTER 1

PLAIN FILM RADIOGRAPHY

1. **How do diagnostic x-rays differ from other kinds of electromagnetic radiation?**
    X-rays have higher frequencies and shorter wavelengths than visible light, microwaves, and radiowaves. Diagnostic x-rays typically have energies between 20 and 150 keV. Gamma rays, which are emitted by many agents used in nuclear medicine, have even higher frequencies and shorter wavelengths than x-rays.

2. **What are the components of an x-ray tube?**
    An x-ray tube contains a negatively charged cathode and a positively charged anode. The cathode contains a filament (usually made of coiled tungsten wire) that is the source of electrons. The electrons are accelerated toward the anode. The anode contains the target (most commonly made of tungsten), where x-rays are produced.

3. **How are diagnostic x-rays produced?**
    In an x-ray tube, x-rays are produced when an energetic electron passes close to an atomic nucleus in the anode of the x-ray tube. The attractive force of the positively charged nucleus causes the electron to change direction and lose energy. The energy difference between the initial energy of the electron and the energy of the electron after it changes direction is released as an x-ray photon. This process is called *bremsstrahlung*, which means "braking radiation" in German.

4. **What happens to most of the energy entering the x-ray tube?**
    Most (99%) of the electrical energy entering the tube is converted to heat, and tube heating is often the limiting factor in how much the x-ray tube can be used. About 1% of the electrical energy entering the tube is converted to x-rays.

5. **What are the key parameters that can be manipulated on an x-ray generator?**
    The voltage across the x-ray tube (measured in kilovolts [kV]), the current flowing through the x-ray tube (measured in milliamperes [mA]), and the exposure time (measured in milliseconds [ms]). Current and exposure time can be combined and expressed in milliampere-seconds (mAs).

6. **What happens if kV is increased?**
    X-ray penetration increases, exposure increases (darker film), and contrast goes down. The maximum energy of the x-rays produced is increased. Film contrast is primarily dependent on kV.

7. **What happens if mAs is increased?**
    Increasing mAs means increased film exposure (more x-rays produced), which darkens the film. The maximum energy of the x-rays produced is not changed.

8. **How are plain film radiographs generated?**
The patient is placed between an x-ray tube and a film cassette. The x-ray tube produces x-rays that pass through the human body and are attenuated by interaction with body tissues. The film cassette contains film that is adjacent to fluorescent screens. When the x-rays reach the film cassette, a photochemical interaction occurs between the x-rays and the screen coated with fluorescent particles. The x-rays activate the fluorescent particles to emit light rays. The light rays expose the photographic film, and an image is produced.

9. **What are collimators, grids, and screens? Where are they?**
From the x-ray tube, x-rays pass through a collimator, which consists of lead sheets (Fig. 1-1). Collimators narrow the x-ray beam. X-rays travel through air to the patient and then through a grid, which consists of narrow lead strips separated by plastic. The grid allows passage of x-rays that have passed directly through the patient (and therefore contain useful information) and stops scattered x-rays, which would only contribute to noise and decreased contrast. After passing through the grid, x-rays penetrate the film cassette, which, in standard dual-screen systems, includes an intensifying screen, then the film, and a second intensifying screen. The screens absorb the x-ray photons and emit visible light. The light exposes the film.

Figure 1-1. Apparatus for film/screen radiography.

10. **What is the inverse square law?**
The intensity of the x-ray beam decreases with the square of the distance from the x-ray tube. In other words, if one doubles the distance between oneself and the x-ray tube, x-ray exposure decreases by a factor of 4. This concept is important in determining x-ray exposure and absorbed dose.

11. **What are the advantages and disadvantages of a small focal spot?**
The focal spot is the source of x-rays in the tube. Smaller focal spots produce sharper images, but larger focal spots can tolerate greater amounts of heat. As such, small focal spots are used for mammography (which has few exposures, but very sharp images are required). Large focal spots are used in fluoroscopy (for continuous exposure, but lesser resolution). Regular diagnostic x-rays use focal spot sizes between those used for mammography and fluoroscopy.

12. **What are the five basic densities seen on an x-ray? How do they appear?**
Air, fat, soft tissue, bone, and metal. Air attenuates very little of the x-ray beam, allowing nearly the full force of the beam to darken the film. Thus, air appears black. Bone and metals attenuate a large proportion of the x-ray beam, allowing very little radiation through to blacken the film. Thus, bone and metallic objects appear white on radiographs. Fat and soft tissues attenuate intermediate amounts of the x-ray beam. Thus, they appear somewhere between white and black as a spectrum of shades of gray.

13. **How does computed radiography differ from film/screen radiography?**
In computed radiography, a phosphor plate is used to capture x-ray exposure information. Electrons are trapped in the phosphor layer by the x-ray exposure, and the plate is then "read" by a device that uses lasers to compel the electrons to emit light. This pattern is then electronically stored as a digital image. The ability of the observer to manipulate the brightness and contrast of the digital image is a great advantage of this technique.

KEY POINTS: RADIOGRAPHIC EXPOSURES

1. Increasing voltage (kV) increases the maximum energy of the x-rays produced, decreases the film contrast, and increases exposure, making the film darker.

2. Increasing mAs increases the amount of x-rays produced, does not change the maximum energy of the x-rays produced, and increases exposure, making the film darker.

3. The focal spot is the source of x-rays in the tube.

4. A small focal spot produces sharper images and is used in mammography.

5. A large focal spot can tolerate more heat and is used in fluoroscopy.

14. **How do mammography film/screen combinations differ from those used for chest and abdominal examinations?**
Mammography film/screen combinations are slower than those used for chest and abdominal imaging. This means that mammography film/screen combinations are thinner and have higher spatial resolution.

15. **What is the difference between a posteroanterior (PA) and an anteroposterior (AP) film?**
The names of these views describe the path of the x-ray beam through the patient. In a standing PA chest radiograph, the beam enters the patient from the back and the image is acquired in front of the patient. For acquiring portable chest radiographs, a cassette is placed behind the patient and the x-ray beam is transmitted from the front, creating an AP film. A similar naming convention is followed for all radiographic and mammographic images.

MAMMOGRAPHY

16. **How does mammographic technique (kV and mA) selection differ from that used for chest and abdominal examinations?**
Mammography uses lower kV (for higher image contrast) and higher mA (for shorter exposure times) compared with the technique for chest and abdominal examinations.

17. **What are the two standard views obtained in mammography?**
Medial-lateral oblique (MLO) and craniocaudal (CC). The direction of the x-ray beam is defined by the name of the view. For example, in CC views, the x-ray beam enters the cranial portion of the breast, traverses the breast, and exits on the caudal side of the breast onto the film. By convention, metallic markers indicating view type are placed closest to the axilla—laterally on the CC view and superiorly on the MLO view.

18. **Can any other views be obtained?**
Yes. If an abnormality is seen on only one of the previously described views or if it is seen on both views but needs further characterization or if it is not clear whether an apparent mass is real or just superimposed tissue, additional views are often obtained.

If a lesion is seen on only one of the two standard views (MLO, CC), a 90-degree medial-lateral (ML) view may be helpful to localize the lesion.

Rolled views may be performed in any projection, and tissue can be rolled in any direction desired. This is done to position the area of a potential lesion away from adjacent tissue that may obscure it.

19. **How are spot compression and magnification views used in diagnostic mammography?**
Spot compression views are often obtained to determine whether a density "presses out," meaning that on a compression view it is found to have represented a superimposition of normal breast tissue rather than an actual mass. Magnification views are obtained to better visualize calcifications or to better characterize a mass.

20. **How are women with breast implants imaged with mammography?**
Four views of each breast are done:
- Two CC views, one with the implant in the field of view and one with the implant displaced as much out of the field as possible.
- Two MLO views, one with the implant in the field of view and one with the implant displaced as much out of the field as possible.

21. **What are the two main tissue types in the breast? How do they appear on a mammogram?**
The two main tissues are fibroglandular tissue, which appears bright, and fat, which appears darker.

22. **Why are single screens (rather than dual screens) usually used in mammography?**
Dual-screen systems are more efficient in detecting x-rays and are used for most purposes. The two screens produce more scatter than a single screen, however, and decrease image sharpness. Since sharpness is so important in mammography to characterize calcifications, single-screen systems are used.

FLUOROSCOPY

23. **What is fluoroscopy? How are fluoroscopic images obtained?**
Fluoroscopy uses continuously emitted x-rays and allows real-time visualization of anatomic structures. An x-ray tube located beneath the table emits a continuous x-ray beam that passes through the patient and falls onto a continuously fluorescing screen and image intensifier located above the patient (Fig. 1-2). The fluorescing screen emits a faint light. The emitted light is amplified electronically by an image intensifier, and the image is displayed on a television screen. When an image of interest is identified, a radiograph may be obtained by placing a film between the patient and image intensifier and exposing the film with a pulse of radiation.

24. **Why are image intensifiers used?**
Image intensifiers substantially decrease the amount of radiation needed to produce clinically useful images.

Figure 1-2. A typical C-arm unit for fluoroscopically guided procedures.

25. **How do fluoroscopic conventions differ from radiographic conventions?**
    On fluoroscopy, things that are white on x-rays (like bones or oral contrast) are presented as dark. Things that are dark on x-ray (like air) are presented as white on fluoroscopy.

26. **Discuss the contrast agents used in fluoroscopic studies of the upper and lower gastrointestinal (GI) tract.**
    Barium sulfate is the standard contrast agent for routine fluoroscopic contrast studies of the upper and lower GI tract. "Thin," more fluid suspensions are used for single-contrast studies. "Thick," more viscous suspensions are used for double-contrast (air and oral contrast agent) studies. If perforation of the GI tract is suspected, water-soluble, iodinated contrast such as Gastrografin is used instead of barium because of the high mortality rate from barium peritonitis. Water-soluble agents are quickly resorbed through the peritoneal surface. It should be noted that aspiration of water-soluble agents may result in chemical pneumonitis and should not be used in patients with an increased risk of aspiration.

27. **Why is it important to obtain a scout film before administering contrast in a fluoroscopic study?**
    Objects that appear "white" on a radiograph include contrast agents and calcium. If a white object is seen after contrast administration, it may be either contrast or calcium. The way to differentiate is to see whether it was present on the scout (precontrast) image. If it was present, then it is calcium; if it was not present, then it is contrast. Before administration of a barium enema examination, the scout film may help determine the adequacy of the bowel preparation before the procedure. This helps avoid nondiagnostic examinations due to retained stool.

28. **Name four types of fluoroscopic studies and a possible clinical indication for each.**
    - Esophagram: dysphagia (to rule out stricture or mass)
    - Upper GI study: abdominal pain (to rule out gastric or duodenal ulcer disease)
    - Small bowel follow-through: diarrhea or constipation (to rule out Crohn's disease or other small bowel pathologic conditions)
    - Barium enema: rectal bleeding (to rule out a polyp or mass)

29. **What is digital subtraction angiography?**

    A technique in which a precontrast image is electronically subtracted from an image obtained after intravascular contrast injection. This results in a greater contrast-to-background image because background structures such as bone and soft tissues have been removed.

INTRODUCTION TO ULTRASOUND, CT, AND MRI

E. Scott Pretorius, MD

CHAPTER 2

ULTRASOUND

1. **How is an ultrasound (US) image created?**

   US is an imaging technique that uses sound waves, generally in the range of 2 million–20 million cycles per second (2–20 MHz), well above the frequencies audible to humans or animals. A handheld transducer is applied to the body. This transducer both sends US waves into the body and receives reflected sound waves. The transducer's information is communicated via cable to the US scanner, and the data are rendered on a monitor (Fig. 2-1).

2. **Why is the gel used?**

   US coupling gel (Fig. 2-2) is used to help transmit US waves to and from the transducer. Reflection of sound waves occurs at interfaces where there is a difference in the speed of propagation of sound waves, and, as sound/US waves travel relatively slowly through air, the air-skin interface has potential

Figure 2-1. A US scanner.

Figure 2-2. US transducers, with a bottle of coupling gel. Gel is placed on the skin to facilitate transmission of US waves to and from the transducer.

to reflect a great deal of the waves we would like to use for imaging. Placing US coupling gel between the transducer and skin greatly reduces this effect, and the system is designed so that both the transducer face and the coupling gel have acoustic impedances similar to that of skin.

3. **What makes something bright or dark on US?**
   Sound waves encountering a tissue can be attenuated, reflected, or transmitted by the tissue. Reflected sound waves returning to the transducer are used by the computer to make an image. Sound is generally reflected when waves traveling in one kind of tissue encounter a different kind of tissue, which has different properties of US wave propagation. These are called *acoustic interfaces.*

   Regions with many acoustic interfaces reflect a lot of sound returning to the transducer. These are termed *echogenic* or *hyperechoic* and by convention are viewed as bright areas. Regions with few acoustic interfaces do not reflect many sound waves. These are termed *hypoechoic* and are viewed as dark areas.

4. **What are some things that are hyperechoic?**
   Hyperechoic and *hypoechoic,* of course, are terms that refer to the brightness of an object relative to other things in the image. Air-tissue interfaces reflect a great deal of sound, and such interfaces are markedly hyperechoic. This makes US not useful for identifying an aerated lung and air-filled bowel. Gel is applied to the patient's skin to minimize this effect at the air-skin interface.

   Bone–soft tissue interfaces also reflect a great deal of sound. Imaging inside bone is generally not possible with US.

5. **What are some things that are hypoechoic?**
   Fluid is usually homogenous, and fluid-filled objects such as the urinary bladder, cysts, and large blood vessels are generally very hypoechoic.

6. **What transducer should I choose for the examination?**
   It depends largely on what you are examining. Lower US frequencies penetrate to greater depths, whereas higher US frequencies generally provide higher resolution. For a general examination of the abdomen, which requires large depths to see the liver, pancreas, and spleen, a 3- or 5-MHz transducer is a good choice. For a superficial examination, such as the scrotum or thyroid, a 10-MHz transducer is often used.

7. **What kinds of specialized transducers exist?**
   Endovaginal probes are commonly used for gynecologic examinations and for evaluation of early pregnancies. They are usually 7.5-MHz probes. Endorectal probes are available for prostate imaging. They are generally in the range of 9 MHz.

8. **Why do you ask patients to come with a full bladder for a pelvic US?**
   Fluid in the urinary bladder facilitates transmission of sound waves so that the uterus and ovaries can be better seen using a transabdominal probe. If the bladder is not full, endovaginal examination is more often necessary.

9. **What is the difference between "posterior acoustic enhancement" and "posterior acoustic shadowing?"**
   - *Posterior acoustic enhancement* refers to the increased brightness seen beyond objects that transmit a lot of sound waves. Since fluid-filled cysts transmit a great deal of sound, the area beyond cysts often displays posterior acoustic enhancement.
   - *Posterior acoustic shadowing* has the opposite effect—decreased brightness seen beyond objects that reflect a great deal of sound. Gallstones, which are echogenic, reflect a lot of sound, and shadowing is often seen in the tissue beyond the gallstones.

10. **What is Doppler US?**
Doppler US is used primarily to evaluate flowing blood in blood vessels. It is based on the princi-ple that sound waves originating from a moving source appear to have a different frequency/wavelength than those originating from a stationary source. Echoes returning from blood flowing away from the transducer will appear to have a lower frequency and longer wave-length than the original wave. Similarly, blood flowing toward the transducer will appear to have a higher frequency and shorter wavelength than the original wave.

COMPUTED TOMOGRAPHY

11. **How is a computed tomography (CT) image created?**
The patient lies on a mechanical table that slowly moves through a doughnut-shaped scanner (Fig. 2-3). Inside the scanner, an x-ray emitter rotates around the patient in the axial plane. On the opposite side of the patient, 180 degrees from the emitter, electronic x-ray detectors receive the x-ray beam and calculate how much of the beam was transmitted and how much was absorbed by the patient. The computer then calculates the x-ray absorption of each voxel within the slice and assigns it a numeric value.

Figure 2-3. A multidetector row CT scanner.

12. **What makes something bright or dark on CT?**
Since CT images are created with x-rays, the same things that are bright and dark on plain films are bright and dark on CT. Electron-dense structures, such as metal and bone, stop a large num-ber of x-rays and therefore are bright on CT. Lower electron-density regions, such as air or fat, stop very few x-rays and are rendered as dark.

13. **What is the difference between serial CT and helical (or spiral) CT?**
- In *serial CT scanning,* the emitter/detector whirls 360 degrees around the patient to acquire a slice, the table then moves the patient, and the emitter/detector whirls 360 degrees *the other way* to acquire the next slice.
- In *helical (spiral) scanning,* the emitter/detector array moves around the patient continuously in the same direction, and the table also moves continuously through the scanner while the patient is being imaged. This technologic advance was made possible by the development of the slip-ring gantry, which eliminated the cables that brought power to the emitter/detector and therefore allows it to move continuously in one direction. Helical scanning is generally much faster than serial scanning. All multidetector row scanners are also, by definition, helical.

14. **In helical CT, what is pitch?**
    The longitudinal distance (in millimeters) that the table moves during one revolution of the x-ray tube.

15. **What is the difference between single detector row and multidetector row scanners?**
    Multidetector row scanners have more than one row of x-ray detectors, which allow them to acquire more than one image slice at the same time. Multidetector row scanners are much faster than single detector row scanners. Radiologists have used this technology to acquire ever-greater numbers of thinner and thinner slices, which has led to the emergence of many new CT applications, including CT angiography and CT urography.

16. **What is the Hounsfield scale?**
    A scale that is used to assign voxel values in CT. It extends from −1000 to +1000. The center value, 0 Hounsfield units (HU), is the attenuation of water. Things that absorb more x-rays have greater HU values. Cortical bone is approximately 1000 HU, muscle about 40 HU, gray matter 40 HU, white matter 30 HU, cerebrospinal fluid (CSF) 10 HU, fat −60, and air −1000.

17. **What are *window* and *level*?**
    Once the CT data are acquired and an HU value is assigned to each voxel in a slice, the data can be viewed in different ways. The *window* is a range of HU values that are chosen to be viewed as shades of gray; assigned HU values greater than this range are depicted as white, and values less than this range are depicted as black. The *level* is the HU value that is the center value of the window. Commonly used window/level combinations include those for viewing lung, bone, liver, and the brain.

18. **What is the difference between a pixel and a voxel?**
    A pixel is a single "dot" within a two-dimensional image and has unique coordinates along the "x" and "y" axes of the image. A voxel is a pixel with three dimensions. A voxel that is the same length in all three dimensions is an isotropic voxel.

19. **What is field of view?**
    The width of the image in CT or magnetic resonance imaging (MRI). It is most commonly reported in centimeters.

20. **What is the matrix?**
    "No one can tell you what the matrix is. You have to see it for yourself." *The Matrix* is a movie in which computers control people's perceptions of all things, including, apparently, the common perception that Keanu Reeves *can* act his way out of a paper bag. Without invoking the computer mind-control theory, this perception is otherwise inexplicable.
    In diagnostic imaging, *matrix* size refers to the number of pixels contained on each axis of a CT or MRI slice, such as a square matrix of 512×512 pixels (typical in CT) or a rectangular matrix of 256×192 pixels (common in MRI).

21. **What is the difference between spatial resolution and contrast resolution?**
    - *Spatial resolution* is a measure of the ability of an imaging technique to demonstrate that two nearby objects are, indeed, separate objects. It is measured in "line pairs per millimeter," referring to the ability of a modality to demonstrate that very small pairs of lines are indeed *separate* lines and not a single line. Of the digital cross-sectional modalities, CT has the highest spatial resolution.
    - *Contrast resolution* refers to the ability of an imaging modality to render different objects or tissues as different shades of gray. Of the digital cross-sectional modalities, MRI has the highest contrast resolution.

MAGNETIC RESONANCE IMAGING

22. How is the MR image created?

The patient is placed in a scanner that generates a very strong magnetic field (Fig. 2-4). Hydrogen nuclei have a net magnetic moment and therefore behave like little magnets, aligning themselves either parallel (spin up) or antiparallel (spin down) with the magnetic field. Radiofrequency waves are then pulsed in, which scatter the hydrogen nuclei in all directions. Once the radiofrequency pulse is stopped, the hydrogen nuclei tend to realign themselves along the magnetic field, but this happens at different rates in different tissues. These differential relaxation rates are used to create the MR image.

Figure 2-4. A 1.5-Tesla MRI scanner. Note that the central bore of the scanner is narrower than that of a CT scanner.

23. What are the three basic planes used in imaging?

Axial, sagittal, and coronal (Fig. 2-5). An advantage of MRI over CT is that MRI data can be obtained in any plane. CT data are acquired axially but can be reformatted to generate other planes.

Figure 2-5. The planes (axial, sagittal, and coronal) used for cross-sectional imaging.

24. **What is the difference between T1 and T2?**
    T1 is a measure of relaxation time in the longitudinal plane, and T2 is a measure of relaxation time in the transverse plane.

25. **What are T1- and T2-weighted images?**
    - *T1-weighted images* are created primarily by using data from differential proton relaxation rates in the plane longitudinal to the main magnetic field.
    - *T2-weighted images* primarily make use of data from differential proton relaxation rates in the plane transverse to the main magnetic field.

26. **What is a pulse sequence?**
    A series of instructions that is repeated many times to build up the data to create an MR image.

27. **What are TR and TE?**
    TR is the "time to repetition," or the time it takes to complete one full iteration of a pulse sequence. *TE* is the "time to echo," or the time between the start of a pulse sequence and the acquisition of data from the excited protons. TR and TE are, by convention, reported in milliseconds.

28. **What is a spin-echo pulse sequence?**
    A spin-echo pulse sequence begins with a 90-degree pulse, followed by a 180-degree pulse. After the 180-degree pulse, MRI signal is acquired from the protons. Spin-echo pulse sequences may be used to create T1- or T2-weighted images.

29. **What is the difference between spin-echo imaging and fast spin-echo imaging?**
    Fast spin echo (FSE) is a technique that takes advantage of the fact that, after the 90-degree and 180-degree pulses have been applied, there are multiple "echoes"—bits of MRI signal—that can be acquired. FSE is much faster than conventional spin echo (SE), especially for T2-weighted imaging because it requires going through many fewer iterations of the pulse sequence (fewer TRs) to create the image. In practice, FSE is almost always used instead of SE.

30. **How can I tell the difference between T1 and T2 by looking at the TR and TE?**
    - T1-weighted images have a short TR (less than 1000 ms) and a short TE (less than 20 ms).
    - T2-weighted images have a long TR (more than 2000 ms) and a long TE (more than 40 ms).

KEY POINTS: METHODS OF GENERATING CONTRAST BETWEEN DIFFERENT TISSUES

1. US uses US waves. "Acoustic interfaces," regions in tissues where the speed of the US wave changes, are rendered as bright. Areas that are more internally homogenous (like fluid), without acoustic interfaces, are rendered as dark.

2. CT uses x-rays. Tissues of higher electron density (like bone) stop more x-rays and are rendered as bright.

3. MRI uses magnets and radiowaves. Different sequences of radiowaves (pulse sequences) generate different types of images. MRI has greater contrast than US and CT, and, with different pulse sequences, has multiple different ways of generating contrast between tissues.

31. **How can I tell the difference between T1 and T2 by looking at an image?**
    The best way is to look for fluid, which tends to be hyperintense to virtually everything else on T2-weighted images. On T1-weighted images, fluid is of low intermediate signal. Good places to look for fluid include the urinary bladder and the cerebrospinal fluid (CSF).
    Fat is an unreliable predictor of image weighting. Although fat is brighter than most other tissues on T1, its appearance on T2-weighted images is often manipulated. Fat tends to be relatively hypointense to other tissues on spin-echo T2-weighted images and hyperintense on FSE T2-weighted images. Also, a technique known as "fat saturation" is often used to decrease the signal from fat on T1-weighted images and FSE T2-weighted images. Because of these complexities, fat is an unreliable marker of image weighting.

32. **What kinds of things tend to be bright on T1-weighted images?**
    Fat, hemorrhage, proteinaceous substances, melanin, and paramagnetic agents such as gadolinium chelates.

33. **I see something that is dark on both T1 and T2. What kinds of things do that?**
    Air, flowing blood (on spin-echo or FSE images), and cortical bone. Ligaments, tendons, and other dense fibrous tissues are also usually of low T1, low T2 signal.

34. **How strong is 1.5 Tesla (T)?**
    The earth's magnetic field is about 0.5 gauss. Since 1.5 T is equal to 15,000 gauss, the magnetic field of such a scanner is 30,000 times the strength of the earth's magnetic field.

35. **Are low-magnetic-field open scanners as good as high-field scanners?**
    No. In general, low-field (0.5 T and lower) scanners require longer imaging times to produce poorer images. With good surface coils and a lot of imaging time, open scanners can often produce good images of stationary body parts such as joints, the spine, and the brain. For imaging applications requiring high resolution (breast imaging) and/or rapid imaging, such as abdominal MR, magnetic resonance angiography (MRA), and dynamic gadolinium-enhanced MR studies, low-field scanners are markedly inferior to high-field systems.

36. **What is the difference between spin-echo images and gradient-echo images?**
    Spin-echo images start with a 90-degree pulse, followed by a 180-degree refocusing pulse. Gradient-echo sequences use pulses of less than 90 degrees and do not have 180 degrees refocusing pulses. TR and TE are often very short, and gradient-echo sequences usually are used for acquiring T1-weighted images. Because these images can be obtained very rapidly, they are the most common type of image to be acquired after rapid gadolinium injection and are used for performing contrast-enhanced MRA.

37. **What kinds of images are acquired before and after gadolinium chelate administration?**
    Gadolinium chelates that are used as contrast agents for MRI primarily shorten T1 relaxation times, thereby making things appear more hyperintense on T1-weighted images. Precontrast and postcontrast images, therefore, are T1-weighted images. T1-weighted spin-echo imaging is often performed in regions where longer imaging times are acceptable, such as the brain. For the abdomen and pelvis, however, where imaging must be completed in a breath-hold, T1-weighted gradient-echo images are almost exclusively used.

38. **Why is it important that the precontrast image and the postcontrast image have the same imaging parameters?**
    Nothing can be changed on the scanner between the acquisition of the precontrast image and the postcontrast image. The reason is that, unlike CT, there is no absolute scale of "brightness" and "darkness" on MRI. The only way to know whether something enhances on

MRI is to compare its signal on the postcontrast image with its signal on the identical precontrast image. One cannot, for example, compare signal intensities between two images acquired with different TRs.

39. What are contraindications to MRI?

Patients with implanted electronic devices such as pacemakers, defibrillators, neurostimulators, and cochlear implants should not be placed in the magnetic field. A patient who is dependent on a pacemaker for cardiac pacing may die in the scanner if the device malfunctions. Even if the patient is not dependent on the device for survival, the battery life will be shortened by exposure to the field.

Extreme claustrophobia is a relative contraindication to MRI. Such patients may need to be sedated for examination. In some case, low-field imaging on an open scanner may be able to be used instead.

40. Who should not receive gadolinium chelates?

Patients with a prior true allergic response to gadolinium chelates, including hives, bronchospasm, and anaphylaxis, should not be injected. True allergic response is very rare, on the order of 1 in 200,000 injections. The most common side effects of these agents are mild headache and a metallic taste.

Pregnant patients should not receive gadolinium chelates. Many of the agents are known to be able to cross the blood-placental barrier, and their effect on the fetus is unknown.

CHAPTER 3

INTRODUCTION TO NUCLEAR MEDICINE

Linda Kulzer Petrovich, MD, and E. Scott Pretorius, MD

1. **How is a nuclear medicine test performed?**

   A radiopharmaceutical agent, which is radioactively tagged compound, is administered to a patient. Many radio-pharmaceutical agents act like analogs of natural biologic compounds and localize to specific organs. Photons are emitted from the radiopharmaceutical agent in the patient, and a gamma camera is used to detect the tracer distribution. An image is then created by a computer system (Fig. 3-1).

Figure 3-1. Line drawing demonstrating the flow of information of a typical nuclear medicine study, such as a bone scan, obtained with a gamma camera.

2. **What is the difference between the x-rays used in plain films and computed tomography (CT) and the gamma rays used in nuclear medicine?**

   X-rays are produced from the interaction of bombarding photons or electrons within an atom. Gamma rays are produced when an unstable nucleus transitions to a more stable state.

   Diagnostic x-ray imaging is referred to as "transmission imaging." This term is used because images are formed as x-ray photons from an external source traverse tissue and emerge to form the image. Nuclear medicine is referred to as "emission imaging" because photons are emitted from inside the patient and subsequently detected by the gamma camera imaging system.

3. **How does nuclear medicine differ from other imaging modalities used in radiology such as plain film, ultrasound, CT, and magnetic resonance imaging (MRI)?**

   X-rays, ultrasound, CT, and MRI produce anatomic images with very high spatial resolution. Therefore a viewer can see anatomy very well, but function generally is not assessed. Nuclear medicine studies sacrifice spatial resolution, but in return, offer information about organ function.

4. **What are some common clinical indications for performing nuclear medicine imaging?**

   ■ To rule out pulmonary embolism, a ventilation-perfusion scan may be performed.
   ■ To evaluate for acute cholecystitis, a hepato-iminodiacetic acid (HIDA) scan may be performed.

KEY POINTS: HOW NUCLEAR MEDICINE DIFFERS FROM OTHER IMAGING MODALITIES

1. Radiopharmaceutical agents are administered to the patient before imaging.

2. Images are indicative of the functional status of an organ.

3. The spatial resolution in nuclear medicine is less than that of x-rays, ultrasound, CT, and MRI.

4. Photons are emitted from the patient and detected by a gamma camera.

5. The total time for a nuclear medicine test may range from minutes to days, depending on the half-life and distribution of the radiopharmaceutical agent.

- To detect potential a gastrointestinal bleed, a bleeding scan may be performed.
- To evaluate for osteomyelitis, a three-phase bone scan may be performed.

5. **What radiopharmaceutical agents are used in a ventilation-perfusion scan?**
   A ventilation-perfusion scan attempts to identify an aerated lung that is not perfused. The scan therefore consists of two parts: a ventilation phase where the aerated lung is imaged and a perfusion phase that maps blood flow to the lungs. The two sets of images are compared for discrepancies. For the ventilation portion of the study, xenon-133 and technetium (Tc)-99m diethylenetriaminepentaacetic acid (DTPA) are the most commonly used agents. For the perfusion portion of the study, Tc-99m macroaggregated albumin (MAA) is used.

6. **How is a ventilation-perfusion scan performed?**
   The ventilation portion is performed using either radioactive gas (xenon) or radioactive aerosol (Tc-99m DTPA). When radioactive gas is used, the study is accomplished in three phases: single breath/wash-in phase, equilibrium phase, and washout phase. For studies that use radioaerosols, the radiopharmaceutical agent is placed in a special nebulizer system and the patient breathes through the mouthpiece until sufficient radioaerosol is delivered to the lungs. The Tc-99m remains in the lung long enough to obtain multiple views with a gamma camera. Tc-99m MAA is injected into a peripheral vein to assess perfusion. The particles travel to the right side of the heart and then to the lungs, where they are filtered or trapped in the pulmonary vascular bed. The emissions from the trapped particles are then imaged with a gamma camera.

7. **How are the results of a ventilation-perfusion scan interpreted?**
   If an acute pulmonary embolism is present, the thrombus in the blood vessel will prevent radiotracer from reaching the portion of lung supplied by the vessel, thus a perfusion defect will result. An acute thrombus, however, will not prevent air from being distributed to the lung via bronchi, thus the results of the ventilation scan will be normal. This combination of a perfusion defect without a corresponding ventilation defect is called a *mismatch*. The results of a ventilation-perfusion scan are classified as low, intermediate, or high probability for a pulmonary embolism. The classification is based on the number and size of defects, with higher numbers and sizes resulting in greater probability that an embolus is present.

8. **What radiopharmaceutical agent is used in an HIDA scan?**
   Tc-99m–labeled iminodiacetic acid (IDA) compounds. They share biologic activity with bilirubin and are therefore also taken up, transported, and excreted by hepatocytes.

9. **How is an HIDA scan performed?**
   The patient is required to fast for at least 4 hours but not longer than 24 hours. If the test is performed after a recent meal, the gallbladder may still be contracted and this could lead to false-positive test results. After a prolonged fast, the gallbladder may be filled with concentrated bile and this may also lead to false-positive test results by preventing tracer accumulation in the gallbladder. Tc-99m IDA is injected into a peripheral vein, followed by immediate imaging of the right upper quadrant.

10. **How are the results of an HIDA scan interpreted?**
    Because the tracer behaves like bilirubin, it should be taken up by hepatocytes and excreted into the bile ducts. Thus the liver should be visualized first, followed by visualization of the bowel and gallbladder. The appearance of tracer in the bowel and gallbladder by 60 minutes after administration is defined as normal. Nonvisualization of the gallbladder by 60 minutes is diagnostic of acute cholecystitis because this implies a functional obstruction of the cystic duct. False-positive results can be caused by chronic cholecystitis, hepatic insufficiency, and by fasting for less than 4 hours or more than 24 hours as previously described.

KEY POINTS: COMMON CLINICAL INDICATIONS FOR A NUCLEAR MEDICINE STUDY

1. To rule out pulmonary embolism (ventilation-perfusion scan)

2. To rule out acute cholecystitis, bile duct obstruction, or biliary leak (HIDA scan)

3. To rule out lower GI bleed (Tc-99m sulfur colloid or Tc-99m–labeled red blood cells)

4. To rule out infection (bone scan, indium-111–labeled white blood cells, gallium 67)

5. To evaluate for metastatic disease (bone scan, PET scan)

6. To evaluate for thyroid pathologic conditions (iodine-123)

7. To evaluate for renal pathologic conditions such as obstruction, hypertension, reflux, and transplant (Tc-99m–labeled compounds)

---

11. **What radiopharmaceutical agents are used for a gastrointestinal (GI) bleeding scan?**
    Tc-99m sulfur colloid or Tc-99m–labeled red blood cells. Tc-99m–labeled red blood cells are more difficult to prepare but have the advantage of a longer plasma half-life and are therefore able to detect a GI bleed over a longer period.

12. **How do you tell whether the results of the bleeding scan are positive?**
    An abnormal radiotracer hot spot appears and conforms to bowel anatomy. The activity should increase over time and move through the GI tract. Because blood acts as an intestinal irritant, movement can be rapid and bidirectional.

13. **What are some indications for performing a renal scan?**
    Renal scans have a variety of clinical applications, including evaluating renal transplants, differentiating between obstructed and dilated collecting systems, and diagnosing reflux and renovascular hypertension.

14. **What are the four major renal functions that can be evaluated with radionuclide imaging?**
Renal scans are helpful in evaluating blood flow to the kidney, glomerular filtration, tubular function (resorption and secretion), and drainage of the collecting systems.

15. **What are the main radiopharmaceutical agents used in renal scans? How do they differ?**
Tc-99m DTPA is a glomerular agent, meaning that it is cleared primarily by glomerular filtration and is neither reabsorbed nor secreted by the renal tubules. Thus it can be used to measure the glomerular filtration rate. Tc-99m mertiatide (MAG3) is a tubular agent, meaning that its mechanism of renal clearance is solely tubular secretion. Tc-99m dimercaptosuccinic acid (DMSA) is a cortical agent, meaning that it binds to tubular cells in the renal cortex, making possible static imaging of the renal parenchymal cortex.

16. **What three main factors should be examined when interpreting a renal scan?**
Blood flow, radiotracer uptake, and radiotracer excretion.

17. **What radiopharmaceutical agents are used in thyroid imaging?**
Iodine 123 is the diagnostic agent of choice for imaging the thyroid. The iodine is administered orally. It is then absorbed from the GI tract and trapped and organified (incorporated into thyroglobulin molecules) in the thyroid. Tc-99m pertechnetate is used if imaging has to be performed within 1 hour or if the patient is not able to ingest orally. Iodine 131 is used for whole body scans after thyroidectomy for thyroid cancer and for therapeutic purposes.

18. **Describe the appearance of Graves' disease, thyroiditis, and tumor on a nuclear imaging study.**
Graves' disease is manifested by an enlarged gland that demonstrates diffusely increased uptake. *Thyroiditis* appears as diffusely decreased uptake. *Thyroid cancer* tends to appear as a focal area of decreased activity (a solitary cold nodule) rather than demonstrating increased activity on a nuclear medicine study.

19. **What radiopharmaceutical agents are used in bone scanning?**
Tc-99m–labeled diphosphonates are injected intravenously to perform a bone scan. The radiotracer distribution is representative of osteoblastic activity as well as regional blood flow to bone. Dynamic blood flow imaging is performed immediately after the injection of radiotracer. Static imaging is performed 2–4 hours after injection and is indicative of osteoblastic activity.

20. **What are the two types of bone scans that can be performed? What are the indications for each?**
Focal three-phase imaging and whole body imaging. Focal-three phase imaging is used to differentiate cellulitis from osteomyelitis. The three phases are the flow phase (1 minute after injection), the blood pool (5 minutes after injection), and the skeletal phase (2–4 hours after injection). Both cellulitis and osteomyelitis will have increased uptake in the first two phases of the bone scan; however, only osteomyelitis demonstrates increased activity in the third phase.
Whole body imaging consists of static images obtained 2–4 hours after injection. It is used for detection of metastatic and metabolic diseases and bone dysplasia.

21. **If one is concerned about an infection outside the skeletal system, what nuclear imaging studies can be performed?**
Indium (In)-111–labeled white blood cells and gallium 67 citrate can be used to detect occult infection. To label white cells with In-111, the cells must be removed from plasma. Blood is taken

KEY POINTS: MAIN RADIONUCLIDES USED IN NUCLEAR MEDICINE

1. Tc-99m (most common)

2. Iodine-123

3. Gallium 67

4. Thallium 201

5. In-111

6. FDG (for PET imaging)

from the patient, labeled, and then reinjected. Imaging is performed 24 hours after the injection. The normal distribution of white blood cells is spleen, liver, and bone marrow. Activity seen outside the normal expected distribution is evidence of a focus of infection. Gallium, the other agent useful in locating sources of infection, binds to iron-binding molecules. Its normal distribution is liver and bone marrow. It is excreted by the kidneys for the first 24 hours and through the large bowel after 24 hours. As with an In-111 white blood cell scan, activity seen outside the expected normal organs of uptake is evidence of infection.

22. **What is a PET scan?**
PET stands for *positron emission tomography*. A tracer that emits positrons is injected into the patient. After the positrons are emitted from the nucleus of an atom, they travel through surrounding tissue and collide with electrons. This collision between positrons and electrons is called *annihilation* and produces gamma rays. The gamma rays are detected by a PET scanner and analyzed by a computer to form an image.

23. **What radiopharmaceutical agent is used in PET scanning? What type of pathologic conditions can it detect?**
Fluorine 18 fluorodeoxyglucose (FDG). This is a radionuclide combined with glucose, which is the currency of metabolism for both malignant and benign cells. However, because malignant cells tend to grow and metabolize glucose faster than healthy tissue, malignant cells will use more of the tracer. PET scans use the difference in metabolism to differentiate normal from abnormal tissue.

24. **What types of cancer are best detected on PET scan?**
PET scans can be used to detect malignant tumors, determine cancer stage, and judge the effectiveness of cancer treatment. They are most often used in patients with head and neck tumors, colorectal cancer, lymphoma, melanoma, and lung cancer.

CHAPTER 4

COMPUTERS IN RADIOLOGY

William W. Boonn, MD

1. **What is PACS?**
    PACS stands for *picture archiving and communication system*. On the most basic level, PACS integrates image acquisition modalities, workstation displays, the image archiving system, and the underlying network.

2. **How are PACS images stored?**
    The PACS archive traditionally has been composed of short- and long-term storage. Short-term storage usually is composed of redundant array of inexpensive (or identical) disks (RAID) arrays (*see* question 3) that provide quick access to image data. After a certain amount of time (which depends on the size of the short-term archive but can vary from 3 to 30 days), images from the short-term archive are moved to the long-term archive, which is usually composed of magnetic tape or magneto-optical media. Images cannot be viewed directly from the long-term archive. Instead, images need to be "fetched" from the long-term archive and copied back to the short-term archive before being viewed on a workstation. This compromise was made because of the high cost of RAID storage. Recently, the cost of RAID storage has decreased enough so that several PACS archives are now being designed as "always online" systems. These new systems are composed only of RAID arrays, which essentially place all images in the short-term archive and eliminate the need for fetching.

3. **What is a RAID?**
    A RAID is a group of hard disks and a system that sorts and stores data in various forms to improve data-acquisition speed and provide improved data protection. To accomplish this, a system of levels (from 1 to 5) "mirrors," "stripes," and "duplexes" data onto a group of hard disks.

4. **What is image compression?**
    Image compression is the process of reducing image file size using various mathematical algorithms. Compression is usually expressed as a ratio (e.g., 10:1). A 10-megabyte (MB) file that is compressed at a ratio of 10:1 will have a final size of 1 MB. Generally, as compression ratios increase, file sizes decrease; however, a price is inevitably paid in decreased image fidelity.

5. **What is the difference between lossy and lossless compression?**
    Encoding an image is a process that converts a raw image (e.g., the original radiograph) into a more compact coded file. Decoding converts the coded file to a decoded image. If the raw image and the decoded image are the same, the compression method is considered *lossless*. If there is a difference between the raw image and the decoded image, then the method of encoding and decoding is considered *lossy*. Lossless compression can usually achieve ratios of 2:1 or 3:1. Lossy compression, on the other hand, can achieve much higher compression ratios; however, overcompression may destroy fine detail, making the image unacceptable for diagnostic purposes.

6. **What is RIS?**
    RIS stands for *radiology information system*. The RIS is a system responsible for the workflow within a radiology department. These tasks include patient scheduling and tracking, billing, and handling of radiology reports.

7. What is HIS?

HIS stands for *hospital information system*. The HIS manages patient demographics; insurance and billing; and often other clinical information systems, including laboratory results, physician orders, and electronic medical records.

8. What is DICOM?

DICOM stands for *Digital Imaging and Communications in Medicine*. It is a standard that establishes rules that allow medical images and associated information to be exchanged between imaging equipment from different vendors, computers, and hospitals. For example, a computed tomography (CT) scanner produced by vendor *A* and a magnetic resonance imaging (MRI) scanner from vendor *B* can send images to a PACS from vendor *C* using DICOM as a common language. In addition to storing image information, other DICOM standard services include query/retrieve, print management, scheduling of acquisition and notification of completion, and security profiles.

9. What determines image storage size?

Image size, generally expressed in megabytes, is determined by spatial resolution and bit depth. Spatial resolution for a two-dimensional (2D) image is defined by a matrix of horizontal and vertical pixels. For example, a single image in a typical CT scan will be composed of a matrix of 512 vertical pixels $\times$ 512 horizontal pixels, whereas a chest radiograph image might have a matrix size of 2500 vertical pixels $\times$ 2000 horizontal pixels. For a given anatomic area of interest, images with a larger matrix size have greater spatial resolution.

Bit depth is defined by the number of shades of gray within the image, where 2^n equals shades of gray and n equals bit depth. As an example, an image with a bit depth of 1 will have 2 shades of gray (pure black and pure white). A 6-bit image contains 64 shades of gray; 7-bit, 128 shades; 8-bit, 256 shades; and 12-bit, 4096 shades. Most diagnostic-quality digital images in MR, CT, and computed radiography/digital radiography are displayed in 10 or 12 bits.

The file size of an imaging study also depends on the number of images in that study. A chest radiograph may have two images (posteroanterior and lateral), whereas a CT scan of the abdomen may have 50 images. With the advent of multidetector row CT scanners, it is now possible to acquire thinner slices in much less time, often resulting in much larger studies. This capability also allows images to be reconstructed in different planes. All of this contributes to an increased number of images and, overall, larger study sizes for storage. A CT angiogram may contain 500 to 1000 images or more.

10. How large are these studies?

Table 4-1 shows approximate matrix and file sizes for various imaging modalities. These values will vary depending on bit depth, number of images acquired, and compression technique.

11. What is teleradiology?

Teleradiology is the process of sending digital radiology images over a computer network to a remote location (this can be across town or across the globe) for viewing and interpretation. The American College of Radiology publishes a set of guidelines and standards for teleradiology that include minimum display requirements, security and privacy provisions, and documentation standards.

12. What is IHE?

Integrating the Healthcare Enterprise (IHE) is an initiative undertaken by medical specialists and other care providers, administrators, information technology professionals, and industry to improve the way computer systems in health care share information. IHE promotes coordinated use of established communications standards such as DICOM and HL7 (*see* question 13) to address specific clinical needs that support optimal patient care. Systems developed in

TABLE 4-1. APPROXIMATE MATRIX AND FILE SIZES FOR VARIOUS IMAGING MODALITIES

	Image Matrix		Per Study Basis			
			Images		Size (MB)	
Modality	X	Y	Avg.	Range	Avg.	Range
Computed radiography (CR)	2000	2500	3	2–5	30	20–50
Digital radiography (DR)	3000	3000	3	2–5	54	40–90
Film digitizer	2000	2500	3	2–5	30	20–50
CT	512	512	60	40–300	32	20–150
Multidetector row CT	512	512	500	200–1000	250	100–600
MRI	256	256	200	80–1000	25	10–150
Digital mammography	3000	3000	6	4–8	100	75–150
Ultrasound	640	480	30	20–60	20	10–40
Nuclear medicine	256	256	10	4–30	1	0.5–4
Digital fluoroscopy (without digital subtraction angiography [DSA])	1024	1024	20	10–50	20	10–50
Digital fluoroscopy (with DSA)	1024	1024	150	120–240	450	360–720

accordance with IHE communicate with one another better, are easier to implement, and enable care providers to use information more effectively.

13. **What is HL7?**
Health Level 7 (HL7) is the standard used by most RIS and HIS to exchange information between systems. It was designed for sending notifications about events in a health system (e.g., a patient is admitted) and transmitting information (e.g., laboratory data and radiology reports). It was not designed to handle image information; that role is primarily served by DICOM.

KEY POINTS: COMPUTERS IN RADIOLOGY

1. The storage size for a given image is determined by the spatial resolution and bit depth of the image.

2. DR systems eliminate the plate and cassette completely and acquire digital images directly, using flat-panel detectors.

3. RIS and PACS are essential elements of digital radiology.

14. **How are conventional radiographs integrated into an all-digital PACS?**
There are three methods. The first method is to obtain a conventional radiograph on film and digitize the image using a scanner. In fully digital environments, this method is usually reserved

for digitizing "outside" films or films from settings where digital acquisition has not yet been implemented, such as in the operating room. The second and third methods for acquiring digital radiographs are computed radiography (CR) and digital radiography (DR).

15. **What is the difference between CR and DR?**
CR systems use a stimulable phosphor screen or plate, usually contained in a cassette, which is exposed in a manner similar to that of conventional radiographs. This produces a latent image on the plate. After exposure, the plate is scanned with a laser spot-scanning mechanism and photomultiplier tubes, and this produces a digital image. The plate is then "erased" using fluorescent lamps and reused. A major advantage of CR over conventional screen-film systems is increased exposure latitude. It allows radiographs that may have been overexposed or underexposed to be processed to produce diagnostic images.

DR systems eliminate the plate and cassette completely and acquire digital images directly, using flat-panel detectors.

16. **What is three-dimensional reconstruction?**
Three-dimensional (3D) reconstruction is the process of analyzing a 2D data set and displaying it in three dimensions using various postprocessing techniques and algorithms. The most common 3D reconstructions are multiplanar reformat (MPR), maximum intensity projection (MIP), surface shaded display (SSD), volume rendering (VR), and virtual intraluminal endoscopy (also called "virtual fly-through").

MPR processes images acquired in one plane (e.g., an axial CT) and reconstructs the image in other planes (sagittal, coronal, or oblique) so that one may view and scroll through images from multiple perspectives. Curved MPR is another algorithm that is more commonly used in angiographic studies in which curved structures (e.g., the aorta or other blood vessels) are viewed in a single plane. This algorithm is helpful for studying vascular stenosis and aneurysms.

17. **What are the differences between MIP, SSD, and VR?**
   - *MIP* processes a volume of data and assigns a value to each voxel along a line to the viewer's eye. Only the maximum voxel value along that line is displayed. This technique is commonly used in CT and MR angiography, where vascular structures (usually containing contrast and thus having high voxel values) can be separated from background structures and be better visualized.
   - *SSD* reconstructions, also known as *surface shading*, are images in which apparent surfaces of anatomic structures are determined and shaded according to local orientation of the surface with respect to a virtual lighting source. Advantages of this method are better 3D rendering of the shape and positioning of structures; however, SSD images generally require more user intervention to achieve optimal images.
   - *VR* displays all of the 3D data at once, using voxel intensities to determine the transparency of each structure. High–voxel-intensity structures are more opaque, whereas low–voxel-intensity structures are more translucent. The user can assign colors to particular voxel intensities (e.g., red for soft tissues, white for bone density, and yellow for fat density) to create more realistic 3D images. The major disadvantage of VR reconstruction is the need for powerful computing resources.

18. **What is voice recognition (or speech recognition)?**
Voice recognition is the process by which a computer system recognizes spoken words and converts them to text. Comprehending human languages falls under a different field of computer science called *natural language processing*.

Early systems required that the speaker speak slowly and distinctly and separate each word with a short pause. These systems were called *discrete speech systems*. More recently, *continuous speech systems* have become available that allow the user to speak more naturally.

19. What are the advantages and disadvantages of voice or speech recognition relative to conventional dictation/transcription?

There are several *advantages* to voice recognition over conventional dictations for radiology reporting. Report turnaround time is vastly reduced, overall cost is decreased (since transcriptionists are no longer required), and users who take advantage of text macros can dictate standard reports in less time.

The *disadvantages* include erroneous reports because of poor recognition of the speech of certain individuals (sometimes due to lack of training) and difficulty in recognizing similar sounding words (e.g., "hypodense" vs. "hyperdense"). Poor recognition and inefficient use of macros often result in increased dictation time and frustration on the part of the radiologist, which is usually remedied with better training and support.

BIBLIOGRAPHY

1. Dreyer K, Mehta A, Thrall J: PACS: A Guide to the Digital Revolution. New York, Springer-Verlag, 2002.
2. Horii SC: Primer on computers and information technology. Part four: A nontechnical introduction to DICOM. Radiographics 17(5):1297–1309, 1997.
3. Liu B, Cao F, Zhou M, et al: Trends in PACS image storage and archive. Comput Med Imaging Graph 27:165–174, 2003.
4. Ratib O, Ligier Y, Bandon D, Valentino D: Update on digital image management and PACS. Abdom Imaging 25(4):333–40, 2000.
5. Siegel EL, Kolodner RM: Filmless Radiology. New York, Springer-Verlag, 1999.

SCREENING MAMMOGRAPHY

Susan P. Weinstein, MD

CHAPTER 5

1. **What is a screening mammogram?**
   Screening mammogram is a radiographic examination of the breasts performed for early detection of breast cancer in asymptomatic women.

2. **When should an average woman start getting mammograms?**
   This topic has been controversial. The American College of Radiology recommends that women begin getting mammograms at age 40 and annually thereafter.

3. **Are there instances when screening should start earlier than 40?**
   Patients with a history of Hodgkin's disease treated with radiation or those with a strong family history of breast cancer may be candidates for earlier screening. In women treated for Hodgkin's disease, surveillance may begin 10 years after chest wall/mediastinal radiation exposure. For patients with a history of a first-degree relative with breast cancer, screening should begin 10 years before the age at which the relative was diagnosed. If the relative was diagnosed after age 50, there will be no impact on the screening recommendation. However, if the relative was diagnosed at an age earlier than 50, the woman should begin screening before the age of 40.

4. **How many views are obtained for a routine mammogram?**
   Four views. Craniocaudal (CC) and mediolateral oblique (MLO) views of each breast are obtained. In some patients, more than four images may be needed to adequately visualize all of the breast parenchyma.

5. **Which view visualizes the most breast tissue?**
   The MLO view.

6. **Which portion of the breast is better visualized on the CC view than on the MLO view?**
   The medial breast.

7. **How should a film screen mammogram be hung?**
   The CC views are hung next to one another, and the MLO views are hung adjacent to each other (Fig. 5-1). The films are hung with the labels in the upper corner. On the CC views, the labels are placed adjacent to the lateral breast. On the MLO views, the labels are placed adjacent to the superior breast. The comparison films are hung in the same manner above the current study.

8. **How old should the comparison films be?**
   If the patient has multiple sets of prior films, we like to compare with the studies that are 2 years old. The reason is that early changes from breast cancer can be subtle, and the changes will be easier to detect over the 2-year interval.

Figure 5-1. Screening mammogram hung for viewing. From the viewer's left, the images are (A) the left MLO view, (B) the right MLO view, (C) the left CC view, and (D) the right CC view. The comparison films are typically hung above the current study.

9. **What if there are comparison films elsewhere? Do we need to get them?**
   If the mammogram results are considered to be negative, no. Studies have shown that it is not cost-effective and does not improve patient care to obtain comparison films for studies with normal results. If there is an abnormal finding, an attempt should be made to get the prior studies from the outside institution.

10. **What is the incidence of screening-detected breast cancer?**
    In a population that has never been screened, the incidence is about 6–10/1000. In a population that is routinely screened, the incidence drops to about 2–4/1000.

11. **What is the reported sensitivity of screening mammography?**
    False-negative interpretation (mammograms that are interpreted as negative but a cancer is present) is usually reported to be in the range of 83–95%. The sensitivity seems to decease as the glandularity of the breast tissue increases.

12. **What is the difference between a screening mammogram and a diagnostic mammogram?**
    A screening mammogram is performed on asymptomatic patients as part of routine annual surveillance. A diagnostic mammogram is performed when the patient has a history of breast cancer or presents with a breast-related complaint/symptom.

13. **Are there other types of breast cancer screening modalities? Which are used in everyday clinical practice?**
    Digital mammography is similar to film screen mammography, but the images are acquired in a digital form. After acquisition, image processing is possible with the digitized images. The images can be printed and viewed as hard copies like film screen mammography or reviewed on a computer monitor. Two full-field systems have been approved by the Food and Drug Administration and are used in clinical practice.
    Screening breast ultrasound consists of an ultrasound examination of both breasts in asymptomatic women. No blinded, randomized, controlled trials have been performed to date. The true sensitivity and specificity of screening sonography are not known. An examination with negative results may lead to a false sense of security. False-positive results may lead to unnecessary biopsies. Also, screening ultrasound is operator-dependent. Currently, the clinical role of screening ultrasound is being investigated by multicenter research protocols.
    Screening magnetic resonance imaging (MRI) probably will not be used in everyday clinical practice, given the lack of availability, high cost, and variable specificity leading to many

false-positive interpretations. However, MRI screening has shown to be promising in very high-risk patients. More research needs to be done to assess its potential role in the screening setting. Currently, MRI screening should be performed only under a research protocol.

Positron emission tomography (PET) scans are not used in the screening setting due to limited availability, high cost, and low image resolution. No studies to date have evaluated the role of PET scans as a screening tool.

KEY POINTS: SCREENING MAMMOGRAPHY

1. Annual screening mammography should begin at age 40.

2. Mammography is still the best screening test to detect subclinical breast cancer.

3. The sensitivity of mammography is in the range of 83–95%.

4. An individual's risk of developing breast cancer increases with increasing age.

5. Most breast cancers occur in women with no family history of the disease.

14. **Is digital mammography better than film screen mammography in detecting breast cancer?**
    The answer is unknown. Thus far, the two major studies, the International Digital Mammography Development Group Digital Mammography Pilot Study and Colorado/Massachusetts Full-Field Digital Mammography Screening Trial, have shown no statistically significant difference in cancer detection. The largest digital trial to date, the multi-institutional Digital Mammography ACRIN Trial, has closed patient accrual, but the final results are pending.

15. **Is there an age at which breast cancer screening should stop?**
    In the United States, there are no guidelines for when screening should stop. In other countries, the recommended age at which screening should stop ranges from 59 to 74 years.

16. **What is batch reading of screening mammograms?**
    This is the most efficient way to read screening mammograms. The films are hung on a multiviewer, and multiple films are read at a time. This approach increases efficiency.

17. **What are some of the risk factors for developing breast cancer?**
    Some of the risk factors include female gender, first-degree relative with breast cancer, personal history of breast cancer, history of atypia such as atypical ductal hyperplasia and lobular carcinoma in situ on biopsy, early menarche, late menopause, nulliparous status, late first-term pregnancy (>30), and increasing age.

18. **True or false: Most breast cancers occur in women with a family history of breast cancer.**
    False. About 20% of breast cancers occur in patients with a positive family history. About 75–80% of breast cancers are sporadic.

19. **True or false: With increased use of breast cancer screening, the incidence of breast cancer has been declining.**
    False. The incidence of breast cancer has been steadily rising since the 1980s. This rise has been partly attributed to early detection due to breast cancer screening with mammography. As more

women start to get annual screening, detection increases. However, increased detection with screening does not entirely account for the overall increased incidence.

20. **It has been said that 1 in 8 women has a risk of developing breast cancer. Does a 40-year-old woman have the same risk as an 80-year-old woman?**
No. The 1 in 8 risk of developing breast cancer refers to an overall lifetime risk if the woman lives to age 85. Therefore, given identical circumstances, a 40-year-old does not have the same risk as an 80-year-old person. The National Cancer Institute (NCI) gives an overall risk given the age of the patient (Table 5-1).

TABLE 5-1. AGE-RELATED INCIDENCE OF BREAST CANCER	
Age	Risk
30–40	1 of 252
40–50	1 of 68
50–60	1 of 35
60–70	1 of 27
70+	1 of 8

Data from National Cancer Institute Surveillance, Epidemiology, and End Results Program, 1997–1999. In Ries LA, Eisner MP, Kosary CL, et al (eds): SEER Cancer Statistics Review, 1973–1999. Bethesda, MD, National Cancer Institute, 2002.

21. **What is the risk of getting breast cancer by age 70 in a patient with the BRCA1 gene?**
About 85%.

22. **How much radiation does a woman receive from a routine screening mammogram?**
The amount of radiation is 0.2 rads (2 mGray) for two views of one breast. This is equivalent to the amount of radiation a person would get on a plane ride from the East to the West Coast.

23. **How is the patient who is being screened informed of test results?**
Usually, by a letter sent in the mail. There are two potential results. The patient may be informed that her mammogram was normal. Alternatively, the patient may be informed of the need for additional evaluation, which may be in the form of additional imaging or obtaining the patient's prior mammograms for comparison.

24. **What happens if additional imaging evaluation is needed based on findings on the screening mammogram?**
The patient is sent a letter advising her that additional evaluation is needed. In addition, at our institution, a coordinator calls the patient to schedule the necessary appointment.

25. **What is the call-back rate? What should the call-back rate be for a radiologist?**
The call-back rate is the percentage of the screening cases that the radiologist recommends for additional imaging evaluations. The rate should be 10% or less.

26. **Which is true: The breast is a modified skin gland, fatty tissue, muscle, or lymphatic structure?**
The breast tissue is derived from ectodermal origin and is a modified skin gland.

27. How does accessory breast tissue form? Where is it most commonly located?
Breast tissue development begins at about 6 weeks of gestation and originates from ectodermal elements. The "milk line" extends from the groin region to the axillary region. Most of the potential breast tissue atrophies except in the fourth intercostal region, where "normal" mammary tissue eventually develops. The lack of appropriate regression results in accessory breasts anywhere along the "milk line."

BIBLIOGRAPHY

1. Gardenosa G: Breast cancer: An overview. In Gardenosa G: Breast Imaging Companion, 2nd ed. Philadelphia, Lippincott Williams & Wilkins, 2001, pp 1–11.

2. Heywang-Kobrunner SH, Dershaw DD, Schreer I: Mammography. In Heywang-Kobrunner SH, Dershaw DD, Schreer I: Diagnostic Breast Imaging, 2nd ed. New York, Thieme, 2001, pp 14–86.

3. Kopans D: Epidemiology, etiology, risk factors, survival, and prevention of breast cancer. In Kopans D: Breast Imaging, 2nd ed. Philadelphia, Lippincott-Raven, 1998, pp 29–54.

4. Mushin AI, Kouides RW, Shapiro DE: Estimating the accuracy of screening mammography: A meta-analysis. Am J Prev Med 14:143–153, 1998.

5. Shapiro S, Coleman EA, Broeders M, et al: Breast cancer screening programs in 22 countries: Current policies, administration and guidelines. Int J Epidemiol 27:735–742, 1998.

CHAPTER 6

DIAGNOSTIC MAMMOGRAPHY

Susan P. Weinstein, MD

1. **What are the indications for a diagnostic mammogram?**
   Some of the indications for a diagnostic mammogram include history of breast cancer, breast lump, nipple discharge, focal breast pain, and follow-up for a previously evaluated mammographic finding (BIRADS category 3 lesion [*see* question 3]).

2. **How are diagnostic patients informed of results?**
   The routine views are performed with additional views as needed. Sonography may also be performed if indicated. The imaging evaluation is completed while the patient is present, and the patient is informed of the results before she leaves. At our institution, the physician discusses the results with the patient.

3. **What is BIRADS?**
   The Breast Imaging Reporting and Dictation System (BIRADS) lexicon was developed by the American College of Radiology to provide a clear and concise way to report the mammographic results. A BIRADS category is reported at the end of every mammogram report and summarizes the results of the mammogram (Table 6-1).

TABLE 6-1. BIRADS LEXICON	
BIRADS Category	**Definition**
1	Normal mammogram. The patient should return in 1 year for her annual mammogram.
2	Benign finding on the mammogram. The patient should return in 1 year for her annual mammogram.
3	A finding is present, but there is a high likelihood of benignity (>98%). A short-term follow-up is recommended in 6 months. Normally, the follow-up is performed over a total of 2 years.
4	A finding is present, and a biopsy is warranted.
4a	Low likelihood of malignancy.
4b	Intermediate likelihood of malignancy.
4c	Moderate likelihood of malignancy.
5	A finding is present, and a biopsy is recommended. There is a high likelihood of malignancy (>95%).
6	Confirmed malignancy.
0	Indicates that the imaging evaluation is incomplete. Additional evaluation or prior films are needed for comparison.

4. **What types of mammographic changes may be seen after breast conservation?**
    There may be persistent distortion and edema. Other findings include skin thickening and trabecular thickening.

5. **Does mammography have a very high sensitivity in detecting recurrent breast cancer after breast conservation?**
    The sensitivity of mammography in detecting recurrent tumor is limited by the post-therapy changes seen on the mammogram. Mammography will not detect recurrence about one third of the time. Therefore, physical examination plays an important role in evaluating the patient after breast conservation.

6. **What is the incidence of recurrent breast cancer in a patient after breast conservation?**
    The risk of recurrence is about 1–2% per year. At 5 years, the risk of recurrence is about 5–10%.

7. **True or false: In patients who develop recurrence after breast conservation, survival rates are about the same as for patients who had a mastectomy as the initial treatment.**
    True. Recurrence after breast conservation does not seem to affect the overall survival rate for patients with breast cancer.

8. **What are contraindications to breast conservation?**
    Multicentric cancer; size of cancer relative to breast size, resulting in poor cosmesis; first- or second-trimester pregnancy; history of prior radiation therapy to the chest or mediastinum; and active collagen vascular disease.

9. **In a patient who is planning to have breast conservation, when is it necessary to obtain a postbiopsy mammogram shortly after a successful excisional biopsy?**
    If the malignancy was associated with calcifications on the mammogram, a postbiopsy mammogram should be obtained to ensure that all the suspicious microcalcifications have been removed.
    For breast cancers that present as a mass on the mammogram, a postbiopsy mammogram is not needed. The decision to re-excise should be based on the histologic margins. Due to the postbiopsy changes in the surgical bed, it would be difficult to differentiate between postbiopsy changes and residual tumor.

10. **True or false: In a patient with a history of breast cancer, it is beneficial to get a mammogram more frequently than once a year.**
    False. No studies have demonstrated the benefit of increased frequency of screening. We recommend mammography once a year.

11. **How do you hang a mammogram of a patient who has had a mastectomy?**
    The craniocaudal (CC) and mediolateral oblique (MLO) views should be hung on the appropriate side on the light box. The old films should be hung in mirror image.

12. **What is a 6-month follow-up? How long is the follow-up performed for BIRADS category 3 lesions?**
    Six-month follow-up is performed for BIRADS category 3 lesions (after an appropriate imaging evaluation). The follow-up is performed for a total of 2 years at 6-month intervals.

13. **How is the mastectomy bed evaluated?**
    We do not recommend routine imaging evaluation of the mastectomy bed. No studies have shown the benefit of routine imaging evaluation of the surgical bed. Instead, clinical evaluation

is recommended. If there is a palpable area of concern on the physical examination, sonography should be performed as the next step in the evaluation.

14. **What types of surgical reconstruction are available after a mastectomy?**
There are various types of tissue flaps, such as transverse rectus abdominis musculocutaneous (TRAM) flaps and latissimus dorsi flaps. Alternatively, breast implants may be used for reconstruction. Breast implants may be used with or without a subcutaneous mastectomy.

15. **True or false: After a benign breast biopsy, significant residual changes are usually visible on a mammogram.**
False. After a benign breast biopsy the breast tissue usually heals with few residual changes. Infrequently, distortion may persist.

16. **For all breast biopsies, approximately what percentage of the pathology results should be malignant?**
The positive predictive value for all breast biopsies should be approximately 25–40%. This rate is considered acceptable.

17. **A 47-year-old woman presents with a palpable breast mass and negative mammogram results. What should be done next?**
The next step in the evaluation should be a directed sonographic evaluation of the area of palpable concern. If a mass is present, a biopsy should be recommended.

18. **If sonography results are negative, what should be done next? What percentage of the time can a cancer be missed on both sonography and mammography?**
If the ultrasound results are negative, clinical management is advised. Depending on the literature, the negative predictive value of combined mammography and sonography is 95–100%. That is, with both negative studies, a cancer may be missed 5% of the time or less.

19. **What types of nipple discharge are considered suspicious and warrant additional imaging evaluation? What should be the imaging work-up of suspicious nipple discharge?**
Nipple discharge that is spontaneous, bloody, clear, or serosanguineous is considered suspicious. The first step in the evaluation should be a mammogram. The mammogram results may be normal or show a finding.
    The next step may be a galactogram. The involved ductal orifice is cannulated, and a catheter is inserted. A small amount of contrast is injected into the ductal system until resistance is felt. A mammogram is then obtained to look for filling defects that may be the cause of the discharge (Fig. 6-1). Magnetic resonance imaging (MRI) may also have a role in the evaluation of nipple discharge.

Figure 6-1. An image from a galactogram in a patient presenting with bloody nipple discharge. Contrast is seen filling a ductal system. A lobulated filling defect is marked with an *asterisk*. Biopsy revealed a papilloma.

20. **What are the benign types of nipple discharge?**
    The typical benign discharge may be greenish, brownish, or milky in color. Bilaterality and discharge arising from multiple ductal orifices are also benign characteristics.

KEY POINTS: DIAGNOSTIC MAMMOGRAPHY ✔

1. The BIRADS categories (*see* Table 6-1) are essential for reporting results of diagnostic mammography.

2. Diagnostic mammography is indicated for women with a specific breast-related problem that needs to be evaluated. Screening mammography is indicated for asymptomatic patients.

3. In patients who have had breast conservation, the postbiopsy changes may limit the sensitivity of mammography.

4. In a patient presenting with a palpable breast mass, if the mammogram results are negative, the imaging evaluation should not stop at that point. Directed sonographic evaluation is necessary to complete the evaluation.

21. **In a patient with one of the suspicious types of nipple discharge, what is the likelihood that the discharge is due to cancer?**
    About 10%.

22. **What is the most common etiology for bloody nipple discharge?**
    Benign papillomas.

23. **What are the most common histologic types of breast cancer?**
    Invasive ductal carcinoma, intraductal (DCIS) carcinoma, and invasive lobular carcinoma. Subtypes of ductal carcinoma are medullary, mucinous, papillary, and tubular. Less common histologic types of breast cancer include sarcoma and lymphoma.

24. **Is lobular carcinoma in situ (LCIS) a form of cancer? What is the significance of LCIS?**
    LCIS has no clinical or mammographic correlate. It is a histologic diagnosis. It is not a cancer but is considered a risk lesion. In a woman previously diagnosed with LCIS, the risk of developing breast cancer in either breast is about 33%.

25. **What is the differential diagnosis for a red swollen breast?**
    The differential diagnosis includes infection, inflammatory breast cancer, history of prior radiation, and lymphatic or vascular obstruction. The history of prior radiation should be easy to corroborate with the patient. Patients with infection and inflammatory breast cancer can present with similar histories: red, swollen, tender breast. Imaging should be performed to exclude a mass or an abscess. If the patient's symptoms do not improve with treatment (usually antibiotics), inflammatory breast cancer should be excluded.

26. **Is there such a thing as a mammographic emergency?**
    Probably the only breast imaging-related emergency is an abscess that needs to be drained, but this problem can usually be managed clinically. If a fluctuant mass is present, it can be drained by palpation. Otherwise, if there is clinical concern of an abscess, the patient can be treated

symptomatically. Patients are usually in too much pain to get a mammogram anyway; if they undergo imaging, an ultrasound examination is usually performed.

27. **How many views are obtained in a patient with breast augmentation?**
   At our institution, four routine views (CC and MLO views) and four implant-displaced views are obtained. (At some institutions, an implant-displaced ML view may also be obtained.) On the four routine views, the breast implant is imaged. Therefore, the glandular tissue is not well compressed. The implant-displaced views are obtained with the implant pushed back so that the breast tissue can be compressed. Usually the presence of the breast implants limits the visualization of the posterior breast tissue.

28. **Where can the implants be placed in the breast?**
   They can be placed retropectorally, behind the pectoralis muscle. Alternatively, they can be placed in the retroglandular position, or in front of the muscle.

29. **What types of implants are available?**
   Currently, the only types of implants on the market in the United States are saline-filled implants. In the past, silicone implants were also used. Silicone implants are currently being reevaluated, and they may return to the market in the near future.

30. **What is the most sensitive imaging evaluation for implant rupture?**
   MRI is the gold standard. Ultrasound may be used to evaluate for rupture as well, but the examination is operator dependent. Rupture may be contained within the fibrous capsule surrounding the implant (intracapsular) or may extend outside the fibrous capsule (extracapsular). Although mammography will detect extracapsular rupture, it is limited in the evaluation of intracapsular rupture, the more common form of rupture.
   Some of the MRI findings of implant rupture are the linguine sign (most reliable), the keyhole sign, and the noose sign.

31. **A male patient presents with a breast lump. How should the patient be imaged? What is most common etiology for a breast lump in a man?**
   For a man presenting with a breast lump, we usually recommend a bilateral mammogram. Sometimes sonography may be needed if there is dense tissue in the area of the breast lump on the mammogram. The most common etiology for a breast lump in a man is gynecomastia. Usually this is bilateral, although typically asymmetric (Fig. 6-2).

32. **What is the etiology of gynecomastia?**
   There is a long differential diagnosis for gynecomastia. In babies and in teenagers, it is most commonly due to hormonal influences. Transplacental maternal hormones are responsible in babies. In teenagers, the hormonal changes of adolescence may be responsible. However, other pathologic processes should be excluded. A few of the more common etiologies for gynecomastia are marijuana use, certain types of medications, liver dysfunction, and androgen deficiency. Finally, hormone-secreting tumors should be excluded.

Figure 6-2. An MLO view of a male patient who presented with breast pain. There is glandular tissue seen in the subareolar region consistent with gynecomastia.

33. **Do men get breast cancer? What is the frequency?**
     Yes, but male breast cancers are very uncommon, accounting for
     less than 0.5% of all breast cancers (Fig. 6-3).

34. **True or false: Breast cancer can present in the
     following ways: calcifications, masses, architectural
     distortion, and density.**
     True for all of the above, although benign lesions may also present
     as any of the above categories.

35. **The following terms are commonly used to describe
     calcifications. Classify the terms as describing benign,
     indeterminate, or malignant calcifications.**
     a. Popcorn
     b. Centrally lucent
     c. Amorphous
     d. Heterogeneous
     e. Indistinct
     f. Round
     g. Milk of calcium
     h. Linear, branching
     i. Rodlike
     j. Eggshell
     k. Dystrophic
     l. Pleomorphic
     Benign: a, b, f, g, i, j, k; *indeterminate:* c, e; *malignant:* d, h, l.

36. **Figures 6-4 through 6-9 show images of calcifications.
     Classify them as benign or malignant calcifications.**

Figure 6-3. An MLO view of a male patient who presented with a breast lump. There is a lobulated, circumscribed mass seen in the subareolar region. Note the mass is definitely masslike, unlike the changes of gynecomastia seen in Figure 6-2. Biopsy showed invasive carcinoma.

Figure 6-4.

Figure 6-5.

Figure 6-6. (A) CC view. (B) ML view.

Figure 6-7.

Figure 6-8.

Figure 6-9.

Answers: Figures 6-4 and 6-5 display malignant calcifications. Figures 6-6, 6-7, 6-8, and 6-9 are different types of benign calcifications: Figure 6-6 is milk of calcium; Figure 6-7 shows round calcifications; Figure 6-8 shows popcorn calcifications; and Figure 6-9 shows secretory calcifications.

BIBLIOGRAPHY

1. Bassett LW: Imaging of breast masses. Radiol Clin North Am 38:669–692, 2000.

2. Dennis MA, Parker SH, Klaus AJ, et al: Breast biopsy avoidance: The value of normal mammograms and normal sonograms in the setting of a palpable lump. Radiology 219:186–191, 2001.

3. Dershaw DD: Breast imaging and the conservative treatment of breast cancer. Radiol Clin North Am 40:501–516, 2002.

4. Gardenosa G: The male breast. In Gardenosa G: Breast Imaging Companion, 2nd ed. Philadelphia, Lippincott Williams & Wilkins, 2001, pp 401–412.

5. Kaiser JS, Helvie MA, Blacklaw RL, Roubidoux MA: Palpable breast thickening: Role of mammography and US in cancer detection. Radiology 223:839–844, 2002.

6. Nakahara H, Namba K, Watanabe R, et al: A comparison of MR imaging, galactography and ultrasonography in patients with nipple discharge. Breast Cancer 10:320–329, 2003.

7. Orel SG, Dougherty CS, Reynolds C, et al: MR imaging in patients with nipple discharge: Initial experience. Radiology 216:248–254, 2000.

8. Soo MS, Rosen EL, Baker JA, et al: Negative predictive value of sonography with mammography in patients with palpable breast lesions. Am J Roentgenol 177:1167–1170, 2001.

BREAST ULTRASOUND AND BREAST PROCEDURES

Susan P. Weinstein, MD

1. **What are the labeled structures on the ultrasound (US) image in Figure 7-1?**
   (A) Skin; (B) subcutaneous fat; (C) glandular tissue; (D) fat; (E) muscle; and (F) rib.

2. **What type of transducer should be used to perform breast sonography?**
   A linear array transducer. This should be at least 7 MHz, ideally 10 MHz or greater.

3. **What are the indications for breast sonography after mammographic evaluation?**
   - To further evaluate a palpable abnormality
   - To characterize a mammographic finding/abnormality

4. **In what situations would you not perform a mammogram but go directly to breast sonography in evaluating patients with palpable breast masses?**
   In patients who are younger than 30 and in pregnant patients. For all other patients, mammography should be obtained first.

Figure 7-1. US image of normal breast tissue.

5. **What are some suspicious sonographic lesion features?**
   Markedly hypoechoic appearance, posterior acoustic shadowing, angular margins, spiculations, microlobulations, taller than wide, and ductal extension. Although these features are usually seen in malignant lesions, there is an overlap and benign masses may also exhibit some of these findings (Fig. 7-2).

6. **What are some benign sonographic lesion features?**
   Benign sonographic features include absence of malignant features,

Figure 7-2. A highly suspicious hypoechoic lobulated solid mass with irregular margins in a woman who presented with a palpable breast mass. Biopsy revealed invasive carcinoma.

well-circumscribed mass, ellipsoid shape, and hyperechogenicity. Even though these features are typically seen in benign lesions, again some malignant masses may exhibit some of these features. Well-circumscribed cancers include invasive ductal, medullary, and colloid cancers (Fig. 7-3).

Figure 7-3. A 26-year-old woman presented with a palpable mass. US evaluation shows a benign-appearing, well-circumscribed oval mass. The US findings are consistent with a benign mass such as a fibroadenoma.

7. **What types of biopsy procedures may be performed to evaluate breast lesions?**
   - *Fine needle aspiration (FNA)* is readily available and needs no special equipment. Overall, it is less traumatic than the other two types of biopsies.
   - *Core biopsy* can be done under US guidance or stereotactic mammographic guidance. US-guided core needle biopsy is used to biopsy US-visible masses. Biopsies performed under sonography tend to be faster than stereotactic biopsies (BBST). At our institution, we reserve the stereotactic method to biopsy calcifications, although solid masses may also be biopsied using this method. Percutaneous core biopsies are less expensive and traumatic than surgical biopsies. The false-negative rates are similar to open biopsies.
   - *Needle localization with excisional biopsy* is the gold standard. To confirm removal of the lesion, a specimen radiograph is obtained.

8. **What are the relative disadvantages of FNA, core needle biopsy, and needle localization/excision?**
   - *FNA:* The results are dependent on the skill of the person performing the procedure and the cytopathologist. There can be a high percentage of unsatisfactory aspirates (20–30% of cases). Invasive versus in situ cancer cannot be differentiated on FNA. The false-negative rate for image-guided FNA is not known.
   - *Core needle biopsy:* Tissue displacement may occur during the biopsy, resulting in misinterpretation of intraductal carcinoma as invasive carcinoma. Inversely, cancer can occasionally be understaged.
   - *Needle localization with excisional biopsy:* This is the most expensive and most traumatic of all the biopsies.

9. **After core biopsy, how can one be certain that the lesion of interest was actually what was sampled?**
   After a stereotactic biopsy, a specimen radiograph is used to confirm that the appropriate area was sampled. Real-time visualization during the US-guided biopsy confirms that the appropriate area of concern was biopsied.

10. **What is stereotaxis?**
    A technique used to localize breast lesions for biopsy. A digital image of the lesion is taken on the stereotactic machine, the scout image. Two views are then taken at +/−15 degrees from the original 0-degree scout image. From the three views, the machine calculates the Z axis, which is the depth the needle needs to be placed to biopsy the lesion.

KEY POINTS: US/INTERVENTIONAL PROCEDURES

1. For optimal imaging evaluation, at least a 7-MHz transducer (ideally 10 MHz or greater) should be used to perform breast sonography.

2. In addition to doing the percutaneous breast biopsy, the radiologist's role includes evaluating the pathology results for concordance with the imaging findings.

3. If atypical ductal hyperplasia is present on pathologic evaluation of a percutaneous biopsy specimen, excisional biopsy should be recommended.

11. **In what circumstances would stereotactic biopsy be difficult to perform?**
    - Lesions in the subareolar location
    - If the breast tissue compresses to less than 2.5 cm
    - Lesions that are very posterior in location
    - If the calcifications are indistinct and difficult to see

12. **In what circumstances would a US-guided biopsy be difficult to perform?**
    - Lesions that are very small and close to the skin surface
    - Lesions behind the nipple
    - Lesions close to the chest wall

13. **What is discordance in relation to percutaneous biopsies?**
    When a percutaneous breast biopsy is performed, one of the radiologist's roles is to make sure the histologic diagnosis is concordant, or makes sense with the imaging appearance. If the imaging appearance is highly suspicious and the pathologic results are benign, this may suggest a discordance.

14. **In what situations or histologic diagnosis should an excisional biopsy be recommended after a percutaneous breast biopsy?**
    When there is pathologic imaging discordance, excisional biopsy should be recommended. When atypical ductal hyperplasia (ADH) is present on pathologic evaluation, excisional biopsy should also be recommended. When ADH is present, 20–56% (14 G needle) and 0–38% (11 G needle) of the time, cancer is present on excisional biopsy. More controversial pathologic diagnoses include papillary lesions, radial scars, atypical lobular hyperplasia, and lobular carcinoma in situ. Some advocate excisional biopsy for these lesions as well.

BIBLIOGRAPHY

1. Gardenosa G: Breast ultrasound. In Gardenosa G: Breast Imaging Companion, 2nd ed. Philadelphia, Lippincott Williams & Wilkins, 2001, pp 159–184.

2. Gardenosa G: Terminal duct. In Gardenosa G: Breast Imaging Companion, 2nd ed. Philadelphia, Lippincott Williams & Wilkins, 2001, pp 231–268.

3. Liberman L: Percutaneous image-guided core breast biopsy. Radiol Clin North Am 40:483–500, 2002.

CHAPTER 8

BREAST MRI

Mark Rosen, MD, PhD

1. How is breast magnetic resonance imaging (MRI) performed?

The patient is required to lie on her stomach in the prone position. The breasts are placed into openings or wells that house the receiver coils (devices that detect emitted MRI signal from the body). Prone positioning helps minimize the motion of the breast during respiration. Dependent positioning of the breast also helps to extend the breast away from the chest wall and allows for mild compression of the breast, further minimizing unwanted motion during the MRI examination.

2. Is contrast required for breast MRI?

For an MRI examination performed only to define the integrity of breast implants, no contrast is required. Breast MRI examinations performed to evaluate known or potential breast cancer require the administration of a gadolinium-based MRI contrast agent via a peripheral IV.

3. What scanner capabilities are required for breast MRI?

Breast MRI is generally performed on high–field strength scanners (i.e., ≥1.0 T). Even though breast MRI examinations at lower field strengths of open MRI systems are feasible, most radiologists use greater field strengths (≥1.0 T) of closed MRI systems. The scanning at greater magnetic field strength allows for substantial improvement in image quality and diagnostic accuracy.

Breast MRI also requires the use of a dedicated breast receiver coil. Since the strength of emitted MR signals is quite weak, optimal MRI requires placing the detector coil as close as possible to the anatomy of interest. Specialized receiver coils for breast MRI have been designed that allow one to place the coil immediately against the surface of the breast (Fig. 8-1).

Figure 8-1. Breast coil as used at the University of Pennsylvania MRI Center. The patient is placed prone on the coil with the breasts dependently positioned in the wells. The lateral plates *(long arrows)* can be adjusted for mild compression and stabilization of the breast. Two medial MR receiver coils *(short arrows)* are found within the unit. Two lateral receiver coils *(arrowheads)* are attached once the patient is positioned properly.

4. What are the indications for breast MRI?

Breast MRI is performed either for evaluation of the integrity of breast prostheses (implants) or for evaluation of breast cancer. Breast cancer evaluation can further be subdivided into screening, diagnosis, staging, and post-therapy monitoring. Often, a patient may undergo breast MRI for a combination of reasons, such as staging the local extent of known cancer in one breast while simultaneously screening for an occult cancer in the other breast.

5. **What pulse sequences are required for breast MRI?**
   The pulse sequences used to create the different MR images in a breast MRI examination depend on several factors, including the capabilities and performance of the MR system used and the type of information (e.g., implant evaluation or cancer identification) sought by the referring doctor. In addition, the imaging techniques used by a particular MRI center reflect the experience and preferences of the local radiologists at that center. At our institution, for example, breast MRI is performed in the sagittal plane and includes T1 spin echo, fat-saturated T2 fast spin echo (FSE), and fat-saturated three-dimensional T1-spoiled gradient echo. The latter sequence is performed once before and several times after IV gadolinium administration.

6. **What are the components of the female breast?**
   The mature female breast is divided into the following components: glandular elements (ducts and lobules), fibrous supporting structure (Cooper's ligaments), and surrounding adipose tissue. Blood vessels and, occasionally, lymph nodes are also found within the breast. Anatomically, the breast is bounded anteriorly, inferiorly, and medially by skin. Posteriorly, it is bounded by the chest wall (pectoralis major and minor muscles, ribs, and intercostal muscles). Superiolaterally, the glandular breast tissue variably extends into the axilla, where adipose tissue, major blood vessels, and lymph nodes reside.

7. **How is the breast organized anatomically?**
   The breast is divided into 8–20 segments, each of which is supplied by a major lactiferous duct. The ducts extend from the nipple, each communicating with a separate nipple orifice. The lactiferous duct subdivides into numerous ductules, each of which ramifies into several lobules. A terminal ductule and its associated lobules are classified together as a terminal ductule-lobular unit (TDLU). It is within the TDLU that the majority of breast cancers develop.

8. **What is the normal appearance of the breast on MRI?**
   On MRI, one can distinguish between the fatty adipose tissue and the fibroglandular elements, or parenchyma, on the basis of signal intensity. On T1-weighted imaging, the fat is bright, whereas the parenchyma is intermediate-dark (Fig. 8-2, *A*). The appearance of the breast on T2-weighted imaging depends on whether one uses fat suppression. Most radiologists use fat suppression on T2-weighted imaging. On fat-suppressed T2-weighted imaging, breast tissue is intermediate-bright (Fig. 8-2, *B*). This fat suppression eliminates or reduces the high signal intensity of fat in order to highlight the bright signal of fluid in ducts or cysts or the bright signal intensity of certain masses, such as lymph nodes or fibroadenomas.

BREAST CANCER DETECTION ON MRI

9. **How is contrast material used in MRI for breast cancer detection?**
   Gadolinium-based contrast agents shorten the T1 relaxation time of neighboring water protons, which leads to a relative increase in signal intensity of perfused tissue after IV injection of gadolinium contrast. The degree of brightening (enhancement) depends on the amount of gadolinium that enters the tissue, which in turn is related to the amount of blood flow that the tissue receives. Since breast cancers are heavily dependent on blood flow for growth, they tend to enhance markedly after gadolinium contrast administration.

10. **What is the appearance of breast cancer on MRI?**
    Breast cancer is depicted as an enhancing mass or an enhancing region of the breast after contrast administration (Fig. 8-3). In some patients, cancers may enhance less prominently (Fig. 8-4). In such cases, identification of the cancer requires close comparison between the unenhanced and enhanced T1-weighted images or the use of computer-generated subtraction images. Occasionally, a cancer will enhance minimally or not at all. This is especially true of

Figure 8-2. (A) Sagittal T1-weighted image of a normal breast. The fat within the breast is bright, and the fibroglandular elements are intermediate-dark (*P* = pectoralis major, *p* = pectoralis minor, *L* = lung). (B) Sagittal FSE T2-weighted image with fat saturation, at same location as (A). The suppressed fat is now dark on this image, and the fibroglandular elements are variably intermediate-bright. Higher signal intensity is seen in small cysts *(arrows)* and in peripheral veins *(arrowhead)*.

Figure 8-3. (A) Breast cancer on T1-spoiled gradient recalled echo image (TR = 7.7 ms, TE = 1.8 ms). The cancer *(arrow)* is isointense to the background glandular tissue. (B) After gadolinium administration, the cancer is seen as an avidly enhancing mass. The contrast-enhanced images also help depict the irregular and spiculated borders of the mass.

purely intraductal cancers, also known as *ductal carcinoma in situ (DCIS)*. However, in most studies, the sensitivity of MRI for invasive breast cancer is found to be at or near 100%.

11. **Do all enhancing abnormalities in the breast represent cancer?**
     No. Even though MRI is very sensitive for detecting breast cancer, it is less specific. This is because many other breast entities can be enhancing. Many benign masses, such as

Figure 8-4. Subtly enhancing cancer (invasive lobular carcinoma) demonstrated on contrast-enhanced T1-weighted spoiled GR imaging before (A) and after (B) contrast administration. The cancer is shown as an irregular region of glandular-type intensity, with enhancement mildly greater in degree than that of the surrounding glandular tissue. This enhancement *(arrows)* is much more apparent in the computer-generated subtraction (postcontrast minus precontrast) image (C).

fibroadenomas, papillomas, or radial scars, will also enhance after gadolinium administration. Proliferative breast changes, such as fibrocystic disease or ductal hyperplasia, may also enhance after gadolinium administration. Even normal breast parenchyma may enhance after contrast administration, especially in premenopausal women or those receiving hormone replacement therapy.

12. **What are the characteristic features of malignant breast masses?**
As is true in mammography, most cancers in MRI are depicted as spiculated or irregular focal masses. Benign masses that may enhance on MRI, such as lymph nodes and fibroadenomas, are more often round or oval with smooth margins. However, some cancers are also depicted as smoothly marginated enhancing masses on MRI. Therefore, careful evaluation of the morphology of enhancement (e.g., homogeneous vs. heterogeneous) may be required to differentiate benign from malignant enhancing masses.

13. **Do all breast cancers appear as focal enhancing masses on MRI?**

No. Certain cancers, especially invasive lobular carcinoma or cancers that are largely intraductal, may present as an ill-defined region of enhancement, rather than as a focally enhancing mass. Pure DCIS may present as linear or branching enhancement along the margins of a duct. However, regional enhancement is not specific and can be seen in benign breast disease (e.g., fibrocystic disease). Enhancement that is markedly more intense than that of surrounding breast parenchyma and that follows a segmental or ductal distribution or that features "clumping" (grouping of distinct foci of solid enhancement greater than 5 mm) is more often indicative of an underlying malignancy (Fig. 8-5).

Figure 8-5. Grouped clumped enhancement *(arrows)* on a subtraction postgadolinium T1-weighted spoiled GR image. Several, large, grouped foci of avid enhancement are seen in a background of milder regional and ductal enhancement. Biopsy revealed DCIS. Two rim-enhancing cysts are noted inferiorly *(asterisks)*.

14. **How is kinetic enhancement information used in breast MRI?**

Breast cancers tend to enhance earlier and more intensely than do benign enhancing entities. Furthermore, this early enhancement of breast cancers will often be followed by a "washout" phase, in which the degree of enhancement decreases several minutes after the initiation of contrast enhancement. Benign lesions tend to enhance more gradually than malignancies do and in general will demonstrate sustained or increasing enhancement for at least 4–5 minutes after contrast administration.

15. **Can T1- or T2-weighted images be used to identify breast cancer?**

There is considerable overlap in the appearance of breast cancer and benign breast parenchyma on T1- and T2-weighted images. As such, neither T1- nor T2-weighted images in and of themselves are useful for breast cancer detection. However, T1- and T2-weighted images may be useful for improving diagnostic specificity. The demonstration of intralesional fat on T1-weighted images can help confirm the diagnosis of certain benign enhancing lesions, such as a breast hamartoma. Other benign lesions, such as lymph nodes or fibroadenomas, tend to demonstrate marked hyperintensity on T2-weighted imaging, distinguishing them from most cancers, which are isointense to parenchyma on T2-weighted imaging.

16. **Does MRI detect cancers that cannot be seen on mammography?**

MRI has been shown to detect cancers that are occult on mammography and physical examination. MRI is especially helpful in women with dense breasts, in whom mammography is known to be less sensitive. In women with axillary nodal metastases and negative mammogram results, MRI is often successful in identifying the site of primary malignancy. In patients with newly diagnosed cancer, MRI can be used to demonstrate the true extent of an infiltrative malignancy (e.g., invasive lobular cancer) or to detect unsuspected additional malignant foci (multifocal/multicentric cancer).

KEY POINTS: MRI BREAST CANCER DETECTION

1. IV contrast is required for all breast cancer detection by MRI.

2. MRI is nearly 100% sensitive for invasive breast cancer but is less sensitive for DCIS. MRI can detect foci of cancer that are occult on mammography and physical examination.

3. Cancer detection requires identification of foci or regions of abnormal enhancement.

4. Differentiation of benign from malignant enhancement requires evaluation of both lesion morphology (e.g., borders) and enhancement kinetics.

5. MRI is most useful for evaluating indeterminate mammographic findings, staging known cancer, and identifying occult cancer in high-risk women.

6. Currently, MRI is not believed to be cost-effective as a screening modality for the general population.

17. **Should breast MRI be used for routine screening and diagnosis for breast disease?**
    No. Given the relatively low specificity of breast MRI and the propensity for false-positive findings, most experts recommend that MRI be used only in well-defined applications. Indiscriminate use of MRI as a screening modality in the general population will undoubtedly lead to increased medical costs, as well as unnecessary follow-up examinations and biopsies with little overall benefit to the population as a whole. However, in certain selected groups of women at a particularly high risk for breast cancer, such as BRCA1 or BRCA2 mutation carriers, screening MRI may be cost-effective. MRI also has been successfully used at the time of breast cancer diagnosis as a screening modality to identify coexisting occult cancers in the contra-lateral breast.

18. **When should diagnostic breast MRI be performed?**
    Breast MRI may be indicated when a breast abnormality cannot be completely characterized through the use of traditional imaging modalities (mammography and sonography), such as a suspicious abnormality found on mammography that is sonographically occult and can only be visualized in one mammographic projection. Other indications for breast MRI include: staging MRI to fully define the local extent of histologically proven cancer, follow-up examination after breast conservation therapy when postoperative or postradiation changes may obscure or mimic local tumor recurrence, or documenting the local tumor response to preoperative (neoadjuvant) chemotherapy.

19. **How can suspicious lesions that are identified only by breast MRI be biopsied?**
    When a suspicious breast lesion is identified by MRI, it is imperative to correlate the findings with those of mammography and ultrasound. Often, an MRI abnormality will have a corresponding mammographic finding. In other cases, an abnormal MRI result may be used to guide a directed sonographic study to locate a previously unidentified solid abnormality. When a suspicious abnormality on MRI cannot be identified on other imaging modalities, an MR-guided biopsy procedure is required. MR-guided needle localization and core biopsy can be performed with specialized MR-compatible equipment.

IMPLANT EVALUATION BY MRI

20. What are the components of a breast prosthesis?

There are two broad categories of breast implants: saline-only implants and silicone-containing implants. All implants (including saline-only implants) have a thin elastomer shell, generally derived from a silicone polymer. Saline implants often contain an access port that allows for injection of additional saline into the lumen, since these implants are also used as tissue expanders. Silicone implants may be single-lumen or dual-lumen, usually with a silicone-containing inner lumen surrounded by a saline-containing outer lumen.

21. How does one distinguish between silicone and saline implants on MRI?

Because both silicone and saline are hypointense on T1-weighted imaging and hyperintense on T2-weighted imaging, differentiation between the two requires more sophisticated MRI. More heavily T2-weighted sequences (with echo times on the order of 200 ms) accentuate slight differences in the T2 relaxation times of these substances (Fig. 8-6, *A*). Frequency-selective water saturation can effectively eliminate the signal intensity of saline while preserving the bright silicone signal on T2-weighted images (Fig. 8-6, *B*). More advanced imaging methods can be used to create images with signal contribution from only one moiety or the other.

Figure 8-6. (A) Normal appearance of a silicone implant on MRI. Sagittal heavily T2-weighted FSE (TR = 5016 ms, TE = 202 ms) image demonstrates an intact single-lumen silicone implant. *Dark lines* extending into the center of the implant are normal radial folds of the outer elastomer shell. The silicone is intermediately high in single intensity, and fluid condensation within the radial folds *(arrow)* is brighter than silicone. (B) Silicone-only imaging on MRI. Sagittal short tau inversion recovery image (TR = 4600 ms, TE = 105 ms) with frequency-selective water suppression yields an image in which only silicone contributes bright signal intensity. This sequence is useful for demonstrating extracapsular ruptures with extravasation of free silicone into the breast or chest wall.

22. What is the normal MR appearance of a breast implant?

The normal breast implant is oval or ellipsoid in shape. An outer fibrous capsule will form as part of the normal tissue response to the implant. On T2-weighted MRI, the lumen of the implant should be uniformly bright with no internal debris. Infolding of the outer implant shell is not uncommon and will manifest as radially oriented protrusions ("radial folds") into the lumen of the implant. This is a common appearance of the normal implant and is not a sign of implant rupture. Condensation of fluid outside the implant shell but within the fibrous capsule is also a common phenomenon and should not be viewed as a sign of rupture.

23. **What are the different types of implant rupture?**
Gel bleed, contained (intracapsular) rupture, and extracapsular rupture. These categories refer to the degree of disruption of both the elastomer shell of the implant and the external fibrous capsule that develops around it.

24. **What is gel bleed?**
Gel bleed refers to transudation of small amounts of silicone gel through tiny perforations, or microtears, of the outer elastomer shell. Gel bleed is diagnosed by visualization of a small amount of silicone gel external to an otherwise intact elastomer shell but contained within the external fibrous capsule. The term *gel bleed* is reserved for MR evaluation of silicone implants. It is impossible on MRI to distinguish between saline extrusion through a microtear of the elastomer shell and normal fluid condensation between the elastomer shell and the fibrous capsule.

KEY POINTS: IMPLANT EVALUATION

1. Breast implants can be saline-only, silicone-only, or a combination of saline and silicone (dual-lumen).

2. MRI is the most accurate imaging test for evaluating implant integrity.

3. Implant rupture is divided into three categories of increasing severity: gel bleed, intracapsular rupture, and extracapsular rupture.

4. Depiction of free silicone in the breast tissue is the hallmark of extracapsular rupture.

25. **Describe the appearance of a "contained" implant rupture.**
Contained rupture can occur in either saline or silicone implants. In contained rupture, there is complete or near complete separation of the elastomer shell from the fibrous capsule and fragmentation of the elastomer shell. However, the contents of the implant lumen (saline or silicone) remain contained within the external fibrous capsule. The hallmark of contained rupture on MRI is the "linguine sign" (Fig. 8-7), in which strands of the remnant elastomer shell float freely in the contents of the implant lumen. These are identified as dark linear strands on T2-weighted images.

26. **What are the MRI findings of extracapsular rupture?**
Extracapsular rupture refers to rupture of the external fibrous capsule. For either silicone or saline implants, extracapsular rupture can be diagnosed when there is gross deformity or collapse of the fibrous capsule. For silicone-containing implants, extracapsular rupture is diagnosed whenever free silicone is identified within the extracapsular soft tissues of the breast or within axillary

Figure 8-7. Axial T2-weighted FSE image of a silicone implant with contained (intracapsular) rupture. The silicone is contained by the outer fibrous capsule that develops within the breast after implant placement. The fragmented strands of the outer elastomer shell of the implant can be seen floating freely within the contained silicone, like strands of linguine *(arrows)*.

lymph nodes. When one seeks to identify the presence of free silicone within breast tissue, one must separate not only silicone and saline signals, but also those of breast parenchyma and fat. Silicone-only imaging sequences are therefore essential for detecting free silicone in the breast or axilla.

BIBLIOGRAPHY

1. Berg WA, Caskey CI, Hamper UM, et al: Single- and double-lumen silicone breast implant integrity: Prospective evaluation of MR and US criteria. Radiology 197(1):45–52, 1995.

2. Gilles R, Guinebretiere JM, Lucidarme O, et al: Nonpalpable breast tumors: Diagnosis with contrast-enhanced subtraction dynamic MR imaging. Radiology 191(3):625–631, 1994.

3. Harms SE, Flamig DP, Hesley KL, et al: MR imaging of the breast with rotating delivery of excitation off resonance: Clinical experience with pathologic correlation. Radiology 187(2):493–501, 1993.

4. Heywang SH, Wolf A, Pruss E, et al: MR imaging of the breast with Gd-DTPA: Use and limitations. Radiology 171(1):95–103, 1989.

5. Hochman MG, Orel SG, Powell CM, et al: Fibroadenomas: MR imaging appearances with radiologic-histopathologic correlation. Radiology 204(1):123–129, 1997.

6. Kaiser WA, Zeitler E: MR imaging of the breast: Fast imaging sequences with and without Gd-DTPA. Preliminary observations. Radiology 170(3 Pt 1):681–686, 1989.

7. Kinkel K, Hylton NM: Challenges to interpretation of breast MRI. J Magn Reson Imag 13(6):821–829, 2001.

8. Kuhl CK, Klaschik S, Mielcarek P, et al: Do T2-weighted pulse sequences help with the differential diagnosis of enhancing lesions in dynamic breast MRI? J Magn Reson Imag 9(2):187–196, 1999.

9. Kuhl CK, Schmutzler RK, Leutner CC, et al: Breast MR imaging screening in 192 women proved or suspected to be carriers of a breast cancer susceptibility gene: Preliminary results. Radiology 215(1):267–279, 2000.

10. Lee SG, Orel SG, Woo IJ, et al: MR imaging screening of the contralateral breast in patients with newly diagnosed breast cancer: Preliminary results. Radiology 226(3):773–778, 2003.

11. Liberman L, Morris EA, Dershaw DD, et al: MR imaging of the ipsilateral breast in women with percutaneously proven breast cancer. Am J Roentgenol 180(4):901–910, 2003.

12. Monticciolo DL, Nelson RC, Dixon WT, et al: MR detection of leakage from silicone breast implants: Value of a silicone-selective pulse sequence. Am J Roentgenol 163(1):51–56, 1994.

13. Morris EA, Schwartz LH, Dershaw DD, et al: MR imaging of the breast in patients with occult primary breast carcinoma. Radiology 205(2):437–440, 1997.

14. Nunes LW, Schnall MD, Orel SG, et al: Correlation of lesion appearance and histologic findings for the nodes of a breast MR imaging interpretation model. Radiographics 19(1):79–92, 1999.

15. Orel SG, Schnall MD, LiVolsi VA, Troupin RH: Suspicious breast lesions: MR imaging with radiologic-pathologic correlation. Radiology 190(2):485–493, 1994.

16. Orel SG, Schnall MD, Powell CM, et al: Staging of suspected breast cancer: Effect of MR imaging and MR-guided biopsy. Radiology 196(1):115–122, 1995.

17. Rovno HD, Siegelman ES, Reynolds C, et al: Solitary intraductal papilloma: Findings at MR imaging and MR galactography. Am J Roentgenol 172(1):151–155, 1999.

18. Schneider E, Chan TW: Selective MR imaging of silicone with the three-point Dixon technique. Radiology 187(1):89–93, 1993.

19. Teifke A, Hlawatsch A, Beier T, et al: Undetected malignancies of the breast: Dynamic contrast-enhanced MR imaging at 1.0 T. Radiology 224(3):881–888, 2002.

CARDIAC IMAGING

Sridhar R. Charagundla, MD, PhD, and Harold I. Litt, MD, PhD

1. **What forms the borders of the heart on the frontal posteroanterior (PA) or anteroposterior chest radiograph?**
   The chest radiograph represents an important first step in the imaging work-up of cardiovascular disease. Analysis of the cardiac silhouette can yield valuable information about chamber enlargement. For example, the right heart border is composed of the right atrium. This becomes bulbous when the right atrium is enlarged. Superiorly, the left heart border is composed of three convexities (called the "three moguls"), which, from superior to inferior, are the aortic knob, main pulmonary artery, and left atrial appendage. Inferiorly, the left heart border is composed of the left ventricle (lateral wall and apex).

2. **What forms the borders of the heart on the lateral chest radiograph?**
   Superiorly, the posterior heart border is composed of the left atrium. Inferiorly, the posterior heart border is composed of the left ventricle. The anterior heart border is composed of the right ventricle; inferiorly, this abuts the posterior aspect of the sternum (Fig. 9-1).

3. **What are signs of left atrial enlargement on the chest radiograph?**
   Chamber enlargement can be identified, in general, by increased prominence of convexity of the corresponding heart border. In particular, left atrial enlargement causes a posterior bulging of the superior-posterior heart border. On the frontal chest radiograph, signs of left atrial enlargement include enlargement of the left atrial appendage, "splaying" of the carina and elevation of the left mainstem bronchus, and a "double density" projecting over the central portions of the heart, sometimes extending over toward the right (Fig. 9-2).

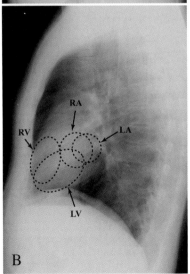

Figure 9-1. Normal PA (A) and lateral (B) chest radiographs with location of cardiac chambers outlined (*LA* = left atrium, *RA* = right atrium, *RV* = right ventricle, *LV* = left ventricle).

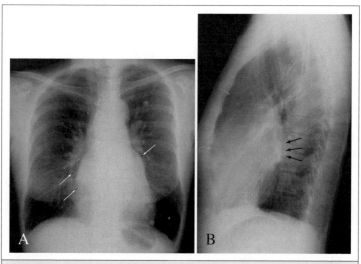

Figure 9-2. Left atrial enlargement *(arrows)* on PA (A) and lateral (B) chest radiographs. Note the "double density" projecting over the right heart, the enlarged left atrial appendage (the "third mogul"), and the convexity of the superior-posterior heart border.

KEY POINTS: CHEST X-RAY EVALUATION OF CARDIAC CHAMBER SIZE

1. Right atrium: right heart border on frontal view.

2. Right ventricle: anterior heart border on lateral view.

3. Left atrium: posterior-superior heart border on lateral view.

4. Left ventricle: left inferior heart border on frontal view.

4. **What are signs of right ventricular enlargement on the chest radiograph?**
   On the frontal radiograph, right ventricular enlargement can cause rounding of the left heart border (obscuring the normal shadow created by the left ventricle) and uplifting of the cardiac apex. On the lateral radiograph, right ventricular enlargement can displace normal retrosternal aerated lung (fill in the "anterior clear space"), although this is a notoriously unreliable finding (Fig. 9-3).

5. **What are common causes of an intra-atrial mass?**
   The most common cause is thrombus. Patients with indwelling central venous catheters are at risk for developing right atrial thrombus, and patients with atrial fibrillation are at increased risk for developing left atrial thrombus. Deep venous thrombi of the extremities can migrate to the right atrium before causing a pulmonary embolism (*see* Figs. 11-1 and 11-2). Other causes of clot in the atria include hypercoagulable states and tumors that invade the inferior vena cava and propagate as "tumor thrombus" into the right atrium (e.g., renal cell carcinoma, adrenal carcinoma, and hepatocellular carcinoma). The most common primary atrial neoplasm is a myxoma (Fig. 9-4).

Figure 9-3. Right ventricular enlargement *(arrows)* on PA (A) and lateral (B) chest radiographs. Note the rounded, uplifted left heart border and the extra density in the retrosternal clear space.

6. **What are the types of atrial septal defect (ASD)? Which chambers/vessels become enlarged with an ASD?**

ASDs are classified as ostium primum, ostium secundum, or sinus venosus defects, depending on their position in the septum. Secundum defects are the most common, and sinus venosus defects are often associated with partial anomalous pulmonary venous return.

A defect in the interatrial septum creates a communication between the left and right atria. Usually, since the left atrium has slightly higher pressures, the direction of flow through the septal defect is left to right. This results in increased flow through the right atrium, right ventricle, and pulmonary arteries and can ultimately cause enlargement of any or all of these structures. The left atrium should be normal in size.

7. **What are the types of ventricular septal defects (VSDs)? Which chambers/vessels become enlarged with a VSD?**

The most common VSDs are classified as muscular, membranous, or supracristal, depending on their location in the muscular or membranous septum or in the outflow tract. A defect in the interventricular septum creates a communication between the ventricles, resulting in blood flowing from the left ventricle into the right ventricle. This results in right ventricular, pulmonary arterial, and left atrial enlargement.

8. **What is a patent ductus arteriosus (PDA)? Which chambers/vessels become enlarged with a PDA?**

A PDA is a persistent communication between the aorta and main pulmonary artery just beyond the origin of the left subclavian artery. Flow is directed from the aorta into the pulmonary artery, causing enlargement of the pulmonary arteries, left atrium, and left ventricle.

9. **What is the most sensitive imaging technique for the detection of myocardial infarction?**

Cardiac MRI with delayed postgadolinium imaging ("viability study") is the most sensitive imaging technique. Echocardiography can detect areas of myocardial wall thinning or abnormal myocardial contraction. Cardiac single photon emission computed tomography (SPECT) can detect areas of nonviable myocardium. However, MRI has greater specificity than echocardiography and far greater spatial resolution and sensitivity than SPECT. Acute or chronic myocardial infarction demonstrates accumulation of gadolinium in a delayed fashion (10–15 minutes after administration), probably due to a combination of increased vascular permeability and enlargement of the extracellular space. The percentage of the myocardial thickness demonstrating delayed enhancement correlates inversely with the likelihood of return of function of that segment of myocardium after a revascularization procedure.

10. **How long after myocardial infarction does a ventricular aneurysm develop?**
    A ventricular aneurysm develops in the setting of remote prior myocardial infarction. Areas of the heart muscle that have undergone infarction ultimately become thin and fibrotic; these weak areas of myocardium can balloon out over time due to chronic exposure to systemic blood pressure. Ventricular aneurysms usually have a wide mouth, and may undergo mural calcification, resulting in a characteristic curvilinear density on chest radiographs (Fig. 9-5).

11. **How long after myocardial infarction does a ventricular pseudoaneurysm develop?**
    Infarcted myocardial tissue undergoes a predictable sequence of histologic changes. As the tissue undergoes necrosis, it becomes mechanically weak and is prone to rupture. This most commonly occurs approximately 3–7 days after the infarction. Myocardial rupture most often occurs in the ventricular free wall but can also occur in the interventricular septum (causing a left-to-right shunt) or in a

Figure 9-4. Intra-atrial thrombus (A, *arrow*) and intra-atrial myxoma (B and C, *arrows,*). Contrast-enhanced CT image (A) shows a filling defect in the anterior aspect of the left atrium, representing thrombus. This patient had undergone heart transplant. Gradient-echo (B) and T2-weighted spin-echo (C) MR images show a mass in the left atrium that is hyperintense on T2-weighted images and represents a myxoma.

papillary muscle (causing mitral regurgitation). If the myocardial rupture is contained, a ventricular pseudoaneurysm forms. These characteristically have a narrow mouth, since they essentially represent rupture through a small hole in the myocardium. Myocardial pseudoaneurysms are generally considered to be unstable because they themselves may rupture (*see* Fig. 9-6).

12. **What are some imaging findings of chronic (constrictive) pericarditis?**
Chronic (constrictive) pericarditis can be caused by cardiac surgery, radiation, or tuberculosis; however, most cases are idiopathic. Patients commonly present with right heart failure.

Figure 9-5. True ventricular aneurysm. Contrast-enhanced CT image shows marked thinning *(arrow)* of the myocardium at the left ventricular apex, a characteristic location for a true ventricular aneurysm.

Imaging findings include pericardial thickening (> 3 mm), pericardial calcification, and abnormal motion of the interventricular septum. None of these findings is pathognomonic. In the appropriate clinical setting and with invasive or noninvasive hemodynamic findings suggesting constriction or restriction, demonstration of thickened pericardium by magnetic resonance (MR) or CT is sufficient to make the diagnosis of constrictive pericarditis.

Figure 9-6. Ventricular pseudoaneurysm. PA chest radiograph (A) and contrast-enhanced CT image (B) show a pseudoaneurysm *(arrows)* arising from the posterior-inferior portion of the left ventricle. In this case, there is extensive mural calcification, indicating that the pseudoaneurysm is old.

13. **In a patient with an abnormal electrocardiogram (ECG) finding and a family history of sudden death, cardiac MRI shows a dilated right ventricle with abnormal wall motion and a normal left ventricle. What is the most likely diagnosis?**
Arrhythmogenic right ventricular dysplasia or cardiomyopathy (ARVD/ARVC) is a disease of unknown etiology, characterized by fatty or fibrous infiltration of the myocardium. It is a common cause of sudden death and may be familial. Diagnosis is made through a combination of clinical, imaging, electrocardiographic, and pathologic findings. MRI is a useful test for

evaluating right ventricular morphology, composition, and function. Suggestive findings on MRI include dysfunction, dilation, or thinning of the right ventricular wall, aneurysms of the right ventricle, and fatty infiltration of the right ventricular wall. Treatment consists of placement of an implantable cardioverter defibrillator. It is important to realize that the diagnosis of ARVD should not be made on the basis of imaging findings alone.

14. **How is "bright blood" MRI accomplished? Why is it used?**
    As its name implies, "bright blood" imaging is an MRI technique whereby flowing blood has high signal compared with tissue. This is accomplished through the use of gradient-echo imaging. Bright blood imaging techniques are useful because they are fast and have high spatial resolution; they are commonly used for depicting blood vessels, cardiac chambers, and valve leaflets. Turbulent blood flow causes dark "jets" in bright blood images, allowing the detection of valvular stenosis or incompetence.

15. **How is "dark blood" MRI accomplished? Why is it used?**
    "Dark blood" imaging is an MRI technique whereby the blood signal is suppressed. This can be done with spin-echo or inversion recovery imaging. By reducing the signal from blood, myocardial tissue and vessel walls stand out from the background and can be seen in great detail. Dark blood imaging techniques are useful for detailed analysis of myocardial morphology and composition, cardiac anatomy, and vascular anatomy.

16. **How is cine imaging accomplished? Why is it used?**
    Cine imaging portrays the heart in motion. Images are acquired during all phases of the cardiac cycle and require synchronization with the electrocardiographic signal. In MRI, this is accomplished with gradient-echo imaging (note that these images are therefore bright blood). Cine imaging is necessary to evaluate cardiac function and can be used to detect wall motion abnormalities, calculate ejection fraction, and study the motion of valve leaflets.

17. **Which congenital coronary artery anomalies can cause sudden death?**
    Normally, the right and left main coronary arteries arise from the aorta at the right and left sinuses of Valsalva, respectively. Anomalous origin of the coronary arteries occurs rarely (about 1% of cardiac catheterizations). Sudden death is associated with the left main coronary artery arising from the right sinus (particularly when the artery courses between the aorta and pulmonary artery), the right coronary artery arising from the left sinus, or a single coronary artery. The left main coronary artery may also arise from the pulmonary trunk; this anomaly tends to present earlier, with congestive heart failure or sudden death (Fig. 9-7).

18. **What are the standard planes for cross-sectional cine cardiac imaging?**
    The oblique orientation of the heart with respect to the body axis requires special planes of imaging. The "four-chamber" view of the heart captures all four cardiac chambers in a single image and also includes the tricuspid and mitral valves. The "short-axis" view of the heart is perpendicular to the four-chamber view and allows accurate measurement of septal thickness and ventricular free wall thickness. In the short-axis view, the left ventricle is depicted in cross section and appears almost circular. Standard axial images also are commonly used. Coronal images are sometimes used to evaluate the diaphragmatic surface of the heart (Fig. 9-8).

19. **What is the most common malignancy of the heart and pericardium?**
    Metastatic disease. Lung cancer, lymphoma, breast cancer, and melanoma can all involve the heart or pericardium. Lung cancer is the most common primary tumor of patients with cardiac metastases; however, melanoma is the most likely tumor to spread to the heart. Primary tumors of the heart are rare, and primary malignant tumors of the heart are exceedingly rare.

Figure 9-7. Normal and aberrant coronary arteries. Contrast-enhanced CT coronary angiography demonstrates normal origins *(arrows)* of the right coronary artery (A) and left main coronary artery (B). In another patient, the study shows the left main coronary artery *(arrow)* (C) arising from the right coronary artery.

20. **What are some causes of dilated cardiomyopathy?**
    Cardiomyopathies are diseases that involve primary dysfunction of the heart muscle. This broad collection of diseases can be divided on a pathophysiologic basis into dilated, hypertrophic, and restrictive subtypes, with some overlap occurring between these categories. A few causes of dilated cardiomyopathy include ischemia, viral infection (especially coxsackie B virus and cytomegalovirus), and toxic exposure (e.g., cocaine, alcohol, and doxorubicin).

21. **What is Eisenmenger's syndrome?**
    Small left-to-right shunts, such as ASDs and VSDs, are commonly asymptomatic early in life and may go undetected. Over time, the right side of the cardiopulmonary circulation responds to the increased volume with pulmonary arterial hyperplasia. This ultimately leads to elevated pulmonary vascular resistance and a rise in right-sided pressures (pulmonary hypertension). When right-sided pressures exceed left-sided pressures, the left-to-right shunt switches and becomes a right-to-left shunt. Dyspnea, fatigue, and cyanosis then develop. This syndrome usually presents in young adulthood.

22. **What are some noninvasive methods of coronary artery imaging?**

    Imaging the coronary arteries is a major part of evaluating ischemic heart disease. Traditionally, this has been performed through cardiac catheterization, a procedure that requires arterial puncture. Newer technologies promise noninvasive, cross-sectional imaging of coronary artery patency and offer the potential to characterize coronary artery plaque. MRI, using bright blood, dark blood, and gadolinium-enhanced techniques, can image vessel patency and determine lipid content in coronary plaques. Coronary CT angiography can image vessel patency, potentially with a higher spatial resolution than MRI, and measure coronary calcification.

Figure 9-8. Standard views for cardiac MRI. Bright blood gradient-echo MR images demonstrate the four-chamber (A) and short-axis (B) views.

23. **What are some diseases that affect valvular function? How can they be diagnosed with imaging?**

    The aortic, pulmonic, mitral, and tricuspid valves can become stenotic, incompetent, or both. A chamber draining through a stenotic valve experiences a pressure load; if this chamber is a ventricle, it responds with muscular hypertrophy. However, if this chamber is an atrium, it responds with enlargement. A chamber draining through an incompetent (regurgitant) valve experiences a volume load and responds with enlargement (whether it is an atrium or a ventricle). Echocardiography and MRI can measure chamber size and velocity and direction of blood flow across a valve orifice, thereby detecting and quantifying valvular disease.

24. **What is the differential diagnosis of a regional wall motion abnormality?**

    A wall motion abnormality indicates a portion of myocardium that has abnormally reduced contractility. This usually occurs on the basis of previous or ongoing ischemia and suggests heart muscle that is acutely ischemic, dead, stunned, or hibernating. Acutely ischemic myocardium cannot contract properly because of inadequate blood flow and poor energy supply. Infarcted myocardium will not contract and may eventually exhibit "paradoxical" motion, where it balloons out during systole instead of thickening. When a portion of heart muscle remains viable after a temporary episode of ischemia, it can become "stunned," where wall motion abnormality persists due to chemical changes in the myocardium that resolve over time. Finally, ischemic myocardium can down-regulate its own contractility to match its energy demands with energy supply; this is termed *hibernating* and may signify tissue at risk for becoming infarcted.

25. **What portions of the heart are supplied by the right coronary, left anterior descending, and circumflex arteries?**
     The left anterior descending (LAD) artery supplies the left ventricular apex and the anterior portion of the interventricular septum. The right coronary artery (RCA) supplies the posteroinferior wall of the left ventricle and the posterior portion of the interventricular septum. The circumflex artery (LCX) supplies the lateral wall of the left ventricle (Fig. 9-9).

Figure 9-9. Coronary vascular territories. Bright blood gradient-echo MR images with coronary vascular territories delineated on vertical long-axis (A) and short-axis (B) views.

BIBLIOGRAPHY

1. Bomma C, Rutberg J, Tandri H, et al: Misdiagnosis of arrhythmogenic right ventricular dysplasia/cardiomyopathy. J Cardiovasc Electrophysiol 15(3):300–306, 2004.

2. Kimura F, Sakai F, Sakomura Y, et al: Helical CT features of arrhythmogenic right ventricular cardiomyopathy. Radiographics 22(5):1111–1124, 2002.

3. Manning WJ, Pennell DJ (eds): Cardiovascular Magnetic Resonance. New York, Churchill Livingstone, 2002.

4. Troughton RW, Asher CR, Klein AL: Pericarditis. Lancet 363(9410):717–727, 2004.

CHAPTER 10

CTA AND MRA OF THE AORTA

Andrew J. Kapustin, MD, and Harold I. Litt, MD, PhD

1. **How are aneurysms and pseudoaneurysms different?**
   An aneurysm (also known as a "true aneurysm") is dilation of a vessel in which all three layers of the vessel wall remain intact. A pseudoaneurysm (also known as a "false aneurysm") is a contained rupture and implies disruption of at least part of the aortic wall (i.e., the intima and/or media), with intact adventitia. Pseudoaneurysms are therefore potentially highly unstable lesions. They are often post-traumatic or iatrogenic (Fig. 10-1).

2. **What is a mycotic aneurysm? Which imaging findings help suggest the diagnosis?**
   One might think mycotic means "related to fungus," but *mycotic aneurysm* refers to an aneurysm caused by any type of infection, usually bacterial. Imaging features that may suggest the diagnosis are rapid change in size, adjacent inflammation, perivascular gas, eccentric (*see* Fig. 10-1), or saccular, configuration, or lack of atherosclerotic calcification.

3. **What is an inflammatory aneurysm?**
   Inflammatory aneurysms are much less common than atherosclerotic aneurysms. They are a form of retroperitoneal fibrosis associated with aortic aneurysms. These aneurysms are surrounded by extensive inflammation and fibrosis that often lead to complications such as ureteral obstruction. Some believe that the surrounding fibrosis is a result of microscopic leakage of the aneurysm causing a severe secondary inflammatory response, whereas others espouse a viral or immune-reaction related etiology.

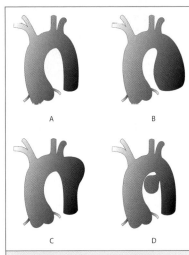

Figure 10-1. Types of aortic aneurysm. (A) Normal configuration of thoracic aorta. (B) Fusiform aneurysmal dilation of the descending thoracic aorta. Fusiform aneurysms are common in atherosclerosis. (C) Eccentric, or saccular, aneurysm of descending thoracic aorta, perhaps caused by infection. (D) Pseudoaneurysm, a contained rupture. In true aneurysms, all three layers of the vessel wall are intact. In pseudoaneurysms, the intima and/or media have been disrupted, leaving intact adventitia.

4. **How is aortic dissection different from aortic transection?**
   A dissection is caused by a tear of the intima, creating a false channel or lumen within the wall of the artery. Flowing blood then *dissects* along the course of the aorta, extending the false lumen longitudinally and into branch vessels. The classic presentation is "ripping" back or chest pain.
   Aortic transection (perhaps better referred to as "traumatic aortic injury") occurs in trauma patients. The entire aortic wall is injured or *transected*, leading to hemorrhage or pseudoaneurysm formation. Transection is usually a focal injury, and imaging should focus on the region of interest,

usually in the chest. Dissections extend for some distance and therefore require more extensive imaging of the entire aorta and its branch vessels.

5. **In the setting of blunt trauma, where do aortic injuries most commonly occur?**
    The overwhelming majority of injuries seen by radiologists occur at the aortic isthmus, which is just distal to the take-off of the left subclavian artery. Most believe this is due to asymmetric aortic fixation at this location, leading to shear stress. Radiologists less commonly see injuries to the ascending aorta since many patients with this type of injury die before reaching the hospital.

KEY POINTS: COMMON TERMS ASSIGNED TO AORTIC PATHOLOGIC CONDITIONS

1. Aortic aneurysm: dilation of the aorta, but all three levels of the aortic wall remain intact.

2. Pseudoaneurysm: a contained aortic rupture, with disruption of at least one layer of wall.

3. Dissection: a tear in the intima, with propagation of this tear along the aortic long axis.

4. Transection: traumatic aortic injury, with compromise of at least a portion of the aortic wall. Most patients with transection die before reaching a hospital.

---

6. **How are traumatic aortic injuries diagnosed?**
    Clinical suspicion and/or chest x-ray findings should be enough to send a patient with an unstable condition to surgery. If the patient's condition is relatively stable, most now recommend CTA, preferably with a multidetector computed tomography (CT) scanner. Catheter angiography, once the mainstay of diagnosis, is now most useful for problem-solving when CTA is nondiagnostic or equivocal.

7. **Name the chest x-ray findings of a thoracic aortic pathologic condition.**
    Primary signs include an enlarged or enlarging aorta, an indistinct aortic contour, and displacement of intimal atherosclerotic calcifications (in aortic dissection). Secondary signs, indicating mass effect from an aneurysm or hematoma, include mediastinal widening; displacement of adjacent structures such as the trachea, the left mainstem bronchus, or a nasogastric tube in the esophagus; an "apical cap," or mediastinal hematoma extending above the lung apex; or pleural or pericardial effusion (can be hemorrhagic but is more commonly exudative fluid secondary to the adjacent acute aortic process).
       Note that many of these findings are not specific for aortic pathologic conditions. Even mediastinal hematoma in the setting of trauma is not specific because it may be secondary to venous rather than arterial injury.

8. **What are the two classification schemes for aortic dissection?**
    The Stanford classification categorizes dissections into those involving the ascending aorta regardless of involvement of the descending aorta and those involving the descending aorta only:
    ■ Type A: Ascending aorta is involved with or without descending aortic involvement
    ■ Type B: Descending aorta only
    The DeBakey classification denotes three categories of aortic dissection: singular involvement of the ascending or descending aorta or involvement of both ascending and descending aortas. The mnemonic for this system is BAD:
    ■ Type 1: *B*oth ascending and descending
    ■ Type 2: *A*scending only
    ■ Type 3: *D*escending only
       Note that the descending aorta is defined as distal to the take-off of the left subclavian artery.

9. **How are dissections that involve the ascending aorta managed differently from those that involve the descending aorta only?**
Dissections involving the ascending aorta (Stanford type A and DeBakey types 1 and 2) are surgical emergencies because mortality is significantly greater in medically managed patients (approximately 90% in the first 3 months) compared with surgically treated patients. This high mortality rate is mostly due to hemopericardium causing tamponade, acute aortic regurgitation, or involvement of coronary artery origins causing myocardial infarction. Descending aortic dissections are usually treated medically (antihypertensive agents) because morbidity and mortality are greater with surgery than with medical management. However, complicated descending aortic dissections may require surgical or endovascular intervention.

10. **Which lumen is usually larger in aortic dissection: the true or false lumen?**
Approximately 90% of the time, the false lumen is larger than the true lumen.

11. **Describe other "acute aortic syndromes" that are often called variants of aortic dissection.**
Penetrating atherosclerotic ulcer (PAU) is a focal tear of intima caused by ruptured plaque, leading to focal ulceration into the aortic wall. It is different than a dissection because a dissection is not focal, but rather propagates along the length of the vessel. *Intramural hematoma (IMH)* is a term that describes hemorrhage into the wall of the vessel. IMH may occur without an intimal tear, such as secondary to rupture of the vasa vasorum or small blood vessels in the wall of the aorta. This is usually secondary to hypertension but can be caused by trauma. Alternatively, IMH may be associated with an intimal tear, such as secondary to a PAU (Fig. 10-2).

WARNING: These terms can become extremely confusing because one form of an aortic pathologic condition can lead to another. In part because of this confusion in terminology, there are numerous controversies in the surgical literature regarding prognosis and management of the "dissection variants."

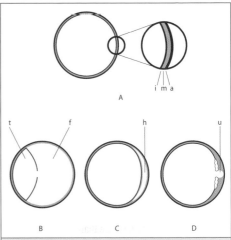

Figure 10-2. Aortic wall anatomy and pathologic conditions. (A) The layers of the aortic wall: *i* = intima; *m* = media; *a* = adventitia. (B) Aortic dissection, between the intima and media: *t* = true lumen; *f* = false lumen. (C) *h* = intramural hematoma. (D) *u* = penetrating atherosclerotic ulcer.

12. **What is the best imaging modality for diagnosing each of these conditions?**
CT and MRI are the two best modalities for evaluating these conditions. CT (particularly multidetector CT) is generally preferred because it is faster (important in patients with an unstable condition) and has better spatial resolution. MRI is often used for problem-solving in patients with a stable condition or in patients who cannot tolerate iodinated contrast. Ultrasound also has been used, but it cannot visualize the entire aorta and therefore misses the extent of disease or associated complications. At this time, the main indication for use of catheter angiography for these conditions is treatment of complications.

13. **How can these conditions be distinguished on axial MR or CT images?**
    A dissection flap will most often be a line across the vessel, separating the true lumen from the false lumen (Fig. 10-3). IMHs usually appear as a crescentic region of high attenuation or signal intensity with smooth borders. The presence of an irregular luminal border with peripheral low attenuation may reflect ulcerated atherosclerotic plaque or thrombus.

Figure 10-3. (A) Axial CTA image demonstrates aortic dissection, with differential flow in the true lumen *(long arrow)* and false lumen *(short arrow)*. (B) Oblique sagittal maximum intensity projection reformatted image demonstrates this to be a type B dissection, beginning just distal to the take-off of the left subclavian artery *(arrow)*. The dissection flap is indicated by *arrowheads*.

14. **What is the utility of precontrast imaging when performing CTA or MRA of the aorta?**
    Subacute hemorrhage has higher attenuation than flowing blood on noncontrast CT and high signal intensity on precontrast T1-weighted MRI. These findings can be easily obscured in the presence of intravenous contrast; therefore, precontrast imaging is mandatory to detect the presence of IMH.

15. **How large must the thoracic and abdominal aortas be to be called aneurysmal?**
    Any artery dilated by more than 50% of its normal size is called *aneurysmal*. Therefore, most define aortic aneurysm as 4 cm in the thoracic aorta and 3 cm in the abdomen. Note that the aorta should normally decrease in size as it extends distally, and any focal dilation should be considered abnormal.

16. **When is an abdominal aortic aneurysm (AAA) usually repaired?**
    Surgical repair of an AAA is generally considered for aortas larger than 5 cm or for aortas that are symptomatic or display rapid growth.

17. **What is Laplace's law? How is it relevant to aortic aneurysms?**
    Laplace's law states that the larger the radius of a sphere, the greater the wall stress. In regard to aneurysms, this means that as an aneurysm increases in size, the stress on the aortic wall also increases. Therefore, the aneurysm becomes more prone to rupture with increasing size.

18. **Can the overall size of an aortic aneurysm be determined by catheter angiography?**
No. Often there is an extensive mural thrombus in an aneurysm, and a large aneurysm can therefore have a normal-sized lumen. Only the lumen is opacified by catheter angiography, and therefore the outer size of the aneurysm cannot be determined by this method.

19. **How is the size of the aorta most accurately measured on CT or MRI?**
Drawing a line perpendicular to the course of the aorta is required for accurate measurement of the aortic diameter. Note that this is often different than the cross section of the aorta commonly seen on axial CT and MR images because these images are axial to the patient's *body*, not axial relative to the *aorta*. Accurate measuring, especially of a tortuous vessel, often requires multiplanar or three-dimensional reformatting (Fig. 10-4).

Figure 10-4. (A) Oblique sagittal volume-rendered CTA image of a tortuous aorta demonstrates the proper way to measure a tortuous aorta. An imaginary line is drawn down the center of the long axis of the vessel, and the transverse diameter is measured perpendicular to that line. Measurements such as this must be made using multiplanar or three-dimensional reformatting to compensate for vessel tortuosity. (B) Axial CT image from same study as in (A) demonstrates how reliance on axial images can result in overestimation of aortic size. At this level, the tortuous aorta is flowing roughly in the axial plane and therefore appears much more dilated than it actually is.

20. **Name two methods of repairing aneurysms. Compare their advantages and disadvantages.**
Surgical repair and endovascular stent-graft. *Surgical repair* is a more definitive treatment, requiring no imaging follow-up, and has known long-term durability. *Endovascular repair* is newer; therefore, long-term data are not yet available. Because of potential complications of endovascular repair, follow-up imaging and reintervention often are required. However, many patients with aortic aneurysm are not surgical candidates because of co-morbidities such as cardiopulmonary disease. Endovascular repair is preferred for these patients. Controversy exists as to whether it is better for all patients.

21. **What criteria are used to determine whether an aortic aneurysm can be treated by endovascular technique?**
   - The relationship of the aneurysm to the origins of other vessels: In the abdomen, the relationship of the aneurysm to the renal arteries is paramount since the angiographer would not want to occlude the origin of these arteries with a stent graft.
   - The luminal size of the common and external iliac arteries: Since the stent-graft is delivered to the aorta via a femoral artery approach, the angiographer needs a vessel large enough to accommodate the size of the delivery system (currently 6–8 mm).
   - The length of the aneurysm and whether it extends into the iliac arteries: This determines the size and type of stent-graft used.

22. **Why is follow-up imaging of stent-grafts needed?**
   Follow-up imaging is performed to look for complications and reevaluate the size of the aneurysm after endovascular repair. Ideally, the aneurysm sac will gradually decrease in size after repair. Complications include migration of the stent-graft, hemorrhage, infection, and endoleak.

23. **What are endoleaks? What imaging technique is used to find them?**
   An *endoleak* is defined as residual blood flow in the "aneurysm sac" (in other words, between the native aortic wall and the wall of the stent-graft). This complication is subcategorized based on the origin of the blood flow to the aneurysm sac. Type II endoleaks are the most common and are related to reversed flow into the aneurysm sac from collateral vessels such as the inferior mesenteric artery or lumbar arteries. Screening for endoleaks is usually performed with CTA or MRA. An appropriate protocol requires precontrast images and postcontrast arterial phase and delayed phase images since endoleaks may only be identified on delayed imaging.
   CT and MR cannot always delineate the type of endoleak. Catheter angiography can be used to better define an endoleak. Many endoleaks can be repaired percutaneously.

24. **How do aortic coarctation and pseudocoarctation differ?**
   Aortic coarctation is a hemodynamically significant stenosis of the aorta, most commonly seen just distal to the take-off of the left subclavian artery. Pseudocoarctation mimics coarctation, as there is an apparent focal narrowing of the proximal descending aorta. However, this narrowing is due to buckling of a tortuous aorta and does not result in a hemodynamically significant pressure gradient across the area of narrowing. Therefore, rib notching due to collateral intercostal arteries is seen in true coarctation not in pseudo-coarctation.

25. **What is a "bovine" aortic arch?**
   Most people have three large arteries originating from the aortic arch: the innominate (brachiocephalic artery), the left common carotid artery, and the left subclavian artery. The most common variant of aortic arch anatomy is termed a *bovine arch,* in which there are two vessels that arise from the aorta. The more proximal of these is a common trunk of the innominate artery and left common carotid artery. The more distal vessel is the left subclavian artery. This anatomic variant is of no clinical significance, except when planning aortic surgery.

BIBLIOGRAPHY

1. Coady MA, Rizzo JA, Elefteriades JA: Pathologic variants of thoracic aortic dissections. Cardiol Clin North Am 17(4):637–657, 1999.
2. Coady MA, Rizzo JA, Goldstein JL, Elefteriades JA: Natural history, pathogenesis, and etiology of thoracic aortic aneurysms and dissections. Cardiol Clin North Am 17(4):615–635, 1999.

3. Creasy JD, Chiles C, Routh WD, Dyer RB: Overview of traumatic injury of the thoracic aorta. Radiographics 17(1):27–45, 1997.

4. Debakey ME, McCollum CH, Crawford ES, et al: Dissection and dissecting aneurysms of the aorta: Twenty-year follow up of 527 patients treated surgically. Surgery 92(6):1118–1134, 1982.

5. Dyer DS, Moore EE, Mestek MF, et al: Can chest CT be used to exclude aortic injury? Radiology 213(1):195–202, 1999.

6. LePage MA, Quint LE, Sonnad SS, et al: Aortic dissection: CT features that distinguish true lumen from false lumen. Am J Roentgenol 177:207–211, 2001.

7. Macedo TA, Stanson AW, Oderich GS, et al: Infected aortic aneurysms: Imaging findings. Radiology 231:250–257, 2004.

8. Manning WJ, Pennell DJ (eds): Cardiovascular Magnetic Resonance. New York, Churchill Livingstone, 2002.

9. Thurnher S, Cejna M: Imaging of aortic stent-grafts and endoleaks. Radiol Clin North Am 40(4):799–833, 2002.

CTA OF THE PULMONARY VASCULATURE

Milan Sheth, MD, and Harold I. Litt, MD, PhD

CHAPTER 11

1. **What are the primary methods for imaging for pulmonary embolus (PE)?**
   There are three main methods of pulmonary arterial imaging. One is pulmonary arteriography, which is accomplished by inserting a catheter under fluoroscopic guidance into the pulmonary artery and injecting contrast to directly visualize the pulmonary arteries. Nuclear ventilation/perfusion (V/Q) examinations compare the location of radiolabeled ventilated particles to radiolabeled injected particles to help infer the presence of PE. Lastly, there is computed tomography pulmonary angiography (CPA), which involves injecting contrast into a vein and using computed tomography CT to evaluate the pulmonary arteries.

2. **What plain film findings may suggest PE?**
   A chest radiograph is usually the first imaging modality used for a patient with suspected PE. The results of the chest film may be negative or have nonspecific findings such as pleural effusions and atelectasis, but occasionally the film can have a wedge-shaped peripheral opacity, referred to as a *Hampton's hump*. An area of lucency due to decreased perfusion that is termed *Westermark's sign* also may be seen.

3. **What are the advantages of CTA over other methods in the evaluation of PE?**
   One important advantage over both catheter pulmonary arteriography and V/Q nuclear medicine scans is that CTA may be used to diagnose other causes of the patient's symptoms, such as a pleural effusion or atelectasis. Unlike arteriography, CTA is noninvasive and therefore safer. CTA also takes less time to perform. CTA has several advantages over nuclear V/Q imaging. For example, it is less dependent on patient cooperation. In addition, nuclear V/Q examinations may have up to a 60–70% indeterminate rate, especially in patients with underlying lung disease or other co-morbidities, which limit specificity.

4. **How do you perform a CTA for PE?**
   The technique for performing a CTA optimally involves the use of a multidetector row CT scanner. Contrast is injected at a high rate into a peripheral vein. Scanning is timed to obtain optimal contrast opacification of the pulmonary arteries. Then, thin-section axial CT images of 1–2 mm-thickness are obtained throughout the chest.

KEY POINTS: CTA

1. Multidetector row CTA has become the first-line imaging examination for evaluation of suspected PE.

2. CTA has greater specificity than a V/Q scan.

3. CTA has greater availability and safety than pulmonary angiography.

5. **What are the direct CTA findings of PE?**

   The most specific finding of a PE is a partial or complete intraluminal filling defect in a pulmonary artery (Fig. 11-1). It should be present on at least two contiguous sections. Abrupt cut-off of the artery also indicates a PE.

6. **What are the indirect findings of PE?**

   A pulmonary artery with an embolus may be slightly enlarged. Parenchymal findings, such as wedge-shaped opacities denoting areas of infarction and atelectasis, sometimes can be seen as well. Areas of decreased perfusion can manifest as wedge-shaped hyperlucency.

Figure 11-1. Axial image from pulmonary CTA examination demonstrates bilateral pulmonary emboli, which are visualized as intraluminal filling defects in the pulmonary arterial system *(arrows)*.

7. **How can acute PE be distinguished from chronic PE on CTA?**

   It may be difficult to differentiate acute from chronic PE. In fact, chronic PE may be complicated by superimposed acute PE. Acute pulmonary emboli are often seen as central filling defects as opposed to chronic emboli, which are more peripheral. This is easy to remember because the peripheral appearance of chronic PE is due to an acute clot in a vessel that recanalizes over time. Chronic emboli can also calcify, whereas acute emboli do not. Long-standing pulmonary emboli are more likely than acute emboli to cause pulmonary hypertension, leading to right heart enlargement and enlargement of the main and central pulmonary arteries (Fig. 11-2). Lastly, increased mediastinal collateral vessels can be seen in some cases of chronic pulmonary emboli.

Figure 11-2. Axial CTA image demonstrates bilateral chronic pulmonary emboli *(short arrows)*. Although these emboli have not calcified, the main pulmonary artery *(long arrow)* is enlarged, indicating pulmonary hypertension.

8. **What are other uses for CT in PE?**

   CT also can be useful in evaluating the lower extremity venous system for thrombosis, using the same contrast bolus, by imaging several minutes after the PE study. Lower extremity sonography is generally used to evaluate lower extremity veins, but CT has several advantages. One is that it is not operator dependent, unlike ultrasound. CT can be used to evaluate for clot in areas that are not accessible to ultrasound or difficult to evaluate. This includes the deep pelvic veins (a common source of thrombus that may embolize to the lungs) and the region around the adductor canal. Ultrasound can be of limited value in patients who are obese or have had recent surgery. Within certain limitations, CT may be a better choice than ultrasound in these situations.

9. **What is a pulmonary arteriovenous malformation (AVM) and what symptoms can it cause?**

   A pulmonary AVM is an abnormal communication between the pulmonary artery and a draining vein, causing blood to bypass the pulmonary capillary bed before returning to the left heart.

AVMs may be asymptomatic, but they can present with a wide range of clinical symptoms. Symptoms result from the loss of two essential physiologic functions of the lungs. Hypoxia may occur due to shunting, and paradoxical emboli, stroke, or brain abscess may occur due to the loss of the "filter" effect of the lung. Pulmonary AVMs may cause vague symptoms such as chest pain and dyspnea on exertion due to shunting of deoxygenated blood. With severe shunting, high-output cardiac failure can result from right-to-left shunting.

10. **What is orthodeoxia?**
    Orthodeoxia is a term used to describe position-dependent oxygen desaturation. Most pulmonary AVMs occur in the lower lobes. Shunting of blood and desaturation are maximum when blood flow to the lung bases is greatest. Patients with large pulmonary AVMs in the lower lobes will have larger shunts and lower oxygen saturation when standing. When lying down, blood is redirected toward the lung apices, and the shunt fraction and desaturation may decrease.

11. **What pulmonary AVMs are associated with what hereditary disorder?**
    Even though pulmonary AVMs are often isolated, they can be associated with hereditary hemorrhagic telangiectasia (HHT), which is also known as Osler-Weber-Rendu disease. HHT is a genetic disorder that causes vascular malformations that can lead to multiple pulmonary AVMs. It is characterized by telangiectasias of the skin and mucosal linings, epistaxis, and AVMs in various internal organs such as the brain and liver. It is wise to screen family members of patients who present with pulmonary AVMs so that they can receive treatment.

12. **You are asked to start a peripheral IV line in a patient with a known pulmonary AVM. What special precautions should you take?**
    Patients with pulmonary AVMs lack the "filter" function performed by the pulmonary capillary bed. This predisposes patients to paradoxical emboli from both endogenous and exogenous sources. Air or other material accidentally introduced into the venous system could pass through the shunt and cause a stroke. Care must be taken that all venous lines are free of air and that filters are used to prevent paradoxical emboli.

13. **What are the imaging characteristics of a pulmonary AVM on plain film and CT?**
    On plain film, pulmonary AVMs appear as serpiginous or nodular densities that can connect to the hilum. On CT, they appear as a homogeneous noncalcified nodule that has a vascular connection with an enlarged feeding artery and draining vein (Fig. 11-3). On dynamic images, the malformation enhances in a sequential manner from the feeding artery to the malformation to the vein.

14. **What is partial anomalous pulmonary venous return (PAPVR)?**
    PAPVR occurs when part of the pulmonary venous system drains directly into the systemic circulation. It can occur in isolation or be associated with either atrial septal defect or a hypogenetic lung. When it is associated with atrial septal defect (usually a sinus venosus defect), the right upper lobe will drain into the superior vena cava.

Figure 11-3. Axial CTA image demonstrates a pulmonary AVM, with feeding artery and draining vein *(arrows)* associated with the lesion.

When it occurs with a hypogenetic lung, it is a component of congenital pulmonary venolobar syndrome known as *scimitar syndrome.*

15. **What is scimitar syndrome? What are its associated imaging findings?**
Scimitar syndrome is a hypogenetic lung (almost exclusively on the right) that is drained by an anomalous vein. This anomalous vein can drain into many structures including the infradiaphragmatic inferior vena cava (IVC), suprahepatic IVC, portal vein, or right atrium. The chest x-ray will demonstrate a small right lung with a tubular opacity paralleling the right heart border (called the *scimitar*). Magnetic resonance imaging and CT better demonstrate the course and nature of the abnormal vascular anatomy.

16. **What is the most common primary tumor of the pulmonary artery?**
Tumors associated with the pulmonary vascular system are exceedingly rare. Angiosarcomas are most common. These are rare tumors and sometimes can be difficult to distinguish from occlusive PE since both fill the lumen of the pulmonary artery.

CHAPTER 12

CTA AND MRA OF THE PERIPHERAL AND VISCERAL VASCULATURE

Maxim Itkin, MD, and Harold I. Litt, MD, PhD

1. **What are computed tomographic angiography (CTA) and magnetic resonance angiography (MRA)?**
   CTA and MRA are methods to image blood vessels noninvasively using CT or MR. To make vessels visible, iodine-based contrast material (for CTA) or gadolinium chelate contrast material (for MRA) is injected through a peripheral IV and images are acquired at peak vascular enhancement.

2. **When is peak contrast enhancement?**
   Contrast is injected intravenously as a bolus at a rate 2–4 mL/sec. The concentration of the contrast at a specific location changes with time, according to an enhancement curve. The maximum concentration in proximal systemic arteries usually occurs 20–30 seconds after beginning the injection. Peak opacification occurs at different time points at different parts of the body. To scan vessels at optimal enhancement, the scanning table moves to image the appropriate body part. This is a technique referred to as "bolus chase."

3. **How do we know the time of peak contrast enhancement?**
   The time of peak enhancement varies from patient to patient and is influenced by factors such as patient size, cardiac output, and contrast injection site. Although timing may be estimated, the peak opacification time is usually determined for each patient in order to obtain consistent results. This can be performed by injecting a "test bolus," a small amount of contrast (20 mL for iodine-based CT contrast), and measuring the opacification curve at the most proximal point upstream to the area of interest (usually somewhere in the aorta) by scanning at the same location every 1–2 seconds. The time between start of the injection and peak enhancement determines the scan delay. Another method, called "bolus tracking," measures the enhancement (or MR signal intensity) at a given point every 1–2 seconds during the main contrast injection until a threshold enhancement is reached, and then scanning begins.

4. **What images are obtained during a CTA or MRA study?**
   CTA images are acquired in the axial plane. Although experienced radiologists can interpret these images, it is easier to diagnose vessel pathologic conditions by creating an image in a plane that allows the long axis of the vessel to be viewed. To view vessels in this perspective, axial images are transferred to a special workstation where the physician or a specially trained technologist performs reconstructions. There are several main modes of image reconstruction. Multiplanar reformatting (MPR) allows reconstruction of the image along any oblique plane or a curve. Maximum intensity projection (MIP) (Fig. 12-1) is a method in which only the brightest pixel at a given location in a volume of tissue is displayed. Images obtained with this method appear similar to a conventional angiogram. Shaded surface display (SSD) (Fig. 12-2) shows data in a three-dimensional (3D) representation using only pixels that are on the surface of objects.
   Volume-rendering (VR) techniques use advantages of both MIP and SSD methods, preserving all image data and displaying them as a 3D representation. This is achieved by assigning different transparencies to tissues with different opacification (Fig. 12-3).

Figure 12-1. Coronal MIP image of a dynamic, gadolinium-enhanced 3D MRA demonstrates a normal aorta and normal bilateral renal arteries. The patient has had right lower pole partial nephrectomy.

Figure 12-2. Coronal SSD image of CTA data set demonstrates a patent femoral-femoral bypass *(arrow)*. The left common iliac and external iliac arteries are occluded.

One of the important advantages of MRA is the ability to acquire images in any plane. MRA acquisitions can be performed in the plane along the course of vessels (usually coronal for the legs), which may decrease the volume of tissue that needs to be covered by the examination. The data then can be reformatted and displayed similar to that of CTA data.

5. **When should one choose MRA versus CTA for a runoff examination?**
Both methods have advantages and disadvantages, and sometimes they are complementary. CTA has a shorter acquisition time and higher resolution, especially when new 16- or higher-channel

Figure 12-3. Coronal VR image of CTA data set demonstrating the kidneys, renal veins, and inferior vena cava.

machines are used. An arterial scan from the diaphragm to the toes takes 60 seconds, and the whole study, including preparation and positioning, lasts only about 10 minutes. MRA is a much longer study and requires the patient to lie still in the magnet for the entire examination. This requirement may be problematic for claustrophobic patients or for those with an unstable condition. MRA is the study of choice for patients with contraindications to iodinated contrast, such as a contrast allergy or renal insufficiency. However, CTA can be performed when MRA is contraindicated, as in patients with pacemakers. One advantage of CTA over MRA is the ability to obtain images with fewer artifacts when the patient has metal intravascular stents. Generally, both methods are acceptable substitutes for catheter angiography, and each institution has to tailor its own policy according to available resources and expertise.

6. **What do intravascular stents look like on MRA and CTA?**

   There are two main types of intravascular stents: balloon expandable, made from stainless steel, and self-expandable, made from a special alloy called NITINOL. The first type of stent is paramagnetic and creates strong MRI artifacts that prevent imaging of the underlying vessel. NITINOL stents are made from a diamagnetic material that creates fewer artifacts. Both stainless steel and NITINOL stents cause minimal artifacts in CTA and therefore usually do not obscure the underlying vessel.

7. **What is the definition of a hemodynamically significant artery stenosis?**

   Different arterial distributions can tolerate different degrees of stenosis, depending on the metabolic activity of the target organ and the availability of collateral blood supply. On CTA and/or MRA, most authors define "significant stenosis" as a diameter reduction of >75%, although a more conservative definition is >50%. Pressure gradients cannot be measured on CTA and MRA. Even though quantitative measurements of the degree of stenosis are important, the presence of clinical symptoms should be the major determinant in the decision to treat an arterial lesion. Sequential subcritical stenoses result in a pressure drop that approximates the sum of each stenosis. Additional signs of hemodynamically significant stenosis are poststenotic dilation of a vessel and delayed enhancement of the target organ.

8. **What is the best way to measure the degree of a stenosis?**

   The most accepted way is to measure the ratio of the diameter of the stenosis to a "normal-appearing" vessel segment. This method was adopted from the technique used to measure stenoses during conventional angiography. Although well established, this method may lack precision because it uses a 2D representation of a 3D object to estimate a stenosis. It also relies on the ability to select a "normal" segment of vessel to use as a reference. This may be problematic because even normal vessels taper distally and it may be difficult to find an area adjacent to a stenosis that is not aneurysmal or affected by poststenotic dilation. CTA and MRA offer the unique opportunity to evaluate the stenosis precisely, by measuring the decrease in cross-sectional area. With the development of more automated vessel analysis tools, measurements of cross-sectional area will become the gold standard.

KEY POINTS: MEASURING DEGREE OF VESSEL STENOSIS

1. Most accurate method: compare cross-sectional area of stenotic lesion segment to that of a normal segment of the vessel.

2. Most commonly used method: compare linear diameter of stenotic lesion segment to that of a normal segment of the vessel.

9. **What is the distribution of peripheral vascular disease in different age groups?**

   In general, young smokers have more proximal disease involving the iliac vessels. Older patients, especially those with diabetes, have more distal disease involving the infrapopliteal vessels. This is important because patency rates after treatment of proximal disease using both endovascular and surgical methods are significantly greater.

10. **What is meant by "single, two, or three vessel" runoff?**

   Normally there are three infrapopliteal vessels: the anterior tibial, posterior tibial, and peroneal arteries. The number of these calf vessels that are continuously patent from the origin to the ankle defines the number of runoff vessels. A higher number usually corresponds to a better prognosis after surgery or endovascular procedures.

11. **What structures separate the superficial femoral from the popliteal artery and the external iliac from the common femoral artery?**
    The superficial femoral artery becomes the popliteal artery after entering the adductor (Hunter's) canal. The external iliac artery becomes the femoral artery immediately after the take-off of the deep circumflex iliac artery.

12. **On an anterior projection, which thigh vessel takes a more medial course: the superficial femoral artery or the deep femoral artery?**
    The normal course of the superficial femoral artery is medial to that of the deep femoral artery (Fig. 12-7).

13. **Why are angiographic studies performed on potential renal donors?**
    Donor kidney harvesting is often performed using a minimally invasive laparoscopic approach. The surgeon's field of view is limited, so precise information concerning the location, size, and number of renal arteries and veins is required before surgery. This is extremely important because of the variability of the renal vasculature in humans.

14. **What is the prevalence of accessory renal arteries in the general population?**
    Approximately 30% of people have accessory renal arteries (Fig. 12-4). Identification of the number, location, and size of the renal arteries is vital. Significant post-transplant complications may result if even a small vessel that supplies the ureter is accidentally sacrificed. Larger arteries that supply the renal pelvis or significant portions of renal parenchyma must be preserved, sometimes necessitating complicated reconstructive surgery.

Figure 12-4. Multiplanar reformatted MIP image of the renal arteries in a potential kidney donor, showing left upper pole accessory artery *(long arrow)* as well as main left renal artery *(short arrow)*.

15. **What is the most common left renal vein anatomic variant?**
    Generally, renal veins have more consistent anatomy than renal arteries. Knowledge of the venous anatomy before laparoscopic surgery is important to prevent vascular injury and bleeding. The left vein is longer than the right vein, which is one reason why the left kidney is preferred for transplantation. The most common left renal vein anatomic variant is a circumaortic renal vein, which occurs in 5–7% of the population. With this anatomic variant, the left renal vein forms a ring around the aorta. The anterior segment of the ring connects with the inferior vena cava (IVC) at the expected level of the left renal vein, and the posterior segment connects with the IVC below the insertion of the anterior segment. A retroaortic left renal vein is less common and occurs in 2–3% of people.

16. **What are the secondary imaging signs of renal artery stenosis?**
Delayed parenchymal enhancement and an overall reduced kidney size. A difference of more than 1–2 cm in renal length is considered significant.

17. **Can fibromuscular dysplasia (FMD) be diagnosed using MRA or CTA?**
Currently, the gold standard for the diagnosis of FMD is still conventional arteriography. The main findings of FMD are subtle intimal changes, resulting in a beaded appearance to affected vessels. The resolution of MRA is not sufficient for diagnosis. CTA, using 16- and 64-channel scanners, shows promise for detecting FMD, but it is not considered reliable enough at this time to accurately diagnose FMD.

18. **What are the collateral pathways between the superior mesenteric artery (SMA) and inferior mesenteric artery (IMA) and the celiac artery and the SMA?**
There are two collateral pathways that connect the SMA and IMA: the arc of Riolan proximally and the marginal artery of Drummond distally. The main collateral pathways between the celiac artery and the SMA are through the common hepatic artery, gastroduodenal artery, and pancreatico-duodenal arteries. The arc of Buhler is a direct connection between the SMA and celiac artery.

19. **Can ostial SMA or celiac artery occlusion result in mesenteric ischemia?**
Because of the extensive collaterals between the three main mesenteric vessels, occlusion of just one of these three vessels usually does not cause symptoms. Severe stenosis of at least two of the vessels is necessary for symptomatic mesenteric ischemia (Fig. 12-5).

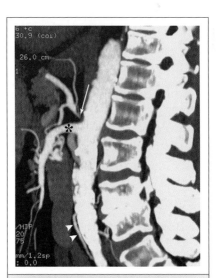

Figure 12-5. Sagittal MPR image of CTA data set demonstrates complete occlusion of the celiac artery at its origin *(arrow)* and patent superior mesenteric *(star)* and inferior mesenteric *(arrowheads)* arteries.

20. **Identify each of the vessels shown in Figure 12-6.**

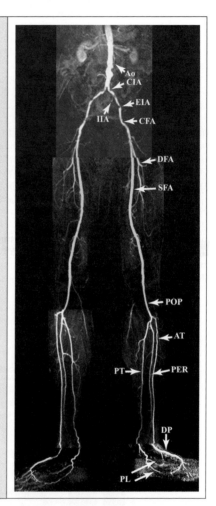

Figure 12-6. Coronal subtracted MIP-projection image from a multistation, gadolinium-enhanced bolus chase runoff examination. The patient had claudication, and there are bilateral stenoses of the common iliac and external iliac arteries *(arrows)*. (Ao= aorta, CIA = common iliac artery, EIA = external iliac artery, IIA = internal iliac artery [not shown on right in this patient], CFA = common femoral artery, DFA = deep femoral artery, SFA = superficial femoral artery, POP = popliteal artery, AT = anterior tibial artery, PT = posterior tibial artery, PER = peroneal artery, DP = dorsalis pedis, PL = medial and lateral plantar arches.)

21. **What is the median arcuate ligament? What is its significance?**
The median arcuate ligament is formed from fibers derived from the medial edge of both left and right diaphragmatic crus during their ascent anterosuperiorly. The median arcuate ligament may occasionally cause a stenosis of the proximal celiac axis because of extrinsic compression. The clinical significance of the resulting narrowing is uncertain. The finding is often made incidentally in asymptomatic patients. Furthermore, severe celiac stenosis and even celiac occlusions are often well tolerated. The diagnosis of celiac compression can be made by imaging during inspiration and expiration. The degree of stenosis is dependent on the phase of the respiratory cycle, often becoming less pronounced during inspiration.

Figure 12-7. Coronal subtracted MIP-projection image of the thigh station from a gadolinium-enhanced bolus chase runoff examination demonstrates occlusion of the left superficial femoral artery. The left deep femoral artery (LDFA) is patent and gives rise to tortuous collateral (COL) vessels that reconstitute the distal left superficial femoral artery (LSFA) just above the knee joint. The right superficial femoral artery (RSFA) and deep femoral artery (RDFA) are patent.

WEBSITE

http://www.ctisus.org

BIBLIOGRAPHY

1. Manning WJ, Pennell DJ (eds): Cardiovascular Magnetic Resonance. New York, Churchill Livingstone, 2002.

PLAIN RADIOGRAPHS OF THE ABDOMEN

Stephen E. Rubesin, MD

CHAPTER 13

1. What is a "flat plate" of the abdomen?

Flat plate of the abdomen is a historical term that refers to a past method of radiography when radiographs were recorded on flat "plates" of glass coated with an emulsion sensitive to x-rays. This examination also has been termed a "plain abdominal radiograph," "plain film of the abdomen," "abdominal plain film," and "KUB." The term *KUB* refers to the kidney, ureters, and bladder. The term *KUB* is not preferred because the ureters are not visible on the plain radiograph and other organs are visible. The term "plain film of the abdomen" is not accurate if the image is recorded on either a phosphor plate or directly by electronic means, stored electronically, and displayed on a monitor or plasma screen. No "film" is involved. Therefore, the preferred terms are *plain radiograph of the abdomen* or *plain abdominal radiograph*.

2. What structures are visible on a plain radiograph?

Structures are demonstrated on a plain radiograph due to differential attenuation of the x-ray beam by air, fat, soft tissue, calcium, and various metals. Therefore, the edge of an organ composed of soft tissue will be demonstrated only where it interfaces with fat of the retroperitoneum or mesenteries, gas within the lumen of the adjacent bowel, or gas within the intraperitoneal or retroperitoneal spaces. Interfaces are best demonstrated when the x-ray beam is tangential to the interface. Calcium density is detected in bones or abnormal calcifications, such as gallstones or kidney stones, or within vessel lumina or vascular walls.

The inferior edge of the liver may be demonstrated. The soft tissue of the spleen may be outlined by air in the stomach and gas in the splenic flexure of the colon. The kidneys and lateral border of the psoas muscles are outlined by retroperitoneal fat. A moderately distended urinary bladder may be outlined by pelvic fat. Portions of the uterus may also be outlined by pelvic fat. The stomach is defined by its rugal folds. Air and fluid in a nondistended stomach is a normal finding. The duodenal bulb may be demonstrated by air. Small intestine is identified by its thin, transverse folds (valvulae conniventes). The colon is defined by its haustral sacculations (Fig. 13-1). A small amount of gas may be present in nondistended small intestine. Gas may outline the nondependent portions of the colon, in particular, the transverse colon.

Figure 13-1. Coned-down image of left upper quadrant obtained with the patient in standing position. Air density *(a)* varies from black to gray. Bone density is demonstrated in the lower left ribs *(small black arrow on left 11th rib)*. The colon is identified by its air-filled haustral sacculations *(large black arrow)*, interfaced with adjacent soft tissue density. The interhaustral folds of the descending colon are thick *(white arrow)* in this patient diagnosed with fulminant colitis ("toxic megacolon"). The interhaustral fold density is representative of soft tissue density.

3. **What is an anteroposterior (AP) radiograph?**
The standard plain abdominal radiograph is obtained with the patient in a recumbent position, lying on his or her back, and is termed a *supine radiograph*. The x-ray tube is anterior (superior) to the patient, and the radiographic image capture device is posterior (inferior) to the patient. Thus, the x-ray beam travels from anterior to the patient to be captured posterior to the patient. By convention, this is termed an *anteroposterior radiograph*.

4. **What is a lateral decubitus radiograph?**
The term *decubitus* means lying down. Without qualification, it is therefore meaningless. A "decub" is obtained with the patient lying with his or her left or right side down. Therefore, a right lateral decubitus radiograph is an image obtained with the patient lying with his or her right side down, the x-ray tube oriented in a horizontal position on one side of the patient, and the image capture device (usually a "cassette") oriented perpendicular (upright) to the tube on the other side of the patient. To prevent any confusion, the best terms are "right-side down decubitus" and "left-side down decubitus" views.

5. **What is the purpose of an image obtained with the patient in a lateral decubitus or erect position?**
Images obtained with the patient in an erect position (chest x-ray or abdominal image) or images obtained with the patient in a lateral decubitus position are used to demonstrate air-fluid levels in the gastrointestinal tract or free intraperitoneal gas (Fig. 13-2). These views are important in patients with suspected perforation or bowel obstruction. An erect view is used in patients who can stand; decubitus views are performed in patients who are unable to stand.

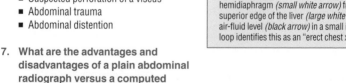

Figure 13-2. Radiograph of the chest obtained with the patient standing. A large amount of free intraperitoneal gas separates the right hemidiaphragm *(small white arrow)* from the superior edge of the liver *(large white arrow)*. An air-fluid level *(black arrow)* in a small intestinal loop identifies this as an "erect chest x-ray."

6. **What are some of the indications for an abdominal plain radiograph?**
   ■ Acute or subacute abdominal pain
   ■ Suspected calculus in any viscus
   ■ Suspected obstruction or adynamic ileus
   ■ Suspected perforation of a viscus
   ■ Abdominal trauma
   ■ Abdominal distention

7. **What are the advantages and disadvantages of a plain abdominal radiograph versus a computed tomography (CT) scan?**
A *plain abdominal radiograph* is a low-cost procedure that is relatively easy to perform with relatively inexpensive radiographic equipment. A radiograph requires little cooperation from the patient. The radiation dose is small. A *CT scan* is a high-cost procedure that also requires little cooperation from the patient. CT equipment is expensive and delivers a relatively high radiation dose to the patient. Given the rapid speed of new CT scanners, the time that a patient is lying on the radiographic tabletop is nearly equal for both a plain film of the abdomen and CT scan. An abdominal film requires no patient preparation. There is about a 1-hour preparation time for a CT that uses both IV and oral contrast.

CT has far greater contrast resolution than a plain film and is far superior in demonstrating abnormal calcifications or fluid/gas patterns in the viscera or peritoneal space. CT is tremendously superior at demonstrating the solid organs. The plain radiograph has better spatial resolution than CT does, in particular, the overview scout image of a CT scan (variously termed *scanogram, topogram,* etc.). Thus, a plain film provides an overall "big picture" for bowel obstruction superior to a CT. This advantage is greatly surpassed, however, by CT's demonstration of individual bowel loops, fluid-filled bowel loops, and bowel wall thickness and enhancement patterns.

8. **In the era of fast CT scanners, what is the role of the plain radiograph?**
    Plain radiographs are helpful when patients require serial studies, such as patients undergoing decompression for small bowel obstruction or follow-up for resolution of postoperative adynamic ileus. Plain radiographs are also helpful in determining positions of various tubes placed in the abdomen. If there is any question, however, that a tube tip is not within its expected location, a contrast study must be performed.

    Plain radiographs may be of value in intensive care patients who are too seriously ill to move. The physicians have to balance the risk of patient transport from the intensive care unit to the CT scanner and the greater information obtained by a CT with the mediocre diagnostic capability but safety of an abdominal film obtained with portable radiographic equipment.

    In situations that require extreme speed, a CT scan without the use of either oral or IV contrast still provides much more information than a plain abdominal radiograph.

9. **Why is the term *free air* a misnomer?**
    Gas in the stomach is initially similar in composition to atmospheric air swallowed by the patient. Once various digestive processes occur, the gas in the luminal organs no longer has the same composition as atmospheric air. For example, carbon dioxide is generated when acid secreted by the stomach combines with bicarbonate secreted by the pancreas. Both oxygen and carbon dioxide are resorbed in the small bowel. Only nitrogen is not absorbed. Colonic gas also reflects gas such as methane produced by bacterial fermentation.

    Gas in the peritoneal cavity is trapped in various crevices of the organs and mesenteries. Therefore, a patient should be positioned in an erect or decubitus position for about 10 minutes before a radiograph is obtained to look for "free intraperitoneal gas."

10. **What are the best patient positions to detect free intraperitoneal gas on a plain radiograph?**
    Free intraperitoneal gas is best demonstrated on an erect chest x-ray centered over the diaphragms (see Fig. 13-2). As little as 1 mL of gas may be detected under the curve of a hemidiaphragm. A left-side down lateral decubitus view to demonstrate air above or under the liver edge is a second best choice.

11. **What percentage of supine radiographs demonstrates free intraperitoneal gas?**
    In some patients, an erect chest, erect abdominal, or lateral decubitus radiograph is not possible and an image can only be obtained with the patient in a supine position. A supine abdominal radiograph will demonstrate free intraperitoneal gas in about 60% of patients with free intraperitoneal gas.

12. **What is Rigler's sign?**
    Rigler's sign is named after a famous radiologist, Leo Rigler, who described a sign of pneumoperitoneum. Normally, gas outlines only the luminal side of a bowel loop. The soft tissue side of the bowel is not visible as a sharp edge because there is no difference in contrast attenuation between the soft tissue of bowel wall and the remainder of the abdomen. However, when free

intraperitoneal gas abuts a gas-filled loop of bowel, gas will surround both sides of the bowel wall. If the interfaces of gas and bowel wall are perpendicular to the x-ray beam, the bowel wall will be visible and appear as a thin stripe of soft tissue (Fig. 13-3).

13. **In what quadrant is free intraperitoneal gas best detected?**
    Signs of free intraperitoneal gas are most commonly seen in the right upper quadrant, as either lucency over the liver; curvilinear, triangular, or linear streaks of gas outlining the edge of liver near the porta hepatitis; or gas outlining the falciform ligament (Fig. 13-4).
    Other signs of free intraperitoneal gas include a curved lucency under the mid-diaphragm resembling a "cupola," gas trapped in the interhaustral folds (the triangle sign), and air in the pelvis outlining the lateral umbilical folds (Fig. 13-5).

14. **A coned-down image of the right upper quadrant is presented. What structure is outlined by gas in Figure 13-6? Where is the gas located?**
    Gas in the retroperitoneal space usually results from iatrogenic causes or gas-forming infections. Gas originates in the following retroperitoneal structures: the second through fourth portions of the duodenum; pancreas and distal common bile duct; ascending and descending colon and rectum; kidneys, ureters, and urinary bladder; and abdominal aorta and its branches. Gas rarely arises in the retroperitoneal adrenal glands.

15. **What is the most common noniatrogenic cause of pneumobilia?**
    Gas in the biliary tree, or pneumobilia, usually results from communication of bowel with the biliary tree not a gas-forming infection. The most common cause of pneumobilia is probably endoscopically or surgically performed sphincterotomy or a choledochoenteric anastomosis. In patients who have not undergone iatrogenic interventions, the most common cause of pneumobilia is a penetrating duodenal ulcer. Other etiologic factors include choledochoduodenal or cholecystoduodenal fistula due to gallstones eroding into the duodenum.

16. **What is Rigler's triad?**
    The combination of gas in the biliary tree; small bowel dilation; and a calcified, ectopic gallstone is a triad of findings described by Rigler and also has been termed *gallstone ileus*. This triad is

Figure 13-3. Rigler's sign of free intraperitoneal gas. Radiograph of abdomen obtained with the patient in the supine position. The outer walls of small bowel are normally not visible. Free intraperitoneal gas outlines the outer wall of a loop of small intestine *(white arrow)* and the proximal sigmoid colon *(black arrow).*

Figure 13-4. Falciform ligament sign of free intraperitoneal gas. The falciform ligament *(black arrows)* and inferior edge of the liver *(white arrow)* are outlined by free intraperitoneal gas.

Figure 13-5. Free intraperitoneal gas in the pelvis in this coned-down image of the pelvis obtained with the patient in the supine position. Radiolucent free intraperitoneal gas outlines the lateral umbilical folds (left fold identified by *long arrow*) and inferior left *(short arrow)* and right paracolic gutters.

Figure 13-6. What structure is outlined by gas? The kidney is outlined by gas in the retroperitoneum. An ovoid lucency outlines the kidney *(thick arrows)*. Lobules of perirenal fat appear as 0.5- to 1-cm lucencies surrounded by rings of soft tissue *(thin arrow)*. This retroperitoneal gas was the result of perforation of the rectum at endoscopy.

seen in fewer than one half of patients in whom a gallstone erodes into the bowel and causes an obstruction in either the distal ileum or sigmoid colon, the narrowest areas of small and large bowel, respectively. The triad is uncommon in patients in whom a gallstone erodes into bowel because only a small percentage of gallstones are calcified; obstruction is not always present; and the fistula may close, resulting in lack of biliary air.

17. What does the linear form of pneumatosis imply?

Pneumatosis is gas in the intestinal wall. Linear streaks of gas (Fig. 13-7) or tiny bubbles (Fig. 13-8) within the small or large intestinal wall suggest ischemia, but not necessarily irreversible necrosis. In patients with ischemia, bowel does not contract normally and therefore dilates. Ischemia is one of the most common causes of severe small bowel dilation. Edema or blood in the bowel wall associated with ischemia may appear as nodular soft tissue densities resembling "thumbprints."

Rounded air collections in bowel wall may be due to benign causes of rents in the mucosa, termed *pneumatosis cystoides intestinalis* or *benign pneumatosis coli*. The gas-filled blebs are most commonly detected in the colon and are associated with various clinical conditions such as scleroderma, steroid use, and celiac disease.

Figure 13-7. Linear form of pneumatosis. This coned-down image obtained from a radiograph with the patient in the supine position shows linear streaks of gas *(arrows)* within the smooth-surfaced walls of small intestine. Soft tissue within the lumen of the bowel represents both fluid and debris composed of blood and sloughed cells ("the small bowel feces sign"). The patient was hypotensive. Ischemia with transmural necrosis was found at surgery.

18. In what portions of the gastrointestinal tract is normal gas located when the patient is radiographed in a supine position?

Gas collects in nondependent portions of the gastrointestinal tract. When the patient is lying in a supine position, the gastric antrum and transverse colon are the most anterior portions of the gastrointestinal tract. When the patient lies in a prone position, the gastric fundus, ascending and descending colon, and midrectum are the most nondependent portions of the gastrointestinal tract. Therefore, an air-filled transverse colon less than 5–7 cm in diameter is a normal finding on a supine radiograph.

19. What does the term *ileus* mean?

Ileus is Greek, meaning "to wrap" or "to roll." The term initially was used to describe patients "doubled-over" with abdominal pain. The term later was used to describe bowel dilation.

The term *ileus*, meaning dilation, needs a qualifier to imply either atony or obstruction. *Mechanical ileus* means bowel obstruction. The terms *adynamic ileus, paralytic ileus,* or *functional ileus* describe diminished bowel contraction or peristalsis, not obstruction, with accumulation of air and fluid in the intestinal lumen.

20. Which study is superior in diagnosing small bowel obstruction: plain radiograph or CT?

Before the advent of CT, plain abdominal radiographs (Fig. 13-9) and barium studies were used to diagnose small bowel obstruction. However, CT has become the imaging modality of choice in patients with suspected small bowel obstruction. CT is superior in diagnosing the presence, location, and etiologic factors of small bowel obstruction. The value of plain radiographs is in follow-up of the resolution or progression of small bowel obstruction in patients who do not undergo surgery.

Figure 13-8. Pneumatosis coli. (A) This coned-down image from an x-ray obtained with the patient in the supine position demonstrates small (1–2 mm) irregularly shaped bubbles of gas overlying the descending colon. Where the colonic wall is demonstrated in profile, the bubbles of gas *(arrows)* are shown to be located in the colonic wall. This hypotensive patient had infarction in the portion of colon that is at the transition of arterial supply between the superior mesenteric artery and inferior mesenteric artery (the "watershed zone"). (B) This axial image from a CT scan of the abdomen shows curvilinear air density between the contrast-filled lumen of the descending colon and the soft tissue of the colonic wall *(arrows)*.

21. What are the pitfalls of plain radiograph diagnosis of small bowel obstruction?

A small bowel loop is identified on plain abdominal radiography by intraluminal air outlining valvulae conniventes. If a small bowel loop is completely filled with fluid, it cannot be identified on a plain abdominal radiograph. Therefore, plain abdominal radiography will miss fluid-filled loops, will underdiagnose small bowel obstruction, and will not be able to estimate the level of obstruction accurately. In contrast, CT can identify fluid-filled bowel loops just proximal to the obstruction that plain radiography cannot identify.

The clue to an obstruction is a transition between dilated small bowel proximal to an obstructing lesion and collapsed small bowel distal to the obstruction (see Fig. 13-9). False-negative diagnoses may be made with both CT and plain abdominal radiography when bowel is not dilated due to vomiting, nasogastric tube/long tube decompression, or when an examination is performed before fluid can accumulate proximal to the obstruction. False-positive diagnosis of obstruction is not infrequent by either CT or plain abdominal radiography. False-positive diagnoses may be made in patients with an adynamic ileus predominantly involving the small intestine (Fig. 13-10). In all, plain film radiography will detect about 80% of small bowel obstructions.

22. What modality is able to diagnose an obstruction complicated by ischemia?

Ischemia may occur when the mesentery is twisted during a closed loop obstruction, compromising venous return and arterial inflow. Ischemia may also occur during any obstruction in which luminal dilation results in venous congestion. CT is the best radiologic modality to identify ischemia. CT diagnosis depends on identification of a thick-walled bowel that either does not enhance or has a mural stratification pattern due to marked submucosal edema (Fig. 13-11). In some patients, there is increased attenuation of bowel wall on unenhanced scans due to intramural hemorrhage. Congestion in the mesentery is seen.

Figure 13-9. Closed-loop small bowel obstruction with ischemia. This plain abdominal radiograph obtained with the patient in the supine position shows that the mid small intestine is disproportionately dilated. The loops are "radially arranged" *(thick arrows)*, with their mesenteric origin in the right lower quadrant. Normal valvulae conniventes are 1–2 mm thick. The small bowel folds are markedly thickened, about 4–5 mm *(thin arrows)*.

Figure 13-10. Adynamic ileus mimicking small bowel obstruction. This plain abdominal radiograph obtained with the patient in the erect position shows that the mid small intestine is disproportionately dilated. Air-fluid levels *(large arrows)* are seen in the small intestinal lumen. The nondistended colon is identified by its haustral sacculations. Air-fluid levels are also present in the colon *(small arrow)* and are a clue that this patient had (bacterial) enteritis with a hypersecretory state.

KEY POINTS: RADIOLOGY OF THE GASTROINTESTINAL TRACT ✓

1. Plain radiographs of the abdomen have been replaced by CT, ultrasound, and MRI in patients with acute clinical problems.

2. Plain radiographs are helpful to demonstrate the location of various tubes as well as for evaluation of ICU patients or patients who require serial studies.

3. The first examination the radiologist should obtain for a patient with suspected small bowel obstruction is a CT.

4. Free intraperitoneal gas is detected in a supine plain radiograph in 60% of patients with perforation.

5. Linear pneumatosis is highly suggestive of ischemia.

23. **Can CT demonstrate adhesions?**
    CT diagnosis of small bowel obstruction relies on identification of the transition zone between dilated and nondilated bowel. CT can identify causes of obstruction that have bulk, such as primary carcinomas or metastases, and CT can demonstrate external hernias. CT identifies extrinsic inflammatory processes such as appendicitis or diverticulitis that may secondarily obstruct small bowel. However, CT diagnosis of adhesions as a cause of obstruction is a

Figure 13-11. Small bowel ischemia shown by comparison of plain radiograph and CT. (A) This coned-down image of the left upper quadrant from a plain radiograph of the abdomen obtained with the patient in the supine position shows a mildly dilated loop of small intestine with thick valvulae conniventes *(small arrows)*. Smooth, 1-cm nodules *(large arrows)* seen on the mesenteric border of a second left upper quadrant loop are examples of "thumbprinting" due to severe submucosal edema (in this case) or hemorrhage. (B) This axial image from a CT scan of the abdomen at the level of the upper sacrum shows two loops of ileum with a mural stratification pattern ("target sign") *(large arrows)*. High attenuation contrast and bubbles of gas are seen within the ileal lumen surrounded by a thick band of fluid attenuation in the submucosa surrounded by high attenuation in the muscularis propria. Ascites is present in the paracolic gutters (left paracolic gutter identified by *open arrow*). The mesentery supplying these abnormal loops is engorged and of fluid attenuation *(m)* in comparison to the normal fat attenuation of normal small bowel mesentery *(small arrow)* of nonischemic loops.

presumptive diagnosis only, made when no identifiable cause of obstruction is seen at the transition zone.

24. **In what situations are barium studies most helpful for the diagnosis of small bowel obstruction?**
    Barium studies are superior to CT in diagnosing low-grade or intermittent small bowel obstructions. The site of obstruction is identified more reliably by a barium study than with CT. Barium studies are superior in determining whether a stricture in a patient with Crohn's disease is functionally obstructive. Barium studies also are superior to CT in demonstrating intraluminal tumors as a cause of intussusception/obstruction.

25. **What is the most common form of colonic volvulus?**
    Sigmoid volvulus accounts for about three fourths of cases of colonic volvulus (Fig. 13-12). Radiographically, an inverted U-shaped loop of dilated colon extends far out of the pelvis into the upper abdomen. If the inner walls of the ascending and descending portions of the sigmoid loop are apposed to each other, a thick soft tissue stripe is seen radiating toward the pelvis. This has been described as resembling a "coffee bean." The colon and even the small intestine proximal to the twist also are dilated.

26. **What patient groups have a greater incidence of sigmoid volvulus?**
    Patients with elongated, dilated sigmoid colons are predisposed to sigmoid volvulus. Sigmoid volvulus is common in parts of the world (such as Africa) where people have high-fiber diets, bulky stools, and large colons. In the United States, sigmoid volvulus is common

Figure 13-12. Sigmoid volvulus. (A) This plain radiograph of abdomen shows a markedly dilated sigmoid colon *(S)*. A thick soft tissue stripe *(arrows)* is seen between adjacent limbs of the dilated sigmoid colon, representing the walls of two adjacent loops coapted together. This overall appearance is said to resemble a "coffee bean" (radiologists are a very imaginative group of individuals). (B) This overhead image from a subsequent single contrast barium enema shows a smooth narrowing *(arrow)* distal to a massively dilated sigmoid colon *(S)*. Once the obstruction has been demonstrated, the radiologist does not fill the colon with barium because barium can form concretions in the colon behind a colonic obstruction. (Barium will not form concretions in an obstructed small intestine.)

in patients who are either bedridden or who are taking medications that cause colonic hypomotility; thus, patients in nursing homes and mental institutions are at the most risk for sigmoid volvulus.

27. **In what quadrant of the abdomen does the cecum lie in a patient with cecal volvulus?**
    The ascending colon is fused to the retroperitoneum in most people. In patients in whom the right colon has incompletely fused to the retroperitoneum, the ascending colon can twist on its mesentery and become obstructed. The colon proximal to the twist, in particular the cecum, becomes dilated and is located in the mid left abdomen or in the left upper quadrant. This condition is poorly termed a *cecal volvulus,* when, in reality, it is an ascending colon volvulus.

28. **What percentage of gallstones are calcified?**
    About 15% of gallstones are radiopaque on plain abdominal radiography (Fig. 13-13). Calcification is detected in about 30–40% of gallstones on CT. CT detects about 80% of gallstones, either calcified or not (Fig. 13-14). Cholesterol calculi appear as low attenuation filling defects, often floating in bile. Ultrasound detects about 95% of gallstones.

    Gallstones are an example of concretions formed in the abdomen. The calcification

Figure 13-13. Calcified gallstones. This coned-down image from an abdominal radiograph performed with the patient in the supine position demonstrates numerous 2- to 3-mm, polygonally shaped, calcified, "faceted" gallstones *(arrow)*.

usually occurs around a central nidus of organic or inorganic foreign matter, thrombus, focal pus, or cellular debris. The calcification occurs within the lumen of tubular structures, such as blood vessels, biliary tree, or ureters, or within a hollow viscus, such as the gall-bladder or urinary bladder. Concretions may have a round, ovoid, branched, or spiculated shape.

Figure 13-14. Noncalcified gallstones. This axial image at the level of the gallbladder from an abdominal CT scan demonstrates three noncalcified gallstones *(arrows).* The periphery of the stones has a higher attenuation than that of the surrounding bile. Tiny bubbles of air attenuation are seen in two of the stones, representing trapped nitrogen gas.

29. **A plain radiograph of the abdomen is obtained in a patient who has a palpable abdominal mass (Fig. 13-15). What is your diagnosis?**
There is a curvilinear calcification in the midabdomen centered at the L2 vertebral body level. A diagnosis of a calcified abdominal aortic aneurysm is made. Linear or curvilinear calcifications are seen in tubular or cystic structures. In the walls of tubes, such as blood vessels, the bile duct, the ureter, and the vasa differentia, the calcifications are usually discontinuous and of varying thickness. If a tubular structure is seen en face, a thick, discontinuous ring of calcification may be detected. This type of calcification is typical of arterial calcifications, in particular, atherosclerotic calcification.

Calcifications in the walls of cysts appear as a curvilinear rim of calcification. This rim is often

Figure 13-15. This plain radiograph of the abdomen obtained with the patient in the supine position shows a discontinuous ring of curvilinear calcification *(arrows)* surrounding a soft tissue mass (11 cm in diameter) in the midabdomen. This proved to be a saccular abdominal aortic aneurysm. This is an example of vascular calcification due to atherosclerosis.

incomplete. A wide variety of lesions gives this appearance, including renal cysts and renal cell carcinoma, aneurysms of the aorta and other major vessels, echinococcus cysts in the liver or spleen, pancreatic pseudocysts, adrenal cysts, mesenteric cysts, mucinous tumors of the appendix, and cystic tumors of the ovaries. Calcification of the gallbladder wall in chronic cholecystitis (porcelain gallbladder) has a similar appearance.

The location of an abnormality is a clue to the location of a calcification in the abdomen detected on plain film radiography. CT will demonstrate the organ of origin and the cause of a calcified mass in most cases.

Figure 13-16. Calcific pancreatitis due to chronic alcohol abuse. This coned-down view of the upper abdomen demonstrates dense clumps of calcification *(arrows)* to the right of the L2 vertebral body. These calcifications are not in the pancreatic parenchyma but are within dilated pancreatic ducts.

30. **A coned-down view of the upper abdomen (Fig. 13-16) is obtained in a man with chronic abdominal pain. What is your diagnosis?**
Dense, sharply angulated clumps of calcium are confined to a 4-cm area just to the right of the L2 vertebral body. A diagnosis of calcific pancreatitis is made.

Calcifications in abdominal masses and inflammatory processes have a variety of shapes and sizes. Calcifications in mucin-producing tumors appear amorphous or punctate. Intraductal calcifications in patients with alcoholic pancreatitis appear as small clumps overlying the pancreas (see Fig. 13-16). Mottled, slightly irregular, ovoid masses of calcification are typically seen in calcified lymph nodes. Uterine leiomyomas are the most common pelvic tumor to calcify. These tumors may have a peripheral rim, central whorled, or clumplike calcification (Fig. 13-17).

Figure 13-17. Calcified uterine leiomyomas. This plain radiograph of the abdomen demonstrates a large calcified mass *(arrows).* Four round calcified masses are confluent in the midline. The calcifications are dense and punctate, but some are said to resemble "popcorn." This is the type of calcification typically seen in uterine leiomyomas.

31. **A patient has a palpable abdominal mass (Fig. 13-18). What organ is enlarged?**
CT, MRI, and ultrasound are now the modalities of choice in the work-up of a palpable abdominal mass. If gynecologic disease is suspected, an ultrasound of the pelvis or MRI is the preferred examination. For upper abdominal masses, CT or MRI is indicated.

Figure 13-18. Plain abdominal radiograph obtained with the patient in the supine position demonstrates a large (25-cm) mass *(arrows)* in the left upper quadrant that deviates the splenic flexure of the colon *(S)* medially. This mass is an enlarged spleen in a patient with leukemia.

BIBLIOGRAPHY

1. Baker SR, Cho KC (eds): The Abdominal Plain Film with Correlative Imaging, 2nd ed. Stamford, CT, Appleton & Lange, 1998.

2. Baker SR, Cho KC: Abdominal calcifications. In Gore RM, Levine MS (eds): Textbook of Gastrointestinal Radiology, 2nd ed. Philadelphia, W.B. Saunders, 2000, pp 178–187.

3. Messmer JM: Gas and soft tissue abnormalities. In Gore RM, Levine MS (eds): Textbook of Gastrointestinal Radiology, 2nd ed. Philadelphia, W.B. Saunders, 2000, pp 157–177.

4. Miller RE, Nelson SW: The roentgenologic demonstration of tiny amounts of free intraperitoneal gas: Experimental and clinical studies. Am J Roentgenol 112:574–585, 1971.

5. Williams SM: Abdomen: Normal anatomy and examination techniques. In Gore RM, Levine MS (eds): Textbook of Gastrointestinal Radiology, 2nd ed. Philadelphia, W.B. Saunders, 2000, pp 144–156.

CHAPTER 14

THE UPPER GI TRACT

Stephen E. Rubesin, MD

1. **What organs are studied during an upper gastrointestinal (GI) series?**
   The morphology and motility of the esophagus, stomach, and duodenum.

2. **What organs are studied during a pharyngoesophagram?**
   The radiologist evaluates the motility of the oral cavity, pharynx, and esophagus and the morphology of the pharynx, esophagus, and gastric cardia. The radiologist records oral, pharyngeal, and esophageal motility either via a VCR (video), DVD recorder, or on film ("cine"). Film has been almost completely replaced as the recording medium for motility because of increased radiation exposure, cost, and difficulty of film processing.

3. **What organ is demonstrated in Figure 14-1?**
   Figure 14-1 shows a normal lower thoracic esophagus. The esophagus is a muscular tube within the mediastinum. The esophagus is usually collapsed unless distended by liquid or solid food; swallowed air; or, in this image, swallowed air and barium. In this patient, swallowed high-density barium coats the mucosa. The swallowed carbon dioxide (effervescent agent) and swallowed air distend the lumen of the esophagus. The mucosa of the esophageal tube seen in profile appears as a white line *(arrows)*. The mucosal surface is seen en face, "etched in white" by the barium. The mucosal surface of the normal esophagus is smooth and varies from white to gray (representative mucosa identified by *S*). Normal structures in the mediastinum push on the distended esophagus, manifested as alterations of the normal straight tubular contour of the esophagus. These indentations are identified as *(a)*, the bottom of the aortic arch; *(b)*, the left mainstem bronchus; and *(l)*, the left atrium.

4. **What organs are shown in Figure 14-2? Identify the numbered parts of the organs as labeled.**
   This image is a double contrast image of the stomach and duodenum. See the figure legend for the answers.

5. **What curvatures do the *black* and *open arrows* in Figure 14-2 identify?**
   The *black arrows* identify the lesser curvature of the stomach; the *open arrows* identify the greater curvature.

Figure 14-1. Normal esophagus (*see* question 3 for description).

6. **Why does the gastric fundus appear white in Figure 14-2, whereas the antrum appears gray?**
   Barium sulfate absorbs and scatters x-rays, but air does not. Therefore, x-rays passing through barium are blocked and do not reach the film. X-rays easily pass through GI structures filled with

air and expose the film. The relatively exposed areas of the film appear as shades of black; the relatively unexposed areas of the film appear as shades of white. The heavy barium falls to the lowest or most "dependent" portion of the stomach. This image was obtained with the patient recumbent, back against the fluoroscopic tabletop (a "supine" radiograph). The gastric fundus is posterior to the gastric antrum; therefore, barium falls into the gastric fundus when the patient lies in a supine position. As barium absorbs more x-rays than air, the gastric fundus appears "white." In this radiograph, the anteriorly located gastric antrum is filled with air and is also "etched in white" by a thin layer of barium. Most of the x-rays, but not all, pass through the antrum, partially exposing the film. Therefore, the gastric antrum appears "gray," not black as a purely air-filled structure would appear.

Figure 14-2. Normal stomach (*1* = gastric fundus, *2* = gastric body, *3* = gastric antrum, *4* = pylorus (pyloric channel), *5* = duodenal bulb, and *6* = second portion of duodenum).

Today, most radiographs are not obtained using real film as the recording medium, but they use some type of image capture device. The relative exposures on the image capture device are digitized and then are assigned gray scale values, from white to black. The images are then displayed on a monitor or flat panel. Depending on the radiologist, large exposures are either assigned "white" or "black" values. In the United States, barium is usually assigned a "white" value; in Japan, barium often is assigned a "black" value.

7. **Two images of the esophagus are presented in Figure 14-3. What is your diagnosis?**
   This is a semiannular carcinoma of the esophagus. The tumor originated on the side of contour irregularity and has begun to spread circumferentially. The wall opposite the tumor is smooth and uninvolved by the tumor but has been pulled inward by the desmoplastic tumor. The barium pool in Figure 14-3, *A*, demonstrates the contour of a luminal organ but obscures mucosal detail. The air contrast image in Figure 14-3, *B*, reveals the luminal contour in profile, as does the barium pool. The air contrast image also reveals the mucosal surface en face. In this case, the air contrast image demonstrates the surface and the edge of the semiannular cancer.

8. **What does "single contrast" mean?**
   A single-contrast study of a GI structure means that one contrast agent is used, such as a suspension of barium sulfate, an ionic water-soluble contrast agent such as diatrizoate meglumine (Gastroview/Gastrografin), or a nonionic water-soluble contrast agent such as Omnipaque.
   Figure 14-4 is an example of a single-contrast image obtained with the patient swallowing barium while lying in a prone position. A column of "thin" barium fills the distal esophageal lumen. The radiologist examines the luminal contour in profile for abnormalities that either protrude into the lumen or protrude outside of the expected luminal contour of the organ. The radiologist also looks for abnormalities en face. Large protrusions into the lumen displace the barium column, allow x-rays to pass through the esophagus, and appear as radiolucent "filling defects" in the barium column. Large protrusions outside the luminal contour fill with barium and, when seen en face, appear as a "double density" of barium.

Figure 14-3. Air contrast versus the barium pool. (A) Spot radiograph of the esophagus performed while the patient drinks high-density barium in an erect position shows a pool of barium (with an air-barium level, *open arrow*) in the mid-esophagus. A region of focal circumferential narrowing, 3 cm in length, is present. The narrowing appears smooth on one wall *(white arrow)* and has an irregular contour on the opposite wall *(black arrows)*. (B) Spot radiograph performed seconds later after the barium pool has passed through the esophagus shows the same circumferential narrowing with a smooth contour on one side and an irregular contour on the other. However, the mucosal surface is now seen en face as well, revealing focal mucosal nodularity *(open arrow)* and barium etched lines *(arrows)* that disrupt the normal smooth surface of the esophagus and outline the outer margin of a mass.

In this patient there is a small hiatal hernia *(h)*. At the esophagogastric junction, a thin, smooth, symmetric ringlike narrowing, 3 mm in height, is seen in profile as a shelflike indentation of the luminal contour *(white arrows)*. En face, the ring is manifested as a thin radiolucent filling defect in the barium column *(open arrow)*. This is a Schatzki ring, a narrowing that commonly causes dysphagia with solids.

9. What does "double contrast" mean?

A double-contrast study means that the radiologist uses two contrast agents to examine the organs in question. For example, a double-contrast upper GI series uses an effervescent agent that creates carbon dioxide to distend the luminal organs and high-density barium to "scrub and paint" the mucosa. This study is also known as an "air contrast upper GI series" or a "biphasic upper GI series."

Figure 14-4. Schatzki ring demonstrated by single contrast esophagogram (*see* question 8 for explanation).

Figure 14-5 is an example of a double-contrast image of the distal stomach. Rugal folds are seen as radiolucent filling defects in the barium pool *(white arrow)* and as parallel barium etched lines *(black arrows)*. Rugal folds are composed of mucosa and submucosa and are most prominent along the greater curvature of the stomach. The normal gastric antrum *(A)* has few, if any, rugal folds in most patients.

Figure 14-5. Normal distal stomach (see question 9 for description).

10. **What are some of the clinical indications for performing an upper gastrointestinal study (upper GI)?**
    Heartburn, dysphagia, or odynophagia referred to a substernal location; upper abdominal pain or discomfort; upper GI bleeding; and vomiting.

KEY POINTS: RADIOLOGY OF THE UPPER GI TRACT ✓

1. Single-contrast GI examinations:
   - Use "thin barium" or water-soluble Gastroview (no gas used).
   - Are easier to perform in sick patients who cannot turn.
   - Can detect bowel obstruction, perforation, or fistulas.
2. Double-contrast GI examinations:
   - Use high-density barium and air/carbon dioxide.
   - Require patients to turn.
   - Are more sensitive than single-contrast examinations for detecting mucosal abnormalities.

11. **What are some of the clinical indications for performing a video/DVD pharyngoesophagram?**
    Dysphagia or odynophagia referred to the head, neck, and suprasternal regions; history of globus sensation; chronic cough; aspiration pneumonia or cerebrovascular accident; dribbling

from the mouth; abnormal tongue motions; and history of surgery or radiation of the tongue, palate, pharynx, or larynx.

12. **What is the preparation for an upper GI or pharyngoesophagram?**
Each hospital or outpatient facility has its own preparation routines for these studies. These preparations should be available from the radiologists. At our institution, for example, a handout describing the examination and explaining the preparation (see the following) is available to all referring doctors:
1. Nothing by mouth after 9 PM.
2. Eliminate or decrease the dose of insulin in insulin-dependent diabetics the morning of the examination.
3. No antacids or Pepto-Bismol on the morning of the examination.
4. Patients should wear dentures or other swallowing appliances.
5. If patients have solid food dysphagia, they should bring a type of food that causes dysphagia.
6. After the examination, patients are encouraged to drink liquids and may take a laxative if additional radiologic tests are scheduled or if there is a history of colonic hypomotility.

13. **What are contraindications to a barium study of the upper GI tract?**
- Known or suspected perforation (*see* question 14).
- Inability to swallow. In this instance, an examination of the stomach and small bowel may be performed by sending the patient to fluoroscopy with a nasogastric tube placed in the stomach.

14. **What type of contrast agent should be requested first in patients with suspected upper GI perforation?**
In patients with known or suspected perforations of the pharynx, esophagus, or duodenum, an ionic water-soluble contrast agent such as diatrizoate meglumine (Gastroview or Gastrografin) should be used initially. This type of agent is readily absorbed from the soft tissues of the neck, mediastinum, and peritoneal cavity. This type of agent, if aspirated, has the theoretical potential of causing pulmonary edema because it is hyperosmolar and will draw fluid into the lungs. Therefore, if aspiration is a likely possibility, the radiologist may start with a nonionic water-soluble contrast agent that is either only mildly hyperosmolar or iso-osmolar. Other radiologists will start with barium if a perforation of the pharynx or esophagus is suspected and there is a high risk of aspiration, since barium in the soft tissues of the neck or mediastinum is relatively harmless. Barium entering the peritoneal cavity from a gastric or duodenal perforation can potentially cause barium peritonitis. This situation is not as serious, however, as barium entering the peritoneal space from a colonic perforation. The combination of barium and feces entering the peritoneal space during a barium enema has a much greater likelihood of causing peritonitis and has a high mortality rate.

15. **When is a single-contrast upper GI series performed?**
Double-contrast examinations focus on demonstrating mucosal detail. Single-contrast examinations focus only on the big picture to detect obstruction, perforation, abnormal motility, or fistulae. A single-contrast examination is performed to detect a complication along a staple/suture line, at an anastomosis, or near a wound; to evaluate an organ as it passes through a surgically created tunnel; or to identify a rent in a mesentery. A single-contrast examination also may be performed to evaluate emptying of surgically created pouches after surgery for morbid obesity and in conjunction with a small bowel follow-through examination.

16. **What portion of the GI tract is demonstrated in Figure 14-6?**
For the answer, see the figure legend.

17. **What portion of the GI tract is demonstrated in Figure 14-7?**
For the answer, see the figure legend.

18. **What are the indications for a small bowel follow-through?**
A small bowel follow-through may be performed whenever small bowel disease is suspected. The patient drinks a large volume (750–1000 mL) of thin barium, and a single-contrast examination of the esophagus, stomach, and small intestine is performed.

Barium filling of the small intestine is limited by gastric emptying at the pylorus. Thus, the radiologist is unable to distend all the loops of small intestine either quickly or at the same time. A small bowel follow-through is also limited by the normal 30–120-minute transit time from the pylorus to the ileocecal valve. The radiologist cannot stand in the fluoroscopic suite for 1–2 hours and watch the barium flow down the small intestine. Therefore, the radiologist examines the patient at 15–30-minute intervals, palpating loops of small intestine when they are optimally distended with barium. A small bowel follow-through relies on fluoroscopically obtained spot films, not overhead images.

Water-soluble contrast is used if a perforation is strongly suspected. A water-soluble contrast study of the small bowel is often suboptimal, however, as the hyperosmolar water-soluble contrast draws fluid into the lumen and prevents fluid resorption. Thus, water-soluble contrast is diluted and the images are very difficult to interpret. If a gastric or proximal small bowel leak is suspected, a water-soluble upper GI tract and proximal small bowel follow-through will usually suffice. If a

Figure 14-6. Spot radiograph of the duodenal bulb *(B)* and second portion of the duodenum *(2)* obtained during a double-contrast upper GI series. The folds of the duodenum (folds of Kerckring) *(arrow)* cross the duodenum, except at the level of the papilla of Vater.

Figure 14-7. Close-up from an overhead obtained during a small bowel follow-through examination. Many loops of small intestine are demonstrated. Two loops are well distended *(thin arrows)* and demonstrate that the valvulae conniventes lie perpendicular to the longitudinal axis of the small bowel. Some loops are partially collapsed and the valvulae conniventes overlap each other, giving the folds what has been described as a "feathery" *(thick arrow)* appearance. Some loops overlap and no morphologic detail is demonstrated *(open arrow)*.

mid to distal small bowel leak is suspected, a computed tomography (CT) scan may be the better initial test. If a very distal small bowel leak or anastomotic leak is suspected in a patient with an ileocolic anastomosis, a water-soluble contrast enema is probably the best choice of examination.

19. **Figure 14-8 is an overhead image obtained from what type of study? What organ is being imaged?**
    For the answer, see the figure legend.

Figure 14-8. Overhead radiograph from an enteroclysis, or small bowel enema. During this examination, a tube is passed through the patient's mouth or nose, down the throat, through the esophagus, around the stomach, through the duodenum, and past the ligament of Treitz. Passage of the tube *(arrows)* eliminates the pylorus as a rate-limiting factor of barium passage into the small bowel. In this particular case, the radiologist has injected both medium-density barium to coat the mucosa and methylcellulose to distend the lumen. A double-contrast (but not air contrast) image is obtained. The jejunum *(J)* is in the left upper quadrant, and the ileum *(I)* in the right lower quadrant. An enteroclysis may be performed as a single-contrast study with low-density barium or as a double-contrast study using barium and either air or methylcellulose to distend the lumen.

20. **What layers of bowel appear in the valvulae conniventes?**
    Valvulae conniventes (plicae circulares, folds of Kerckring) are composed of mucosa and submucosa. These folds increase the surface area of the small bowel. The villi of the intestine are just at the radiographic limits of resolution.

21. **What are the indications for enteroclysis (small bowel enema)?**
    Small bowel enemas are difficult to perform and often are uncomfortable for the patient. They are superior, however, to small bowel follow-through examination for demonstrating short lesions and the valvulae conniventes. Indications include the following:
    - Unexplained anemia or GI bleeding. A patient should have a normal upper or lower endoscopy or normal double-contrast upper GI and barium enema before enteroclysis.
    - Malabsorption.
    - Demonstration of skip lesions in a patient with known Crohn's disease.
    - Suspected tumor of any kind.

22. **What is the preparation for enteroclysis?**
    Residual fluid and feces should be removed from the small intestine and right colon. The patient should not eat past 9 PM. Bisacodyl tablets are given with water at 10 PM the night before the examination to stimulate the right colon to contract. The patient does not drink fluids after midnight. Insulin-dependent diabetic patients do not take their morning dose of insulin. Other hospitals request that a full barium enema preparation be administered (*see* question 9 in Chapter 15).

23. **Figure 14-9 is a spot radiograph of the terminal ileum in a young man with chronic diarrhea. What disease does this patient have?**

    Figure 14-9 is an image obtained during a "per-oral pneumocolon." This is a specialized air contrast examination of the distal ileum, terminal ileum, cecum, and ascending colon. The patient undergoes a barium enema preparation the day before the examination to empty the terminal ileum and colon of feces. The patient then undergoes a routine small bowel follow-through examination. At the end of that examination, the per-oral pneumocolon study is performed. The patient receives 1 mg of glucagon intravenously to relax the colon, ileocecal valve, and small intestine. Air is then insufflated into the rectum via a small soft catheter, such as a Foley catheter. The radiologist then distends the colon with air and attempts to reflux the terminal ileum with air. Air refluxes into the terminal ileum in most patients (85%), enabling double-contrast images of the terminal ileum that are superior to those obtained during small bowel follow-through examination alone.

    A per-oral pneumocolon study may be of value to demonstrate subtle mucosal changes of Crohn's disease and to evaluate the right colon and ileocecal valve if these areas were not seen at either endoscopy or barium enema.

Figure 14-9. Spot radiograph of the terminal ileum shows numerous aphthoid ulcers demonstrated en face as 2–5 mm punctate or slightly elongated collections of barium surrounded by radiolucent halos *(thin arrows)*. In profile, the aphthoid ulcers appear as 2–4 mm punctate barium collections *(open arrow)* protruding outside the expected luminal contour. In patients with chronic diarrhea, demonstration of aphthoid ulcers in the terminal ileum strongly suggests a diagnosis of Crohn's disease. (Reproduced with permission. From Rubesin SE, Bronner M: Radiologic-pathologic concept in Crohn's disease. Gastrointest Radiol 1:27–55, 1991, Fig. 8.)

24. **Figure 14-10 is from a double-contrast esophagogram performed in an immunocompromised patient with acute odynophagia. What is your diagnosis?**
    For the answer, see the figure legend.

25. **Figure 14-11 is an image performed during an esophagogram while the patient lies prone and rapidly drinks thin barium. The patient had long-standing dysphagia for solids and chronic heartburn. What is your diagnosis?**
    Endoscopy and barium studies diagnose reflux esophagitis in about 40% of patients with biopsy-proven reflux esophagitis. Endoscopy has the ability to obtain biopsy specimens, whereas an upper GI series is more accurate in the diagnosis of gastroesophageal reflux itself, since only a small percentage of patients (10%) who have gastroesophageal reflux have reflux esophagitis. An upper GI will detect gastroesophageal reflux in about 50–70% of patients who have pH probe-proven gastroesophageal reflux. Barium studies are superior to endoscopy in the diagnosis of reflux-induced strictures because subtle tapered strictures are easily missed at endoscopy.

Figure 14-10. Spot radiograph of the esophagus obtained during a double-contrast upper GI examination shows numerous 1–4-mm, elongated radiolucent filling defects aligned longitudinally *(top arrow)*. The intervening mucosa is smooth and normal. In profile, the filling defects are shown to be mildly elevated plaques *(bottom arrow)*. These small, elevated plaques are almost pathognomonic for *Candida* esophagitis. A double-contrast esophagogram has 90–95% sensitivity for detecting *Candida* esophagitis in immuno-compromised patients.

Figure 14-11. There is a long (4-cm), tapered narrowing of the distal esophagus *(thick arrows)* with an 8-mm luminal diameter. A small hiatal hernia is present, as the *thin arrow* identifies the top of a gastric fold and, therefore, the esophagogastric junction is above the diaphragm. This is a classic reflux-induced stricture.

26. **Figure 14-12 shows two images of the lesser curvature of the stomach from a double-contrast upper GI series performed in a young patient with 1 week of abdominal pain. What is your diagnosis?**
A double-contrast upper GI can be used to confidently diagnose an ulcer as a benign gastric ulcer in two thirds of patients with ulcers. In the remaining one third of patients, ulcers are either equivocally benign and need endoscopic biopsy or are frankly malignant.

27. **Figure 14-13 is an image of the gastric antrum from a double-contrast upper GI series performed in a 52-year-old woman with anemia. What is your diagnosis?**
For the answer, see the figure legend.

Figure 14-12. (A) A 6-mm focal barium collection *(arrow)* is seen en face. No mass effect is seen. (B) When the barium collection is viewed in profile, the collection protrudes from the expected luminal contour *(large arrow)*. A thin lucency *(small arrow)* crosses the collection at its interface with the luminal contour. These are findings of a benign gastric ulcer. The ulcer niche (crater) is filled with barium *(large arrow)* and protrudes outside the expected contour of the stomach. No mass or mucosal nodularity is seen to indicate that a tumor is present. As the ulcer extends into the soft submucosal fat, it spreads laterally, burrowing under the mucosa. The undermined mucosa is manifested as the lucency *(small arrow)* crossing the edge of the ulcer, termed a "Hampton's line."

Figure 14-13. Coarsely lobulated, nodular folds radiate toward a central barium collection *(u)*. Compare a normal sized fold *(open arrow)* with an enlarged, lobulated fold *(black arrow)*. The radiographic findings are that of a malignant tumor, proved at surgery to be an adenocarcinoma.

28. Figure 14-14 is a close-up of the distal greater curvature of the stomach obtained during a double-contrast upper GI series performed in a patient with abdominal pain and rheumatoid arthritis. What is your diagnosis?
   For the answer, see the figure legend.

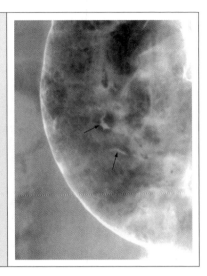

Figure 14-14. In the gastric antrum, there are two thin, serpentine barium collections surrounded by radiolucent halos. These are the radiographic findings of erosive gastritis. Erosions are most commonly caused by nonsteroidal anti-inflammatory agents, but also may be caused by alcohol, viral infection, hypotension, or iatrogenic trauma (electrocautery). Linear erosions, as depicted in this figure, are usually related to nonsteroidal anti-inflammatory agent use. This patient with rheumatoid arthritis was taking aspirin.

29. **A coned-down image of the gastric fundus obtained during a double-contrast upper GI series is demonstrated in Figure 14-15. What is your diagnosis?**
For the answer, see the figure legend.

Figure 14-15. A small (6-mm) area of increased density is etched in white *(thick arrow)*. A subtle ring shadow *(thin arrow)* is seen centrally. These are the radiographic findings of a pedunculated polyp seen en face. The head of the polyp *(thick arrow)* is manifested as the outer barium-etched ring. The pedicle of the polyp *(thin arrow)* is etched in white and is seen toward the center of the polyp. The biopsy specimen showed this was a hyperplastic polyp.

30. **A coned-down image of the gastric fundus obtained during a double-contrast upper GI series in presented in Figure 14-16. What is your diagnosis?**
Figure 14-16 demonstrates the typical appearance of a submucosal mass. A smooth-surfaced tumor protrudes into the lumen. The tumor has an abrupt interface with the normal adjacent contour manifested, in profile, as sharp angulation with the lumen and, en face, as a ring shadow or sharp-edged barium pool. Central ulceration is demonstrated in about 50% of submucosal masses. The most common submucosal mass in the stomach is a gastrointestinal stromal tumor (GIST). Lymphoma, granular cell tumor, and metastases are other common submucosal masses.

Figure 14-16. There is a 4-cm, smooth-surfaced mass *(large arrows)* protruding into the stomach. The mass has sharp angles to the luminal contour *(arrowheads)*. There is a sharp line between the obliquely oriented tumor and mucosal surface *(thin arrows)*. These are the classic findings of a submucosal (extramucosal) mass. This proved to be a GIST.

31. Figure 14-17 is an image of the gastric antrum from a double-contrast upper GI series performed in a 43-year-old man with anemia. What is your diagnosis?
    For the answer, see the figure legend.

Figure 14-17. A mass is demonstrated in profile as focal loss of the mucosal contour of the greater curvature of the gastric antrum with an area of soft tissue density *(double arrow)* protruding into the lumen. En face, the mass appears as numerous lobulated barium-etched lines *(large arrows)* disrupting the mucosal surface. The mass has a central ulceration *(small arrow)* that is not filled with barium because it originated from the anterior wall and greater curvature. These radiographic findings are typical of a mass of mucosal origin, in this case an adenocarcinoma. Compare the nodular surface of this mucosal tumor with the smooth surface of the submucosal tumor in Figure 14-16.

32. An elderly man complains of early satiety. A spot radiograph of the stomach from a double-contrast upper GI series is provided (Fig. 14-18). What is your diagnosis?
    For the answer, see the figure legend.

Figure 14-18. A long, circumferential, tapered narrowing of the distal gastric body and proximal gastric antrum is present (between *arrows* on the greater and lesser curvatures). The mucosal surface is only focally nodular *(open arrow)*. These are the radiographic findings of "linitis plastica," proved in this case to a signet-ring cell adenocarcinoma of the stomach broadly infiltrating the submucosa. Carcinomas of the stomach may spread longitudinally in the submucosal fat. If a desmoplastic (scirrhous) response occurs, large portions of the stomach may be narrowed. The most common causes of long gastric narrowings include adenocarcinoma, metastatic breast cancer, and corrosive ingestion.

33. **Figure 14-19 is a spot radiograph of the lower stomach obtained from a double-contrast upper GI series in a man who has had 4 months of abdominal discomfort. What is your differential diagnosis?**
For the answer, see the figure legend.

Figure 14-19. Rugal folds are composed of mucosa and submucosa. Therefore, rugal fold enlargement indicates a pathologic condition in the mucosa and submucosa. Radiographically, normal rugal folds are smooth, about 5 mm in size, and slightly more undulating along the greater curvature. Normal rugal folds also diminish in size from the gastric fundus to the antrum. A well-distended gastric antrum usually does not have rugal folds. In this image, the folds of the gastric antrum and body are markedly enlarged, lobulated, sometimes smooth *(white arrows)* and sometimes nodular *(black arrow)*. The differential diagnosis includes tumor of the mucosa (adenocarcinoma) or the submucosa (lymphoma) or hyperplasia of a component of the mucosa (Ménétrier's disease [i.e., hyperplasia of the surface foveolar cells]). This cannot represent parietal cell hyperplasia seen in Zollinger-Ellison syndrome because parietal cells are not located in the gastric antrum and the folds are larger than those typically seen in Zollinger-Ellison syndrome. This patient had lymphoma of the stomach.

34. **A young man complains of acute right upper quadrant pain. A spot radiograph from a double-contrast upper GI series is presented (Fig. 14-20). What is your diagnosis?**
Ulcers in the duodenal bulb are invariably benign. Barium examinations are very effective (95%) at detecting acute duodenal bulb ulcers in patients who do not have scarring and sacculations related to chronic scarring. In about 20% of patients with recurrent ulcer disease, however, small ulcers may be missed in scarred or sacculated duodenal bulbs.

Figure 14-20. A 6-mm barium collection *(large arrow)* is seen in the duodenal bulb. Smooth folds *(thin arrows)* radiate to the margin of the collection. These are the radiographic findings of an acute, benign ulcer of the posterior wall of the duodenal bulb. Sacculation of the superior fornix of the duodenal bulb *(s)* reflects the scarring process radiating to the ulcer.

35. **Figure 14-21, *A*, is a coned-down image of the mid small intestine obtained in man with unexplained heme-positive stool. Figure 14-21, *B*, is an axial image from a CT scan that was performed several days later. What is your differential diagnosis?**

    Enteroclysis (small bowel enema) is the best radiologic test for demonstrating most small bowel tumors. Enteroclysis is relatively poor at demonstrating arteriovenous malformations, however. In patients with known metastatic melanoma, enteroclysis can be performed if there is a clinical question of small bowel metastases (Fig. 14-22).

Figure 14-21. (A) A large (6-cm) barium-filled cavity *(large arrows)* protrudes from the mesenteric side of the small intestine. Lobulated folds are seen on the mesenteric side of the bowel *(open arrows)*. (B) A mass *(arrows)* is seen in the right mid abdomen. Centrally, a cavity *(c)* is filled with contrast, debris, and air. These are the radiographic findings of a cavitary tumor originating in the small intestine. Highly cellular tumors, such as lymphoma or metastatic melanoma, or highly vascular tumors, such as GIST, are the most common cavitary masses in the small intestine. This patient had a malignant GIST.

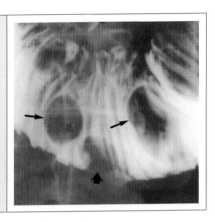

Figure 14-22. Metastatic melanoma to small intestine. Spot radiograph of the mid small bowel obtained during the single-contrast phase of enteroclysis shows at least five, smooth-surfaced, round/ovoid radiolucent filling defects *(arrows)* in the barium column. These findings are typical of submucosal masses. The most common cause of multiple submucosal masses in the small bowel is metastatic melanoma. Disseminated lymphoma, other hematogenous metastases, or Kaposi's sarcoma may have a similar appearance.

36. **A young man complains of increasing abdominal distention and subacute right lower quadrant pain. Two images from a CT scan are presented (Fig. 14-23). Although a specific diagnosis is not possible, describe what is happening.**
CT is an excellent first examination in patients with vomiting and abdominal distention and a suspected clinical diagnosis of small bowel obstruction. CT is a rapidly performed procedure in comparison with a small bowel follow-through in a patient with an obstruction. The radiologist looks for a transition zone between dilated, fluid-filled bowel and collapsed bowel. CT can detect strictures related to Crohn's disease, primary or metastatic tumors, internal or external hernias, and polypoid tumors causing

Figure 14-23. (A) An axial image at the level of the iliac crests shows moderately dilated loops of ileum. Some ileal loops are completely filled with fluid *(I)* and will not be visible on a plain film; other loops *(L)* have a small amount of intraluminal gas. A collapsed loop of ileum has a mildly thickened wall *(arrow)*. A portion of the small bowel mesentery is hazy *(open arrow)* due to inflammatory stranding of the mesenteric fat. The cecum *(c)* is identified. (B) Axial image caudal to (A) reveals a markedly thick-walled distal small bowel *(thick arrows)*. The mucosal surface *(thin arrow)* is enhancing more than skeletal muscle. The submucosa is of low attenuation. This is a mural stratification pattern (see Chapter 19). A diagnosis of partial small bowel obstruction can be made, manifested as disproportionate dilatation of proximal small bowel, but a specific diagnosis of the cause of bowel wall thickening cannot be made. The cause of the obstruction was demonstrated on small bowel follow-through examination to be Crohn's disease.

intussusception. Unfortunately, CT cannot directly demonstrate adhesions, the most common cause of small bowel obstruction in patients who previously have undergone surgery. CT diagnosis of adhesion is a diagnosis of exclusion; if an abnormality is not seen at the transition zone, a diagnosis of adhesion is made.

37. **A young man complains of experiencing diarrhea for 4 weeks. Figure 14-24 is a spot image of the terminal ileum from a small bowel follow-through. What is your diagnosis?**
For the answer, see the figure legend.

Figure 14-24. Note the long, thin barium collection *(thin white arrows)* on the mesenteric border of the terminal ileum. The collection is paralleled by a radiolucent mound of edema *(black arrows)*. These are the radiographic findings of a mesenteric border ulcer, a radiographic finding that is almost pathognomonic of Crohn's disease. Also present are thick, slightly nodular folds in the terminal ileum *(n)* and a mild stricture of the ileocecal valve *(thick white arrow)*. (Reproduced with permission. From Rubesin SE, Bronner M: Radiologic-pathologic concepts in Crohn's disease. Gastrointest Radiol 1:27–55, 1991, Fig. 4.)

38. **A patient with known Crohn's disease comes to the emergency department with abdominal pain. What is the first radiologic test that should be performed?**
A CT scan will demonstrate an unsuspected complication in about 25% of symptomatic patients with Crohn's disease. Figure 14-25 is such an example.

39. **A middle-aged woman has peripheral lymphadenopathy and heme-positive stool. An image of the terminal ileum and ileocecal valve from the single-contrast phase of a small bowel enema is presented (Fig. 14-26). What are the diagnostic possibilities?**
For the answer, see the figure legend.

40. **A middle-aged woman has foul-smelling yellow stools. A spot image of the proximal jejunum obtained during enteroclysis is presented (Fig. 14-27). The *double arrows* represent 1 inch. What is your diagnosis?**
Diseases that cause malabsorption usually involve the mucosa, submucosa, and lymphatics and mesenteric lymph nodes. Enteroclysis is superior to small bowel follow-through in the work-up of malabsorption because enteroclysis demonstrates the mucosal surface and valvulae conniventes better than a small bowel follow-through.

Figure 14-25. (A) Axial image through the pelvis shows varying degrees of wall thickening in this patient with known Crohn's disease. The thickness of the wall of the terminal ileum varies from normal *(short white arrow)* to mildly thickened *(long white arrow)* to markedly thickened *(long black arrow)*. The wall of the cecum *(C)* is mildly thickened and has a mural stratification pattern. The omental fat *(open arrow)* anterior to the ileum has numerous linear soft tissue strands (the so-called "dirty fat"). (B) An axial image more cephalad in the pelvis shows an unsuspected abscess *(large white arrows)*. There is a 5-cm inhomogeneous mass in the right lower quadrant that has areas of soft tissue, fluid *(black arrow)*, and air attenuation. The surrounding fat has soft tissue stranding. There also is local lymphadenopathy *(small white arrow)*. These images are an example of CT's ability to demonstrate serious complications in patients with known Crohn's disease. (Reproduced with permission. From Rubesin SE, Bartram CI, Laufer I: Inflammatory bowel disease. In Levine MS, Rubesin SE, Laufer I [eds]: Double Contrast Gastrointestinal Radiology, 3rd ed. Philadelphia, W.B. Saunders, 2000, pp 417–470, Fig. 13-47.)

Figure 14-26. The folds of the terminal ileum *(T)*, ileocecal valve *(I)*, medial wall of the cecum *(open arrow)*, and proximal ascending colon *(arrow)* are markedly thickened and slightly lobulated but smooth-surfaced. There are no pathognomonic findings of Crohn's disease (aphthoid ulcers, mesenteric border ulcers, cobblestoning, fissures, fistulas). The folds are much larger than would be seen in Crohn's disease. The two most likely possibilities are lymphoma or carcinoma of the ileocecal valve invading the terminal ileum. This proved to be mantle cell lymphoma of the ileocecal region.

41. **A 35-year-old woman has right lower quadrant pain and diarrhea. The results of the CT scan were normal. A spot radiograph of the distal ileum from a small bowel follow-through is presented (Fig. 14-28). What is your diagnosis?**
Even though CT is excellent at demonstrating disease outside of the small bowel and markedly thickened bowel wall, this imaging modality cannot demonstrate the mucosal surface or subtle wall abnormalities, nor can it be used to make specific diagnoses in most cases.

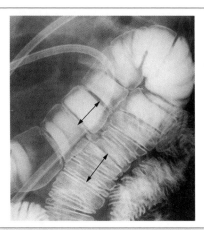

Figure 14-27. There are a diminished number of valvulae conniventes per inch in the more superior loop of the jejunum than in the inferior loop. Only two folds per inch are seen superiorly, whereas about five to six folds per inch are seen inferiorly. Loss of valvulae conniventes indicates that there is a loss of mucosal surface area. These radiographic findings are the macroscopic correlate of villous atrophy seen in gluten-sensitive enteropathy (celiac disease, nontropical sprue). Celiac disease is underdiagnosed in adult patients. Currently, antibodies are found in 95% of patients with gluten-sensitive enteropathy and in about 1 in 200 adults. The role of enteroclysis in symptomatic patients with celiac disease is to exclude development of a complication such as ulcerative jejunoileitis or adenocarcinoma or lymphoma of the small intestine.

Figure 14-28. Note the innumerable uniformly round, radiolucent filling defects (1–2 mm in size) *(arrows)* in the barium column of the distal-most three loops of ileum. Normal smooth mucosa separates these nodules. These findings are characteristic of extensive lymphoid hyperplasia. The causes of extensive lymphoid hyperplasia in the ileum include recent enteric infection and immunodeficiency states such as common variable immunodeficiency and immunoglobulin A deficiency. After the barium study, a diagnosis of common variable immunodeficiency was made.

BIBLIOGRAPHY

1. Gore RM, Levine MS (eds): Textbook of Gastrointestinal Radiology, 2nd ed. Philadelphia, W.B. Saunders, 2000.
2. Herlinger H, Maglinte DDT, Birnbaum BA (eds): Clinical Radiology of the Small Intestine. New York, Springer-Verlag, 1999.

3. Lee JKT, Sagel SS, Stanley RJ, Heiken JP: Computed Body Tomography with MRI Correlation, 3rd ed. Philadelphia, Lippincott-Raven, 1998.

4. Levine MS, Rubesin SE, Laufer I (eds): Double Contrast Gastrointestinal Radiology, 3rd ed. Philadelphia, W.B. Saunders, 2000.

5. Meyers MA: Dynamic Radiology of the Abdomen, 5th ed. New York, Springer, 2000.

CHAPTER 15

THE COLON AND BARIUM ENEMA

Stephen E. Rubesin, MD

ANATOMY

1. **Identify the parts of the colon, numbers 1 through 8, in Figure 15-1. What structures are identified by the *open* and *white arrows*?**
   See the figure legend for answers.

2. **What are haustra?**
   The longitudinal muscle layer of the colon is divided into three thick bands, termed the *teniae coli.* There is a paucity of longitudinal muscle between the three tenial bands. Haustra are sacculations of colon protruding between the three rows of teniae coli (Figs. 15-2 and 15-3). At the edges of the haustral sacculations, folds, termed *interhaustral folds,* radiate toward the teniae coli. Thus, the colon is identified by its haustral sacculations and interhaustral folds on any radiologic study, whether plain radiograph, computed tomography (CT), magnetic resonance imaging (MRI), or barium enema. Rounded, air-filled pockets are seen in a nondependent (anterior) position. Fluid- or contrast-filled rounded sacculations are seen on the dependent (inferior) surface.

   Haustra are relatively fixed structures in the right and transverse colon. Haustra are intermittently seen structures in the descend-

Figure 15-1. Overhead radiograph from double-contrast barium enema demonstrates the following portions of the colon: 1 = cecum, 2 = ascending colon, 3 = hepatic flexure, 4 = mid-transverse colon, 5 = splenic flexure, 6 = descending colon, 7 = sigmoid colon, and 8 = rectum. The terminal ileum *(white arrows)* and the appendix *(open arrow)* are identified.

ing and proximal sigmoid colon, depending on the stage of colonic contraction. The left colon may intermittently appear "ahaustral," depending on the degree of colonic contraction.

Whereas the edge of the colon has a sacculated appearance, the edge of the small bowel is relatively straight, only altered by its thin valvulae conniventes. Valvulae conniventes are thinner than interhaustral folds and cross the entire lumen of the bowel, whereas interhaustral folds cross about one third of the colonic diameter when see in profile. Seen en face, the interhaustral folds may falsely appear to cross the entire lumen of the colon.

Figure 15-2. Haustra on CT. Axial image through the lower abdomen demonstrates the three rows of haustral sacculations *(arrows)* in the ascending colon. The feces (f) in the ascending colon have a mottled appearance of air *(black);* soft tissue appears *gray,* and the contrast appears *white.* Feces are not seen in the mid small intestinal loops.

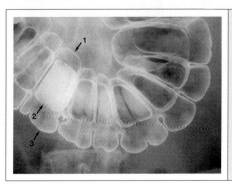

Figure 15-3. Spot radiograph of the transverse colon from a double-contrast barium enema shows three rows of haustral sacculations (edges of three haustra are identified by *black arrows*). The more dependent haustral row is partially filled with barium.

TECHNIQUE

3. **Figure 15-4 is from what type of examination?**
   A double-contrast (or air-contrast) barium enema uses two contrast agents to image the colon. A medium-density, medium-viscosity barium suspension is instilled into the colon via a rectal tube. This barium scrubs residual feces and fluid into the suspension, then coats the mucosal surface with barium. Air (or carbon dioxide) is then insufflated via the rectal tube to distend the colon and render it "translucent." The end result is that the mucosal surface is "etched" in white by barium and the colonic walls are widely separated. Spot radiographs and overhead images are then obtained.

   A colonic hypotonic agent (1 mg of glucagon IV) is routinely administered at our hospital, for example. Other hospitals only use glucagon if there is colonic spasm, excessive patient discomfort, or inability to retain the contrast. In other countries, an anticholinergic agent (e.g., hyoscine-*N*-butylbromide [Buscopan]) may be used to induce colonic hypotonia.

4. **In what position is the patient lying tabletop of the fluoroscope in Figure 15-1?**
   Air-barium levels are the clue to the patient's position. Barium is heavier than air; therefore, barium identifies the "down" side of the patient. The air-barium levels show that the patient is lying with his or her left side down. The x-ray tube is positioned in a "cross-table lateral position," so the x-ray beam parallels the tabletop. Thus, this image is termed a *left side down decubitus view.*

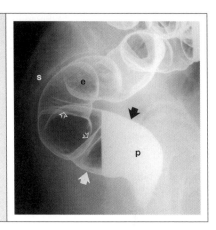

Figure 15-4. Spot radiograph of the rectum from a double-contrast barium enema study. The patient lies in a prone position and the x-ray beam is "shot" across the patient, termed a "cross-table" image. The mucosal detail is seen en face in air contrast (e) but obscured by the barium pool (p). The radiologist looks at the contour of the colon both in the barium pool *(black arrow)* and in the air *(white arrow)*. Two of the valves of Houston are identified *(open arrows)*. The proximal and mid rectum parallel the sacrum (s).

5. **What type of patient is capable of undergoing a double-contrast barium enema?**
A patient has to be able to hold the barium and air in his or her colon; therefore, anal sphincter tone must be normal. The patient must be able to roll around the tabletop of the fluoroscope; therefore, he or she must be strong enough to roll over in bed. The radiologist must be able to communicate with the patient. If the patient does not speak the same language as the radiologist, a translator must be provided. The patient must have enough mental acuity to be able to understand and respond to the following commands: "Don't breathe/breathe," "Turn left/turn right," and "Hold the barium in your rectum."

6. **Figure 15-5 is an image from what type of examination?**
This is a spot radiograph from a single-contrast barium enema. This type of examination uses one contrast agent: low-density barium. Under fluoroscopic control, the colon is filled with barium. Spot radiographs and overhead images of the entire colon are obtained. Postevacuation spot radiographs or overhead images are also obtained.

Figure 15-5. Spot radiograph of the ascending colon from a single-contrast barium enema. The radiologist evaluates the contour and the barium column. In this patient, the luminal contour has normal sacculations, but there is a 1.5-lobulated radiolucent filling defect *(thick arrow)* connected to a smooth tubular filling defect *(thin arrow)*. This is the typical appearance of a pedunculated polyp in a single-contrast examination. Barium in the interstices of the lesion indicates its villous or tubulovillous nature. The polyp proved to be a tubulovillous adenoma. (Reproduced with permission from Rubesin SE, Stuzin N, Laufer I: Tumors of the colon. Semin Colon Rect Surg 4:94–111, 1993, Fig. 6, *B*.)

7. **What are the indications for a double-contrast barium enema?**

   Any time colonic disease is suspected and a patient has no contraindications for barium enema, this examination can be performed. Indications for double-contrast barium enema include rectal bleeding, diarrhea, abdominal pain, screening for colorectal neoplasia, or involvement of the colon by extracolonic inflammatory or neoplastic masses.

8. **What are the indications for a single-contrast barium enema?**

   A single-contrast barium enema may be performed in patients with suspected fistula, high-grade colonic obstruction, or Hirschsprung's disease. If a distal small bowel obstruction is suspected, a single-contrast barium enema with reflux of barium into the distal ileum to the point of obstruction may be performed as a complementary study to CT.

9. **What is your hospital's preparation for a barium enema?**

   Each hospital has its own preparation for a barium enema that should be available from the Department of Radiology. Preparations generally include (1) a period during which solid food is limited in an effort to reduce undigested material reaching the colon, (2) an oral laxative, and (3) a medication that induces colonic contraction.

   The preparation at the Hospital of the University of Pennsylvania, for example, includes:
   - Clear liquids only the day before the examination.
   - 10–16 oz of magnesium citrate at 5 PM the day before the examination.
   - At least three to four 8-oz glasses of water throughout the day of the examination.
   - Four 5-mg bisacodyl tablets taken with 8 oz of water the evening before the examination.
   - Nothing by mouth after midnight until after the examination.
   - A bisacodyl suppository the morning of the examination.
   - Reduction or elimination of insulin the morning of the examination.
   - After the examination, patients are encouraged to drink water and take laxatives if they have colonic hypomotility.

   At our hospital, for example, we do not use large-volume colonic lavage agents that are used for colonoscopy because they leave large amounts of fluid in the colon that degrade barium coating of the mucosa.

10. **What patients may require more than the standard barium enema preparation?**

    A 2-day preparation may be necessary in immobile or bedridden patients, patients with hypomotility disorders such as diabetes or hypothyroidism, postoperative patients, or patients taking opiates or drugs with anticholinergic side effects.

11. **What are the contraindications for a barium enema?**
    - Known or suspected colonic perforation. If a perforation is suspected, CT or an enema using a water-soluble contrast material should be used.
    - Fulminant colitis ("toxic megacolon") or any severe colitis (*see* Fig. 13-1).
    - A recent procedure that has potentially created a hole in the colonic mucosa. A barium enema should be postponed for 1 week if a large forceps biopsy at rigid sigmoidoscopy, a snare polypectomy, or hot biopsy has been performed. A biopsy taken with small forceps via a flexible endoscope is not a contraindication.
    - The clinician should alert the radiologist if a patient has a latex allergy, so all products containing latex can be removed from the fluoroscopic suite and the room can be cleaned before a procedure.

12. **What are the contraindications for the use of IV glucagon?**

    Patients with known or suspected insulinoma or pheochromocytoma should not receive IV glucagon.

13. **What patients should be scheduled early in the day?**
    - Patients with latex allergy should be scheduled first in the day, after the room has been cleaned.
    - Insulin-dependent diabetic patients, patients with hypoglycemia, or other patients who require breakfast should be scheduled as early in the day as possible.

14. **What are the complications of a barium enema?**
    - The examination may fail to image the entire colon if the patient has colonic spasm or poor sphincter tone and is unable to retain barium or air.
    - Distention of the colon may cause the patient to complain of cramps but rarely produces syncope.
    - Colonic perforation occurs in about 1 in 40,000 examinations. Perforation is usually retroperitoneal and related to distention of a rectal balloon. If a free intraperitoneal perforation occurs, it is usally in a patient who has severe colitis or ischemia. In contrast to the rarity of barium enema perforation, perforation occurs in about 1 in 1000 colonoscopies.
    - Rarely, barium impaction occurs in patients who have colonic hypomotility, such as bedridden patients, patients taking narcotics or other drugs that cause hypomotility, and diabetic patients. Barium impaction can be prevented, in part, by having patients take oral laxatives after the procedure.
    - Allergic reactions to the barium, glucagon, or colonic preparation are rare but have been reported. Although allergic reactions to latex in barium enema balloons have previously occurred, the manufacturers have removed latex from balloon tips.
    - Rarely, patients develop myocardial ischemia during barium enema.

15. **Is there a need for antibiotic prophylaxis before administration of a barium enema?**
    There is conflicting evidence regarding bacteremia during barium enema. Routine antibiotic prophylaxis is probably not necessary, except in patients with susceptible cardiac lesions who have a history of endocarditis or a prosthetic valve.

16. **What patients need a preparation for a CT scan?**
    Patients undergoing abdominal CT on an emergent basis do not have time to undergo an overnight preparation. Oral contrast is administered about 1 hour before CT in most patients. An effervescent agent (gas), water, or another fluid attenuation oral agent (e.g., methylcellulose) is administered to patients in whom the biliary tree or the head of the pancreas is the target region. In the future, if it is possible for patients with acute gastrointestinal bleeding to be studied with a CT angiography, high-attenuation oral contrast will not be administered so that hypervascular lesions of the bowel can be more easily detected.

    Most hospitals do not require colonic and distal small bowel cleansing before nonemergent CT scans. However, some nonemergent patients may benefit from colonic cleansing before CT, including patients with weight loss, lower gastrointestinal bleeding, chronic abdominal pain, diarrhea, or abdominal distention.

17. **What is the most important radiographic predictor of malignancy arising in a polyp?**
    Size; the larger the polyp, the greater the chance of malignancy. The amount of villous change is a much less important factor. About 1% of tubular adenomas smaller than 1 cm are malignant (Fig. 15-6); 10% of tubular adenomas 1–2 cm are malignant, and 35% of tubular adenomas larger than 2 cm are malignant. About 10% of villous adenomas smaller than 2 cm are malignant, and about 50% of villous adenomas larger than 2 cm are malignant. The presence of a pedicle longer than 1 cm means that a pedunculated polyp has a greater than 95% chance of benign behavior, regardless of the histology in the head of the polyp.

Figure 15-6. Spot radiograph of the splenic flexure demonstrates two polyps. The small polyp resembles a "hat." The "top of the hat" *(open arrow)* is the top of the polyp. The "brim of the hat" *(thin black arrow)* is barium trapped between the mucosa and the polyp as it is retracted by its stalk. This was a tubular adenoma. The second polyp has a more worrisome morphology, that of an umbilicated, sessile polyp. A small barium collection *(thick black arrow)* fills a central umbilication or ulceration. The edge of the polyp is coated by barium (or "etched in white") *(white arrow).* This polyp was a tubulovillous adenoma.

18. **What does fine lobulation of the surface of a polyp mean?**
    Barium enters the interstices between fronds of a polyp *(see* Fig. 15-5), and the greater the number of lobules, the greater the amount of villous change in a polyp. A polyp with more than several lobules is in the spectrum of tubulovillous to villous adenoma (Fig. 15-7) and therefore has a slightly greater risk of malignancy.

Figure 15-7. Adenocarcinoma arising in a villous adenoma of the ascending colon. Spot radiograph from a double-contrast barium enema shows a 4-cm area of polygonal nodules with barium filling the interstices between tumor lobules. The flat nature of the tumor is evident in profile where the luminal contour is neither pushed in nor excavated out *(small arrows).* Adenocarcinoma is present where the lesion disrupts the luminal contour *(large arrows).* This flat lesion has been termed a "carpet lesion" by some authors. (Reproduced with permission from Rubesin SE, Laufer I: Pictorial glossary. In Gore RM, Levine MS [eds]: Textbook of Gastrointestinal Radiology, 2nd ed. Philadelphia, W.B. Saunders, 2000, pp 44–65, Fig. 5-20.)

19. **What percentage of colonic cancers is out of reach of the flexible sigmoidoscope?**
    Over the past four decades, the distribution of colon cancers has shifted toward the right colon (Fig. 15-8). About 40–50% of colonic cancers are out of reach of the flexible sigmoidoscope. This is why screening for colonic carcinoma requires a total colonic examination, either by colonoscopy or double-contrast barium enema.

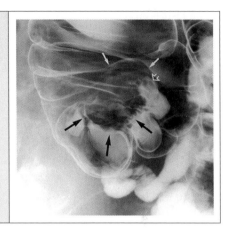

Figure 15-8. Polypoid carcinoma of the inferior lip of the ileocecal valve invading the terminal ileum. Spot radiograph of the cecum from a double-contrast barium enema shows a 3-cm finely lobulated mass *(black arrows)* expanding the contour of the inferior lip of the ileocecal valve. The normal-sized and smooth superior lip of the ileocecal valve is labeled *(white arrows)* for comparison. The lumen of the ileocecal valve *(open white arrow)* is nodular, indicating tumor spread into the ileum.

20. **Which of the following morphologic shapes is the most common form of symptomatic colonic carcinoma: polypoid, carpet, plaquelike, or annular?**
    About 50% of advanced cancers in symptomatic patients are annular cancers. When an annular cancer is seen radiographically (Fig. 15-9), there is a 98% chance of serosal invasion, a 50% chance of lymph node metastasis, and about a 15% chance of liver metastasis.
    Polypoid cancers are most commonly found in the rectum or cecum. Polypoid cancers have a better prognosis: 55% of patients have serosal invasion and 25% have lymph node metastasis.

Figure 15-9. Annular adenocarcinoma of the rectum. Spot radiograph from the single-contrast phase of a double-contrast barium enema shows a 5-cm-long, circumferential narrowing of the proximal rectum. The lesion has abrupt "shelflike" margins *(large black and white arrows)* and an irregular surface *(open arrows)*. This has been called an "apple core" lesion, but this is a misnomer because the tumor represents the part of the apple that has been eaten away, and the lumen would be the "apple core."

21. **What is the most common cause of colonic intussusception in adults?**
    Colonic cancers are the most common cause of colonic intussusception in adults. Less likely causes include adenomas and lipomas.

22. **Hyperplastic polyps are found most commonly in what part of the colon?**
    Hyperplastic polyps are small (< 5 mm), smooth, surface polyps most commonly found in the rectum on the crest of folds. Unlike adenomatous polyps, hyperplastic polyps are not premalignant.

23. **Figure 15-10 is an image from a CT scan through the mid abdomen. What is your diagnosis?**
   The diagnosis is lipoma (*see* Fig. 15-10 legend for discussion). Lipomas are most commonly found in the right colon as a sessile or broadly pedunculated smooth-surfaced mass (Fig. 15-11). On CT, the mass is shown to be composed of fat. These tumors change size and shape with palpation and varying degrees of colonic distention.

Figure 15-10. Axial CT through the mid abdomen shows a 4-cm polypoid mass in the right colon. Four lobules of fat attenuation *(open arrows)* are found in the contrast-filled lumen of the ascending colon. This is a lipoma. (Compare the CT attenuation of the lipoma with the retroperitoneal fat [r].) Increased attenuation of the greater omentum *(white arrows)* was due to nearby diverticulitis. The lipoma was an incidental finding. The mesenteric fat adjacent to the ascending colon shows stranding due to adjacent right-sided diverticulitis. (Reproduced with permission from Rubesin SE, Laufer I: Tumors of the colon. In Levine MS, Rubesin SE, Laufer I [eds]: Double Contrast Gastrointestinal Radiology, 3rd ed. Philadelphia, W.B. Saunders, 2000, pp 357–416, Fig. 12-62.)

Figure 15-11. Spot radiograph of the cecum from a double-contrast barium enema shows a smooth-surfaced 2-cm polypoid lesion *(white arrow)* arising from the superior lip of the ileocecal valve. This is the typical smooth appearance of a colonic lipoma on barium enema. The appendix is identified *(black arrow)*.

24. **What tumors commonly spread to the intraperitoneal space?**
   Cancers of the ovary are the most common type of tumor that spread to the peritoneal space in women. In both sexes, cancers of the colon, pancreas, and stomach are the primary tumors that most frequently spread to the intraperitoneal space. Hepatocellular carcinomas spread to the peritoneal space, but they are less common in the United States compared with Asia or Africa.

25. **What is the most common finding of intraperitoneal metastasis on CT?**
   Ascites is seen in about 70% of patients with intraperitoneal metastasis on CT (Fig. 15-12). The intraperitoneal implants are seen less commonly. Implants are more easily detected on the peritoneal surfaces of the diaphragm, liver, and omentum than in bowel. Barium enemas are helpful in determining the extent of colonic involvement and where to perform a colostomy in a patient with intraperitoneal implants.

Figure 15-12. CT demonstrating adenocarcinoma of the splenic flexure with intraperitoneal metastasis. A 4-cm soft tissue mass *(thick arrow)* focally obliterates the lumen of the splenic flexure. Local lymphadenopathy is present *(thin black arrow)*. Ascites *(black "a")* surrounds the tip of the right lobe of the liver (l). Ascites is also present in the left paracolic gutter *(white "a").* A soft tissue mass *(open arrows)* infiltrates the greater omentum, representing omental metastasis, the so-called omental "cake."

26. **What are the differences in distribution between ulcerative colitis and Crohn's disease?**
Ulcerative colitis (Table 15-1) is left-sided colonic disease, beginning at the anorectal junction and extending continuously and retrogradely a variable distance (proctosigmoiditis, left-sided colitis, pancolitis) (Fig. 15-13). Ulcerative colitis symmetrically involves a bowel segment (Fig. 15-14).

    Crohn's disease involves the colon and terminal ileum in 55% of patients. Terminal ileal involvement alone is seen in 14% of patients. Terminal ileal and distal small bowel involvement alone is seen in 13% of patients. Pure colonic involvement is seen in about 15% of patients. Crohn's disease is discontinuous, having patchy involvement both locally and between loops, called "skip areas." Crohn's disease is asymmetric, first involving the mesenteric side of bowel.

TABLE 15-1. COMPARISON OF CROHN'S DISEASE AND ULCERATIVE COLITIS

Crohn's Disease	Ulcerative Colitis
Right-sided	From rectum, extends proximally
Discontinuous	Continuous
Asymmetric	Symmetric
Terminal ileal changes in 85% of patients	Backwash ileitis in 10% of patients
Aphthoid ulcers	Mucosal granularity
Ulcers on background normal mucosa	Ulcers on background mucosal granularity
Severe perianal disease	Colon cancer in larger percentage of patients
Sinus tracks and fistulae	Sclerosing cholangitis in larger percentage of patients
Abscess	

27. **Aphthoid ulcers are characteristic of which chronic inflammatory bowel disease?**
Crohn's disease (Fig. 15-15). They are also seen in patients with acute diarrheal states such as yersiniosis, amebiasis, and viral (cytomegalovirus/herpes) infection. An aphthoid ulcer results from breakdown of the mucosa above an inflamed lymph aggregate in the lamina propria or submucosa.

Figure 15-13. Ulcerative colitis. Overhead radiograph from double-contrast barium enema shows that the transverse, descending, and sigmoid colon and rectum have a tubular configuration. The colon is narrowed and the haustral sacculations have disappeared. The rectum is narrowed and the valves of Houston are gone. In this patient the ascending colon appears normal. (Reproduced with permission from Rubesin SE, Bartram CI, Laufer I: Inflammatory bowel disease. In Levine MS, Rubesin SE, Laufer I [eds]: Double Contrast Gastrointestinal Radiology, 3rd ed. Philadelphia, W.B. Saunders, 2000, pp 417–470, Fig. 13-10, *A*.)

Figure 15-14. Ulcerative colitis on CT. Axial image through the pelvis shows that the rectum is narrow and has a "target sign." The mucosa enhances with IV contrast *(arrow "m");* the submucosa is low attenuation *(arrow "s");* and the muscularis propria is soft tissue attenuation *(arrow "p")*. The urinary bladder (u) and seminal vesicles (s) are identified.

Figure 15-15. Aphthoid ulcers in Crohn's disease of colon. Spot radiograph of the splenic flexure from a double-contrast barium enema shows numerous 2–3-mm punctate and stellate barium collections surrounded by radiolucent halos. Several aphthoid ulcers are identified in profile *(white arrows)* and en face *(black arrows)*. Note that a large portion of the mucosa is smooth and normal. (Reproduced with permission from Rubesin SE, Bartram CI, Laufer I: Inflammatory bowel disease. In Levine MS, Rubesin SE, Laufer I [eds]: Double Contrast Gastrointestinal Radiology, 3rd ed. Philadelphia, W.B. Saunders, 2000, pp 417–470, Fig. 13-30.)

The other characteristic findings in Crohn's disease include mesenteric border ulcers and criss-crossing knifelike clefts resulting in cobblestoning (*see* Table 15-1). Pathologically, granulomas are detected in 25–70% of patients.

The characteristic radiographic findings in ulcerative colitis are granular mucosa (Fig. 15-16), ulcers on a background of inflammatory granularity, shortening of the colon, and loss of haustration.

Figure 15-16. Ulcerative colitis. Spot radiograph of the splenic flexure from a double-contrast barium enema shows innumerable diminutive radiolucencies surrounded by linear and punctate barium collections. This very fine mucosal nodularity has been described as "granular mucosa." Note that it involves the entire surface of the bowel. The colon is tubular in shape without haustration. (Reproduced with permission from Rubesin SE, Bartram CI, Laufer I: Inflammatory bowel disease. In Levine MS, Rubesin SE, Laufer I [eds]: Double Contrast Gastrointestinal Radiology, 3rd ed. Philadelphia, W.B. Saunders, 2000, pp 417–470, Fig. 13-1, *B*.)

28. **What is the first radiographic study that should be performed in symptomatic patients with Crohn's disease?**
    CT, primarily to exclude an intra-abdominal abscess and to demonstrate the cause of "separated bowel loops," whether abscess, inflammation, or "fibrofatty proliferation." Note that fat does not creep or proliferate, so "fibrofatty proliferation" is a misnomer. Prominent fat may be related to retraction of fat due to inflammation spreading along lymphatic and venous channels.

29. **What is the most common form of colitis in an outpatient older than 50 years?**
    Ischemic colitis. The most common causes of ischemic colitis are low-flow states such as congestive heart failure, shock, or arrhythmia. Occlusion of large vessels due to atherosclerosis or embolism infrequently causes colonic ischemia because the colon is fed by large collateral arterial arcs (arc of Riolan, marginal artery of Drummond).

    Ischemia may occur in any part of the colon; however, it commonly involves the distal transverse colon and descending colon (Fig. 15-17) because these regions are the sites of transition between the blood supply from the superior mesenteric and inferior mesenteric arteries, respectively. The splenic flexure region is known as the "watershed" area of the colonic arterial supply.

30. **A woman with a history of cervical cancer now has rectal bleeding (Fig. 15-18). What is the most likely diagnosis?**
    Radiation-induced stricture (*see* Fig. 15-18 legend for discussion). Radiation acutely causes necrosis to the bowel walls. With time, blood vessels and lymphatics are obliterated, resulting in chronic ischemia with mucosal atrophy, fibrosis, and occasional stricture formation. Radiation-induced changes in the rectum, sigmoid colon, and pelvic ileum are common causes of gastrointestinal bleeding or obstruction. Radiation-induced colitis and enteritis are most commonly encountered in patients who have been irradiated for cervical or prostatic carcinoma.

Figure 15-17. Ischemic colitis in a patient with 6 days of left upper quadrant pain and bleeding. *A,* Spot radiograph of the splenic flexure from a double-contrast barium enema shows diffuse narrowing of the lumen, loss of the normal haustral pattern, and fine nodularity of the mucosa *(arrows). B,* CT axial image through the upper descending colon shows a mural stratification pattern in the splenic flexure *(top white arrow)* and descending colon *(bottom white arrow).* The low attenuation of the submucosa represents submucosal edema related to ischemia. Compare the thickness and attenuation of the wall in areas of ischemia to the wall of the normal ascending colon *(open arrow).* (*A,* reproduced with permission from Rubesin SE, Bartram CI, Laufer I: Inflammatory bowel disease. In Levine MS, Rubesin SE, Laufer I [eds]: Double Contrast Gastrointestinal Radiology, 3rd ed. Philadelphia, W.B. Saunders, 2000, pp 417–470, Fig. 13-71.)

Figure 15-18. Spot radiograph of the rectum from the single-contrast phase of a double-contrast barium enema shows a 10-cm-long, focal narrowing of the distal sigmoid colon and proximal rectum. The margins of the stricture are tapered. The contour is irregular; the mucosa is nodular *(open arrows),* and focal ulceration *(arrows)* is present. Clips present in the pelvis indicate prior surgery. In conjunction with the clinical history provided, a diagnosis of a radiation-induced stricture can be made. If no clinical history was available, a stricture due to Crohn's disease, lymphogranuloma venereum, or a rare infiltrating carcinoma could give a similar radiographic appearance.

31. **What form of colitis is sometimes detected when CT is performed to exclude an intra-abdominal abscess in hospitalized patients with fever and leukocytosis?**
    Clostridium difficile colitis (pseudomembranous colitis) may be first detected on CT in patients with atypical clinical histories and nonspecific endoscopic findings or when an abscess is to be excluded. The colonic wall has a thick, nodular contour (Fig. 15-19). Wall thickening may be of low attenuation.

Figure 15-19. Colitis related to cytotoxin produced by *C. difficile*. Axial CT image through the upper pelvis in a febrile, postoperative patient reveals thickening of the walls *(white arrow)* and interhaustral folds *(black arrows)* of the descending and tortuous sigmoid colon.

32. **Neutropenic colitis (typhlitis) most commonly involves what part of the colon?**
    CT may demonstrate typhlitis in the cecum and ascending colon or distal small intestine in neutropenic patients, in particular those with right lower quadrant pain and diarrhea. Wall thickening, pericolic fat stranding/fluid, and focal perforation may be detected in neutropenic patients with leukemia, lymphoma, AIDS, organ transplants, or aplastic anemia.

33. **What are colonic diverticula?**
    Colonic diverticula are protrusions of mucosa and submucosa through areas of colonic wall weakness (Fig. 15-20), primarily where the end arteries perforate the colonic wall (on the mesenteric side of the antimesenteric teniae). The diverticula protrude into the pericolic fat, separated from the pericolonic fat by a thin layer of longitudinal muscle. "Diverticulum" is the singular form; "diverticula" is the plural form. "Diverticuli" and "diverticulae" are incorrect plural forms.

Figure 15-20. Diverticulosis of the colon. Coned-down image of the splenic flexure from a left side down decubitus overhead from a double-contrast barium enema reveals numerous diverticula. Some barium-filled diverticula are seen in profile *(thick black arrow)*. Most diverticula seen en face have a small pool of barium on their dependent surface resembling a meniscus *(thin black arrow)*. Other diverticula are devoid of a barium meniscus and are only depicted as barium-etched ring shadows *(open arrow)*. Note that the normal haustral sacculations and interhaustral folds are preserved.

34. **Describe the distribution of diverticula.**

   In patients with diverticulosis, diverticula are found in the sigmoid colon in 90% of patients, in the descending colon in 30%, throughout the colon in 16%. Isolated right-sided diverticula, although uncommon in the United States (about 4% of patients), are not uncommon in Japan. Appendiceal diverticula are found in 0.2–2% of patients.

35. **What is the primary muscle abnormality in diverticular disease?**

   The longitudinal muscle layer of the colon is primarily divided into three bands, termed the *teniae coli.* In diverticular disease, elastin deposits between normal muscle fibers in the teniae coli. Macroscopically, the teniae coli are shortened and thickened, resulting in overall shortening and straightening of the colon and redundancy of the circular muscle fibers and mucosa. The circular muscle forms thick, 180-degree bands of muscle that cross the colon. This "bunching" together of the circular muscle layer and the mucosa of the colon occurs particularly in the sigmoid colon. For lack of a better name, the longitudinal muscle abnormality has been termed circular muscle "thickening," "hypertrophy," or "bunching." The term *diverticular disease* implies circular muscle bunching (Fig. 15-21). The term *diverticulosis* implies presence of diverticula with or without circular muscle bunching.

Figure 15-21. Diverticular disease of the sigmoid colon. *A,* Spot radiograph from a single-contrast barium enema shows circular muscle thickening and diverticulosis of the sigmoid colon. The lumen has a "zigzag," "accordion-like," or "concertina-like" appearance created by thick folds of circular muscle and redundant mucosa protruding into the lumen. The diverticula *(long arrows)* are small, barium-filled, saccular protrusions outside of the expected luminal contour. Representative circular muscle folds are identified *(open arrows).* The height of one thick, circular muscle fold is identified by the *double arrow. B,* Axial CT image of a different patient with diverticular disease shows a thick, undulating wall *(open arrows)* in the sigmoid colon, the CT demonstration of circular muscle "bunching." Barium- and air-filled diverticula are present *(arrows).*

36. **An elderly patient presents with acute left lower pain. The clinical concern is diverticulitis. What examination should be performed?**

   CT of the abdomen is the first study that should be performed in most adults with acute left lower abdominal pain. An ultrasound should be the first examination to be performed, particularly in women of childbearing age, if the clinician suspects disease originating in the ovaries or uterus.

37. **One image from a CT scan in a patient with acute left lower quadrant abdominal pain is presented (Fig. 15-22). What is your diagnosis?**

   An abscess abuts the sigmoid colon, a finding suggestive of diverticulitis. CT is somewhat superior to barium enema in the diagnosis of diverticulitis. CT demonstrates the presence and size of the pericolic abscess and is superior in diagnosing other complications of diverticulitis (liver abscess, venous thrombosis, small bowel obstruction). CT is also slightly safer than contrast enema. A small percentage (<1%) of patients with diverticulitis have perforation with communication with the peritoneal space. CT is inferior to barium studies in diagnosing a perforated colon cancer as the cause of the pericolic abscess. Some patients with subacute abdominal pain will undergo barium enema. The contrast findings of diverticulitis (Fig. 15-23) are the demonstration of air or contrast outside of the expected luminal contour and the extrinsic inflammatory effect the pericolic abscess has on the colon. Both CT and contrast enema are superior to endoscopy in the diagnosis of left lower quadrant pain.

Figure 15-22. Axial CT through the pelvis reveals a 3 × 4-cm heterogeneous mass *(arrow)* adjacent to the sigmoid colon (S). Fluid attenuation and air bubbles are seen centrally in the pericolic mass. A thick rind of soft tissue is at the periphery of the pericolic mass. The findings are that of a pericolic abscess in a patient with diverticulitis. No colonic wall thickening or intrinsic colonic mass is present to suggest a perforated colonic carcinoma. A right pelvic renal transplant (K) is also present.

Figure 15-23. Diverticulitis. Spot radiograph of the sigmoid colon from a double-contrast barium enema shows several small barium-filled tracks *(open arrow)* forming a flame-shaped collection *(large arrow)* in the pericolic space. The wall of the adjacent sigmoid colon has a spiculated contour (spicule represented by *small arrow*). (Reproduced with permission from Rubesin SE, Laufer I: Diverticular disease. In Levine MS, Rubesin SE, Laufer I [eds]: Double Contrast Gastrointestinal Radiology, 3rd ed. Philadelphia, W.B. Saunders, 2000, pp 471–493, Fig. 14-24.)

38. **A young woman complains of left lower quadrant pain (Fig. 15-24). What is your diagnosis?**
Endometriosis involving the sigmoid colon. Disease in the peritoneal space falls to the rectovesical space in men and to the rectouterine space (pouch of Douglas) in women. This is most commonly seen with intraperitoneal metastases from the colon, pancreas, or stomach in men or ovarian cancer in women. Pelvic diseases can also invade the rectosigmoid colon: primary tumors from the ovary, cervix, or prostate or abscesses related to the ovaries, appendix, or colon. Barium studies and CT are superior to endoscopy in diagnosing extrinsic disease involving the colon.

39. **What are the advantages and disadvantages of virtual colonoscopy?**
Virtual colonoscopy is easier for a radiologist to perform. A technologist or nurse gives the patient IV glucagon and inserts a catheter into the rectum, insufflating air or carbon dioxide into the colon. A technologist performs the examination. The radiologist does not have to perform fluoroscopy, wear a lead gown, or take time to perform the procedure. The radiologist only reads the images. Virtual colonoscopy may be more comfortable for the patient.

Figure 15-24. Spot radiograph from a double-contrast barium enema shows spiculation of the inferior border of the sigmoid colon *(arrows)*. The colon is tethered, manifested as smooth thin folds *(open arrow),* toward the inferior contour. These are the findings of disease extrinsic to the colon. This young woman has endometriosis.

Barium enema digital spot images are about 5–10 times the resolution as CT images. A CT is of higher radiation dose. CT is the equivalent of a three-dimensional single-contrast barium enema. It is not used to study the en face mucosal detail. During a barium study, the colonic mucosa is viewed both in profile and en face. During a barium enema, the radiologist turns the patient to achieve proper luminal distention. Virtual colonoscopy is performed in the prone and supine positions and does not achieve controllable optimal distention of each loop.

Double-contrast barium enemas are relatively inexpensive. Virtual colonoscopy is more expensive than barium enema and, as of 2005, was not reimbursable from insurance companies.

40. **What is defecography?**
Defecography is an examination that records a patient defecating a thick, stool-like barium paste. This is a dynamic examination recorded on videotape or DVD recorder. Defecography is also known as "voiding proctography" and is often performed in conjunction with cystography.

41. **What types of symptoms are the indications for defecography?**
Patients complaining of incontinence, painful defecation, incomplete defecation, or constipation may benefit from defecography.

42. **What happens to a patient during defecography?**
The patient ingests a moderate volume of barium (500 mL) to opacify the small intestine. If the patient is a woman, a small amount (3–5 mL) of thick barium is instilled into the vagina to opacify the vagina. A tiny lead marker (such as a nipple marker used in chest radiography) is placed on the perineal body. Thick barium paste that mimics soft, formed stool is instilled into the rectum. The patient then sits on a commode and defecates. The radiologist takes images before, during, and after defecation. The radiologist demonstrates the relationships between the small intestine, vagina, and rectum during defecation.

43. **What abnormalities are detected during defecography that are not identified during endoscopy or barium enema?**
Defecography can demonstrate rectocele, enterocele (Fig. 15-25), abnormal anal sphincter opening, abnormal "relaxation" of the puborectalis muscle of the pelvic floor, abnormal rectal squeeze, and varying degrees of prolapse of the rectal or anal tissue either through the anal canal or vagina (Fig. 15-26).

Figure 15-25. Development of enterocele during defecation. *A,* Lateral image of the pelvis at the beginning of defecation shows barium in the small bowel (S), rectum (R), and vagina *(short black arrow).* The anal sphincter *(white arrow)* is opening normally while the patient defecates paste *(long black arrow).* *B,* Lateral image of the pelvis at the end of defecation shows residual barium static in a small rectocele (R). Several barium-filled loops of small intestine (E) have dipped deep into the pelvis between the vagina *(thin arrow)* and collapsed rectum *(thick arrow).* This is an enterocele. Enteroceles typically appear at the end of defecation or during straining after defecation.

Figure 15-26. Development of rectocele prolapsing through the vagina during defecation. *A,* Lateral image of the pelvis at the beginning of defecation shows a mild bulging of the anterior wall of the rectum (R), representing the beginning of rectocele formation. Note that the anal canal has not completely opened and the impression of the puborectalis muscle *(thick arrow)* still is present. The vagina *(thin arrows)* bulges slightly forward. An *arrowhead* identifies a metallic marker on the perineal body. *B,* Lateral image of the pelvis at the end of defecation. The puborectalis impression has normally disappeared *(thick arrow).* The anal canal (a) remains open. Both the vagina *(long arrows)* and a large rectocele (R) now prolapse out of the vaginal introitus. An *arrowhead* identifies a metallic marker on the perineal body.

KEY POINTS: BARIUM ENEMA

1. Know or have access to your institution's preparation instructions for barium enema.

2. Contraindications for barium enema include suspected perforation, fulminant colitis (toxic megacolon), recent polypectomy/deep biopsy, and latex or barium allergy.

3. A patient with latex allergy should be the first patient scheduled in the morning, after the fluoroscopic room has been cleaned; diabetic patients should be scheduled early in the day.

4. Know the difference between a double-contrast and single-contrast barium enema and what types of patients are capable of undergoing a double-contrast barium enema.

5. A CT scan is the examination of choice in patients with suspected diverticulitis.

BIBLIOGRAPHY

1. Cunnane ME, Rubesin SE, Furth EE, et al: Small flat umbilicated tumors of the colon: Radiographic and pathologic findings. Am J Roentgenol 175:747–749, 2000.

2. McCarthy PA, Rubesin SE, Levine MS, et al: Colonic cancer: Morphology detected with barium enema examination versus histopathologic stage. Radiology 197:683–687, 1995.

3. Rubesin SE, Bartram CI, Laufer I: Inflammatory bowel disease. In Levine MS, Rubesin SE, Laufer I (eds): Double Contrast Gastrointestinal Radiology, 3rd ed. Philadelphia, W.B. Saunders, 2000, pp 417–470.

4. Rubesin SE, Laufer I: Tumors of the colon. In Levine MS, Rubesin SE, Laufer I (eds): Double Contrast Gastrointestinal Radiology, 3rd ed. Philadelphia, W.B. Saunders, 2000, pp 357–416.

5. Rubesin SE, Laufer I: Diverticular disease. In Levine MS, Rubesin SE, Laufer I (eds): Double Contrast Gastrointestinal Radiology, 3rd ed. Philadelphia, W.B. Saunders, 2000, pp 471–494.

CHAPTER 16

MRI AND CT OF THE LIVER AND BILIARY TRACT

Evan S. Siegelman, MD

1. **What sequences should be obtained when performing a magnetic resonance (MR) examination of the liver?**
   A generic MR protocol would include axial T1-weighted images, axial T2-weighted images (echo time [TE] range, 80–120 ms), and heavily T2-weighted images (TE >180 ms). Contrast-enhanced images are useful for characterizing indeterminate focal liver lesions, evaluating the hepatic vasculature, and detecting potential complications of liver cirrhosis.

2. **List the MR contrast agents approved by the U.S. Food and Drug Administration (FDA).**
   There are three subtypes of FDA-approved MR contrast agents. Gadolinium chelates are the most commonly used MR contrast agent. Their pharmacokinetics are similar to those of the iodinated agents used in computed tomography (CT). However, gadolinium chelates have a lower incidence of allergic reactions, are not associated with nephrotoxicity, and require smaller injection volumes than iodinated agents.

   Two other types of MR contrast agents are available that have delayed uptake within the liver. Manganese-DPDP is incorporated into hepatocytes and is excreted into the biliary system. Enhanced liver parenchyma and bile will have high signal intensity on delayed T1-weighted images. Enhanced imaging can be used to increase detection of nonhepatocellular lesions and to perform functional MR cholangiography (Fayad et al., 2003). Superparamagnetic iron oxide is incorporated into Kupffer cells of the liver and can be used to detect and characterize focal liver lesions. One potential disadvantage of these two latter agents is that dynamic imaging cannot be performed with them.

KEY POINTS: DIFFERENTIAL DIAGNOSIS OF HEPATOCELLULAR LESIONS

1. Focal nodular hyperplasia

2. Hepatic adenoma

3. Focal steatosis or focal sparing of steatosis

4. Regenerating nodule

5. Hepatocellular carcinoma

3. **Why does the liver have high signal intensity on T1-weighted images?**
   It is hypothesized that abundant intracellular protein and/or paramagnetic substances, such as copper or zinc, result in the relatively high T1 signal intensity of liver. Most focal liver lesions are hypointense to normal liver on T1-weighted images. Thus, T1-weighted images are useful for liver lesion detection. Focal lesion characterization is usually established with the use of T2- and contrast-enhanced images.

4. **Can T1-weighted images characterize focal liver lesions as hepatocellular in origin?**
Yes. There are two ways. First, if a focal liver lesion is isointense or hyperintense to surrounding liver parenchyma, then it is likely hepatocellular in origin (Fig. 16-1, Table 16-1). Focal liver lesions that are not hepatocellular in origin are usually hypointense to liver on T1-weighted images. Second, if chemical shift imaging reveals loss of signal intensity within a liver mass, then it has been characterized as lipid-containing and in almost all cases is also hepatocellular in nature.

5. **What is the most commonly depicted benign hepatocellular lesion?**
Focal nodular hyperplasia (FNH) is the most common benign hepatocellular lesion, with a prevalence of nearly 1% of the population (Hussain et al., 2004). FNH is most often detected on CT and MR in younger asymptomatic women. FNH is not considered a neoplasm but instead is defined as a regenerative lesion composed of benign hepatocytes. The etiology of FNH is not fully understood. It is hypothesized that FNH is a reactive response of normal liver parenchyma that forms around a vascular malformation.

6. **What are the imaging findings of FNH?**
The MR findings of FNH can be divided into two regions: the periph-

Figure 16-1. MR depiction of focal nodular hyperplasia (FNH) in an asymptomatic woman. T1-weighted image (A) shows a well-circumscribed mass that has components that are isointense with surrounding liver. A central hypointense scar *(arrow)* is present. Arterial (B) and delayed phase (C) enhanced images show immediate marked enhancement of the FNH *(curved arrow)*, and the delayed image reveals lesion washout and interval enhancement of the scar *(arrow).*

eral regenerative tissue and the central scar (*see* Fig. 16-1). The peripheral portion of FNH has components that are isointense to liver on T1-weighted images in most lesions. On T2-weighted images, most FNH lesions have signal intensity in between that of liver and spleen. Thus isointensity to spleen on T2-weighted images is not diagnostic of malignancy (*see* question 17). During dynamic contrast-enhanced imaging, FNH shows marked arterial phase enhancement and variable rates of subsequent washout of contrast. The central scar of FNH shows low T1 signal intensity and high T2 signal intensity and does not enhance during the arterial phase of contrast enhancement, but does enhance variably during delayed imaging.

The enhanced CT findings of FNH are similar to those on MR. The lesion itself shows intense hyperattenuation during the arterial phase of enhancement, with variable degrees of washout on subsequent phases. The central scar remains hypoattenuating on dynamic imaging but fills in on delayed scanning. CT is less specific than MR in being able to characterize focal lesions as hepatocellular, based on relative attenuation.

KEY POINTS: DIFFERENTIAL DIAGNOSIS OF LIPID-CONTAINING LIVER LESIONS

1. Hepatic adenoma
2. Hepatocellular carcinoma (especially well-differentiated subtype)
3. Focal steatosis
4. All other conditions are uncommon

TABLE 16-1. MR APPEARANCE OF LESIONS OF HEPATOCELLULAR ORIGIN

	T1	T2 (TE = 80 ms)	T2 (TE = 180 ms)	Postcontrast	Other
Focal fat/focal fatty sparing	Iso	Iso	Iso	Iso	Regions of fatty infiltration lose signal on chemical shift imaging
Focal nodular hyperplasia	Iso	Iso	Iso	↑↑↑ in arterial phase	Homogeneous for lesion size Central scar
Adenoma	Iso to ↑	Iso to ↑	Iso	↑↑ in arterial phase	Oral contraceptive use
Regenerative nodule	Iso to ↑	Iso	Iso	Iso	Cirrhosis
Hepatocellular carcinoma	Iso to ↓	Iso to ↑	Iso	↑↑ in arterial phase	Cirrhosis

Iso = roughly isointense to liver, ↑ = increased signal relative to liver, ↓ = decreased signal relative to liver.

7. **What is the second most common benign hepatocellular mass?**
   Hepatic adenoma, which is a true neoplasm. Hepatic adenoma is most commonly found in young women, especially those who take birth control pills. The incidence of hepatic adenoma has decreased in recent decades with modifications of the estrogen and progesterone content of oral contraceptives. Hepatic adenoma is treated with surgical resection because of the risk of bleeding, especially with lesions that are >3 cm and located in the subcapsular portion of the liver.

8. **How does one distinguish between hepatic adenoma and FNH at imaging?**
   Most FNH lesions reveal a central scar, but hepatic adenomas do not. FNH enhances to a greater extent and in a more homogeneous pattern than hepatic adenoma. On MRI, hepatic adenoma

may show hyperintense components on T1-weighted images secondary to either intratumoral hemorrhage or lipid. Depicting loss of signal intensity on opposed-phase chemical shift imaging can show the presence of lipid. High signal intensity that persists on a fat-suppressed T1-weighted image represents intratumoral hemorrhage. FNH lesions do not hemorrhage and only rarely contain lipid. Hepatic adenomas are, on average, twice the size of FNHs and are more likely to be multiple.

9. **What are the two most commonly encountered benign liver lesions?**
    Hepatic cysts and hemangiomas. Both lesions have been reported to be present in up to 15–20% of the adult population (Carrim and Murchison, 2003; Vilanova et al., 2004).

KEY POINTS: MRI OF THE LIVER

1. On T2-weighted images, the signal intensity of liver metastases is similar to that of the spleen, whereas liver cysts and hemangiomas are relatively isointense to cerebrospinal fluid.

2. Most liver lesions are hypointense to liver on T1-weighted images. Lesion isointensity to liver on a T1-weighted image suggests that it is hepatocellular in origin.

3. Metastatic disease is rare in a cirrhotic liver. A focal liver lesion in a cirrhotic liver that shows arterial phase enhancement or is isointense to spleen on T2-weighted images should be considered hepatocellular carcinoma until proven otherwise.

4. Chemical shift imaging of the liver is invaluable in diagnosing hepatic steatosis and depicting the presence of lipid within some hepatocellular neoplasms.

10. **What are the CT and MR imaging features of hepatic cysts?**
    The majority of hepatic cysts are composed of simple serous fluid and therefore have the CT and MR signal intensity characteristics of simple fluid: very low signal intensity on T1-weighted images, very high signal intensity on T2-weighted images, and persistent high signal intensity on heavily T2-weighted (TE >180 ms) images. Cysts reveal fluid attenuation on CT. Cysts do not enhance after contrast on either CT or MR.

11. **How are hemangiomas differentiated from cysts on MR and CT?**
    Hemangiomas have T1 and T2 signal intensity similar to that of cysts. A simplified explanation is that as blood enters the enlarged cavernous vessels of a hemangioma, its velocity decreases such that it mimics stagnant fluid. Thus, hemangiomas and cysts can have similar appearances on T1- and T2-weighted images.
    On heavily T2-weighted images, hemangiomas remain hyperintense to liver and spleen but become slightly hypointense relative to relatively simple fluid (e.g., within hepatic cysts or cerebrospinal fluid). On dynamic enhanced CT or MR, hemangiomas show a discontinuous peripheral nodular enhancement that fills in centripetally with time (Table 16-2).

12. **Are there atypical patterns of hemangioma enhancement on CT and MR?**
    Yes. Smaller hemangiomas may appear homogenously hyperintense during the arterial phase of enhancement. This has been attributed to limitations of temporal resolution, not the spatial resolution of either CT or MR. To differentiate such a smaller hemangioma from a hypervascular malignancy, one could perform a portal or delayed phase scan.

TABLE 16–2. MR APPEARANCE OF NONHEPATOCELLULAR LESIONS

	T1	T2 (TE = 80 ms)	T2 (TE = 180 ms)	Postcontrast	Other
Cyst	↓↓	↑↑↑	↑↑↑	No enhancement	
Hemangioma	↓↓	↑↑↑	↑↑	Interrupted peripheral nodular enhancement Progressive	
Metastasis	↓↓	↑↑	↑	Continuous rim enhancement Washout	Multiplicity
Abscess	↓↓	↑↑	↑	Wall only Regional hyperemia and/or edema	Fever, chills

Iso = roughly isointense to liver, ↑ = increased signal relative to liver, ↓ = decreased signal relative to liver.

13. **What is nonalcoholic fatty liver disease (NAFLD)?**

NAFLD comprises a spectrum of disorders. The most common subtype of NAFLD is uncomplicated steatosis that affects 20–30% of adult Americans. Risk factors include obesity and diabetes.
Steatosis is defined histologically by the presence of excess lipid within hepatocytes. Patients with
steatosis are usually asymptomatic but may present with mild right upper quadrant pain or mildly
elevated transaminases.

Approximately 10% of individuals with NAFLD may progress to develop nonalcoholic steatohepatitis (NASH). NASH is a histologic diagnosis and to date has not been characterized with
noninvasive imaging. Up to one third of patients with NASH may progress to cirrhosis. NASH is
now thought to be the leading cause of cryptogenic cirrhosis.

14. **What are the imaging features of steatosis (fatty infiltration)?**

Ultrasound can suggest a diagnosis of steatosis with limited specificity and sensitivity by revealing increased liver echogenicity. Unenhanced CT or chemical shift MR can confirm the presence
of hepatic steatosis (Fig. 16-2). CT diagnosis is made when the unenhanced CT attenuation of
liver is >10 Hounsfield units less than that of the spleen. The MR diagnosis of steatosis is established by showing loss of signal intensity on an opposed-phase T1-weighted image when compared with a corresponding in-phase image.

15. **What are the imaging features of liver cirrhosis?**

Cirrhosis is defined as the presence of regenerating nodules and surrounding fibrosis. Both CT
and MR can show the presence of regenerating nodules. On MR, benign regenerative nodules
have relatively high signal intensity on T1-weighted and low signal intensity on T2-weighted
images, which is similar to normal liver. Preferential atrophy of the medial segment left lobe and
anterior segment right lobe results in an appearance that has been described as the "empty gallbladder fossa sign." Caudate lobe and lateral segment left lobe hypertrophy can also be present
in cirrhotic livers. Extrahepatic findings of cirrhosis that reflect the presence of portal hypertension include splenomegaly, varices, and ascites.

Figure 16-2. CT and MR images of hepatic steatosis. Nonenhanced CT image (A) reveals that the liver has lower attenuation than that of the spleen *(S)*. Corresponding-phase (B) and opposed-phase (C) T1-weighted gradient-echo images show normal high-signal intensity liver *(L)*, low-signal intensity spleen *(S)* in (B), and variable loss of hepatic signal intensity in (C), which is characteristic of steatosis. Subtraction image (in-phase – opposed-phase) (D) depicts voxels that have both lipid and water protons as high signal intensity. The variable signal within the liver *(L)* reflects the distribution of steatosis. Normal vertebral body marrow *(M)* contains both fatty and nonfatty elements and thus shows signal on this image.

16. **What are the imaging features of hepatocellular carcinoma (HCC)?**

Regenerative nodules obtain their blood supply from the portal vein. As regenerative nodules progress into dysplastic nodules and subsequently to HCC, the portal venous supply decreases and the hepatic arterial supply increases. Thus, a lesion that enhances during the arterial phase in a cirrhotic liver is suggestive of HCC. However, focal arterial phase enhancement is not specific for HCC. Hepatic "pseudolesions" have been reported that are depicted as small foci of arterial phase enhancement. Unlike HCC, on follow-up examinations, the foci either disappear or become smaller (Shimizu et al., 2003). These hepatic pseudolesions in the cirrhotic liver may be secondary to arterial-portal shunts and/or altered intrahepatic flow dynamics.

Other imaging features that may be indicative of HCC include lesion multifocality, tumor thrombus in adjacent branches of the portal vein, and the presence of contrast washout on the venous phase of imaging (Carlos et al., 2003). An additional MR imaging feature of HCC is lesion Isointensity to spleen on T2-weighted images (Fig. 16-3). Whereas T2 isointensity to spleen suggests metastatic disease in patients with established extrahepatic primary tumors, liver metastases to a cirrhotic liver is rare.

17. Describe the CT and MR imaging appearances of metastatic disease.

Suggestive imaging features of liver metastases include multifocality, internal heterogeneity, and ill-defined margins. History of a known primary tumor or findings of extra-hepatic metastatic disease would increase the likelihood that coexistent liver lesions are malignant. Hepatic metastases commonly show rim enhancement on both CT and MR. An insensitive but specific finding of hepatic malignancy on portal or delayed phase imaging has been termed the *peripheral washout sign.* This refers to the appearance of decreased attenuation (CT) or signal intensity (MRI) within the periphery of a lesion. Peripheral washout is hypothesized to occur because of increased tumor angiogenesis within the growing outer margins of tumors that fosters both increased entry and egress of extracellular contrast agents.

MR can characterize many liver metastases without the use of contrast. Metastatic disease appears isointense to spleen on both moderate and heavily T2-weighted images (Fig. 16-4), whereas benign cysts and hemangiomas appear hyperintense to spleen. Gadolinium enhancement can help further characterize indeterminate lesions and evaluate for extrahepatic metastatic disease.

18. What MR techniques are used to perform magnetic resonance cholangiopancreatography (MRCP)?

MRCP techniques use heavily T2-weighted sequences where bile and pancreatic juices have high signal intensity. These T2-weighted techniques do not selectively "enhance"

Figure 16-3. MR depiction of multifocal HCC in a man with hepatitis C. T2-weighted fast spin echo image (A) reveals liver lesions *(arrows)* that have components that are isointense to spleen *(S).* Arterial (B) and portal phase (C) T1-weighted images show arterial phase enhancement and subsequent washout within the hepatomas *(arrows).* Additional hepatomas are revealed in (B) and (C) *(curved arrows)* that were not well depicted in (A).

the bile. Any other fluid within the same slice or volume (e.g., cerebrospinal fluid, urine, succus entericus) will also be depicted as high signal intensity. T2-weighted MRCP techniques include thin section imaging (usually obtained in the axial or coronal planes) or single-projection coronal imaging that evaluates a 20–60-mm slab of tissue. The latter is an ideal technique to obtain a rapid overview image of the biliary system, which can reveal the presence of duct dilation or any suspect transition. The thin section images can better reveal the presence of stones.

19. **What are the advantages and disadvantages of MRCP compared with endoscopic retrograde cholangiopancreatography (ERCP)?**

Unlike ERCP, MRCP does not require sedation or bowel intubation, uses no ionizing radiation, and does not result in potential postprocedural pancreatitis. Potential advantages of ERCP include the ability to biopsy suspect lesions, remove obstructing stones, and stent biliary strictures.

Figure 16-4. MR illustration of hepatic metastases in a woman with breast cancer. T2-weighted fast spin echo image shows multiple liver lesions *(arrows)* that are isointense to spleen *(S)*. The presence of capsular retraction *(curved arrow)* along the margin of the right metastases is commonly identified in women with metastatic breast cancer who have been treated with chemotherapy. However, the presence of retraction is not predictive of therapeutic response (Fennessy et al., 2004).

BIBLIOGRAPHY

1. Carlos RC, Kim HM, Hussain HK, et al: Developing a prediction rule to assess hepatic malignancy in patients with cirrhosis. Am J Roentgenol 180:893–900, 2003.

2. Carrim ZI, Murchison JT: The prevalence of simple renal and hepatic cysts detected by spiral computed tomography. Clin Radiol 58:626–629, 2003.

3. Fayad LM, Holland GA, Bergin D, et al: Functional magnetic resonance cholangiography (fMRC) of the gallbladder and biliary tree with contrast-enhanced magnetic resonance cholangiography. J Magn Reson Imag 18:449–460, 2003.

4. Fennessy FM, Mortele KJ, Kluckert T, et al: Hepatic capsular retraction in metastatic carcinoma of the breast occurring with increase or decrease in size of subjacent metastasis. Am J Roentgenol 182:651–655, 2004.

5. Hussain SM, Terkivatan T, Zondervan PE, et al: Focal nodular hyperplasia: Findings at state-of-the-art MR imaging, US, CT, and pathologic analysis. Radiographics 24:3–17; discussion, 18–19, 2004.

6. Ito K, Mitchell DG, Siegelman ES: Cirrhosis: MR imaging features. Magn Reson Imaging Clin North Am 10:75–92, vi, 2002.

7. Neuschwander-Tetri BA, Caldwell SH: Nonalcoholic steatohepatitis: Summary of an AASLD Single Topic Conference. Hepatology 37:1202–1219, 2003.

8. Shimizu A, Ito K, Koike S, et al: Cirrhosis or chronic hepatitis: Evaluation of small (≤ 2-cm) early-enhancing hepatic lesions with serial contrast-enhanced dynamic MR imaging. Radiology 226:550–555, 2003.

9. Siegelman ES, Rosen MA: Imaging of hepatic steatosis. Semin Liver Dis 21:71–80, 2001.

10. Tchelepi H, Ralls PW, Radin R, Grant E: Sonography of diffuse liver disease. J Ultrasound Med 21:1023–1032; quiz, 1033–1024, 2002.

11. Vilanova JC, Barcelo J, Smirniotopoulos JG, et al: Hemangioma from head to toe: MR imaging with pathologic correlation. Radiographics 24:367–385, 2004.

CHAPTER 17

CT AND MRI OF THE SPLEEN

E. Scott Pretorius, MD

1. **What are the magnetic resonance (MR) signal characteristics of the normal spleen?**
   The normal spleen is slightly hypointense to the liver on T1-weighted images and slightly hyperintense to the liver on T2-weighted images.

2. **What is the difference between white pulp and red pulp?**
   The spleen is composed of two tissue types, termed the *white pulp* and the *red pulp,* that are not distinguishable on unenhanced computed tomography (CT) or MR imaging. The white pulp represents lymphatic reticuloendothelial cells and lymphoid follicles.

   The vascular red pulp is composed of two distinct circulatory systems, one with slow flow and one with rapid flow. The open circulation of the spleen contains a slow flow filtration system through which abnormal and aged red blood cells, platelets, and granulocytes are cleared from the blood stream. The closed, or direct, circulation supplies the splenic parenchyma that is exposed to more rapid blood flow.

3. **Why does the normal spleen look so bizarre in the arterial phase?**
   During the arterial phase of contrast enhancement the spleen appears as alternating, wavy bands of high and low CT attenuation or MR T1 signal intensity. This has been termed the *arciform* enhancement pattern and is due to variable rates of flow within the two compartments of the red pulp. Variation from this pattern is suggestive of diffuse splenic disease. After 1 minute, the distribution of contrast within the spleen rapidly equilibrates, and there is homogenous, intense enhancement of the entire spleen (Fig. 17-1).

Figure 17-1. Axial postcontrast T1-weighted gradient-echo images in the arterial phase (A) and in the portal venous phase (B) demonstrate normal splenic enhancement. In the arterial phase, the spleen displays alternating bands of high and low signal (or, on CT, high and low attenuation). In a more delayed phase, the spleen enhances homogenously.

4. **What is an accessory spleen?**
   An accessory spleen is a separate body of normal splenic tissue, with identical CT attenuation and/or MR signal of the normal spleen. It is seen in 10–25% of patients, usually within the splenic hilum or near the pancreatic tail.

5. **What is the differential diagnosis of splenomegaly?**
   The normal spleen is less than 13 cm in craniocaudad dimension. Splenic volume is a more accurate reflection of splenic size, and mean human adult splenic volume is approximately 215 mL. Causes of splenomegaly include cirrhosis with portal hypertension, leukemia/lymphoma, infections such as Epstein-Barr virus, thalassemia, granulomatous diseases including sarcoid, storage diseases such as Gaucher's, and myeloproliferative diseases.

6. **What is the most common cause of a small spleen?**
   Sickle cell disease resulting in splenic autoinfarction is the most common cause of a small or absent spleen.

7. **What does splenic iron deposition look like on MRI?**
   The presence of iron within the spleen results in low T1, low T2 signal relative to normal splenic tissue. Small foci of iron, termed *Gamna Gandy bodies,* result from intraparenchymal hemorrhage in cirrhotic patients with portal hypertension. Diffuse iron overload in the spleen is most commonly due to repeated transfusion. In contrast, genetic (primary) hemochromatosis, which results from a genetic abnormality that leads to excess iron absorption from the gut, classically affects the liver, pancreas, and myocardium but spares the spleen.

8. **What are causes of splenic calcifications?**
   Histoplasmosis is the most common cause in the United States. Other causes include tuberculosis, brucellosis, infarct, cyst wall calcifications, and *Pneumocystis carinii* pneumonia.

9. **What is the CT/MRI appearance of splenic segmental infarction?**
   Splenic segmental infarction is depicted on contrast-enhanced CT or MRI as a wedge-shaped, peripheral region of marked hypoenhancement or nonenhancement. Causes of splenic infarction include bland emboli, septic emboli, pancreatitis, and sickle cell disease.

10. **What abdominal organ is most commonly injured in blunt trauma to the abdomen?**
    The spleen is the most commonly injured organ in blunt abdominal trauma, followed by the liver, pancreas, and kidney. Splenic laceration can be managed conservatively in hemodynamically stable patients (Fig. 17-2).

Figure 17-2. Axial postcontrast images in a trauma patient demonstrate splenic laceration (A and B). The hypoenhancing defect *(arrow)* in the spleen has "jagged" sharp edges and is surrounded by high-attenuation hemoperitoneum. The left kidney is also lacerated.

11. **What is a splenic cleft? How can it be differentiated from a splenic laceration?**
Splenic clefts (Fig. 17-3) are congenital, smooth infoldings of the splenic surface, which, in the setting of trauma, may potentially be confused with splenic laceration. Splenic clefts have gently curving, rounded margins, whereas lacerations tend to be associated with abrupt, straight margins and with nearby focal hemorrhage or hemoperitoneum.

12. **What are some nontraumatic causes of splenic rupture?**
Patients with mononucleosis, viral hepatitis, and coagulopathies are at increased risk for splenic rupture.

Figure 17-3. In contrast to Figure 17-2, this patient displays a developmental splenic cleft *(arrow)* with smooth, rounded edges and no surrounding hemoperitoneum.

KEY POINTS: CT AND MRI OF THE SPLEEN

1. On postcontrast images, the normal spleen displays alternating bands of high and low attenuation (CT) or signal (MR) in the arterial phase. The spleen appears more homogeneous in a more delayed phase.

2. Splenic laceration can be differentiated from developmental splenic cleft. Patients with laceration will have a trauma history, display a low-attenuation defect with sharp edges, and have perisplenic hemoperitoneum.

3. Both MR and CT are less specific in the characterization of splenic lesions than they are in the characterization of liver, adrenal, or renal lesions.

13. **What is the most common CT appearance of lymphoma involving the spleen?**
The most common appearance is splenomegaly without focal lesion. If therapy would be altered by a positive result, splenic biopsy may be necessary to establish whether the spleen is affected by infiltrative lymphoma. In some lymphoma patients, one or more hypovascular splenic lesions may be seen, although in delayed postcontrast phases these lesions generally become iso-dense/isointense to the remainder of the spleen.

14. **What is the differential diagnosis of a cystic lesion within the spleen?**
Benign, posttraumatic splenic cysts are the most common focal splenic lesion in the United States. Also in the differential diagnosis are parasitic cyst (which is the most common cause worldwide), congenital epidermoid cyst, and abscess.

15. **What is the differential diagnosis of a noncystic lesion within the spleen?**
Benign lesions include hemangioma, lymphangioma, splenic hamartoma, bacterial abscesses, fungal abscesses, granuloma, lymphoma, and metastatic disease (Fig. 17-4).

16. **Can CT or MRI be used reliably to differentiate noncystic splenic lesions from one another?**
Not really. There is considerable overlap in the CT and MR imaging appearance of focal noncystic splenic lesions. History helps considerably, especially in diagnosing abscesses. In febrile

patients, commonly those with endocarditis, a focal splenic lesion with peripheral enhancement is likely to be a pyogenic abscess. Multiple, very small splenic lesions in an immunocompromised patient are likely to be fungal microabscesses, especially *Candida albicans*.

Metastatic disease to the spleen is not terribly common. Hematogenous spread is the most common route of splenic involvement, and there is virtually always more than one lesion. Approximately one third of melanoma patients will eventually develop splenic metastases. Breast carcinoma and lung carcinoma do not go to the spleen as commonly, but because they are more common tumors, they cause the largest number of splenic metastases.

17. **What is polysplenia?**
Patients with polysplenia have between 2 and 15 nodules of splenic tissue in the right or left upper quadrant. Polysplenia is found in patients with bilateral left-sidedness. Polysplenia is associated with cardiac septal defects (acyanotic), interruption of the inferior vena cava (IVC) with azygous continuation, bilateral trilobed lungs, bilateral hyparterial bronchi (the mainstem bronchus lies below the artery, as is typically seen in the left lung), a midline liver, and a hypoplastic pancreatic body and tail.

Figure 17-4. (A) Coronal T2-weighted image in a patient with colon cancer demonstrates multiple lesions *(arrows)* within the spleen. (B) After contrast administration, these lesions *(arrows)* enhance heterogeneously. These lesions were metastatic carcinoma of the colon.

18. **What is asplenia?**
Asplenia means absence of the spleen and is a feature of patients with bilateral right-sidedness. Asplenia is associated with more severe, cyanotic cardiac defects than is polysplenia. The IVC tends to be on the left side of the body, and the liver will generally be found in the midline. Bilateral bilobed lungs and bilateral eparterial bronchi (the mainstem bronchus lies above the artery, as is typically seen in the right lung) are generally present.

BIBIOGRAPHY

1. Fenchel S, Boll DT, Fleiter TR, et al: Multislice helical CT of the pancreas and spleen. Eur J Radiol 45(Suppl 1): S59–S72, 2003.

2. Novelline RA, Rhea JT, Bell T: Helical CT of abdominal trauma. Radiol Clin North Am 37(3):591–561, 1999.

3. Robertson F, Leander P, Ekberg O: Radiology of the spleen. Eur Radiol 11(1):80–95, 2001.

4. Torres GM, Terry NL, Mergo PJ, Ros PR: MR imaging of the spleen. Magn Reson Imaging Clin N Am 3(1):39–50, 1995.

CHAPTER 18

CT AND MRI OF THE PANCREAS

Wendy C. Hsu, MD, and E. Scott Pretorius, MD

1. **How does a pancreatic protocol CT differ from a routine enhanced abdominal CT study?**
   A CT scan performed with pancreatic protocol takes images of thin sections (1–4 mm) of the pancreas before IV contrast administration, during the arterial phase of contrast enhancement, and during the portal venous phase of contrast enhancement to detect and characterize focal pancreatic lesions. Immediately before the scan, the patient may be asked to drink water, which acts as a "negative" oral contrast agent (i.e., dark relative to the bowel wall and surrounding soft tissue). This distends the duodenum to help to identify it as a structure separate from the pancreatic head.
   A routine enhanced abdominal CT scan is obtained in a single postcontrast phase (the portal venous phase) of enhancement with axial section thickness of 5–8 mm. A positive oral contrast agent is used, so that segments of fluid-filled small bowel are not mistaken for peripancreatic fluid collections. A routine abdominal CT scan is usually adequate for evaluation of diffuse pancreatic disease such as pancreatitis.

2. **What is the normal morphology of the pancreas on CT and MR?**
   The pancreatic acini impart a slightly lobulated contour to the pancreas, and the pancreas is not encapsulated. In anteroposterior dimension, the pancreatic head measures 2–2.5 cm; the pancreatic body and tail measure 1–2 cm. The maximal diameter of a normal main pancreatic duct is about 3 mm in adults, not to exceed 5 mm in the elderly. The duct should taper slightly from head to tail. The main pancreatic duct of Wirsung empties into the duodenum via the major papilla of Vater (also know as the "ampulla"). In patients with pancreas divisum, the accessory duct of Santorini enters the duodenum via the minor papilla. The major papilla is located distal (caudal) to the minor papilla, along the medial aspect of the second portion of the duodenum.

3. **What blood vessels are found near the pancreas?**
   The splenic vein courses posterior to the body and tail of the pancreas. The portal vein confluence (where the splenic vein and superior mesenteric vein join to form the portal vein) lies immediately posterior and to the left of the pancreatic neck.

4. **What is the normal CT attenuation and MR signal intensity of the pancreas?**
   - **CT density:** Soft tissue density is variable. Density may decrease with aging due to fatty replacement as part of the normal aging process.
   - **MR signal intensity:** In the abdomen, the pancreas is the organ with the highest signal intensity on T1-weighted images due to its high protein content. T1-weighted images provide the most contrast between normal pancreas (high T1 signal intensity) and pancreatic disease processes (lower in T1 signal intensity). The addition of fat suppression on T1-weighted sequences eliminates signal of the peripancreatic fat and allows delineation of the contour of the pancreas.

5. **What is magnetic resonance cholangiopancreatography (MRCP)? How does it compare with endoscopic retrograde cholangiopancreatography (ERCP)?**
   MRCP (Fig. 18-1) consists of a series of heavily T2-weighted sequences that depict the pancreatobiliary ducts. Bile and secretions in the pancreatic duct are static or slow moving and appear

intrinsically very high in T2 signal. Signal from the surrounding tissues is markedly suppressed on these types of sequences. MRCP should be performed as part of a complete contrast-enhanced abdominal MRI, so that important information about the surrounding soft tissues is also provided. MRCP is noninvasive and does not require sedation. However, ERCP has therapeutic applications, can directly visualize ampullary lesions, and has better resolution for fine detail.

Figure 18-1. Normal coronal, heavily T2-weighted MRCP image. The normal-caliber pancreatic duct *(arrow)* and intrahepatic/extrahepatic bile ducts are well seen. Note that fluid in the stomach and duodenum is also apparent, which can be a limitation of this type of imaging.

6. **When is MR/MRCP of the pancreas indicated?**
   General indications for MR include (1) contraindications to contrast-enhanced CT, such as allergy to iodi-nated contrast or pregnancy, and (2) equivocal results on another imaging study. MR/MRCP is particu-larly sensitive for assessment of var-ious pancreatic disorders due to its superior soft tissue contrast, greater sensitivity for contrast enhancement, and direct multipla-nar capability. Specific indications include evaluation of ducts and peripancreatic collections in chronic pancreatitis; identification of developmental abnormalities (pancreas divisum and annu-lar pancreas); detection of small (<2 cm) adenocarcinomas, including evaluation of a prominent pancreatic head without focal lesions seen on another imaging modality; characterization of a lesion as fat-containing (e.g., lipoma); evaluation of pancreatic transplant dysfunction and vas-cular complications; determination of the internal architecture of cystic lesions; detection of islet cell tumor; and assessment of organ involvement in genetic hemochromatosis.

7. **What normal or normal variant structures may be seen in the portocaval space?**
   The uncinate process of the pancreas, the portocaval lymph node, and an accessory or replaced right hepatic artery (arising from the superior mesenteric artery).

8. **What are the roles of CT in assessment of acute pancreatitis?**
   Contrast-enhanced CT is the imaging modality of choice for evaluating complications of acute pancreatitis (Fig. 18-2). CT can detect peripancreatic inflammation, pancreatic edema, fluid collections (phlegmon, abscess, pseudocyst, hemorrhage, ascites), necrosis, splenic artery pseudoaneurysm, and splenic venous thrombosis. The presence of abscess or necrosis indi-cates need for intervention, specifically percutaneous drainage for the former and surgical debridement for the latter. A CT staging system for severity exists, but it has not been definitively shown to predict clinical outcome. (Prognosis is still best assessed using clinical staging, such as the Ranson or APACHE II criteria.)
   CT is also used to guide percutaneous drainage procedures and to monitor evolution or resolution of the disease.
   Diagnosis of acute pancreatitis remains a clinical diagnosis based on symptoms and labora-tory values rather than imaging. A normal-appearing pancreas on CT does not exclude acute pancreatitis.

9. **What is the optimal time to perform the initial contrast-enhanced CT for assessment of complications of acute pancreatitis?**
The optimal time appears to be 48–72 hours after acute onset of symptoms, since the areas of lique-faction indicating pancreatic necrosis are better defined. Accurate assessment of the presence and extent of pancreatic necrosis has important implications because it has a high mortality rate and requires surgical debridement (see Fig. 17-5) Earlier scans may show areas of pancreatic hetero-geneity that are not specific for necrosis in the setting of acute pancreatitis.

Figure 18-2. Acute pancreatitis. Axial CT image demonstrates peripancreatic stranding *(arrow)*, a finding of pancreatitis. There are multiple gallstones in the gallbladder, which were the cause of this patient's pancreatitis.

10. **What are imaging findings of chronic pancreatitis?**
Chronic pancreatitis refers to the irreversible damage from repeated episodes of pancreatitis. The CT/MR may reveal an atrophic pancreas with fatty replacement and areas of fibrosis, as well as focal calcifica-tions (Fig. 18-3). Irregular dilation of the main duct and side branches, with or without calculi or focal stricture, can also be seen (Fig.18-4).
    Complications of pancreatitis that can be seen on CT and MRI include pseudocyst formation, splenic vein thrombosis, splenic artery pseudo-aneurysm, pancreatic hemorrhage, and pancreatic necrosis.

Figure 18-3. Chronic calcific pancreatitis. Axial unenhanced CT image demonstrates multiple pancreatic calcifications, which are a common finding in chronic pancreatitis. The pancreatic duct is also dilated, although that is generally better delineated on postcontrast images.

11. **True or false: Pancreatic adenocarcinoma enhances to a greater degree than normal surrounding pancreas during the arterial phase.**
False. Pancreatic adenocarcinoma is a hypovascular tumor due to its fibrotic nature (Figs. 18-5 and 18-6). During the arterial phase of enhancement, the tumor appears darker than the normal enhancing pancreas. This is true on both CT, on which the tumor appears hypodense, and MR, on which the tumor appears hypointense on T1-weighted fat-suppressed postgadolinium imaging. During the portal venous phase, the tumor may become inconspicuous relative to the normal pancreas.

12. **What CT/MR findings determine unresectability of pancreatic adenocarcinoma?**
Surgical excision will not be curative for pancreatic adenocarcinoma if the primary tumor extends directly into adjacent organs (stomach, spleen, colon, adrenal gland) or encases major blood vessels, including the celiac axis, hepatic artery, superior mesenteric artery, main portal vein, or superior mesenteric veins. Distant metastases to the liver or peritoneum also render a tumor unresectable (see Fig. 18-6).

Figure 18-4. Pancreatic duct stones. Axial T2-weighted image demonstrates a greatly dilated pancreatic duct, with atrophy of the pancreatic parenchyma. Several stones *(arrows)* are seen in the duct of this patient with chronic pancreatitis.

Tumor invading the duodenum is considered resectable. Invasion of the gastroduodenal artery does not render a tumor unresectable because this vessel is removed through the Whipple procedure. Because of new surgical techniques such as venous graft interposition, limited short-segment, nonocclusive involvement of the superior mesenteric vein may be considered resectable.

Figure 18-5. Pancreatic adenocarcinoma. Axial contrast-enhanced CT image demonstrates a mass in the body of the pancreas *(single arrow)*, which enhances less than the normal pancreatic head *(twin arrows)*. This is the typical CT appearance of pancreatic adenocarcinoma.

Figure 18-6. Metastatic pancreatic carcinoma. Axial postcontrast CT image demonstrates a hypoenhancing mass *(long black arrow)* that arose from the tail of the pancreas. There is metastatic disease to the left adrenal gland *(white arrow)* and to the liver *(short black arrows)*, which means that this patient's disease is unresectable.

13. **Why is the "double duct" sign important?**

The *double duct sign* refers to obstruction and dilation of both the common bile duct and the pancreatic duct (Fig. 18-7). It is highly suggestive of a pancreatic adenocarcinoma in the head of the pancreas. About 60–70% of adenocarcinomas occur in the head of the pancreas. The double duct sign is not entirely specific for malignancy since focal scarring from chronic pancreatitis can also create this appearance.

Figure 18-7. MRCP "double duct" sign. Coronal heavily T2-weighted MRCP demonstrates dilation of both the pancreatic duct and common bile duct. This "double duct" sign can be caused by ampullary lesions, distal common bile duct lesions, or pancreatic head masses.

14. **What are the three most common types of islet cell tumors?**

Insulinoma, gastrinoma, and nonfunctioning islet cell tumor.

15. **How does an islet cell tumor typically enhance on CT and MRI?**

The majority of islet cell tumors (about 70%) are hypervascular to the pancreas, enhancing greatest during the arterial phase (Fig. 18-8). Liver metastases, if present, are also hypervascular.

Figure 18-8. Islet cell neoplasm. Axial T2-weighted image (A) and axial postcontrast T1-weighted gradient-echo image (B) demonstrate a lesion *(arrows)* in the pancreatic tail. Since the lesion is very hyperintense to the pancreas, it may be mistaken for a cyst on T2. Unlike a cyst, however, it enhances markedly after contrast administration. This is an insulinoma, an islet cell neoplasm.

16. **How do imaging findings at presentation differ for functioning vs. nonfunctioning islet cell tumors?**
Functioning islet cell tumors produce hormones, allowing early diagnosis based on clinical manifestations and laboratory tests. Typically, they are small and homogenous in CT density and MR intensity at presentation. They tend to be hyperintense to the pancreas on T2-weighted images. Nonfunctioning tumors often grow to sizes greater than 5 cm with areas of necrosis before they become clinically apparent. Patients with nonfunctioning tumors generally present with symptoms related to mass effect on the pancreatic duct and adjacent organs.

17. **What is the differential diagnosis of a solid pancreatic mass?**
When a solid pancreatic mass is identified, the two main considerations are pancreatic ductal adenocarcinoma and focal scar from chronic pancreatitis. Islet cell tumor, lymphoma, and metastatic disease are also in the differential diagnosis of a solid pancreatic mass.

18. **What causes diffuse fatty replacement of the pancreas?**
Fatty replacement, either diffuse or patchy, can be a normal finding in older patients. Causes of premature fatty replacement include cystic fibrosis, obesity, steroids, and prior inflammation.

19. **True or false: The pseudocyst is the most common cystic lesion of the pancreas.**
True. The pseudocyst accounts for about 90% of all cystic lesions in the pancreas. Patients often, but not always, recall prior episodes of pancreatitis. In the absence of a clear history of pancreatitis, it may not be possible to distinguish the pseudocyst from a cystic pancreatic neoplasm.

20. **What imaging features favor the diagnosis of serous cystadenoma from a mucinous cystic neoplasm?**
Serous cystadenomas (also known as "microcystic adenomas") (Fig. 18-9) are benign neoplasms that are usually managed conservatively with follow-up imaging. Mucinous cystic neoplasms (also known as "macrocystic neoplasms") (Fig. 18-10) must be surgically removed since mucinous cystadenocarcinomas are malignant and mucinous cystadenomas have malignant potential.
    Serous cystadenomas generally have more than six locules of less than 2 cm each. They may have a central scar, and if they calcify, they

Figure 18-9. Microcystic adenoma. Axial T2-weighted image demonstrates a lesion *(arrow)* of the pancreatic neck composed of numerous small cystic locules divided by fine septations. This is the MR appearance of the benign serous cystadenoma, also known as a microcystic adenoma.

display central "sunburst" microcalcification of the scar. In contrast, mucinous cystic neoplasms generally have fewer than six locules of more than 2 cm each. They do not have central scars, and if they calcify, it is peripheral mural calcification.

21. **What is the most common congenital anomaly of the pancreas?**
Pancreas divisum, which is found in up to 14% of patients on autopsy series. In this anomaly, the dorsal anlage (body) fails to fuse with the ventral anlage (head) such that the larger dorsal duct empties via the smaller minor papilla. This may result in obstructive physiology related to

poor drainage. The shorter ventral duct does not communicate with the dorsal duct and empties via the major papilla. Some believe that divisum predisposes the patient to recurrent pancreatitis, although others believe that the association is incidental.

22. **What genetic disorder results in "bronze diabetes?"**
Primary (genetic) hemochromatosis, which is an autosomal recessive disorder in which abnormal iron metabolism results in deposition of iron in various organs. Pancreatic iron deposition is a late finding in this disease and leads to diabetes. Hyperpigmentation imparts a bronze hue to the skin.

Figure 18-10. Macrocystic neoplasm. Axial T2-weighted image demonstrates a lesion of the pancreatic body and tail *(arrow)*. The locules are larger than those of the benign microcystic adenoma shown in Figure 18-9. Macrocystic cystadenomas are considered to be tumors of low malignant potential.

KEY POINTS: CT AND MRI OF THE PANCREAS ✓

1. Pancreatic adenocarcinoma, which encases the celiac axis, superior mesenteric artery, or portal vein, cannot be surgically resected.

2. On CT and MRI, pancreatic adenocarcinoma generally enhances less than the remainder of the pancreas.

3. Pancreatic islet cell tumors are usually hyperintense to the pancreas on T2-weighted images and tend to enhance more than the remainder of the pancreas after administration of CT or MRI contrast agents.

23. **What are characteristic MR findings in primary hemochromatosis?**
Iron deposition in genetic hemochromatosis is responsible for diffuse low signal intensity on T2-weighted images of involved organs, in particular the liver, heart, and pancreas. The pattern of organ involvement distinguishes primary hemochromatosis from secondary hemochromatosis (hemosiderosis), which is iron deposition caused by multiple blood transfusions. Iron in hemosiderosis is deposited in the reticuloendothelial system and involves the spleen, liver, and bone marrow.

24. **Which pancreatic lesions are associated with von Hippel-Lindau disease?**
Pancreatic epithelial cysts, islet cell tumors, and serous cystadenomas (microcystic adenomas). Characteristic lesions in the central nervous system include cerebellar hemangioblastomas and retinal angiomas. Liver and renal cysts may be identified. Patients with von Hippel-Lindau disease are also at risk for developing renal cell carcinoma and pheochromocytoma.

25. **Pancreatic epithelial cysts may be found in association with which three underlying diseases?**
Von Hippel-Lindau disease, autosomal dominant polycystic kidney disease, and cystic fibrosis.

26. **Which portions of the pancreas are most commonly injured in blunt trauma? Why?**
Neck and body (Fig. 18-11). Pancreatic injuries are uncommon, occurring in 0.5% of patients with abdominal trauma. The mechanism is typically blunt trauma to the mid abdomen, which compresses the neck and body of the pancreas against the underlying spine.

Figure 18-11. Pancreatic laceration. Axial CT image of a motor vehicle accident victim demonstrates hypoenhancement of the pancreatic body *(arrows)* relative to the pancreatic neck. In this patient with hemoperitoneum, this represents traumatic pancreatic laceration.

27. **What are CT imaging findings of pancreatic injury?**
Contrast-enhanced CT is used as a screening modality in patients with abdominal trauma. Imaging findings of pancreatic injury may be subtle, with an ill-defined area of low density in the organ and loss of the acini pattern due to edema. A linear hypodensity in the anteroposterior direction represents a laceration. Disruption of the pancreatic duct can be confirmed on ERCP, or increasingly MRCP, and may result in pseudocyst formation. Pancreatitis, abscess, necrosis, and fistula to other organs may develop.

Pancreatic injuries have a high mortality rate because they are often associated with other life-threatening abdominal injuries. Imaging helps direct therapy, which may include partial pancreatectomy, pseudocyst drainage, or ductal stent placement.

BIBLIOGRAPHY

1. Balthazar EJ: Acute pancreatitis: Assessment of severity with clinical and CT evaluation. Radiology 223:603–613, 2002.

2. Fisher AM, Pickhardt PJ: Pancreas. In Slone RM, et al (eds): Body CT: A Practical Approach. New York, McGraw-Hill, 2000, pp 145–158.

3. Ly JN, Miller FH: MR imaging of the pancreas: A practical approach. Radiol Clin North Am 40:1289–1306, 2002.

4. Semelka RC, Nagase LR, Armao D, Balci NC: Pancreas. In Semelka RC (ed): Abdominal-Pelvic MRI. New York, Wiley-Liss, 2002, pp 373–489.

5. Tamm EP, Silverman PM, Charnsangavej C, Evans DP: Imaging in oncology from the University of Texas M.D. Anderson Cancer Center: Diagnosis, staging and surveillance of pancreatic cancer. Am J Roentgenol 180:1311–1323, 2003.

CHAPTER 19

CT OF THE ACUTE ABDOMEN AND PELVIS

Drew A. Torigian, MD

1. **Why is computed tomography (CT) commonly used for diagnostic purposes in patients with an acute abdomen or pelvis?**
    Accurate and timely diagnosis of life-threatening disease involving the abdomen and pelvis is essential to decrease potential morbidity and mortality. Unfortunately, clinical evaluation is sometimes difficult, and laboratory analysis and plain film radiographic findings are not always useful in diagnosing the disease condition at hand. CT evaluation of the abdomen and pelvis is a reliable, highly accurate, and fast imaging tool in the evaluation of symptomatic patients, and it is most useful in those with a clinical presentation that is unrevealing or confusing. CT allows for direct visualization of anatomic structures in the abdomen and pelvis, along with detection and characterization of the nature and extent of disease, when present.

2. **How does CT work?**
    As a patient is passed through the large bore of the doughnut-shaped gantry of a CT scanner, an x-ray tube rapidly spins circumferentially about the patient while simultaneously emitting a beam of x-ray radiation. At each point along the circumferential path of the tube, the x-ray beam is variably absorbed or attenuated, mainly due to the density and chemical composition of the tissues encountered. The remainder of the beam that is not absorbed and passes through the patient is detected by x-ray detectors and contains data on tissue composition, density, and spatial distribution. This process is repeated at multiple points along the circumferential path of the x-ray tube as it moves around the patient, leading to multiple sets of projection data that are all acquired by the detectors. These raw data are then sent to a computer that reconstructs the information into cross-sectional images of the body part scanned and displays information regarding tissue composition, density, and spatial localization.

3. **When are oral and IV contrast materials for CT administered to patients with an acute abdomen?**
    Oral contrast material distends and opacifies bowel, thereby allowing for better characterization of bowel pathologic conditions and separation of bowel structures from nonbowel structures. IV contrast material aids in the characterization of pathologic lesions and allows for opacification and evaluation of vascular and urothelial structures. Thus, both are generally administered in all patients with an acute abdomen. In patients with a history of IV contrast allergy or elevated creatinine level (generally ≥2), IV contrast material is generally not administered unless the patient has received a corticosteroid preparation or is scheduled to undergo dialysis after the CT examination, respectively. In patients with suspected urolithiasis, unenhanced CT without oral or IV contrast material is generally performed, since unenhanced images are often sufficient for making a diagnosis. In patients undergoing CT angiographic evaluation of the arterial vasculature, oral contrast material is generally not administered because it can obscure normal vessels and vascular pathologic conditions during CT angiographic image reconstruction.

4. **What is the major differential diagnosis for acute abdominopelvic conditions diagnosable on CT?**
    This is a broad but important differential diagnosis:

- **Inflammatory/infectious causes** of acute abdominopelvic pain include acute hepatitis, acute cholecystitis, acute cholangitis, acute pancreatitis, acute pyelonephritis, urolithiasis with hydro(uretero)nephrosis, peptic ulcer disease, infectious enteritis or colitis, diverticulitis, appendicitis, mesenteric lymphadenitis, typhlitis, peritonitis, epiploic appendagitis, and segmental omental infarction.
- **Vascular causes** include solid organ infarction (liver, spleen, kidney, uterine leiomyoma), bowel (mesenteric) ischemia/infarction, hemorrhage into a cyst (hepatic, renal, ovarian), abdominal aortic aneurysm rupture, abdominal aortic dissection or penetrating aortic ulcer, and gonadal torsion.
- **Traumatic causes** include solid organ injury (spleen, liver, kidney, pancreas), hollow organ injury (bowel, bladder), and vascular injury.
- **Other causes** of acute abdominopelvic pain include bowel obstruction, bowel perforation, and ectopic pregnancy.

5. **What is an abscess? What is its CT appearance?**
An abscess is a loculated collection of pus that is typically surrounded by a thick rim of fibrous tissue. On CT, an abscess appears as a loculated fluid collection that may contain debris, protein, or hemorrhage with increased density, sometimes with gas bubbles or septations. An abscess often has a thick enhancing rim of fibrous tissue peripherally. When an abscess arises within a parenchymal organ, multiple small adjacent abscesses ("satellite lesions") are also commonly encountered.

6. **What is acute appendicitis?**
Acute appendicitis is inflammation of the appendix that occurs after luminal obstruction and is one of the most common causes of acute abdominal pain. Patients commonly present with right lower quadrant pain and tenderness, nausea, vomiting, fever, and leukocytosis. Early and accurate diagnosis with CT helps to minimize morbidity and mortality due to appendiceal perforation and prevents unnecessary surgery for nonsurgical conditions that may mimic the clinical presentation of appendicitis. The standard treatment for acute appendicitis is appendectomy.

7. **Describe the CT findings related to acute appendicitis.**
The most specific imaging finding is an abnormal appendix that is typically dilated ≥6 mm and is fluid filled. A calcified appendicolith with periappendiceal fat stranding (appearing as ill-defined hazy increased density of the fat) is also another highly specific CT finding (Fig. 19-1). Other findings include:
- Enhancement of the appendiceal wall
- Thickening of the appendiceal wall, sometimes with a low-density ring of submucosal edema in the wall (the "target sign")
- Reactive thickening of adjacent cecum or small bowel
- Arrowhead-shaped funneling of the cecal apex toward the occluded appendiceal lumen (the "arrowhead sign")
- A curved, soft tissue density between the cecal lumen and an appendicolith, which is representative of an inflamed cecal or appendiceal wall (the "cecal bar sign")
- Periappendiceal fluid
- Thickening and enhancement of the adjacent parietal peritoneum due to focal peritonitis.

Figure 19-1. Acute appendicitis on CT. Note the dilated tubular structure *(T)* containing radiodense appendicoliths *(arrows)* with associated periappendiceal fat stranding in right lower quadrant of abdomen due to inflammation of appendix.

Complications include perforation with abscess formation, small bowel obstruction, and mesenteric venous thrombosis.

8. **What is acute large bowel diverticulitis? What are the CT findings?**

Acute diverticulitis involving the large bowel is inflammation/infection in the setting of large bowel diverticulosis (i.e., the presence of multiple blind outpouchings of the large bowel). This most commonly occurs in patients older than 65 and presents clinically with fever, abdominal pain (often in the left lower quadrant), and leukocytosis. CT findings include pericolonic fat stranding, thickening and enhancement of an inflamed diverticulum, pericolonic gas bubbles due to bowel microperforation (Fig. 19-2), and pericolonic fluid. Potential complications include abscess formation and fistula or sinus tract formation from the affected bowel segments to other bowel segments, pelvic organs, or skin surface.

Figure 19-2. Acute large bowel diverticulitis on CT. Note the hazy increased density *(arrowheads)* associated with pericolonic inflammatory fat stranding about the loop of the transverse colon *(TC),* along with pericolonic gas bubbles *(arrow)* due to bowel microperforation.

9. **Describe acute mesenteric lymphadenitis and the associated CT findings.**

Acute mesenteric lymphadenitis is a self-limited condition due to inflammation of ileal mesenteric lymph nodes, sometimes with associated terminal ileal and cecal inflammation. It often presents with right lower quadrant pain and diarrhea, most often in children and young adults. The most common causative agents include the *Campylobacter jejuni* and *Yersinia* species of bacteria. Characteristic CT findings include a cluster of enlarged right lower quadrant mesenteric lymph nodes, sometimes with thickening of the cecum or terminal ileum, and a normal appearing appendix.

10. **What is neutropenic enterocolitis (typhlitis)? What are the CT findings?**

Neutropenic enterocolitis is acute inflammation of the cecum, sometimes with involvement of the ascending colon, terminal ileum, and appendix, typically seen in patients with immunosuppression, particularly in the setting of leukemia. Treatment is generally with antimicrobial therapy. CT findings include thickening of involved portions of the right colon, terminal ileum, and appendix, sometimes with a target sign due to submucosal edema; inflammatory fat stranding or fluid about affected bowel loops; and gas in the bowel wall (pneumatosis) if there is bowel infarction (Fig. 19-3).

Figure 19-3. Neutropenic enterocolitis (typhlitis) on CT in setting of leukemia. Note the wall thickening of cecum *(thick arrow)* and the terminal ileum and appendix *(thin arrows)* associated with low-density submucosal edema, creating the "target sign." Hazy pericecal inflammatory fat stranding is also present.

11. **Describe primary epiploic appendagitis (PEA) and segmental omental infarction. What are their CT findings?**

    PEA and segmental omental infarction are both self-limited conditions that often present with focal, severe, acute abdominal pain and tenderness and are treated with conservative therapy (e.g., analgesics). PEA is related to torsion, inflammation, and ischemia of an epiploic appendage, and segmental omental infarction is related to spontaneous infarction of a portion of the omentum. CT findings of PEA include a small (1–5 cm), pedunculated, round or oval fat density structure with a soft tissue density rim located adjacent to the serosal surface of the colon (in the expected location of an epiploic appendage), commonly with a high-density central dot or line due to hemorrhagic necrosis or thrombosis of a central vein. Associated inflammatory fat stranding and reactive bowel wall or peritoneal thickening may also be seen. CT findings of segmental omental infarction include a larger (5–10 cm), well-circumscribed focus of fat density with hazy inflammatory fat stranding. Typically, the infarction is located in the right anterolateral aspect of the abdomen between the colon and parietal peritoneum at or above the umbilical level (in the expected location of the greater omentum).

12. **What is acute cholecystitis?**

    Acute cholecystitis is gallbladder wall inflammation due to obstruction of the cystic duct or gallbladder neck. This is most often caused by gallstones (calculous cholecystitis), although in 5–10% of cases, gallstones are not present (acalculous cholecystitis). Acalculous cholecystitis tends to occur in the setting of prolonged illness, such as with prior traumatic or burn injury or with a prolonged intensive care unit stay. Most patients present with right upper quadrant pain and tenderness (Murphy's sign), although in the setting of severe advanced inflammation, diabetes mellitus, or elderly age, these clinical findings may be less severe or absent.

13. **List the CT findings related to acute cholecystitis.**

    CT findings include smooth or irregular gallbladder wall thickening, generally ≥3 mm in thickness (sometimes with decreased density due to edema); gallbladder distention; pericholecystic fat stranding; pericholecystic fluid; gallstones or gallbladder sludge; and adjacent increased enhancement of the liver parenchyma (the "rim sign") due to the inflammatory process (Fig. 19-4). Only about 75% of gallstones are detected on CT, but CT has a sensitivity and specificity for the diagnosis of acute cholecystitis that is greater than 90%. Pericholecystic fat stranding is the most specific CT finding of acute cholecystitis.

Figure 19-4. Acute cholecystitis on CT. Note the distended gallbladder *(G)* with enhancing thickened wall *(arrow)* and associated pericholecystic inflammatory fat stranding.

14. **What is gangrenous cholecystitis, and what are its CT findings?**

    Gangrenous cholecystitis is a severe, advanced form of acute cholecystitis with ischemic necrosis of the gallbladder wall, which is associated with a higher rate of gallbladder perforation. This occurs more commonly in elderly men and in those with preexisting cardiovascular disease. CT findings include marked gallbladder wall thickening and distention, intraluminal membranes, intraluminal hemorrhage, irregularity or absence of the gallbladder wall, and lack of gallbladder wall enhancement. Gas may also sometimes be seen within the gallbladder wall or lumen, and a pericholecystic abscess may be seen with perforation.

15. **Describe emphysematous cholecystitis and its CT findings.**
Emphysematous cholecystitis is a rare, rapidly progressive complication of acute cholecystitis, which is related to gas-forming infection (most often by *Clostridium welchii* and *Escherichia coli*) in the setting of gallbladder vascular insufficiency. Up to 75% of cases occur in men, commonly in those with diabetes mellitus, and are associated with a higher rate of gallbladder perforation. CT findings include gas within the gallbladder lumen or wall (sometimes with involvement of the pericholecystic tissues), along with other CT findings of acute cholecystitis previously described.

16. **What is the treatment for acute, gangrenous, or emphysematous cholecystitis?**
Urgent surgical resection is the treatment of choice before gallbladder perforation occurs. If gallbladder perforation occurs, typically seen on CT as gallbladder contour irregularity, complications of bacteremia, septic shock, bile peritonitis, or abscess formation may occur.

17. **What is acute pancreatitis?**
Acute pancreatitis is pancreatic inflammation due to autodigestion by activated pancreatic enzymes, most commonly a result of alcohol abuse and gallstones. Patients often present with nausea, vomiting, and mid-epigastric pain and have a variable prognosis that is predominantly based on the severity of pancreatitis and the presence of complications.

18. **Describe the CT findings related to acute pancreatitis.**
The pancreas may appear normal in the setting of mild pancreatitis. Findings with increasing severity of pancreatitis include pancreatic enlargement (diffuse or focal); loss of the normal acinar pattern or decrease in density due to edema, haziness of the peripancreatic fat due to inflammation, edema, and/or peripancreatic fat necrosis; peripancreatic fluid collections (sometimes with gas due to fistula formation to adjacent bowel or superinfection); or pancreatic necrosis (seen as segmental or diffuse lack of enhancement of pancreatic parenchyma) (Fig. 19-5). Fluid collections are often present in the anterior pararenal space of the retroperitoneum but may also commonly involve the lesser sac of the peritoneal cavity and the transverse

Figure 19-5. Acute necrotizing pancreatitis on CT. Note the lack of enhancement of the enlarged pancreatic head, neck, and body associated with pancreatic necrosis *(N)* with enhancement of residual portions of non-necrotic pancreatic body and tail *(arrows)*. Peripancreatic fat stranding and minimal peripancreatic fluid surround the pancreas and track along left retroperitoneal fascial planes *(arrowheads)*.

mesocolon. Complications may include pseudocyst formation, hemorrhage, venous thrombosis (most commonly involving the splenic vein and superior mesenteric vein), and arterial pseudoaneurysm formation (often involving the splenic, gastroduodenal, pancreaticoduodenal, hepatic, and left gastric arteries) with subsequent rupture.

19. **What is the CT grading system for acute pancreatitis?**
   - Grade A: normal-appearing pancreas
   - Grade B: pancreatic fullness and/or loss of the normal acinar pattern
   - Grade C: peripancreatic fat stranding

- Grade D: one peripancreatic fluid collection
- Grade E: two or more peripancreatic fluid collections or retroperitoneal gas

20. **List the normal phases of renal enhancement seen on CT.**
The cortices of the kidneys enhance before the medullary pyramids do, and as such, within about 30–45 seconds of IV contrast administration, the corticomedullary phase of enhancement is seen, in which only the renal cortices enhance. A short time later, homogeneous enhancement of the kidneys can be seen during the nephrographic phase of enhancement, when both the cortices and medullary pyramids enhance. Finally, after a few minutes, contrast material that is excreted by the kidneys can be seen within the collecting systems, ureters, and bladder during the delayed or excretory phase of enhancement.

21. **What is acute pyelonephritis? What are the CT findings?**
Acute pyelonephritis is infection of the kidney and often presents with fever, chills, and flank pain and tenderness. It is most often due to ascending retrograde infection via the bladder, ureter, and collecting system with subsequent infection of the renal parenchyma. CT findings may include a normal-appearing kidney; focal areas of striated or wedge-shaped hypodensity in the kidney, resulting in a heterogeneous nephrogram (Fig. 19-6); a "striated nephrogram" on delayed postcontrast images due to stasis of contrast material within edematous tubules; enlargement of the kidney;

Figure 19-6. Acute pyelonephritis on CT. Note the multiple focal areas of striated or wedge-shaped hypodensity in the kidneys *(arrows)*, more severe on the right than on the left, resulting in heterogeneous nephrograms.

perinephric fat stranding; and renal pelvic and ureteral thickening with hyperenhancement. Sometimes, associated hydroureteronephrosis (dilation of the collecting system and ureter), renal infarction, and/or renal or perinephric abscess formation may be seen.

22. **What is emphysematous pyelonephritis? What is its CT appearance?**
Emphysematous pyelonephritis is a severe, life-threatening infection of the renal parenchyma by gas-forming bacteria. This condition most often occurs in diabetic patients and is often seen when there is obstruction of the collecting system. Rapid progression to septic shock may occur, and the overall mortality rate may be as high as 50%. The major CT finding is gas within the renal parenchyma, often with radial orientation within the renal pyramids, sometimes extending into the perinephric space, perinephric fascial planes, or collecting system. Associated findings of acute pyelonephritis, as previously described, are also commonly present, and treatment is typically with nephrectomy.

23. **List the CT findings of urolithiasis along with its associated complications.**
Urinary tract calculi (i.e., liths or stones) may vary in size from less than 1 mm to several centimeters ("staghorn" calculi) and are typically seen as round, oval, or polygonal foci of high radiodensity within the renal parenchyma, collecting system, ureter, or bladder. Only calculi composed of protease inhibitors in patients with HIV infection who take such medications may be radiolucent on CT. When there is obstruction of the ureter by a calculus, which most often occurs at the ureteropelvic and ureterovesical junctions, CT findings may include dilation of the upstream ureter and collecting system, a thickened segment of ureter about the calculus

(the "rim sign"), delayed enhancement of the ipsilateral kidney (the "delayed nephrogram"), perinephric or periureteral stranding, and perinephric fluid or urinoma formation (due to rupture of a calyceal fornix with urine leak) that demonstrates enhancement on excretory phase images. Scanning in the prone position may be useful in differentiating between a recently passed calculus within the urinary bladder and a calculus that is impacted within the ureterovesical junction, since the former will drop to the dependent surface of the bladder and the latter will remain trapped within the ureterovesical junction.

24. **What is pelvic inflammatory disease (PID), and what are its CT findings?**
PID is common and covers a spectrum of infectious diseases involving the reproductive tract of women, including endometritis, cervicitis, salpingitis, and oophoritis, along with some more advanced manifestations of disease. Patients typically present with vaginal discharge, pelvic pain, fever, and leukocytosis. CT findings include subtle mesenteric, omental, and/or pelvic fat stranding with obscuration of normal pelvic fascial planes; thickening of the uterosacral ligaments; pelvic peritoneal or endometrial fluid/gas; hyperenhancement and/or enlargement of the endometrium, cervix, fallopian tubes, or ovaries; thickening of the fallopian tubes, sometimes with dilation by fluid or pus (i.e., hydrosalpinx or pyosalpinx, respectively), and often with ovarian involvement (tubo-ovarian abscess [TOA]); abdominopelvic abscess formation; and perihepatic fat stranding and fluid (Fitz-Hugh–Curtis syndrome) (Fig. 19-7). When an intrauterine device is present, infection by *Actinomyces israelii* is more likely and should be considered in the differential diagnosis.

Figure 19-7. PID on CT. Note the dilated fluid- and gas-filled tubular structure in the left pelvis, which is indicative of pyosalpinx *(P)*; loculated fluid and gas in cul-de-sac of pelvis associated with pelvic abscess *(A)*; heterogeneous enhancement of inflamed uterus *(U)*; and subtle pelvic inflammatory fat stranding *(arrows)*.

25. **List the major causes of bowel obstruction.**
The most common cause of small bowel obstruction is adhesions secondary to prior surgery. Small bowel obstruction due to hernia is the second most common cause. Other causes of small bowel obstruction are volvulus, malrotation, annular pancreas, endometriosis, foreign body, gallstone, bezoar, and Crohn's disease.
   Major causes of large bowel obstruction include adhesions, hernia, colonic or rectal tumor, inflammatory bowel disease, sigmoid or cecal volvulus, intussusception, and fecal impaction.

26. **Describe the CT findings associated with bowel obstruction.**
The major finding is upstream dilation and downstream collapse of bowel with respect to the site of obstruction (i.e., the transition zone) (Fig. 19-8). Other findings may include focal bowel wall thickening; mass; luminal filling defect; luminal narrowing or angulation, tethering, or beaking of bowel at the transition zone; a mixture of particulate material and fluid within upstream dilated small bowel, mimicking the appearance of feces (the "small bowel feces sign"); and gradual dilution of oral contrast material when passing from proximal to distal in dilated bowel upstream to the site of obstruction. Associated findings of bowel ischemia may also be present.

27. **Describe the CT findings associated with bowel ischemia.**

If ischemic change of bowel is present (such as in the case of strangulation of herniated bowel), one may see bowel wall thickening often with a target sign, dilation of bowel, perienteric or pericolonic fat stranding or fluid, delayed hyperenhancement of bowel mucosa, lack of wall enhancement, pneumatosis (gas bubbles in the wall of the bowel), mesenteric or portal venous gas, or free intraperitoneal gas (Fig. 19-9). If bowel ischemia is suspected, one should assess the patency of the celiac artery, superior mesenteric artery, inferior mesenteric artery, portal vein, superior mesenteric vein, and inferior mesenteric vein. When the central superior mesenteric vessels are affected, the entire small bowel, along with the large bowel proximal to the distal third of the transverse colon, tends to be affected. When the central inferior mesenteric vessels are affected, the distal third of the transverse colon, the descending colon, and the sigmoid colon are generally involved.

Figure 19-8. Small bowel obstruction on CT due to incarcerated ventral hernia. (A) Note the proximal dilated loops of small bowel *(D)* and distal collapsed loops of small bowel *(arrows),* indicating the level of obstruction in the small bowel. (B) Also note the loops of small bowel passing through the defect in the anterior abdominal wall, indicative of ventral hernia *(arrowheads).*

28. **List the major causes of bowel ischemia.**
   - **Arterial diseases** that can result in bowel ischemia/infarction include embolic disease, arterial thrombosis, vasculitis, aortic dissection extending into a mesenteric artery, tumor encasement of an artery, or trauma.
   - **Venous causes** of bowel ischemia/infarction include thrombosis, tumor encasement of a mesenteric vein, and trauma.
   - **Vessel hypoperfusion** and **systemic shock** are also important causes of bowel ischemia/infarction.

29. **What is a closed loop bowel obstruction? What are the CT findings?**

A closed loop bowel obstruction is a surgical emergency and is due to obstruction of bowel at two separate locations along its course. This generally arises in the setting of volvulus, hernia, or adhesion formation and can rapidly progress to ischemia, infarction, perforation, sepsis, and death. CT findings include C-shaped or U-shaped loops of dilated bowel, often with a radial configuration and convergence of mesenteric vessels toward a central focus; mesenteric haziness and fluid due to edema; prominent engorged mesenteric vessels; a swirling appearance of the mesentery and vessels adjacent to the transition zone (the "whirl sign"); and beaking and taper-

Figure 19-9. Small and large bowel ischemia on CT. Note the dilated and thick-walled loops of small bowel *(S)* and large bowel *(L)* with associated low-density submucosal edema, creating the "target sign." A large amount of pelvic free fluid *(F)* is also present.

KEY POINTS: CT OF THE ACUTE ABDOMEN AND PELVIS

1. If you visualize imaging findings of active arterial extravasation of contrast material, shock, or abdominal aortic aneurysm rupture on CT, immediately check on the status of the patient, start IV fluids if needed, and get help from your clinical colleagues.

2. Whenever you see findings of bowel obstruction on CT, always evaluate the etiology at the transition zone and exclude the presence of a closed loop obstruction because this constitutes a true surgical emergency.

3. Always evaluate patency of the mesenteric arterial and venous vessels on CT, particularly if the bowel is abnormal in appearance.

4. If traumatic injury to the kidneys, ureters, or bladder is suspected clinically or on the basis of CT findings, be sure to obtain images of these areas during the excretory phase of enhancement to detect urothelial perforation as leakage of contrast-opacified urine.

ing of bowel loops at the sites of obstruction (the "beak sign"), often spatially located in close proximity to each other.

30. **List the major causes of bowel perforation.**
    Major causes of bowel perforation include bowel infarction, obstruction (particularly, closed loop obstruction), severe inflammatory bowel disease, peptic ulcer disease, diverticulitis, foreign body perforation, traumatic or iatrogenic injury, and involvement of bowel by tumor.

31. **What are the CT findings associated with bowel perforation?**
    CT findings include direct visualization of a site of focal disruption in the wall of the bowel; free intraperitoneal air (when there is rupture of an intraperitoneal portion of bowel); free retroperitoneal air (when there is rupture of a retroperitoneal portion of bowel); gas bubbles, focal fluid, or inflammatory changes adjacent to the site of perforation; and leakage of fluid (bowel contents) and oral contrast material into the peritoneum or retroperitoneum (Fig. 19-10). If secondary peritonitis is present, thickening and enhancement of the peritoneum may be seen.

32. **Describe the CT appearance of hemorrhage and active arterial hemorrhage.**
    Hemorrhage may occur in any portion of the abdomen and pelvis and generally appears as either a focal heterogeneous high-density region or fluid collection, sometimes with a dependent

high-density layer and a low-density nondependent layer related to settling of red blood cells (the "CT hematocrit level"). The presence of focal high-density clotted blood in the abdomen or pelvis may serve as an indicator of the source of hemorrhage (the "sentinel clot" sign). However, in patients with anemia, hemorrhage may have similar density to that of simple fluid. Active arterial hemorrhage appears as a round or linear focus of extraluminal contrast material with very high density, similar to that of contrast within arterial vessels, and is often surrounded by unenhanced high-density hemorrhage.

Figure 19-10. Bowel perforation on CT. Note the large amount of free intraperitoneal air *(A)* in the perihepatic space, along with layering enteric fluid contents *(F)* and oral contrast material *(arrow)*. A perforated duodenal ulcer was present more inferiorly (not shown).

33. **Describe the CT findings related to AAA rupture and impending rupture.**

CT findings of AAA rupture include periaortic and retroperitoneal hemorrhage, sometimes with hemoperitoneum (Fig. 19-11), and active arterial hemorrhage, as previously described. Other CT findings of rupture or impending rupture include high-density hemorrhage within the thrombus or wall of an AAA (the "crescent sign"); focal high density; irregular contour, defect, or interruption of atherosclerotic calcification of the aortic wall at the site of rupture; an abnormal shape of an AAA; an undefinable area of the posterior wall of an AAA that follows the vertebral contour of the spine (the "draped aorta sign"); a large size (up to 40% of AAA >5 cm will rupture within 5 years); and a rapid increase in the size of an AAA.

Figure 19-11. AAA rupture with retroperitoneal hemorrhage on CT. Note the extensive high-density fluid within the retroperitoneum associated with hemorrhage *(H)* and surrounding enhancing AAA *(A)* with mural thrombus *(m)*. Note the collapsed inferior vena cava *(arrow)*, indicating the low volume status of the patient.

34. **What are the CT findings associated with shock, and what should one do on seeing these findings?**

CT findings include a small caliber of the aorta and renal arteries (related to hypovolemia and compensatory vasoconstriction), a flattened inferior vena cava (the "flat cava sign"), poor enhancement of a small spleen, persistent enhancement of the kidneys (a "delayed nephrogram"), and diffuse thickening of the small bowel with dilation and patchy enhancement ("shock bowel"). Other findings may include hemorrhage, sometimes with active bleeding. When one sees findings of shock on CT, one should immediately check the patient's condition, start administering IV fluids, and call for assistance from other clinical staff as needed.

35. **List the major CT findings associated with solid organ traumatic injury.**
Contusions, lacerations, infarction, arterial pseudoaneurysm formation, and hemorrhage with or without active bleeding are findings that may be encountered on CT in the setting of solid organ injury.

Contusions appear as focal regions of decreased enhancement, whereas lacerations appear as irregular linear, curvilinear, or branching foci of hypodensity within the parenchyma of a solid organ, sometimes containing gas or high-density hemorrhage (Fig. 19-12). Parenchymal infarction typically appears as focal or diffuse areas of hypodensity due to lack of enhancement, often peripheral in location and wedge-shaped when focal,

Figure 19-12. Traumatic renal laceration with hematoma and active arterial hemorrhage on CT. Note the irregular linear hypodensity within the right kidney, indicative of laceration (between *arrowheads)* with associated perinephric hematoma *(H).* Also note the round focus of very high-density extraluminal arterial contrast material *(arrow)* associated with active arterial hemorrhage.

and commonly with a preserved peripheral rim of enhancement resulting from capsular collateral vascular supply. Arterial pseudoaneurysms generally appear as focal, round, or oval well-circumscribed structures that enhance and washout to a degree similar to that of other arterial vessels, such as the aorta, and may be treated through percutaneous interventional techniques.

36. **Describe the major CT findings related to hollow organ traumatic injury.**
Contusion; ischemia or infarction; hemorrhage, sometimes with active bleeding; and perforation may be seen on CT with hollow organ injury. Contusion of a hollow organ generally appears as wall thickening with patchy enhancement, sometimes with increased density due to intramural hemorrhage, and often with adjacent mesenteric fluid, haziness, or hemorrhage when bowel is the hollow organ involved. The CT findings of bowel perforation have been described previously. With bladder rupture, fluid-density urine may be seen in the extraperitoneal space (with extraperitoneal bladder rupture) or in the peritoneal space (with intraperitoneal bladder rupture) that opacifies with renally excreted contrast material during the excretory phase of enhancement. With rupture of the collecting system or ureter, similar findings of extraluminal fluid-density urine with delayed contrast opacification during the excretory phase of enhancement may be seen in the retroperitoneum.

37. **What are the major CT findings associated with vascular traumatic injury?**
CT findings of vascular injury include an abrupt caliber change of a vessel (indicative of contained rupture or pseudoaneurysm formation); an intimal flap within an arterial vessel; lack of luminal enhancement and enlargement of vessel caliber due to acute thrombosis; active extravasation of contrast material due to active bleeding; high-density hemorrhage either within the wall of a vessel (intramural hematoma) or surrounding a vessel; wall thickening, sometimes with an irregular contour; and secondary signs of solid organ infarction or bowel ischemia/infarction, as previously described.

38. **What is Fournier's gangrene? What is its CT appearance?**

Fournier's gangrene represents necrotizing fasciitis of the perineal, genital, or perianal regions; occurs most often in immunocompromised men; and is due to gas-forming infection, most notably by the *Clostridia* species. CT findings include gas and/or fluid along fascial planes of the lower abdomen, pelvis, and perineum, often with extension into the subcutaneous fat, muscles, or deeper body wall layers; skin thickening or ulceration; inflammatory fat stranding; abscess formation; and lytic destruction of bone if osteomyelitis is present. Treatment is with aggressive fluid resuscitation, broad-spectrum antimicrobial therapy, and early surgical debridement to prevent septic shock and death. Adjuvant hyperbaric oxygen therapy may also be used in some cases.

BIBLIOGRAPHY

1. Balthazar EJ: Staging of acute pancreatitis. Radiol Clin North Am 40:1199–1209, 2002.
2. Bennett GL, Balthazar EJ: Ultrasound and CT evaluation of emergent gallbladder pathology. Radiol Clin North Am 41:1203–1216, 2003.
3. Bennett GL, Slywotzky CM, Giovanniello G: Gynecologic causes of acute pelvic pain: Spectrum of CT findings. Radiographics 22:785–801, 2002.
4. Birnbaum BA, Wilson SR: Appendicitis at the millennium. Radiology 215:337–348, 2000.
5. Boudiaf M, Soyer P, Terem C, et al: CT evaluation of small bowel obstruction. Radiographics 21:613–624, 2001.
6. Ferzoco LB, Raptopoulos V, Silen W: Acute diverticulitis. N Engl J Med 338:1521–1526, 1998.
7. Grayson DE, Abbott RM, Levy AD, Sherman PM: Emphysematous infections of the abdomen and pelvis: A pictorial review. Radiographics 22:543–561, 2002.
8. Kawashima A, Sandler CM, Goldman SM, et al: CT of renal inflammatory disease. Radiographics 17:851–866, discussion 867–858, 1997.
9. Macari M, Balthazar EJ: The acute right lower quadrant: CT evaluation. Radiol Clin North Am 41:1117–1136, 2003.
10. Sam JW, Jacobs JE, Birnbaum BA: Spectrum of CT findings in acute pyogenic pelvic inflammatory disease. Radiographics 22:1327–1334, 2002.
11. Sirvanci M, Tekelioglu MH, Duran C, et al: Primary epiploic appendagitis: CT manifestations. Clin Imaging 24:357–361, 2000.
12. Urban BA, Fishman EK: Tailored helical CT evaluation of acute abdomen. Radiographics 20:725–749, 2000.

V. GENITOURINARY TRACT

INTRAVENOUS UROGRAPHY

Parvati Ramchandani, MD

CHAPTER 20

1. **What is an intravenous urogram (IVU)?**
   An IVU is a radiographic study that provides both anatomic and functional information about the urinary tract. Radiographic contrast is injected intravenously and a series of films are performed to demonstrate the kidneys, ureters, and urinary bladder. Other synonyms used for this study are "intravenous pyelogram" (IVP) and "excretory urogram." Although IVP is probably the most commonly used term for this study, it is inaccurate because *pyelogram* literally means "a study of the renal pelvis." An IVU provides far more information than just an anatomic depiction of the renal pelvis alone. The term *pyelogram* is reserved for retrograde studies in which only the collecting system is visualized.

2. **In what clinical situations is an IVU useful?**
   The major indications for an IVU are to evaluate patients with gross or microscopic hematuria, transitional cell carcinoma, urinary tract stones, and suspected postsurgical or posttraumatic ureteral leaks.

3. **The patient I am seeing in the clinic has gross hematuria. Can I send him to the radiology department for an IVU today?**
   Good-quality IVU requires preprocedural preparation. For most of the indications previously listed, it is better to schedule the study so that the patient can receive a bowel preparation. In emergent situations, such as a suspected ureteral leak, the study can be performed without preprocedural preparation, recognizing that the evaluation of the collecting systems for subtle abnormalities may be suboptimal without the bowel preparation.

4. **What preprocedural preparations are necessary for an IVU?**
   Preprocedural preparations are aimed at cleansing the colon so that overlying bowel contents do not obscure the upper urinary tract. This generally consists of laxatives taken the evening before the study. Patients are also asked to avoid solid food the day before the study and consume a clear liquid diet instead.

5. **When is an IVU contraindicated?**
   - IVU requires the administration of IV contrast and thus should not be performed in patients who have a history of severe allergy to radiographic contrast agents. Severe reactions include bronchospasm, laryngeal edema, or anaphylactic shock. In patients with a history of minor allergic reactions to contrast, such as hives, IVU can be performed after preprocedural preparation with steroids and antihistaminic agents, such as diphenhydramine. Steroid administration should optimally be started at least 12 hours before the procedure for maximal efficacy.
   - Patients with renal insufficiency may suffer further deterioration in renal function after IV contrast administration. Therefore, an IVU is best avoided in such patients, and alternative imaging techniques should be used to evaluate the urinary tract.
   - Pregnancy is a relative contraindication, with the primary concern being radiation exposure to the fetus, particularly in the first and second trimesters of pregnancy. Thus, in all female patients of childbearing age, direct questioning is performed to determine the date of the last menstrual

period and to ascertain whether the patient could be pregnant. If there is concern, a pregnancy test is obtained before performing the study. If an IVU is unavoidable in a pregnant patient, efforts are made to minimize the number of films obtained and thus limit the radiation exposure.

- Patients taking oral hypoglycemic agents, such as metformin (Glucophage), should stop taking the medication at the time of the IVU and not resume it until renal function has been confirmed as being normal to avoid the risk of lactic acidosis. Current guidelines do not require the patient to stop taking the medication before contrast administration.

6. **What radiographic contrast agents are used for an IVU?**
The choice of contrast agent is primarily between the older ionic contrast agents and the newer nonionic contrast agents. Nonionic contrast agents are iso-osmolar and have fewer minor side effects. It is controversial whether major contrast reactions occur less often than with ionic contrast. Because of their iso-osmolar nature, nonionic contrast agents cause less hemodynamic alteration and are better tolerated by patients with cardiac disease.

Ionic contrasts are the older contrast agents and are two to three times less expensive than nonionic contrast agents. However, the hyperosmolar character of these agents leads to a higher incidence of minor reactions such as nausea, hives, and skin flushing. In patients with cardiac disease, there is greater potential for precipitating fluid overload and heart failure with these agents.

At present, most radiology departments in the United States and Europe favor the use of nonionic contrast agents for intravascular use in all patients.

7. **What is the sequence of radiographs for an IVU?**
The procedure begins with two plain radiographs, known as the *preliminary* or *scout films,* that are used to examine the soft tissues, bones, and bowel gas pattern. One radiograph is centered over the kidneys, and the second radiograph views the entire abdomen to the level of the pubic symphysis. Scout radiographs are particularly important for detecting radiopaque urinary tract stones since these stones have the same radiographic density as excreted contrast and are often difficult to visualize once the collecting system is opacified with contrast (Fig. 20-1). In addition to calculi, the scout radiographs are also used to detect renal masses (Fig. 20-2, *A*).

The filming sequence of an IVU is aimed at evaluating the parenchyma for masses and the collecting system for urothelial neoplasms and other abnormalities, such as papillary necrosis.

Figure 20-1. Right renal calculus. *A,* Preliminary radiograph centered over the kidneys shows an opaque calculus in the right kidney *(arrow). B,* Image from an IVU. The stone is largely obscured by the contrast in the right renal pelvis.

Parenchymal evaluation is performed with a series of films called *nephrotomograms*, in which the x-ray tube moves over the patient in an arc with a fixed focal plane that is in sharp focus (Fig. 20-2, *B*). Structures anterior or posterior to the focal point are blurred.

Evaluation of the collecting systems for subtle abnormalities is aided by distention of the collecting system. This requires compressing the abdomen with inflatable balloons so that the ureters are obstructed (Fig. 20-2, *C*). Once the compression is released, contrast floods the ureters, allowing visualization of the entire length of the ureters. A film is also obtained in the upright position, which is very sensitive for showing low grades of obstruction (Fig. 20-2, *D*). An unobstructed collecting system should drain nearly completely on an upright film. Films of the urinary bladder are obtained

Figure 20-2. Films from an IVU from a 78-year-old woman. *A,* Preliminary radiograph demonstrates a rounded density projecting from the lower pole of the left kidney *(arrows),* suggesting the presence of a left renal mass. *B,* Nephrotomogram demonstrates the right kidney to be normal. A mass in the left lower pole is seen well. Ultrasound subsequently showed this to be a simple renal cyst (not illustrated). *C,* Film at 12 minutes after injection with abdominal compression. Note the well-distended collecting systems and ureters, with the ureteral contrast column obstructed by the compression balloons. Urothelial abnormalities are difficult to detect in underdistended collecting systems. *D,* Erect radiograph. There is near-complete drainage of the collecting systems. Note the descent of the bladder below the symphysis pubis *(arrows)* in this elderly woman with a cystocele due to pelvic floor laxity.

with the bladder distended and then after the patient voids. The latter allows a rough estimate of bladder function and is also a sensitive film for demonstrating bladder masses.

8. **How should a patient with hematuria be evaluated?**
   The upper and the lower urinary tract of such a patient should be evaluated for stones, neoplasms, and other abnormalities that may cause hematuria. The upper urinary tract is usually evaluated with an IVU, although there is now growing interest in using computed tomography (CT) for this purpose. The sensitivity and specificity of CT urography as compared with conventional IVU in diagnosing collecting system abnormalities are still unclear and the subject of avid research. CT is much more sensitive than IVU in diagnosing renal parenchymal abnormalities and in detecting small renal masses. Currently, IVU is the best study to evaluate both the renal parenchyma and the collecting system in a patient with microscopic hematuria. The urinary bladder is best evaluated with cystoscopy; all imaging studies are much less sensitive in demonstrating pathologic conditions of the bladder.

9. **What should be done if the IVU suggests the presence of a renal mass?**
   It is difficult to distinguish whether a renal mass represents a benign renal cyst (an extremely common occurrence in patients older than 50) or a renal cell carcinoma on an IVU. Any masses detected on an IVU should be further evaluated and definitively characterized with a cross-sectional technique such as renal ultrasound, precontrast and postcontrast CT, or renal magnetic resonance imaging (MRI).

10. **My patient has presented with diffuse lung metastases and gross hematuria. Should I evaluate him with an IVU to look for a renal malignancy?**
    When looking for a primary renal tumor, CT or MRI is preferable to an IVU because they are more sensitive in detecting small masses. Lesions less than 2–3 cm in size are difficult to detect on an IVU.

11. **Why is an IVU necessary in patients with transitional cell carcinoma (TCC) of the urinary bladder?**
    TCC is 50 times more common in the urinary bladder than in the upper urinary tract. However, TCC is a multifocal process, and upper urinary tract involvement occurs in 3–4% of patients with bladder TCC, either synchronously at the time of bladder cancer diagnosis or in a metachronous fashion. Thus, the upper urinary tract of patients with bladder cancer must be kept under close surveillance, usually with periodic IVUs. Patients with upper urinary tract TCC have a 30–40% incidence of TCC involving the opposite side.

12. **What does TCC look like on radiographic studies?**
    Persistent filling defects in the pyelocalyceal system or the ureters are the most common finding (Fig. 20-3). With larger lesions, there may be obstruction of the ipsilateral collecting system by the tumor mass or blood clot.

13. **What do stones look like on an IVU?**
    Approximately 85% of urinary tract stones are composed of calcium oxalate and are radiopaque on plain abdominal films (see Fig 20-1, *A*). Ten percent of stones are composed of uric acid and are either nonopaque or very faintly opaque on abdominal films. Nonopaque stones are invisible on plain radiographs but are seen as filling defects in the contrast-opacified collecting system. Stones associated with chronic or recurrent infection can grow to fill the entire collecting system and are called "staghorn stones" (Fig. 20-4). Other stone compositions, such as cystine and xanthine, are less common. It is important to remember that all stones, regardless of their composition, are dense on CT and echogenic on ultrasound. The terms *radiopaque* and *nonopaque*, when used to describe urinary stones, only apply to the appearance of stones on plain abdominal radiographs.

Figure 20-3. TCC in the right kidney. *A,* Image from a retrograde pyelogram demonstrates an irregular filling defect in the right renal pelvis and proximal ureter *(arrows).* The collecting system above the mass is dilated. Note the right retrograde catheter *(single arrow)* in place for the contrast injection. A brush biopsy was performed using this catheter later in the study. *B,* CT scan on the same patient demonstrates a large mass in the right renal pelvis *(arrow)* that corresponds to the abnormality seen on the retrograde pyelogram.

14. **Is a filling defect in the collecting system diagnostic of TCC?**
    Certainly not! Other pathologic conditions that can cause a filling defect are nonopaque stones, blood clots, fungus balls in patients with a fungal urinary tract infection, and subepithelial cysts associated with chronic infection or inflammation.

15. **How do I distinguish between these very different pathologic conditions?**
    If a filling defect is detected in the collecting system, a brush biopsy is the next step, so that cytopathologic analysis can be performed. Nonopaque stones are mobile, whereas blood clots are always associated with gross hematuria. Fungus balls occur in immunocompromised patients with a fungal urinary tract infection.

Figure 20-4. Staghorn calculus within the right kidney, occupying a large part of the collecting system *(arrows).* These stones are usually related to chronic urinary tract infection and are composed of ammonium magnesium calcium phosphate.

KEY POINTS: IVU

1. All urinary stones are dense on CT scans, including those that are radiolucent (and therefore undetectable) on plain radiographs.

2. A renal mass detected on an IVU should be further characterized by cross-sectional imaging.

3. Patients with suspected acute renal colic are best evaluated with noncontrast CT rather than an IVU.

16. **My patient has severe flank pain after hiking all day in 100°F weather. What study should I order to exclude renal colic as a cause of his flank pain?**
CT is the diagnostic modality of choice in evaluating patients who are suspected of having acute renal colic due to a stone. No IV or oral contrast administration is necessary. Nearly all stones more than 2–3 mm are visible on CT.

17. **What abnormalities are seen on an IVU in a patient with acute renal colic?**
A stone may be visible on the scout radiograph, although calcified phleboliths in the pelvis can be confounding (Fig. 20-5, *A*). Phleboliths are small calcifications in pelvic veins that may be difficult to distinguish from ureteral stones on plain radiographs (and also noncontrast CT) but should lie outside the opacified ureter on an IVU and excretory phase CT. Obstruction due to a stone will cause a delay in excretion of contrast, as well as delayed drainage of contrast from the collecting system and ureter (Fig. 20-5, *B–D*).

18. **Since CT detects all stones, when is an IVU necessary in patients with urinary tract stones?**
An IVU is helpful in demonstrating the anatomy of the urinary tract in patients with recurrent stones, in patients in whom stone passage is arrested in the ureter, and in patients in whom surgical intervention is being contemplated to treat the stones. In such cases, the study helps identify congenital or acquired abnormalities that may be potentiating stone formation, collecting system damage related to chronic stone disease, and ureteral strictures that may prevent spontaneous passage of stones. Stones that are less than 5–6 mm in size almost always pass spontaneously, whereas larger stones may require surgical intervention.
  IVU may also demonstrate abnormalities, such as medullary nephrocalcinosis, that may be contributing to recurrent stone disease. Clustered calcifications are present in the medullary pyramids in patients with medullary nephrocalcinosis, which can be due to medullary sponge kidney, renal tubular acidosis, or hyperparathyroidism—the latter two diagnoses are made on clinical grounds, but medullary sponge kidney, in which the collecting ducts are dilated and prone to form stones, can be diagnosed only by an IVU.

19. **My patient is 2 days postsurgery for an abdominal tumor, and the surgical drains are putting out a lot of yellow fluid. What should I do?**
Collecting system or ureteral injury can be iatrogenic or related to blunt or penetrating abdominal trauma. A patient such as this can be evaluated either with an IVU or contrast-enhanced CT with imaging in the excretory phase. Both studies will show contrast leakage from the collecting system into the retroperitoneal tissues in the region of injury.

20. **Is there a role for IVU in evaluating patients with abdominal masses?**
An IVU offers information about the retroperitoneum only in an indirect manner. Displacement of the kidney or ureter may suggest the presence of a mass. Therefore, a cross-sectional study such as CT or MRI is the preferable study when a potential mass is being investigated. However,

Figure 20-5. Right ureteral calculus with partial obstruction. *A,* Preliminary radiograph. Multiple calcific densities are seen in the pelvis in this patient with right flank pain. The *long arrow* marks the irregular, right distal ureteral stone. The other densities, including the one marked by the *short arrow,* represent smoothly rounded calcified phleboliths. *B,* Nephrotomogram shows delayed excretion from the right kidney. The left kidney is normal in appearance (compare with Fig. 20-2, *B* with symmetrical excretion on both sides). *C,* Erect radiograph shows a column of contrast in the dilated right collecting system and ureter to the level of the bladder. The stone seen on the preliminary film is obscured on this image. Note the near-complete drainage of contrast from the normal left collecting system. *D,* Postvoid radiograph shows continuing ureteral dilation to the level of the stone *(short arrow).* Note that the other densities seen on the preliminary image are outside of the contrast-filled ureter, indicating that they are phleboliths. Note trouser zipper *(long arrow).*

retroperitoneal masses may be detected on an IVU performed for other reasons (Fig. 20-6). Thus, careful attention should be paid to the course and position of the kidneys and ureters when evaluating an IVU.

Figure 20-6. Left ureteral deviation by a retroperitoneal mass. *A,* Image from IVU shows focal lateral deviation of the left lumbar ureter *(arrow).* This indicates the presence of a retroperitoneal mass and should prompt further imaging to evaluate the retroperitoneum with CT or MRI. *B,* Contrast-enhanced CT scan demonstrates a large retroperitoneal mass *(arrow)* that proved to be a paraganglioma.

21. **What is the role of an IVU in a patient with suspected urinary tract obstruction?**
    If the patient has renal insufficiency with elevation in the serum creatinine level, contrast administration is contraindicated. Renal ultrasound is the best study to evaluate such a patient for a dilated collecting system, which would indicate obstruction. Isotope renal scan may also be useful in this clinical scenario. Nondilated obstructive uropathy is rare.

    In patients with normal renal function and suspected obstruction, renal ultrasound and isotope renal scan remain the mainstays for evaluation. In an occasional patient with equivocal results from other diagnostic tests, an IVU may help. Prompt and symmetric excretion on the two sides and complete drainage of the collecting systems on an erector postvoid radiograph effectively exclude significant urinary obstruction.

    In postoperative patients in whom urinary diversion has been performed, a study in the first few months after surgery serves as a baseline to exclude strictures at the ureteral anastomosis site.

22. **Is an IVU useful in patients with urinary tract infections?**
    In patients with clinically suspected acute pyelonephritis, an IVU has no role in diagnosis because the study results will usually be normal and thus neither confirm nor refute the clinical suspicion.

    In patients with chronic or recurrent urinary tract infections, an IVU may demonstrate a congenital abnormality or an obstructive lesion such as a stricture that may be contributory to the refractory urinary tract infection. Scarring of the parenchyma and calyces may confirm the diagnosis. Reflux nephropathy typically results in polar parenchymal scarring, particularly in the upper poles.

    In infections such as tuberculosis, cavitary changes may be seen in the renal papillae in association with strictures in the infundibula and parenchymal calcifications, which clinch the diagnosis.

BIBLIOGRAPHY

1. Choyke PL, Hricak H, Kenney PJ, et al: The future of research in genitourinary radiology: Through the looking glass—a view from the Society of Uroradiology. Radiology 207:3–6, 1998.

2. Dyer RB, Chen MYM, Zagoria RJ: Intravenous urography: Technique and interpretation. Radiographics 21:799–824, 2001.

3. Smith RC, Verga M, McCarthy S, Rosenfield AT: Diagnosis of acute flank pain: Value of unenhanced helical CT. Am J Roentgenol 166:97–101, 1996.

CHAPTER 21

GENITOURINARY FLUOROSCOPIC EXAMINATIONS

Parvati Ramchandani, MD

1. **What are genitourinary fluoroscopic examinations?**

   These are studies that require "real-time" observation using fluoroscopy so that maximal information is obtained about the anatomy of the structure being studied; some of the studies also provide physiologic information about function. Contrast is injected into the various portions of the urinary tract for these examinations. Some examples are retrograde pyelograms for evaluation of the upper urinary tract, cystogram or voiding cystourethrogram (VCUG) to evaluate the lower urinary tract, retrograde urethrogram (RUG) to evaluate the urethra, and hysterosalpingogram to evaluate the uterus and fallopian tubes.

2. **How are retrograde pyelograms and intravenous urograms (IVU) different? Do they provide the same information?**

   For a retrograde pyelogram, cystoscopy is performed (most often by a urologist) and a catheter is placed into the renal pelvis. Contrast is injected through this catheter under fluoroscopic guidance to evaluate the lumen of the pyelocalyceal system and the ureter for mucosal abnormalities, such as transitional cell carcinoma.

   As discussed in Chapter 20, an IVU requires the IV administration of contrast, and it provides physiologic information about the function of the kidney, in addition to depicting the anatomy of the renal parenchyma and the collecting systems. A retrograde pyelogram only provides anatomic information about the lumen of the collecting system, but the depiction of the anatomy is superior to that seen with an IVU.

   A retrograde pyelogram is performed if the patient cannot receive IV contrast because of renal insufficiency or a history of severe contrast allergy. Retrograde examination can also be performed if the IVU fails to show the entire pyelocalyceal system or ureter or to further evaluate an abnormality seen on an IVU.

3. **What is the difference between a cystogram and a VCUG?**

   A cystogram is tailored to evaluate the urinary bladder alone, whereas a VCUG includes evaluation of the bladder neck and urethra under fluoroscopic observation. Both studies require injection of radiographic contrast into the urinary bladder through either an indwelling bladder drainage catheter or a catheter placed in the urinary bladder solely for the procedure. A cystogram is limited to images of the bladder, whereas in a VCUG, the catheter is removed after the bladder has been distended with contrast, and the patient voids under fluoroscopic observation so that the bladder neck and urethra can also be evaluated.

4. **What are the indications for cystogram and VCUG?**

   These studies can be performed to evaluate the anatomy of the bladder and urethra in patients with voiding dysfunction or recurrent urinary tract infections (UTIs) (Fig. 21-1), to look for a leak or fistula from the bladder after surgery or abdominal trauma (Fig. 21-2), to evaluate vesicoureteral reflux, or to evaluate urinary incontinence.

5. **Is a cystogram sensitive in excluding a leak from the bladder?**

   Yes, but only if the study is performed in the correct manner. It is important to distend the urinary bladder with contrast until a detrusor contraction occurs, which indicates that the bladder capacity has been reached. Otherwise, small leaks may not be demonstrated. There is a great deal of variation in the amount of bladder filling required to produce a detrusor contraction, but most patients require 300–600 mL of contrast to reach this point. A detrusor contraction is recognized by one of the following: (1) the patient voids, (2) there is resistance to injection of contrast through a handheld syringe so that the barrel of the syringe starts to move back, or (3) flow through a contrast-filled bag 35–40 cm above the fluoroscopy table stops or reverses.

6. **A patient is brought to the emergency department with blunt abdominal trauma and pelvic fractures. Does he need both an abdominopelvic computed tomography (CT) scan and a fluoroscopic cystogram?**
Not at all. The bladder can be distended with contrast on the CT table (called a *CT cystogram*) to evaluate for a leak. A CT cystogram is as sensitive a study as a fluoroscopic cystogram, if not more so, in excluding a leak from the urinary bladder. However, before placing a catheter in the urinary bladder in a patient with pelvic fractures, the urethra should be evaluated with a RUG and a catheter advanced through the urethra only if there is no urethral injury. Failure to follow this sequence could cause a partial urethral injury to become a complete urethral disruption.

7. **Why is vesicoureteral reflux (VUR) important? How is it demonstrated?**
VUR in children can cause recurrent UTIs and lead to permanent renal scarring, referred to as *reflux nephropathy*. This can cause complications such as hypertension and renal insufficiency; 10–30% of all

Figure 21-1. Cystogram in a 70-year-old man with complaints of incomplete emptying. There is a large bladder diverticulum (D) arising from the left side of the urinary bladder (B) with a wide neck *(single arrow)*. When the patient voids, contrast (and urine) fills the diverticulum and then flows back into the urinary bladder when voiding stops, accounting for the patient's symptoms of incomplete emptying. The urine stasis in a bladder diverticulum can be associated with the formation of stones or recurrent UTIs. The *double arrows* point to a surgical clip in the pelvis from a previous surgery.

Figure 21-2. VCUG in a 40-year-old woman with vaginal leakage after hysterectomy. There is a fistula *(arrow)* between the posterior aspect of the urinary bladder (B) and the vagina (V). Vesicovaginal fistulas can be a complication of hysterectomy; difficult vaginal delivery, particularly if forceps are used; cesarean section; and gynecologic neoplasms, such as cervical cancer.

cases of end-stage renal disease may be related to reflux nephropathy. In adults, VUR has less clinical significance, although it can be associated with recurrent UTI and, rarely, even flank pain.

VUR is reliably demonstrated by fluoroscopically monitored VCUG. If the bladder is not distended to the point of voiding, VUR may not be demonstrated. In children, radionuclide cystography is an alternative study to minimize the radiation exposure to pelvic organs.

8. **What is a RUG?**
   It is a study used primarily to evaluate the anterior urethra in men (Fig. 21-3). The male urethra is divided into two portions: the posterior urethra, consisting of the prostatic and membranous urethra, and the anterior urethra, consisting of the bulbar and pendulous urethra. The external urethral sphincter, located in the urogenital diaphragm, demarcates the posterior urethra from the anterior urethra. The posterior urethra has smooth muscle that relaxes when the detrusor muscle contracts during voiding and is thus best seen on a VCUG. Although visualized on a VCUG, the anterior urethra is better evaluated by a RUG, which is performed by placing a Foley catheter in the tip of the penis and injecting contrast under fluoroscopic guidance. The urethra is usually opacified only to the level of the external sphincter on a RUG since the sphincter is contracted in the nonvoiding state and contrast cannot flow proximal to it.

Figure 21-3. RUG in a 30-year-old man with history of gonorrhea. *A,* The balloon of the Foley catheter *(arrow)* is in the tip of the penis and has been distended with contrast. The balloon is usually placed in the fossa navicularis, which is an area of natural widening in the glans penis. *B,* The anterior urethra is opacified with contrast. There are multiple strictures *(arrows)* in the penile urethra, typical of inflammatory disease. The bulbar urethra is the urethral segment proximal to the *arrows.* The wide caliber of the proximal bulbar urethra is the normal appearance of this segment of the bulbar urethra.

9. **How is the female urethra evaluated?**
   The entire female urethra is well demonstrated on VCUG (Fig. 21-4). The short length of the female urethra makes a RUG a difficult and unnecessary procedure in women.

10. **What is a loopogram?**
    In patients who have undergone cystectomy (usually performed for muscle-invasive bladder cancer), the ureters are connected to a loop of ileum known as an *ileal conduit*. The ileal conduit is excluded from the intestinal stream and is connected to the

anterior abdominal wall through a stoma; a urinary drainage bag is usually applied to the stoma site. A loopogram is performed to evaluate the conduit and the upper urinary tracts. A catheter is placed in the ileal conduit, and contrast is injected under fluoroscopic guidance until it refluxes in a retrograde fashion into the ureters and the pyelocalyceal systems.

11. **What is a hysterosalpingogram?**
It is a study to evaluate the uterine cavity and the fallopian tubes (Fig. 21-5). After sterile cleansing of the vaginal canal and the exocervix, a cannula is placed in the external cervical os and contrast is injected under fluoroscopic guidance. The procedure is performed in women with primary or secondary infertility and in women with recurrent miscarriages.

Figure 21-4. VCUG in a 34-year-old woman. There is a large pocket of contrast on the posterior aspect of the urethra that represents a urethral diverticulum *(arrows)*. A urethral diverticulum is usually the result of infection in periurethral glands, which decompress into the urethra and result in a communicating cavity. Patients present with postvoid dribbling, perineal discomfort, or recurrent UTIs.

KEY POINTS: GENITOURINARY FLUOROSCOPIC EXAMINATIONS ✔

1. Diagnosing small leaks from the urinary bladder requires adequate distention until a detrusor contraction occurs, regardless of whether the evaluation is performed with CT or fluoroscopy.

2. The anterior urethra in men is better evaluated on an RUG. The posterior urethra in men is better evaluated on a VCUG.

3. In a male patient with pelvic trauma, the urethra should be evaluated with a RUG before placement of a bladder drainage catheter.

4. A retrograde pyelogram is an alternative study to an IVU to evaluate the urothelium in patients in whom IV contrast administration is contraindicated.

5. A hysterosalpingogram is the most useful imaging study to evaluate both the uterus and the fallopian tubes in patients with infertility.

12. **Does a magnetic resonance imaging (MRI) or an ultrasound examination of the pelvis provide the same information as a hysterosalpingogram?**
MRI and ultrasound are excellent at demonstrating the uterus, but both studies are poor at showing the normal fallopian tubes. Dilated fallopian tubes (hydrosalpinx) can be identified on MRI and ultrasound, but abnormality in nondilated tubes is best seen on a hysterosalpingogram (Fig. 21-6).

Figure 21-5. Normal hysterosalpingogram in a young woman with primary infertility. The metal cannula within the external os is seen at the bottom of the figure. The uterine cavity and both fallopian tubes are normal in appearance. There is contrast spilling from both tubes into the pelvic peritoneal cavity, a normal finding.

Figure 21-6. Hysterosalpingogram in a woman with history of pelvic inflammatory disease (PID). Outpouchings of contrast *(arrows)* are seen in the proximal portions of both fallopian tubes, a sequel of prior PID. This is known as *salpingitis isthmica nodosa*, and it is associated with tubal dysmotility and infertility. This diagnosis would be difficult to make with any other imaging modality. The patient was advised to consider in vitro fertilization.

13. **If I have a female patient with a pelvic mass, what study will be helpful in further evaluation?**
Either an MRI or ultrasound will be useful to determine the organ of origin of the mass (gynecologic vs. nongynecologic mass, uterine vs. ovarian origin) and to characterize it further. A hysterosalpingogram has no role in this situation.

14. **What about my postmenopausal patient with vaginal bleeding? Will a hysterosalpingogram be helpful in evaluating the endometrium in this patient?**
Endometrial abnormalities such as endometrial hyperplasia or endometrial cancer can cause perimenopausal/postmenopausal bleeding and are best evaluated by a transvaginal ultrasound or pelvic MRI.

BIBLIOGRAPHY

1. Dunnick NR, Sandler CM, Newhouse JH, Amis ES (eds): Textbook of Uroradiology, 3rd ed. Philadelphia, Lippincott Williams & Wilkins, 2001.
2. Sandler CM, Goldman SM, Kawashima A: Lower urinary tract trauma. World J Urol 16:69–75, 1998.
3. Vaccaro JP, Brody JM: CT cystography in the evaluation of major bladder trauma. Radiographics 20:1373–1381, 2000.

CHAPTER 22

CT AND MRI OF THE KIDNEY

E. Scott Pretorius, MD

1. **What computed tomography (CT) protocol should I use to characterize a focal renal mass?**

    A dedicated renal CT includes both precontrast and postcontrast images since the radiologist needs to compare the appearance of a lesion on these two sets of images to determine whether a lesion displays enhancement. Most CT examinations of the abdomen include only postcontrast images and are therefore not optimal for characterizing a renal mass.

2. **What magnetic resonance imaging (MRI) protocol should I use to characterize a focal renal mass?**

    At the Hospital of the University of Pennsylvania, our preferred protocol is as follows: (1) breath-held, T1-weighted gradient-echo images, in-phase and out-of-phase; (2) axial fat-saturated fast spin echo T2-weighted images; (3) coronal, fat-saturated, three-dimensional T1-weighted gradient-echo images obtained before, during, and after the injection of IV gadolinium contrast; and (4) axial, delayed phase, T1-weighted gradient-echo images of the entire abdomen.

    In the kidneys and elsewhere in the body, it is imperative that, if IV contrast is administered, a set of precontrast images be acquired with parameters (e.g., TR, TE, and flip angle) that are *exactly* the same as those of the postcontrast acquisition. This is the only way that one can determine whether a lesion is enhanced.

3. **What is the normal enhancement pattern of the kidneys on CT and MRI?**

    Because the kidneys receive approximately 25% of cardiac output, the kidneys enhance avidly and rapidly after contrast administration.
    - Early renal enhancement on CT and MRI is termed the *corticomedullary phase,* in which the peripheral renal cortex enhances more than the central renal medulla does (Fig. 22-1, *A*).
    - The corticomedullary phase is followed by the nephrographic phase (Fig. 22-1, *B*), in which the renal cortex and medulla enhance to roughly the same degree. This is generally the best phase in which to detect renal neoplasms.
    - Finally, in the excretory phase, a functioning kidney will excrete the injected contrast material. This material will be bright in the renal collecting system on CT. The T1 appearance of excreted gadolinium chelates will depend on whether the kidney is making diluted or concentrated urine. More diluted gadolinium chelates in urine are bright on T1, due to T1-shortening effects. At higher concentrations, gadolinium chelates may appear very dark on T1-weighted images, as T2 effects predominate (Fig. 22-1, *C*).

4. **What are the expected CT and MRI findings related to renal cell carcinoma (RCC)?**

    Due to the presence of internal necrosis or hemorrhage, the appearance of RCC is variable. The common finding on CT and MRI of RCCs is that they enhance after the administration of IV contrast, and, unlike benign angiomyolipomas, they do not contain macroscopic fat. A solid renal lesion that enhances and does *not* contain macroscopic fat is an RCC until proven otherwise (Figs. 22-2 and 22-3).

5. **What are the risk factors for RCC?**

    Known risk factors include cigarette smoking, exposure to petroleum products or asbestos, hypertension, and obesity. RCC is approximately twice as common in men than in women and

Figure 22-1. Axial T1-weighted gradient-echo images with fat saturation in the *A,* corticomedullary, *B,* nephrographic, and *C,* excretory phase after administration of IV gadolinium chelate contrast agent. Excreted gadolinium chelate *(arrows)* may appear either bright on T1 (if diluted urine) or, as in this case, dark on T1 (if concentrated urine).

Figure 22-2. Axial postcontrast CT demonstrates a large, solid, enhancing renal lesion *(arrow)* that does not contain macroscopic fat. Such a lesion should be removed. This lesion was an RCC.

Figure 22-3. *A,* Axial T2-weighted image and *B,* axial postcontrast T1-weighted gradient-echo image demonstrate a large, enhancing left retroperitoneal mass that arose from the left kidney. This lesion, which did not contain macroscopic fat, was an RCC.

slightly more common in African Americans than in people of European descent. Most RCC patients are older than 40 and tend to be in the seventh or eighth decade of life. Persons with acquired cystic kidney disease, von Hippel-Lindau syndrome, and hereditary papillary renal cancer, and possibly those with tuberous sclerosis, are also at increased risk.

6. **What is the Bosniak system for cystic renal lesions?**
   This important classification system describes features of cystic renal lesions and indicates recommendations for lesion management. Although developed for CT, the morphologic features can be applied to MRI as well. Calcifications within a lesion will likely be best seen on unenhanced CT. Internal soft tissue architecture within a cystic lesion will likely be best depicted on multiplanar MRI.
   - *Class 1* lesions are simple cysts. On CT or MRI, they have a thin or imperceptible wall, have no internal architecture, and do not enhance after contrast administration.
   - *Class 2* lesions may have a single, thin septation or fine mural calcification. Also included in class 2 lesions are CT "hyperdense" cysts, which contain internal protein or hemorrhage and therefore are hyperintense to normal renal parenchyma on T1-weighted images. These benign cysts do not enhance after contrast administration and have variable T2 signal intensity depending on their protein content.
   - *Class 3* lesions have thicker septations, multiple septations, or bulky mural calcifications. Class 3 lesions should be excised.
   - *Class 4* lesions display enhancing, mural, solid nodules and should be excised. The majority of these lesions are RCCs (Fig. 22-4).

7. **What if I cannot tell whether a septation is thin or thick or whether the mural calcification is fine or bulky?**
   Deciding whether a cystic renal lesion is class 2 or class 3 can often hinge on whether an internal septation is judged to be "thin" (class 2) or "thick" (class 3) or whether mural calcification is "fine" (class 2) or "bulky" (class 3). For the rare lesions that are truly indeterminate, class 2F may be

assigned. These lesions are monitored with use of CT or MRI, usually at an interval of 4–6 months.

8. **Is CT or MRI better for characterizing cystic renal lesions?**
This question has no simple answer. Both modalities have proven to be very good at characterizing renal masses. A high-quality MRI performed on a high-field (1.5 Tesla) scanner is, overall, probably better than CT for characterizing renal masses because of the high soft tissue contrast of MRI. However, high-quality MRI is somewhat difficult to perform, given that it requires considerable experience on the part of

Figure 22-4. Coronal postcontrast T1-weighted gradient-echo image with fat saturation demonstrates a cystic left renal lesion with an enhancing mural nodule *(arrow)*. This is a Bosniak 4 cystic RCC.

the technologist and radiologist. A good MRI examination also requires a cooperative patient because the examination necessitates that the patient remain motionless during imaging and perform several breath-holds.

If a patient is not capable of remaining motionless or performing multiple breath-holds, a CT examination is likely to be much better than a motion-filled MRI.

Because IV contrast is necessary to characterize most renal masses, the patient's renal status may be an issue. In general, iodine-based agents (for CT) are not administered to patients with serum creatinine levels greater than 1.5. Gadolinium chelates (for MRI) are considered safe, even for patients with very limited renal function. Patients undergoing dialysis treatment can receive either kind of contrast, provided they undergo dialysis within 24 hours after the study.

9. **What is an angiomyolipoma?**
An angiomyolipoma is a benign hamartoma that, as its name suggests, contains elements of blood vessels (angio-), muscle (myo-), and fat (lipoma). Because of their solid nature and enhancement, angiomyolipomas may be confused with enhancing RCCs. A CT (Fig. 22-5) or MRI (Fig. 22-6) diagnosis of angiomyolipoma is made by identifying macroscopic fat (a region of negative Hounsfield [HU] values on CT, or tissue that follows the signal intensity of body wall fat when the same MR sequence is performed with and without frequency-selective fat saturation).

Figure 22-5. Axial unenhanced CT image demonstrates a fat-density mass *(arrow)* in the left anterior interpolar region. Since this renal lesion contains material that is of fat attenuation, it is a benign angiomyolipoma.

10. **What syndrome is associated with angiomyolipomas?**
Tuberous sclerosis. This syndrome can cause renal cysts and/or renal angiomyolipomas. Tuberous sclerosis probably also puts a patient at a slightly higher risk for RCC. Angiomyolipomas can also occur sporadically in patients without tuberous sclerosis.

11. **How are angiomyolipomas treated?**
They are usually embolized (i.e., deprived of their blood supply) when they grow to be 4 cm or greater. This is performed because larger lesions have a greater risk of hemorrhage.

12. **I see an enhancing renal mass that does not have fat attenuation on CT and does not have fat signal on MRI. What is the differential diagnosis?**
This lesion would be presumed to be an RCC until proven otherwise. Other lesions that could have this appearance include oncocytoma, transitional cell carcinoma, angiomyolipoma without detectable fat, or renal lymphoma.

13. **How is RCC staged with CT and MRI?**
RCC is most commonly staged using the Robson classification. Stage 1 includes tumors that are confined entirely to the kidney. Stage 2 lesions invade the per-inephric fat or the adrenal gland on the same side. Stage 3a includes tumor thrombus in the renal vein or inferior vena cava (IVC); 3b includes a tumor in regional lymph nodes; and 3c involves both regional lymph nodes and the renal vein and/or IVC. Stage 4 RCCs involve distant metas-tases, such as the lung, liver, or bones.

14. **What does renal infarction look like on CT and MRI?**
Patients with embolic disease or injury to the aorta, renal artery, or a renal artery branch can develop segmental renal infarctions. These are wedge-shaped areas of hypoen-hancement that are broader at the periphery of the kidney and narrow near the center of the kidney. In segmental renal infarction, there is often a thin rim of preserved enhancement at the edge of the kidney because this region has a separate arterial supply via the renal capsular artery.

Figure 22-6. Axial T1-weighted gradient-echo images obtained, *A*, in phase, *B*, out of phase *C*, with explicit fat saturation, and, *D*, with explicit water saturation. The right-sided renal lesion *(arrows)* follows the signal of the body wall fat on all pulse sequences, indicating the presence of macroscopic fat within the lesion. This is diagnostic of a benign angiomyolipoma.

15. **What does renal laceration look like on CT?**
    Laceration of the kidney complicates 10–25% of cases of blunt abdominal trauma. In patients with renal cortical laceration, CT will show interruption of the renal cortex with associated subcapsular hematoma.

16. **What findings on a trauma CT indicate that a kidney needs to be surgically repaired?**
    Superficial renal lacerations in patients with a stable condition can be managed conservatively, without surgery. Surgical repair is indicated for deep lacerations with disruption of the collecting system, comminuted renal fractures, and vascular pedicle injuries. Vascular pedicle injuries may include arterial/venous avulsion, intimal flap dissection, or traumatic vessel occlusion.

17. **What is autosomal dominant polycystic kidney disease (ADPCKD)? Is it associated with RCC?**
    As the name implies, this is a slowly progressive, single-gene inherited condition that leads to the formation of multiple renal cysts in the kidneys. Although many people present as adults with symptoms of renal enlargement and renal insufficiency (with associated hypertension and anemia), affected individuals may begin to develop cysts in childhood. Persons with ADPCKD often also develop multiple liver cysts and are at increased risk for developing intracerebral aneurysms. There is no increased risk of RCC.

18. **What is autosomal recessive polycystic kidney disease (ARPCKD)? Is it associated with RCC?**
    ARPCKD usually manifests itself on prenatal sonography or in early childhood. The disease may be fatal in very early childhood, but some patients survive into adolescence. ARPCKD is associated with congenital hepatic fibrosis. There is no increased risk of RCC.

19. **What two genetically inherited syndromes *are* associated with RCC?**
    Von Hippel-Lindau syndrome and the very rare hereditary papillary RCC syndrome are both autosomal dominantly inherited and associated with the development of multiple RCCs. A diagnosis of one of these syndromes often leads to screening of first-degree relatives because they may also carry the disease gene.

20. **What is acquired cystic renal disease? Is it associated with RCC?**
    Acquired cystic renal disease is the term applied to end-stage renal disease in patients who are receiving dialysis and have very small kidneys with multiple cysts. The risk these patients have of developing RCC is six to seven times greater than normal.

KEY POINTS: CT AND MRI OF THE KIDNEY

1. An enhancing renal mass that does not contain macroscopic fat is an RCC until proven otherwise.

2. An enhancing renal lesion with macroscopic fat is a benign angiomyolipoma.

3. Cystic renal lesions that contain thick internal septations, thick mural calcification, or enhancing mural nodules are suggestive of cystic RCCs and should be excised.

21. **Should patients who are undergoing dialysis be screened for RCC?**
    This is controversial. RCCs found in patients with acquired cystic renal disease are often low-grade neoplasms and are therefore of relatively little clinical significance in patients with expected short life spans and multiple co-morbid diseases. If screening is performed, it is

probably best reserved for younger patients or for patients who, other than their renal disease, are in good health.

22. **What are some features that suggest oncocytoma on CT and MRI?**
Oncocytomas are solid, enhancing lesions that may display a central, hypoenhancing scar and tend to be relatively homogeneous for lesion size. Because these findings can also be seen in RCC, oncocytomas cannot be reliably differentiated from RCCs on CT or MRI. Although most exhibit benign behavior, there have been reports of rare metastases from oncocytomas. They are perhaps best thought of as lesions of low malignant potential, and most can be excised with partial nephrectomy.

23. **What are the findings associated with pyelonephritis on CT or MRI?**
The affected kidney is usually enlarged, and there may be stranding in the fat surrounding the kidney. The enhancement of the kidney will often be delayed, relative to the unaffected contralateral kidney. A "striated nephrogram" can usually be seen, especially on delayed phase images, on which the kidney will display alternating bands of high and low CT attenuation or MR signal intensity (*see* Fig. 19-6).

24. **I see a multiloculated cystic lesion that looks like it has herniated into the renal collecting system. What could this be?**
This is likely a multilocular cystic nephroma. This unusual lesion is found in young boys and in older women. As its name suggests, it appears as an agglomeration of multiple cystic spaces. In approximately one third of cases, the lesion can herniate into the renal collecting system.
    Although considered benign, in approximately 7% of cases the multilocular cystic nephroma will undergo sarcomatous degeneration. These lesions are therefore excised.

25. **Are CT and MRI useful in imaging transitional cell carcinoma (TCC)?**
TCC may arise in the epithelium of the renal collecting systems, the ureters, the urinary bladder, and portions of the urethra. Both CT and MRI can detect large masses, but with both modalities, it is difficult to identify small, flat tumors that do not result in proximal hydroureteronephrosis. Intravenous urography (IVU) remains superior to CT and MRI for detecting this type of lesion, although multidetector CT urography and gadolinium-enhanced MR urography are rapidly gaining acceptance as viable alternatives to IVU in imaging patients for suspected TCC.

26. **What are the typical MR signal characteristics of TCC?**
TCC is hyperintense on T1-weighted images and hypointense on T2-weighted images compared with surrounding urine.

27. **What does renal lymphoma look like on CT and MRI?**
Renal lymphoma is usually B-cell lymphoma and is generally a manifestation of widespread systemic disease. The most common initial presentation is a large retroperitoneal mass, surrounding one or both kidneys and possibly the IVC and aorta. It is of low intermediate signal on both T1- and T2-weighted images, similar to that of the spleen or lymph nodes. It enhances weakly after contrast administration.
    After the patient is treated for lymphoma, renal involvement by the disease is often seen as multiple, focal, rounded intraparenchymal masses.

28. **Does metastatic disease go to the kidneys? What does it look like on CT or MRI?**
Yes, metastatic disease can go to the kidneys, although these lesions are usually very small and not of clinical significance. They are seen often on autopsy but usually do not cause clinical morbidity on their own. On CT or MRI, they are seen as multiple, bilateral renal lesions with infiltrative margins.

29. **We were asked to perform a CT (or MRI) examination on a patient who is a potential renal donor. What protocol should we use?**

Either CT or MRI may be used to evaluate a potential renal donor. On CT, a precontrast topogram may be used to evaluate for the presence of renal stones. Multidetector thin-section imaging through the kidneys is performed to detect and evaluate the renal arteries. Delayed phase imaging may be performed to evaluate venous morphology. Finally, an excretory phase topogram can be performed to visualize the renal collecting system and ureters.

On MRI, precontrast T1 gradient-echo and T2-weighted images are acquired, followed by coronal, three-dimensional T1 gradient-echo images acquired in the arterial and venous phases of enhancement. Ten milligrams of furosemide may be given with the gadolinium chelate approximately 5 minutes before the MR urogram is obtained.

30. **We performed a CT (or MRI) examination on a patient who is a potential renal donor. What kinds of things should we include in the report?**

Important information includes renal size; the presence or absence of a renal mass or other renal abnormality; and the number, size, and position of renal arteries, renal veins, and ureters for each kidney.

Renal artery duplication is common; it is found in approximately 30% of all kidneys. The morphology of the left renal vein is more variable than that of the right renal vein. The left renal vein usually passes anterior to the aorta before joining the IVC. In approximately 3% of cases, the left renal vein is retroaortic, and in fewer than 1% of cases, it is circumaortic, meaning that there is a left renal vein that passes anterior to the aorta and a left renal vein posterior to the aorta.

31. **I have an emergency room patient with flank pain. What is the best radiologic test to find renal and ureteral calculi?**

Unenhanced multidetector CT has replaced IVU as the examination of choice for identifying renal and ureteral stones (Fig. 22-7). If a cause for the patient's pain is not found or if a calcific density is identified but it cannot be determined whether the density lies within the ureter, contrast may be given and the abdomen and pelvis scanned again.

Figure 22-7. Axial unenhanced CT images of the *A,* kidneys and *B,* the pelvis, demonstrate the presence of a 1-mm right renal calculus *(arrow)*. The patient's flank pain was due to a right distal ureteral calculus *(B)* *(arrow)*.

32. **What is post-transplant lymphoproliferative disorder (PTLD)?**

PTLD is a spectrum of diseases ranging from benign lymphoid proliferation to malignant lymphoma. PTLD is caused by the Epstein-Barr virus and is seen in transplant patients receiving immunosuppressive medications such as azathioprine (Imuran), muromonab-CD3 (Orthoclone OKT3), and cyclosporine. Greater amounts of immune suppression are associated with higher rates of incidence of PTLD. Liver transplant recipients are at greater risk for PTLD than are renal transplant recipients.

33. **Other than PTLD, what else can go wrong with a renal transplant?**
    Things can go wrong with any of the surgical anastomoses—arterial, venous, and ureteral. Complications include renal artery stenosis, renal artery thrombosis, renal vein thrombosis, and ureteral leak. Patients may also develop pelvic "masses," including urinoma, hematoma, and lymphocele. Finally, the transplant may not function well and may develop acute tubular necrosis or rejection.

34. **What is a horseshoe kidney?**
    When the lower poles of the left and right kidneys are attached to one another, it is called a *horseshoe kidney*. The region of connection, termed the *isthmus*, may be composed of fibrous tissue or functioning renal parenchyma. Horseshoe kidney is more common in patients with Turner's syndrome.

35. **What diseases do patients with horseshoe kidney have a greater risk of acquiring?**
    Patients with horseshoe kidney are at increased risk for ureteropelvic junction obstruction, stone formation, vesicoureteral reflux, infection, trauma, Wilms' tumor, TCC, and RCC.

BIBLIOGRAPHY

1. Israel GM, Krinsky GA: MR imaging of the kidneys and adrenal glands. Radiol Clin North Am 41(1):145–159, 2003.
2. Pretorius ES, Wickstrom ML, Siegelman ES: MR imaging of renal neoplasms. Magn Reson Imaging Clin North Am 8(4):813–833, 2000.
3. Teichman JM: Clinical practice: Acute renal colic from ureteral calculus. N Engl J Med 350(7):684–693, 2004.
4. Thomsen HS: Guidelines for contrast media from the European Society of Urogenital Radiology. Am J Roentgenol 181(6):1463–1471, 2003.

CHAPTER 23

CT AND MRI OF THE ADRENAL GLANDS

E. Scott Pretorius, MD

1. **Where are the adrenal glands?**
   The adrenal glands lie superior to the upper poles of the kidneys and are contained, with the kidneys, within Gerota's fascia. The right adrenal gland lies posterior to the inferior vena cava (IVC), medial to the right lobe of the liver, and lateral to the right diaphragmatic crus. The left adrenal gland lies slightly inferior to the right adrenal gland. It can be found to the left of the aorta and the left diaphragmatic crus, posterior to the splenic vessels.

2. **What do normal adrenal glands look like on computed tomography (CT) and magnetic resonance imaging (MRI)?**
   On CT, the adrenal glands are of soft tissue attenuation and therefore are denser than the surrounding fat. On MRI, the normal adrenal gland has similar signal intensity to that of the kidney on both T1- and T2-weighted images. Both adrenal glands are most commonly shaped like an inverted letter Y or an inverted letter V. Each adrenal gland has a body, medial limb, and lateral limb. Each limb is most commonly 4–6 mm in thickness and should be less than 10 mm in thickness (Fig. 23-1).

Figure 23-1. Axial T1-weighted gradient-echo image after gadolinium administration demonstrates the normal appearance of the adrenal glands *(arrows)*. The limbs of the normal adrenal are less than 10 mm in thickness.

3. **What is the differential diagnosis of an adrenal lesion seen on CT or MRI?**
   The differential diagnosis of an adrenal lesion includes both benign and malignant entities. Benign lesions include adrenal cortical adenomas (which are very common), adrenal cysts, and myelolipoma. Adrenal hemorrhage may mimic a solid lesion. Malignant causes include metastatic disease, which is very common, and adrenal cortical carcinoma. Adrenal pheochromocytomas may exhibit either benign (approximately 90%) or malignant (approximately 10%) behavior. In the absence of a known malignancy, a small (1 cm or smaller), well-circumscribed adrenal lesion is virtually always benign.

4. **What is chemical shift imaging?**
   Chemical shift imaging is an MRI technique that is used to determine whether both lipid and water protons are present with the same small voxel (three-dimensional pixel) of space (Fig. 23-2). T1-weighted gradient-echo images are obtained both "in phase" (meaning that the signals of lipid and water protons are additive and both contribute to the observed signal intensity) and "out of phase" (meaning that the signals of lipid and water protons are destructive to one another; if both are present in a voxel, their signals will tend to cancel each other out). If one therefore compares an in-phase image with an out-of-phase image, there will be less signal on the out-of-phase image in areas that contain *both* lipid and water protons.

Note, however, that in areas that contain all lipid protons and in areas that contain all water protons, the signal will not change between the two images. To see the effect of destructive interference on the out-of-phase image, both kinds of protons must be present.

5. **How can I tell which is the out-of-phase image?**

   The out-of-phase image can be identified by the dark outlines seen at fat-water interfaces (*see* Fig. 23-2, *B*). This is seen, for example, where the kidneys meet the fat that sur- rounds them. This is termed "etch- ing" artifact or "India ink" artifact.

   The TR of the in-phase image and the out-of-phase image should always be the same, so that valid signal comparisons can be made between the two images. At 1.5 Tesla, a TE of 4.4 ms is in phase, and multiples of this time ($2 \times 4.4 = 8.8$ ms) are also in-phase. Other TEs are out of phase. In this example, a TE of 2.2 ms is directly out of phase, and it is here that the maximum chemical shift effect is observed.

Figure 23-2. Coronal T1-weighted gradient-echo images, *A,* in-phase and, *B,* out of phase demonstrate dramatic signal loss in bilateral adrenal lesions *(arrows)* on the out- of-phase image relative to the in phase image. This finding indicates the presence of both fat and water protons in the lesions and is diagnostic of benign adrenal adenomas.

6. **How can MRI be used to show that an adrenal lesion is an adenoma?**

   The presence of intracytoplasmic lipid is very specific for the diagnosis of benign adenoma. About 70% of all adrenal adenomas exhibit the presence of this lipid and are termed "lipid-rich" adenomas. The remainder are termed "lipid-poor" adenomas.

   MRI is very sensitive at detecting intracytoplasmic lipid. T1-weighted gradient-echo images can be obtained both in-phase and out-of-phase. If the signal intensity within the adrenal lesion on the out-of-phase image is 20% less than the signal within the lesion on the in-phase image, this demonstrates that there is intracytoplasmic lipid present, and the lesion is therefore a benign adenoma (*see* Fig. 23-2).

7. **How can unenhanced CT be used to show that an adrenal lesion is an adenoma?**

   Thin-section (5 mm or thinner) unenhanced CT is performed. If the adrenal lesion measures less than 10 Hounsfield units (HU) on unenhanced CT, this is generally accepted as indicating the presence of intracytoplasmic lipid within a benign adenoma (Fig. 23-3, *A*).

8. **Are there any malignant adrenal lesions that can contain intracytoplasmic lipid?**

   Unfortunately, yes. Clear cell renal cell carcinomas often have detectable intracytoplasmic lipid and therefore are of low CT attenuation and display signal loss on chemical shift MRI. If these tumors metastasize to the adrenal gland, the adrenal metastases will mimic adenomas on unenhanced CT and chemical shift MRI.

9. **How can enhanced CT be used to show that an adrenal lesion is an adrenal cortical adenoma?**

   If unenhanced CT does not characterize the adrenal lesion, IV contrast can be given. CT imaging of the adrenal gland is performed both 80 seconds and 10 minutes after contrast administration. Region-of-interest measurements are taken of the adrenal lesion on both the 80-second and 10-minute scan, and a percentage of "washout" is calculated. The percentage of contrast agent washout is equal to [1 − (attenuation at 10 minutes/attenuation at 80 seconds)] × 100%.

   Washout that is greater than 50% is very specific for benign adrenal adenoma. Metastatic disease characteristically displays washout of less than 50% (Fig. 23-3, *B–C*). Interestingly, the presence or absence of intracytoplasmic lipid within an adenoma does not make a lesion more or less likely to display washout.

Figure 23-3. *A,* Axial, unenhanced CT performed in a 73-year-old woman with lung cancer and an adrenal lesion demonstrates that the adrenal lesion measures 3.82 HU. Since this lesion is less than 10 HU, it is a benign adenoma. Postcontrast CT images obtained at 80 seconds *(B)* and 10 minutes *(C)* after contrast administration demonstrate that the lesion measures 105.56 HU at 80 seconds postcontrast and 36.30 HU at 10 minutes postcontrast. Since the washout is greater than 50%, this lesion is confirmed to represent a benign adenoma.

10. **Which is better for imaging the adrenal glands, CT or MRI?**
    This is controversial. It depends a great deal on institutional experience and the level of expertise exhibited by the technologist and radiologist. Chemical shift MRI is easily performed, but some centers may lack experience with this technique. Many adrenal lesions are incidentally discovered on CT, but since neither thin-section unenhanced images nor 10-minute delayed images are part of most abdominal CT protocols, the patient will often have to return for a second study.

11. **What is the difference between a functioning and a nonfunctioning adenoma? Can CT or MRI differentiate these?**
    CT and MRI cannot differentiate functioning adenomas (those that have endocrine activity) from those that are nonfunctioning. Functioning adenomas may result in hyperaldosteronism (Conn's syndrome) or hypercortisolism (Cushing's syndrome).

12. **What is a myelolipoma, and how can CT and MRI be used to show that an adrenal lesion is a myelolipoma?**
    Adrenal myelolipomas are benign adrenal neoplasms composed of fatty tissue and variable amounts of hematopoietic elements. On CT, internal attenuation values of −20 to −30 will be detected within the fatty portions of the lesion. On MRI, there will be elements within the lesion that follow the signal of body wall fat on all pulse sequences. On MRI, it is useful to perform the same sequence (either T1 or a fast spin echo T2) both with and without explicit fat saturation. If the tissue in question is fat, it will be very bright on the non–fat-saturated sequence and will become dark on the fat-saturated sequence.

13. **On MRI, I see an adrenal lesion that does *not* lose signal on chemical shift imaging. Could it still be an adenoma?**
    Yes. It could be a lipid-poor adenoma. However, metastatic disease and other adrenal lesions cannot be excluded in this situation.

14. **What is a collision tumor?**
    A collision tumor is a metastasis to an adrenal gland that also contains an adrenal cortical adenoma. Fortunately, these are not common; however, it is worth remembering that in patients with known malignancies, one should be careful about calling a lesion an adenoma if the lesion contains two distinct parts that display very different CT and MRI characteristics.

15. **How commonly do malignancies spread to the adrenal glands?**
    About 50% of melanomas metastasize to the adrenal glands, and 30–40% of breast and lung cancers and 10–20% of renal and gastrointestinal tumors have adrenal metastases.

16. **How do adrenal cysts form, and what do they look like on CT and MRI?**
    Most adrenal cysts are pseudocysts and form after adrenal hemorrhage. As fluid-containing structures, adrenal cysts are of fluid density on CT and are of high T2-signal intensity on MRI. They do not enhance following contrast administration.

17. **Who gets adrenal hemorrhage?**
    Adrenal hemorrhage can be secondary to extreme stress, trauma, or coagulopathic states. Common causes of coagulopathy include anticoagulant and thrombolytic agent use, systemic malignancies, and sepsis.

18. **How can CT or MRI be used to tell the difference between adrenal hemorrhage and an adrenal mass?**
    Compare precontrast and postcontrast images. Masses are living tissue and will therefore enhance on both CT and MRI. Adrenal hemorrhage will not enhance.

19. **What does pheochromocytoma look like on CT?**
    If the patient has laboratory values indicating an elevated catecholamine level, unenhanced CT is often the first imaging study performed. If an adrenal lesion is identified, this is presumed to represent pheochromocytoma. Approximately 10% of adrenal lesions are calcified on unenhanced CT.
    If an adrenal lesion is not found on unenhanced CT, intravenous contrast can be given. Pheochromocytomas enhance very avidly after contrast administration. Some centers prefer *not* to perform contrast-enhanced CT if pheochromocytoma is suspected because of reported cases of precipitation of hypertensive crisis after administration of iodine agents. MRI can be performed as an alternative.

20. **What is the differential diagnosis of T2-hyperintense adrenal lesions on MRI?**
    Adrenal cysts and pheochromocytoma can both be markedly hyperintense on T2, although many pheochromocytomas will contain regions that are not T2-hyperintense. These two lesions are easily differentiated by administration of IV gadolinium chelate. Cysts do not enhance, and pheochromocytomas enhance avidly on both CT and MRI (Fig. 23-4).

Figure 23-4. *A,* Axial T2-weighted image demonstrates a left adrenal lesion *(arrow)* that is of high T2 signal. This could represent a cyst or pheochromocytoma. *B,* Arterial phase postcontrast T1-weighted gradient-echo MR image demonstrates that the lesion *(arrow)* enhances avidly. These are MRI findings of pheochromocytoma.

21. **My patient has an elevated urine catecholamine level and hypertension, but there is no adrenal lesion on the CT (or MRI). Where else should I look for a pheochromocytoma?**
    Pheochromocytoma can occur anywhere along the sympathetic chain. The organ of Zuckerkandl (near the aortic bifurcation) and the urinary bladder are also important places to look.

22. **What is the pheochromocytoma "rule of tens?"**
    Approximately 10% of pheochromocytomas are bilateral, 10% occur outside of the adrenal gland, 10% are calcified, and 10% are malignant. It is perhaps more useful to remember the "rule of 90s" that this implies. Most pheochromocytomas are unilateral, in the adrenal gland, not calcified, and benign.

23. **My patient has lung cancer. What are the odds that there will be an adrenal lesion at time of presentation?**
    About 10% of patients with carcinoma of the lung will have adrenal metastases at the time the primary tumor is diagnosed.

24. **How can I tell whether a lesion is in the adrenal gland or in the upper pole of the kidney?**
    This can be surprisingly difficult, especially when the lesion is large. MRI has the ability to image directly in any plane, and sagittal or coronal images are often helpful in differentiating an adrenal

lesion from a renal lesion. If CT has been performed, reformatting the data into a sagittal or coronal plane on a workstation is usually helpful.

25.   **Where do the adrenal arteries arise?**
There are usually three main arteries. The superior adrenal artery originates from the inferior phrenic artery, the middle adrenal artery arises directly from the aorta, and the inferior adrenal artery is a branch of the renal artery.

26.   **Where do the adrenal veins drain?**
The right adrenal vein enters directly into the IVC. The left adrenal vein drains into the inferior phrenic vein and then to the left renal vein.

27.   **On CT and MRI, I see an adrenal mass that extends into the left renal vein. Does that help narrow the differential diagnosis?**
Yes. This is a common finding in adrenal cortical carcinoma. Adrenal cortical carcinomas are generally large tumors (>5 cm) that display avid enhancement, particularly at their periphery. Due to internal necrosis and hemorrhage, they often display great internal heterogeneity, both on CT and MRI.

KEY POINTS: CT AND MRI OF THE ADRENAL GLANDS

1. The differential diagnosis of a lesion in the adrenal gland includes adrenal cortical adenoma, adrenal cyst, myelolipoma, pheochromocytoma, metastatic disease, and adrenal cortical carcinoma.

2. There are three ways to show that an adrenal lesion is a benign adenoma: attenuation of less than 10 HU on unenhanced CT, washout of greater than 50% on 10-minute delayed CT, or signal loss of 10–15% on chemical shift MRI.

3. Most pheochromocytomas occur in the adrenal glands and enhance avidly on CT and MRI.

4. CT and MRI cannot differentiate functioning (endocrinologically active) adenomas from nonfunctioning adenomas.

28.   **What are the causes of Conn's syndrome?**
Conn's syndrome, or primary hyperaldosteronism, is caused by an adrenal adenoma in 80% of cases. In the remaining 20% of cases, the cause is adrenal hyperplasia. Patients will have hypertension, an elevated aldosterone level, and low potassium and renin levels. Patients with high aldosterone and renin levels likely have secondary hyperaldosteronism, which is secondary to renal artery stenosis.
In patients with primary hyperaldosteronism, it is important to differentiate between those with adenomas and those with adrenal hyperplasia. Aldosteronomas are treated surgically. Hyperplasia is managed medically. If CT and/or MRI do not reveal an adrenal lesion, then adrenal vein sampling can be performed to exclude the presence of a unilateral, hyperfunctioning aldosteronoma.

29.   **What are the causes of Cushing's syndrome?**
Cushing's syndrome is most commonly (80%) caused by an adrenocorticotropin hormone (ACTH)-producing pituitary adenoma that stimulates excessive cortisol production from the adrenal glands.
About 15% of all cases of Cushing's syndrome involve autonomous, cortisol-producing adenomas. The remainder of cases involve cortisol-producing adrenal cortical carcinomas or ACTH-producing small-cell carcinomas of the lung.

30. **Both adrenal glands look thick, but I do not see a focal mass. What does this mean?**

This is likely adrenal hyperplasia. In adults, this can be seen in any "stress" situation that requires the body to make more cortisol. Congenital adrenal hyperplasia can be seen in neonates. It is a manifestation of a number of genetic disorders that result in an inability to make sufficient cortisol or aldosterone. Affected neonates and infants develop adrenal hyperplasia and often overproduce sex hormones, leading to virilization.

31. **Which of the multiple endocrine neoplasia (MEN) syndromes involve the adrenal glands?**

MEN types IIa and IIb involve pheochromocytomas.
- MEN I (Wermer's syndrome) is characterized by parathyroid hyperplasia, pituitary tumors, and pancreatic islet cell tumors.
- MEN IIa (Sipple's syndrome) is characterized by pheochromocytoma, medullary thyroid carcinoma, and hyperparathyroidism.
- MEN IIb is similar to MEN IIa but without parathyroid involvement and with the presence of multiple mucosal neuromas and ganglioneuromas throughout the gastrointestinal tract.

BIBLIOGRAPHY

1. Korobkin M: CT characterization of adrenal masses: The time has come. Radiology 217(3):629–632, 2000.
2. Mayo-Smith WW, Boland GW, Noto RB, Lee MJ: State-of-the-art adrenal imaging. Radiographics 21(4):995–1012, 2001.
3. Otal P, Escourrou G, Mazerolles C, et al: Imaging features of uncommon adrenal masses with histopathologic correlation. Radiographics 19(3):569–581, 1999.
4. Pena CS, Boland GW, Hahn PF, et al: Characterization of indeterminate (lipid-poor) adrenal masses: Use of washout characteristics at contrast-enhanced CT. Radiology 217(3):798–802, 2000.
5. Siegelman ES: MR imaging of the adrenal neoplasms. Magn Reson Imag Clin North Am 8(4):769–786, 2000.

CHAPTER 24

ULTRASOUND OF THE FEMALE PELVIS

Jeffrey Scott Friedenberg, MD, and Susan E. Rowling, MD

1. **What are the main indications to perform an ultrasound of the female pelvis?**
   Ultrasound is useful in the evaluation of pelvic masses, pelvic pain, and abnormal bleeding. A pelvic ultrasound can also be performed to evaluate for uterine anomalies or to monitor for the development of ovarian follicles in infertility patients.

2. **How is a pelvic ultrasound performed?**
   The typical scanning techniques are transabdominal or endovaginal. We typically begin with a transabdominal scan, which is performed with the patient's bladder full. If we are satisfied with the images and have answered the clinical question, then the study is complete. If additional information can be obtained with an endovaginal examination, the patient is asked to empty her bladder before the examination is performed. Transperineal ultrasound is seldom performed but can be useful in the evaluation of the urethra, vagina, and cervix.

3. **What is the normal ultrasound appearance of the uterus?**
   The uterus has a homogenous myometrium of moderate echogenicity with a central echogenic band representing the endometrial stripe complex. Peripheral arcuate vessels may also be identified. A thin hypoechoic layer may surround the endometrium, particularly in postmenopausal women, and represents the innermost layer of myometrium. During the late proliferative (periovulatory) phase of the menstrual cycle, the endometrial stripe may have a trilaminar appearance, with an echogenic outer layer surrounding two hypoechoic layers separated by a thin echogenic line that represents apposition of the two endometrial layers.

4. **How is the endometrial stripe routinely measured?**
   The endometrial stripe complex is measured in the sagittal plane at its widest point, including both layers, from the most anterior to the most posterior echogenic portions of the stripe. If there is fluid within the endometrial cavity, the fluid is not included in the measurement. Endovaginal sonography is the most accurate way to measure the endometrium.

5. **What is the normal thickness of the endometrium?**
   Endometrial stripe thickness varies depending on the timing of the patient's menstrual cycle. During the menstrual phase, the endometrium typically measures between 1 and 4 mm. In the proliferative phase, the endometrial stripe may measure 4–8 mm, and in the secretory phase, the endometrial stripe may measure between 8 and 16 mm. These numbers do not apply for a postmenopausal woman in whom a thickness of up to 8 mm is considered normal if she is asymptomatic. Abnormal thickening of the endometrium can be a sign of endometrial cancer.

6. **What is the name of the simple cysts identified within the cervix? What is their clinical significance?**
   Cysts within the cervix are called *Nabothian cysts*. They represent dilated or obstructed endocervical glands. They are very common in women of reproductive ages and are usually of no clinical significance. Occasionally, the cysts appear complicated, secondary to hemorrhage or infection. Nabothian cysts can be a cause of benign cervical enlargement if they are large or multiple.

7. **What is the most common tumor of the uterus?**
   Far and away the most common uterine tumors are fibroids (leiomyomas), which are seen in approximately 25% of women. Fibroids are benign tumors of smooth muscle origin that can enlarge under hormonal influence. They are typically heterogeneous masses with posterior shadowing and may contain course calcifications or, rarely, central fluid secondary to necrosis. Fibroids can be subserosal, intramural, or submucosal in location. Large subserosal or intramural fibroids may cause symptoms by exerting pressure on adjacent organs. Submucosal leiomyomas are common causes of abnormal uterine bleeding and may become pedunculated within the endometrial cavity.

8. **What are the most common causes of vaginal bleeding in the postmenopausal woman?**
   Postmenopausal bleeding can occur for a number of reasons, the most ominous of which is endometrial carcinoma. Other causes include endometrial hyperplasia, endometrial atrophy, submucosal fibroids, and endometrial polyps (Fig. 24-1). Even though ultrasound may not definitively diagnose endometrial carcinoma, the purpose of the study is to determine which women will need more invasive testing, such as an endometrial biopsy or hysteroscopy.

Figure 24-1. Endometrial polyp. Sagittal view of the uterus demonstrates focal echogenic thickening of the endometrial stripe. Doppler interrogation demonstrated a single feeding vessel in this lesion that turned out to be an endometrial polyp.

9. **What are the ultrasound findings related to endometrial carcinoma?**
   The main finding of endometrial carcinoma is an abnormally thickened endometrium. Other findings include increased vascularity with multiple feeding vessels and an indistinct interface between the endometrium and myometrium. However, these findings are not specific for endometrial carcinoma, and further imaging and/or tissue sampling is necessary. In an asymptomatic postmenopausal woman not undergoing hormone replacement therapy, the endometrial stripe should not exceed 8 mm. In a woman with postmenopausal bleeding, a biopsy should be considered if the endometrium measures greater than 5 mm. When the endometrium measures 4 mm or less, endometrial atrophy is the most likely diagnosis and no further work-up is necessary.

10. **How can ultrasound help differentiate an endometrial polyp from other causes of endometrial thickening?**
    The most reliable technique to distinguish between these entities is sonohysterography, in which a catheter is introduced into the endometrial canal and approximately 5 mL of saline is infused into the endometrial cavity during endovaginal sonography. An endometrial polyp is a focal endocavitary mass that most commonly appears homogenous and echogenic in texture, but may contain internal cysts, and has either a narrow or broad-based attachment to the endometrium. On color or power Doppler interrogation, the most specific finding of an endometrial polyp is a single central feeding vessel entering from the endometrium.

11. **What is the ultrasound appearance of endometrial hyperplasia?**
    Endometrial hyperplasia is commonly a diffuse process with diffuse thickening of the endometrium, but it may occasionally be asymmetric or focal. The thickening is homogeneous

or contains small cysts. On color Doppler, hyperplasia is relatively hypovascular, unlike cancer, which is typically markedly hypervascular. Sonohysterography helps confirm the diffuse nature of the thickening, which can be adequately sampled with blind biopsy or dilatation/curettage. Alternatively, if a focal abnormality is identified at sonohysterography, hysteroscopy is necessary for biopsy or resection, since focal lesions may be missed at the time of blind endometrial biopsy or dilatation/curettage.

12. **Describe the major congenital uterine anomalies.**

The uterus, cervix, and upper portion of the vagina develop from the fused ends of the müllerian ducts. There are multiple uterine anomalies that result from various degrees of arrested development of the müllerian ducts (agenesis, hypoplasia, or unicornuate uterus), failure of fusion of the müllerian ducts (bicornuate or didelphys uterus) (Fig. 24-2), or failure of resorption of the median septum (septate uterus). When a uterine anomaly is identified, it is important to evaluate the kidneys since associated anomalies, such as renal agenesis or renal ectopia, are common.

Figure 24-2. Uterine didelphys. Transabdominal transverse view of the pelvis demonstrates two distinct, widely separate uterine horns.

13. **What is the role of ultrasound in the diagnosis of uterine anomalies?**

Some uterine anomalies can be accurately diagnosed with ultrasound, such as absent uterus or didelphys uterus, in which there are two widely separated uterine horns and two cervices. However, two-dimensional (2D) ultrasound may not be accurate in the diagnosis of other uterine anomalies. It is difficult to distinguish a bicornuate uterus from a septate uterus, since it may not be possible to assess the external fundal contour of the uterus. A bicornuate uterus should have a deep fundal indentation of 1 cm or greater, whereas a septate uterus has a normal outer fundal contour. Magnetic resonance imaging (MRI) or 3D ultrasound is more accurate in making the appropriate diagnosis and guiding treatment planning.

14. **What are the findings associated with adenomyosis on ultrasound?**

Adenomyosis occurs when there are ectopic endometrial glands within the myometrium. It is a common cause of pelvic pain, menorrhagia, or uterine enlargement (Fig. 24-3). Although MRI is

Figure 24-3. Adenomyosis. There is marked thickening and heterogeneity of the posterior wall of the uterus. No discrete mass is identified to suggest fibroids.

more accurate in the diagnosis of adenomyosis, there are ultrasound findings that are suggestive, such as globular uterine enlargement with asymmetric thickening of the myometrium, heterogeneous myometrium with streaky shadowing, and small myometrial cysts. When compared
with fibroids, adenomyosis is more ill-defined, is noncalcified, and is tender to palpation with the
vaginal probe.

15. **What is the normal ultrasound appearance of the ovary in a premenopausal woman?**
The ovaries appear as ovoid soft tissue structures in the adnexa with a volume of approximately
10 mL. During the follicular phase of the cycle, the ovaries contain a varying number of anechoic
follicles, which can range in size depending on the phase of the cycle. During the periovulatory
phase, there is commonly a dominant follicle that may measure up to 2.5–3 cm. After ovulation,
in the luteal phase, there is commonly a hemorrhagic corpus luteum with internal echoes and a
characteristic rim of increased peripheral blood flow.

KEY POINTS: ULTRASOUND OF THE FEMALE PELVIS

1. Ultrasound is useful in evaluating women with pelvic pain, pelvic masses, and dysfunctional
   uterine bleeding. Ultrasound can also help in the diagnosis of congenital uterine anomalies and
   the evaluation of ovarian follicles in infertility patients.

2. Thickening of the endometrial stripe may be a sign of endometrial carcinoma, and further
   evaluation with hysteroscopy or endometrial biopsy should be performed.

3. Ovarian cysts are very common in premenopausal women, and follow-up of these lesions
   should be based on their size and morphology.

4. Features that can suggest a benign vs. malignant etiology of an ovarian mass depend on the
   age of the patient, morphology of the lesion, size of the mass, and resistive index.

16. **Describe the management of simple ovarian cysts in premenopausal women.**
Simple cysts within the ovary that are anechoic, thin walled, and without septations or solid
components are managed based on their size. Since the normal dominant follicles can range up
to 3 cm (or sometimes greater), simple ovarian cysts smaller than 3 cm in premenopausal
women need no follow-up and typically resolve spontaneously. Cysts greater than 3 cm generally require a 6-week follow-up, which places the patient at a different phase in her cycle. If the
cyst is large or shows interval growth or lack or regression, further evaluation with laparoscopy
may be warranted since many of these lesions represent cystic ovarian neoplasms, such as a
benign serous cystadenomas.

17. **What are the ultrasound findings associated with a hemorrhagic cyst?**
A hemorrhagic cyst is a common finding in a premenopausal woman, particularly in the luteal
phase of the menstrual cycle, and is often associated with acute onset of pelvic pain.
The appearance of the internal blood products varies with the age of the hemorrhage. Acute
hemorrhage may mimic an echogenic mass but can be distinguished from a soft tissue mass
by increased through-transmission and lack of internal blood flow. As the clot lyses and retracts,
there may be an internal reticular pattern of lacelike septations, an internal fluid-fluid level, or a
retracting avascular clot adherent to the wall (Fig. 24-4).

18. **What features of an ovarian mass suggest a benign versus malignant etiology?**
Patient age is important because benign lesions predominate in pre-menopausal women. The size of mass is important, too, because masses smaller than 6 cm are typically benign, whereas malignant masses may be very large, often greater than 10 cm.

Figure 24-4. Hemorrhagic cyst. Endovaginal examination of the ovary demonstrates a complex cystic mass with increased through-transmission, a lacelike pattern, and a retractile clot adherent to the wall. Color Doppler demonstrated the lesion to be avascular.

Lesion morphology may be assessed on ultrasound. Benign lesions tend to be simple cystic masses with thin, smooth walls. Solid masses or complex cystic masses with thick, irregular septations or mural nodules are typically malignant. Finally, Doppler ultrasound findings should be assessed. Malignant masses commonly have increased blood flow to their septations and mural nodules, and they display relatively high diastolic flow, with low resistive indices (<0.4) on pulsed Doppler.

19. **If a woman presents with a palpable mass in the pelvis, but no abnormality is identified on ultrasound, which lesion should be considered? (Hint: This is the most common ovarian neoplasm to occur in women younger than age 50.)**
A dermoid cyst, also known as a "mature teratoma" (Fig. 24-5). Dermoids may be bilateral in 10–15% of patients. They have a variety of appearances on ultrasound, due to components arising from any of the three germ layers. They range from completely cystic to completely echogenic with shadowing. The most specific finding is a cystic mass with an echogenic mural nodule, known as the "dermoid plug," that often contains bone or teeth. Other dermoids have fat/fluid levels or a mesh of floating linear echoes due to hair. Dermoid cysts with prominent posterior shadowing can be difficult to detect with ultrasound because they mimic the appearance of bowel gas or they may be much larger than what is visible on ultrasound, which is termed the "tip-of-the-iceberg" sign.

Figure 24-5. Ovarian dermoid—a complex adnexal mass containing cystic and solid components. Anteriorly, there is a solid nodule *(arrowhead)* within the cystic portion of the lesion; this represents the dermoid plug. Posterior is an echogenic structure with shadowing *(arrow)* that represents a tooth.

20. **What are the findings associated with pelvic inflammatory disease on ultrasound?**
The findings related to pelvic inflammatory disease depend on the severity of the infection. The ultrasound findings may be normal in mild infections or demonstrate fluid within the cul-de-sac,

mild uterine enlargement, or endometrial fluid. More severe ascending infections result in salpingitis with pyosalpinx (dilated fallopian tube with internal debris and thickened hyperemic fallopian tube wall). The diagnosis of tubo-ovarian abscess is made when the dilated, inflamed tube is inseparable from the ovary, forming a complex hypervascular cystic mass.

21. **What is the imaging modality of choice in a patient with suspected endometriosis?**
    MRI is the best modality to evaluate for endometriosis. Ultrasound provides little information in cases with disseminated endometriosis. In the focal form of the disease, ultrasound can detect endometriomas, which often appear as complex cystic adnexal masses with diffuse, homogenous, low-level echoes; increased through-transmission; and calcification in the wall (Fig. 24-6).

Figure 24-6. Endometrioma. Sagittal view of the ovary demonstrates a mass with diffuse, low-level echoes and increased through-transmission.

22. **If a patient presents with infertility, hirsutism, and oligomenorrhea and her pelvic ultrasound displays large ovaries with multiple peripherally based follicles, what is the diagnosis?**
    Stein-Leventhal syndrome (polycystic ovarian disease) (Fig. 24-7). Although this diagnosis is made clinically, the ultrasound finding of enlarged ovaries (e.g., with a volume >18 mL) supports the diagnosis. The ovaries are often rounded in shape, with increased central stroma and multiple, small, peripheral follicles of uniform size, due to the lack of maturation of a dominant follicle and anovulation. Normal ovaries also often have numerous follicles, but the follicles are typically of varying sizes.

Figure 24-7. Polycystic ovarian disease. This ultrasound image demonstrates an enlarged ovary with multiple peripheral follicles and echogenic central stroma.

23. **What are the ultrasound findings associated with ovarian torsion?**
    Although suspected ovarian torsion is a common indication given by emergency department clinicians for emergent pelvic ultrasound, the incidence is rare and the diagnosis often must be made clinically. However, there are certain ultrasound findings that suggest ovarian torsion. In the absence of an underlying cyst or mass, the torsed ovary appears enlarged, edematous, and echogenic with small cortical cysts and absent or diminished blood flow, particularly venous. There may be preserved arterial flow due to the dual blood supply or incomplete occlusion of the artery. Severe pain and free fluid are common.

BIBLIOGRAPHY

1. Davidson KG, Dubinsky TJ: Ultrasound evaluation of the endometrium in postmenopausal vaginal bleeding. Radiol Clin North Am 41:769–780, 2003.
2. Levine D: Female pelvis. In McGahan JP, Goldberg BB: Diagnostic Ultrasound—A Logical Approach. Philadelphia, Lippincott-Raven, 1998, pp 935–964.
3. Levine D: Postmenopausal pelvis. In McGahan JP, Goldberg BB: Diagnostic Ultrasound—A Logical Approach. Philadelphia, Lippincott-Raven, 1998, pp 965–985.
4. Nguyen KT: The ovaries and adnexae. In Sauerbrei EE, Nguyen KT, Nolan RL (eds): A Practical Guide to Ultrasound in Obstetrics and Gynecology. Philadelphia, Lippincott-Raven, 1998, pp 71–103.
5. O'Neill MJ: Sonohysterography. Radiol Clin North Am 41:781–797, 2003.
6. Sauerbrei EE: The non-gravid uterus, vagina, and urethra. In Sauerbrei EE, Nguyen KT, Nolan RL (eds): A Practical Guide to Ultrasound in Obstetrics and Gynecology. Philadelphia, Lippincott-Raven, 1998, pp 33–70.

CHAPTER 25

MRI OF THE FEMALE PELVIS

Gautham Mallampati, MD

1. **Describe the normal location and normal magnetic resonance imaging (MRI) appearance of the ovaries.**
   Each ovary is located within the ovarian fossa. Anteriorly, the ovarian fossa is bounded by the external iliac vessels. Posteriorly, the ovarian fossa is bounded by the internal iliac vessels and ureter. The ovaries demonstrate intermediate signal on T1-weighted images. On T2-weighted images, the ovaries are mildly hyperintense to the uterine myometrium. The zonal anatomy of the ovary can often be delineated on T2-weighted images, with the peripheral cortex mildly hypointense to the higher-signal central medulla. Uncomplicated functional cysts located within the ovary have high T2-weighted and low T1-weighted signal relative to the ovarian stroma.

2. **How can uncomplicated functional cysts be distinguished from cystic ovarian malignancy?**
   Uncomplicated functional (physiologic) cysts do not contain internal solid components or complex fluid. Physiologic cysts have a thin wall and display no internal architecture. Functional cysts usually measure less than 4.5 cm. Features of cystic ovarian malignancy include solid internal components, such as mural nodules (Fig. 25-1). Ovarian malignancies may display internal hemorrhage and necrotic material and generally have more heterogeneous signal characteristics than do physiologic cysts.

3. **What is the significance of a papillary projection with a cystic ovarian structure?**
   A papillary projection is a frondlike structure projecting from the cyst wall into the lumen. Its presence indicates that the cyst is neoplastic (as opposed to a physiologic, functional cyst). Ovarian neoplastic cysts may be either benign or malignant.

4. **What are four benign masses of the ovary that exhibit characteristic MR imaging features?**
   One of the advantages of MRI is its ability to characterize the internal content of masses and thereby narrow the differential diagnosis of masses more precisely than computed tomography (CT) or ultrasound. Mature teratomas (also known as "dermoid cysts"), endometriomas, hemorrhagic cysts, and ovarian fibromas can exhibit MR features that permit benign diagnoses to be made noninvasively.

5. **Describe the content of mature teratomas that gives them a characteristic MR appearance.**
   The diagnosis of mature teratoma is made by identifying macroscopic fat within an ovarian lesion (Fig. 25-2). Fat within an ovarian lesion can be conclusively identified by performing the same T1-weighted sequence, both with and without explicit fat saturation. Macroscopic fat will follow the signal intensity of the body wall fat on all pulse sequences. It will be very bright on T1-weighted images performed *without* fat saturation and dark on the T1-weighted images performed *with* fat saturation.

   Mature teratomas, although benign, are resected because of potential complications, including ovarian torsion, chemical peritonitis if ruptured, and a very low risk for malignant degeneration.

Figure 25-1. Serous cystadenocarcinoma. *A,* T2-weighted image demonstrates a midline cystic mass with a left-sided solid component *(arrow). B,* Precontrast and, *C,* postcontrast fat-saturated T1 images show enhancement of the solid component *(arrow)* of a left ovarian serous cystadenocarcinoma.

6. **What imaging characteristics does a hemorrhagic ovarian cyst share with a dermoid?**
    Both of these lesions most commonly reveal high signal intensity on T1-weighted images. However, unlike a fat-containing mature teratoma, the hemorrhagic cyst will retain its bright signal intensity on T1-weighted images acquired with fat saturation.
    The hemorrhagic cyst is a functional cyst, such as a follicular cyst or corpus luteal cyst, that has been complicated by internal hemorrhage. These lesions, unlike dermoids, tend to resolve with follow-up.

7. **Can MRI be used to distinguish between hemorrhagic cysts and endometriomas?**
    Yes, even though both of these lesions may demonstrate similar appearances on T1-weighted images and fat-saturated T1-weighted images because they both contain blood products.
    These lesions can often be distinguished with the use of T2-weighted images, which are sensitive to internal fluid content. Endometriomas tend to demonstrate low signal intensity on T2-weighted images, a characteristic that has been referred to as "shading" (Fig. 25-3). They are also more commonly multiple and bilateral than are hemorrhagic cysts.

8. **How can MRI aid with the diagnosis of ovarian torsion?**

Although sonography is the first-line imaging method for the evaluation of suspected ovarian torsion, MRI is helpful if ultrasound is nondefinitive. MR findings of torsion include increased ovarian size, increased ovarian T2 signal intensity, deviation of the uterus toward an ipsilateral adnexal mass, and the presence of ascites. A torsed, necrotic ovary will fail to enhance after gadolinium administration.

9. **From what cell types can primary ovarian tumors originate? What are some collective features of ovarian malignancy?**

Cells of epithelial origin account for 85% of ovarian malignancies and 60% of ovarian neoplasms. Sex cord stromal tumors and germ cell tumors account for the remainder of malignancies. The presence of solid internal elements is a common feature of malignancy. Thick (more than 3 mm) internal septations and papillary projections are findings that indicate that a cystic structure is more likely a cystic neoplasm rather than a physiologic cyst. Solid, non-fatty mural nodules; peritoneal metastasis; and ascites are all common features of ovarian malignancy.

10. **What is the role of MRI in pregnancy?**

Ultrasound is the imaging technique of choice for the assessment of the fetus. MRI is thought to be safe for the fetus; however, it is avoided in the first trimester unless it offers a large advantage over other studies and is medically necessary. MRI can be useful for the evaluation of fetal anomalies—most commonly cerebral malformations and complex malformations that are difficult to characterize with ultrasound. Maternal lesions, such as ovarian malignancies, can also be evaluated

Figure 25-2. Mature ovarian teratoma. *A,* T2-weighted signal-shot fast spin echo (FSE) image reveals a high signal intensity mass in the posterior pelvis *(arrow).* *B,* T1-weighted image reveals high signal intensity *(arrow)* within this mass, correlating to either lipomatous or hemorrhagic/proteinaceous content. *C,* T1 sequence with explicit fat saturation. The region *(arrow)* that was hyperintense in *(B)* is now hypointense, indicating that the tissue is fat and not hemorrhage or protein. Fat within an ovarian lesion is diagnostic of a germ cell neoplasm—in this case a benign mature teratoma.

Figure 25-3. Endometrioma. *A*, Coronal T2-weighted single-shot FSE image and, *B*, axial FSE T2-weighted image of the pelvis demonstrate a mass posterior-superior to the uterus *(arrows)* that exhibits relatively low signal; this has been termed "shading." *C*, T1-weighted image shows high signal intensity within this mass *(arrow)*. In the ovary, this could be due to either lipomatous or hemorrhagic content. *D*, Fat-saturated T1-weighted image shows preserved high signal intensity of this endometrioma *(arrow)*; this therefore represents hemorrhagic contents rather than fat.

with MRI. The administration of gadolinium contrast agents is avoided in pregnant patients because they may cross the placental barrier and their effect on the fetus is unknown.

11. **What is the MR imaging appearance of the normal uterus?**
The uterus is composed of a fundus, corpus, and cervix. The corpus and fundus are composed of the endometrium, myometrium, and serosa. The endometrium displays a very high T2-weighted signal. The inner portion of the myometrium, also referred to as the "junctional zone," demonstrates a low signal on T2-weighted images. The outer myometrium and serosa are of intermediate signal intensity. These distinctions become less clear in postmenopausal women. On both CT and MRI, the normal cervix enhances less than the uterine corpus and fundus.

12. **Describe the type of congenital uterine abnormalities and the role of MRI in detecting them.**
Failure of the müllerian ducts to properly develop can result in several different types of uterine anomalies (Fig. 25-4). The septate uterus and bicornuate uterus are the most common abnormalities and are also the most common types to result in infertility. The septate uterus causes spontaneous abortion more commonly than the bicornuate uterus. The treatment for these two abnormalities also differs. The septate uterus can be treated with hysteroscopic resection of the septum. The bicornuate uterus is treated with open surgery.

Figure 25-4. Illustration of müllerian duct anomalies. *A,* Normal uterus. *B,* Arcuate uterus, with a small (<1 cm) depression of the outer contour of the uterine fundus. *C,* Septate uterus, with a thin internal septum but a normal outer contour to the uterine fundus. *D,* Bicornuate uterus, with a deep depression of the outer contour of the fundus; this results from a partial failure of fusion of the müllerian ducts.

MRI can generally distinguish between these two abnormalities. A septate uterus will have a smooth outer contour and a fibrous septum. A bicornuate uterus will display a depression (1 cm or greater) of the outer contour of the fundus; and a thicker, more muscular septum.

13. **Name two benign diseases of the uterine myometrium.**
Uterine leiomyomas (fibroids) and adenomyosis are both benign diseases of the uterine myometrium. Ultrasound is the primary modality for leiomyoma evaluation, although MR can generally provide more definitive lesion characterization and localization. Leiomyomas can occur in submucosal, intramural, and subserosal locations. Submucosal lesions abut the endometrial canal. Intramural lesions are located entirely within the muscular wall of the uterus. Subserosal lesions lie more peripherally, just deep to the outermost layer of the uterus, and can become pedunculated.

Leiomyomas are well-demarcated lesions with low signal intensity on both T1- and T2-weighted images. Leiomyomas usually demonstrate some degree of enhancement after the administration of gadolinium contrast material. Avid leiomyoma enhancement is correlated with favorable symptomatic response of fibroid-related pelvic pain after uterine arterial embolization therapy. Adenomyosis occurs when there is invasion of the myometrium by endometrial tissue. It is manifested by either focal or diffuse areas of junctional zone thickening.

14. **What degree of junctional zone thickness is indicative of adenomyosis?**
The normal junctional zone is less than 8 mm in thickness (Fig. 25-5). When the junctional zone is either focally or diffusely greater than 12 mm in thickness, adenomyosis can be diagnosed

(Fig. 25-6). In adenomyosis, the normally low T2 signal intensity junctional zone can contain islets of focally increased T2-weighted signal intensity. The presence of these areas of signal discrepancy can be used to suggest adenomyosis with an intermediate junctional zone thickness between 8 and 12 mm.

15. **If focal adenomyosis and leiomyomas are both of low-signal intensity on T1 and T2 images, then how are they distinguished?**
Adenomyosis generally displays ill-defined borders, whereas leiomyomas are more commonly well defined on MRI. Focal areas of adenomyosis, or adenomyomas, are usually oval, with the long axis of the lesion parallel to the endometrium. Adenomyomas also demonstrate little mass effect.

Figure 25-5. Normal uterine junctional zone. The junctional zone *(short arrow)* in this patient measures 7 mm and is normal in appearance. Note the small benign Nabothian cyst in the cervix *(long arrow)*.

16. **Name three malignant uterine neoplasms.**
Endometrial cancer, uterine sarcoma, and cervical carcinoma. Endometrial cancer is the most common type of female genital tract cancer. Cervical cancer is the third most common type, following ovarian carcinoma. Uterine sarcomas are rare.

17. **What is the role of MR imaging of endometrial carcinoma?**
MRI is not used in screening for endometrial diseases because benign entities such as endometrial polyps and hyperplasia have a similar MR appearance to early endometrial cancer. MRI can be helpful for the staging of endometrial cancer.
Endometrial cancer most commonly appears as widening of the endometrial stripe. Extension into the myometrium, extension toward the cervix, regional nodal spread, and distant metastases can all be characterized with MRI.

Figure 25-6. Adenomyosis. The junctional zone *(arrow)* in this patient measures 16 mm, indicating diffuse adenomyosis. In addition, note the cystic lesion anterior to the uterus and superior to the bladder, which is a pathologically proven serous cystadenoma.

18. **What is the normal appearance of the uterine cervix on MRI?**
The zonal anatomy of the cervix is best appreciated on T2-weighted images. The epithelium and mucus within the endocervical canal are of high T2 signal. Immediately peripheral to the epithelium is a layer of T2-hypointense stroma. A more intermediate T2 signal layer of smooth muscle is located outside of the fibrous stroma. This layer is contiguous with the outer myometrium of the uterus (Fig. 25-7).

19. **Describe the role of MRI for the evaluation of cervical cancer.**

    Similar to its role in endometrial cancer, MRI is not used for the diagnosis of cervical cancer, but for the staging of disease. MRI can assess for the presence of parametrial invasion and thereby distinguish between early-stage and advanced-stage cancer. Early cancer can be treated with hysterectomy; advanced cancer is initially treated with a combination of chemotherapy and radiation therapy. The presence of parametrial invasion is represented on T2-weighted images by spread of tumor through the low-intensity fibrous stroma, previously described. MRI is also useful for the diagnosis of recurrent cervical cancer.

Figure 25-7. Normal cervical anatomy. The endocervix is hyperintense on this T2-weighted image *(long arrow)* and is surrounded by T2-hypointense cervical stroma and, more peripherally, a more intermediate signal layer of smooth muscle. Note the benign Nabothian cyst *(short arrow)*.

20. **What term is given to the cystic outpouchings of the anterior urethra into the vaginal canal? How do these outpouchings appear on MRI?**

    Cystic outpouchings of the urethra are termed *urethral diverticula*. These diverticula are caused by obstruction of the periurethral glands secondary to recurrent infections. Like other cystic lesions on MRI, these lesions demonstrate bright T2 signal and low T1 signal. MRI is superior to other imaging methods for the evaluation of these lesions when they become symptomatic because it offers valuable anatomic information for surgical planning.

KEY POINTS: MRI OF THE FEMALE PELVIS

1. MRI can accurately characterize many benign lesions of the ovary, including physiologic cysts, mature teratomas (also known as dermoid cysts), endometriomas, fibromas, and hemorrhagic cysts.

2. Findings used to distinguish ovarian cystic neoplasms from simple, physiologic ovarian cysts include thick internal septations; papillary projections; and solid, enhancing, mural nodules.

3. MRI is useful for the staging of ovarian, endometrial, cervical, and vaginal cancers.

4. Uterine leiomyomas and adenomyosis are two benign diseases that have characteristic MRI appearances.

5. Cystic lesions of the female pelvis include ovarian cysts, Bartholin cysts, Gartner duct cysts, and urethral diverticula. All show high T2-weighted signal because they contain fluid. The T1 signal may be variable due to the presence of variable amounts of internal hemorrhage or protein.

21. **What is the difference between the MRI appearance of Bartholin cysts and Gartner duct cyst?**

    Bartholin cysts arise from obstruction of the Bartholin glands, which are located in the distal (inferior) posterolateral vagina. Gartner duct cysts are congenital lesions located in the anterolateral aspect of the proximal (superior) vagina. Both of these lesions show the typical high T2-weighted signal of cysts. The T1-weighted signal may vary if they are complicated with infection or proteinaceous content.

22. **What is the most common primary vaginal malignancy?**
Squamous cell carcinomas comprise the vast majority of vaginal malignancies. MRI is primarily used for tumor staging. The normal vagina demonstrates a normal central area of high T2 signal and low T1 signal that correspond to the mucosal layer and fluid within the canal. Moving outwards from the lumen, the second layer of the vagina is of low signal on both T1- and T2-weighted images and includes the submucosa and muscularis. The most peripheral layer consists of the adventitia, which is of high T2 signal and low T1 signal intensity. Vaginal cancer is best appreciated on T2-weighted images, where the tumors are generally hyperintense to the normal vaginal muscularis. Vaginal malignancies generally demonstrate enhancement.

23. **When is MR imaging of the female pelvis performed both with and without the patient engaging in the Valsalva maneuver?**
MRI of the female pelvis is performed with and without Valsalva routinely for the assessment of pelvic floor laxity. The descent of pelvic organs below the pubococcygeal line, which connects the last joint of the coccyx to the inferior portion of the pubic symphysis, is indicative of pelvis floor laxity.

BIBLIOGRAPHY

1. Chaudhry S, Reinhold C, Guermazi A, et al: Benign and malignant diseases of the endometrium. Top Magn Reson Imag 14(4):339–357, 2003.
2. Pretorius ES, Outwater EK, Hunt JL, Siegelman ES: Magnetic resonance imaging of the ovary. Top Magn Reson Imag 12(2):131–146, 2001.
3. Ryu J, Kim B: MR imaging of the male and female urethra. Radiographics 21(5):1169–1185, 2001.
4. Togashi K: MR imaging of the ovaries: Normal appearance and benign disease. Radiol Clin North Am 41(4):799–811, 2003.

CHAPTER 26

MRI AND ULTRASOUND OF THE MALE PELVIS

Lisa Jones, MD, PhD, and E. Scott Pretorius, MD

1. **What is the anatomy of the prostate gland?**
   The prostate consists of a peripheral gland and a central gland (Fig. 26-1). The central gland is located anterior and superior to the peripheral gland and is the portion of the prostate gland that is most intimate to the urethra. Benign prostatic hyperplasia (BPH) affects the central gland.

   The peripheral gland comprises the posterior and inferior aspects of the prostate. Although cancer can occur in the central gland, most cancers occur in the peripheral gland.

   Perhaps counterintuitively, the more cranial portion of the prostate is termed the "base." The more caudal portion is termed the "apex."

2. **What is the normal size of the prostate gland?**
   Radiologists often estimate the volume of objects by multiplying the anteroposterior (AP), transverse, and longitudinal measurements by one another and then multiplying that result by 0.52, which is pi/6. This is an estimation of the volume of an elliptical object. Expected prostate volume increases with advancing age. A prostate with a volume of greater than 40 mL is considered to be enlarged.

Figure 26-1. Axial line drawing of the prostate and seminal vesicles (A = seminal vesicles, B = central zone of prostate, C = transitional zone of prostate, D = peripheral zone of prostate, E = fibromuscular stroma of prostate). The right ejaculatory duct connects the seminal vesicle to the urethra.

3. **What values of prostate-specific antigen (PSA) are considered normal and abnormal?**
   A normal PSA value is less than 4, and an abnormal value is greater than 10. Values between 4 and 10 are borderline.

4. **Other than prostate cancer, what can elevate PSA?**
   Prostatitis, BPH, prostate infarcts, and biopsy.

5. **Where does BPH usually occur? What does it typically look like on magnetic resonance imaging (MRI)? On ultrasound?**
   BPH usually starts in the transitional zone of the central gland, which is the portion that is most intimate to the urethra. BPH is generally of more heterogeneous signal intensity on T2-weighted images than is the normal gland and can indent the bladder base. On ultrasound, BPH is usually hypoechoic to normal gland.

6. **What is the distribution of prostate cancer within the gland?**
   About 70% of tumors begin in the peripheral gland and the remainder in the central gland.

7. **What is the primary role of ultrasound and MRI in the evaluation of prostate cancer?**
    Ultrasound has low sensitivity for detecting prostate cancer (60–70%) and is not used for screening. It is used to guide random biopsies of the gland. MRI also has inadequate sensitivity for screening purposes and is primarily used to stage cancer patients at clinical risk for extracapsular spread of tumor. Accuracy of MRI for staging is 50–90%.

8. **What is the typical imaging appearance of prostate cancer on transrectal ultrasound and MRI?**
    - *On ultrasound*, prostate cancer appears as a hypoechoic mass in 70% of cases. Its appearance in the remainder of cases is hyperechoic or of mixed echogenicity.
    - *On MRI*, prostate cancer typically is isointense to gland on T1-weighted images and hypointense to the normally high-intensity peripheral zone on T2-weighted images (Fig. 26-2). Central gland malignancy is generally difficult to identify due to the presence of BPH that distorts normal anatomy.

Figure 26-2. Prostate cancer. *A*, Axial T2-weighted MRI. The *arrow* points to the focus of prostate cancer in the normally T2-hyperintense peripheral zone. *B*, T2-weighted sagittal image in another patient shows a low-signal tumor in the normally hyperintense seminal vesicles *(long arrow)*, representing extracapsular spread of tumor *(short arrow)* and nonsurgical disease. The same patient also had lymphadenopathy and osseous metastases.

9. **When should MRI be performed after biopsy? How is postbiopsy hemorrhage differentiated from tumor in the peripheral zone?**
    About 3 weeks after biopsy. At this time, fewer than 50% of patients have residual hemorrhage. Hemorrhage and tumor are distinguished by comparing T1- and T2-weighted images. T1-hyperintense/T2-hypointense areas correspond to postbiopsy hemorrhage. T1-isointense/T2-hypointense areas are more likely to correspond to tumor.

10. **How is prostate cancer staged? How does the cancer stage affect patient management?**
    The American Urological Association stages prostate cancer with the following classification:
    - Stage A: clinically unapparent
    - Stage B: tumor confined to prostate
    - Stage C: tumor extends beyond the capsule (may involve the seminal vesicles)
    - Stage D: metastatic disease to pelvic or distant nodes, bones, soft tissues, or organs

Surgery is generally recommended for patients with stage A and B cases. Stage C (extracapsular extension) cases preclude radical prostatectomy in the younger patient. Patients with stage D cases are treated with palliative radiation/hormonal treatment.

11. **What signs of nonsurgical (stage C or D) disease can be seen on MRI?**
Direct extracapsular spread of tumor nodule into periprostatic fat or neurovascular bundle, direct ascent of tumor up the ejaculatory ducts into the seminal vesicles, lymph node involvement (particularly in obturator and pelvic sidewall chains), and osseous metastatic disease.

12. **Where does capsular penetration most commonly occur?**
At the prostatic apex (inferiorly). Note that an irregular capsular bulge is more likely than a smooth bulge to reflect capsular penetration.

KEY POINTS: PROSTATE CANCER

1. Prostate cancer usually occurs in the peripheral zone.

2. Bone metastases are very unlikely with a PSA of <10.

3. Extracapsular extension indicates nonsurgical disease. Patients are treated with chemotherapy or hormonal therapy.

4. Prostate cancer (hypointense) may be distinguished from postbiopsy hemorrhage (hyperintense) on T1 sequences. Both are generally hypointense on T2.

---

13. **What is hematospermia? What causes it?**
Hematospermia is blood in the ejaculate. It is usually benign before age 40 when it is commonly due to prostatitis or orchitis. In patients older than 40, benign causes still predominate, but 5–10% of cases are related to malignancy. Carcinoma of the bladder and carcinoma of the prostate are most common.

14. **Where do the testicular arteries arise?**
The testicular arteries supply the testes and arise from the aorta near the level of the renal vessels. The normal testes descend from this level into the scrotum.

15. **Describe the normal appearance of the testis and epididymis on ultrasound.**
Each testis is ovoid, homogeneous in echotexture, and measures approximately $3 \times (2–4) \times (3–5)$ cm. Centrally within each testis is an echogenic linear structure, the mediastinum testis, which is an invagination of the surrounding tunica albuginea (Figs. 26-3 and 26-4). The testicles and epididymides should have symmetric vascularity and echotexture. Each epididymis is located posterolateral to the testis and is either isoechoic or slightly hyperechoic to the testis. The epididymis is composed of a head, body, and tail. The epididymal head measures 9–12 mm in diameter and is triangle shaped. The epididymal body and tail are thinner, measuring 2–5 mm in diameter.

16. **How does the testicle appear on MRI?**
T2-weighted images are best for evaluating testicular parenchyma. As on ultrasound, testicular tissue is relatively homogeneous and is very T2 hyperintense to nearby soft tissue structures. The surrounding tunica albuginea is well delineated as a low-T1, low-T2 signal intensity band surrounding each testicle. The mediastinum testis, as an invagination of the tunica, is also hypointense to testicular parenchyma.

17. **What is cryptorchidism? What does the cryptorchid testicle look like?**

Cryptorchidism is incomplete descent of testicle into scrotum. It occurs in 3% of neonates, but many testicles descend by age 1 (prevalence of 1%). The cryptorchid testis is commonly located in or below the inguinal canal and can be found by physical examination, ultrasound, or MRI. In about only 10–20% of cases, the cryptorchid testis is located intra-abdominally, and MRI is the modality of choice for detecting the testis. On ultrasound, the cryptorchid testicle is identified/recognized by the presence of its echogenic mediastinum; it is usually small and hypoechoic relative to a normal testicle. On MRI, the cryptorchid testicle is generally smaller than a normal testicle. It is generally T2 hyperintense, similar to a normally descended organ.

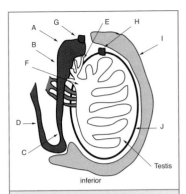

Figure 26-3. Sagittal drawing of the testicle and epididymis (A = epididymal head, B = epididymal body, C = epididymal tail, D = vas deferens, E = efferent ductules, F = rete testis; G = appendix epididymis, H = appendix testis, I = tunica vaginalis, J = tunica albuginea).

18. **What are complications of cryptorchidism?**

Cryptorchid testes are at an 8–30 times increased risk for malignancy, mostly by seminomas. Cryptorchid testes are also more likely to torse. Affected patients also have a higher-than-baseline risk of infertility.

19. **What is testicular microlithiasis? Name diseases commonly associated with microlithiasis.**

Testicular microlithiasis can be seen on ultrasound but generally is not demonstrated on MRI (Fig. 26-5). It refers to minute calcifications (>5 foci per cross-sectional image) associated with cryptorchidism, Klinefelter's syndrome, and pseudohermaphrodism. Although not a premalignant condition, it may be a marker of increased risk for testicular cancer. Yearly ultrasound examinations are recommended at some institutions to screen for tumor.

Figure 26-4. *A,* Sagittal view of epididymis *(arrow)* and superior pole of the testis. *B,* Transverse view of the testis; *arrow* points to the echogenic mediastinum where vessels and ductules enter the testis.

20. **What is the most important question to consider when imaging a palpable scrotal abnormality? Why?**

Is there a mass in the testicle? Most intratesticular masses are malignant. Most extratesticular scrotal masses are benign.

21. **What is the most common cause of a scrotal mass?**

    A spermatocele or an epididymal cyst. Spermatoceles and epididymal cysts are generally indistinguishable on ultrasound, both appearing as anechoic (homogeneously dark) lesions in the epididymis. Epididymal cysts contain simple fluid. Spermatoceles contain spermatozoa. Differentiating epididymal cysts from spermatoceles is rarely of clinical importance.

Figure 26-5. Ultrasound image demonstrates multiple echogenic foci in the testicle, representing testicular microlithiasis.

22. **Do cysts occur in the testicle? Is there anything else in the differential diagnosis?**

    Yes. They have been reported in as many as 10% of testicular ultrasound images, more commonly in the elderly, and are typically located near the mediastinum testis. Testicular cysts are benign. Common mimics of testicular cysts include tunica albuginea cysts and tubular ectasia of the retia testis (Fig. 26-6), which result in multiple, tubular cystic structures in the region of the mediastinum testis (usually bilateral and associated with epididymal cysts and history of vasectomy or epididymitis). Other things to consider in the differential diagnosis are a testicular abscess, which should not appear simple and may contain gas, and a cystic tumor, which is differentiated by a thick wall or solid component.

Figure 26-6. Ultrasound image demonstrates dilation of the rete testis *(arrow)*, a benign condition.

23. **What is the differential diagnosis of a solid testicular mass? Can these be distinguished on ultrasound and MRI?**

    Testicular malignancies are the most common cause. Less common entities include focal orchitis, hematoma, infarction, and rare benign tumors such as the epidermoid inclusion cyst. Most of these entities are not reliably distinguished on ultrasound since small tumors may appear avascular on color Doppler. On MRI, hematoma, infarction, and epidermoid will not enhance. Orchitis can be very difficult to differentiate from tumor using either modality. Reimaging the patient after successful treatment of infection may be useful.

24. **Name the different types of malignant testicular lesions.**

    - *Germ cell tumors* include seminoma (which is overall the most common type), the endodermal sinus (yolk sac), teratoma, embryonal cell, choriocarcinoma, and mixed germ cell types (second most common type).
    - *Stromal tumors* include Leydig cell and Sertoli cell tumors.
    - *Metastatic disease* is most commonly from lymphoma/leukemia. Prostate, lung, melanoma, colon, and renal cell carcinomas also can metastasize to the testicle.

25. **What is most common type of tumor in young adults (20–34 years old)? In children? In older adults (age >50)?**
In young adults, seminoma is the most common. In children, teratomas and yolk sac tumors are the most common. In older adults, lymphoma and metastases are more common than primary germ cell tumors. In men older than 50, lymphoma accounts for 25% of testicular tumors, and it is the most common testicular neoplasm in men older than 60.

26. **Which category of testicular tumors is most common overall?**
Germ cell tumors, which account for approximately 95% of cases.

27. **Germ cell tumors are generally divided according to whether they are seminomatous or nonseminomatous. Why is this distinction important? Describe the general differences between the tumors in these two categories.**
Seminoma has a better prognosis, occurs in an older age group (fourth decade), is more sensitive to radiation, and usually appears as a homogenous hypoechoic intratesticular mass that generally does not invade the tunica albuginea or have cystic components. It does not produce alpha fetoprotein. Any tumor that produces alpha fetoprotein is considered nonseminomatous.

Nonseminomatous germ cell tumors are often of mixed cell type. Relative to seminomas, they have a worse prognosis and are less radiosensitive. Expression of tumor markers depends on constituents. Usually, they are ill-defined inhomogeneous masses, commonly with cystic components, areas of hemorrhage, and calcification or fibrosis. They are more commonly associated with invasion of the tunica albuginea.

28. **Describe the stages of primary testicular tumor.**
 - Stage I: confined to scrotum
 - Stage II: involves lymph nodes inferior to the diaphragm
 - Stage III: has metastasized to extra-abdominal nodes
 - Stage IV: extranodal disease

29. **Describe the spread of primary testicular tumors.**
Primary testicular tumors usually spread along gonadal lymphatics to retroperitoneal lymph nodes, often appearing first at approximately the level of the renal hilum on the left and slightly lower on the right (Fig. 26-7). Inferior iliac and inguinal lymph nodes are usually spared unless the primary tumor has invaded the scrotal skin or epididymis or unless there has been prior surgery (e.g., in recurrent disease after orchiectomy). Hematogenous spread generally occurs after lymphatic spread, usually to the lungs.

Figure 26-7. *A,* Axial CT scan shows retroperitoneal lymphadenopathy *(arrow)* near the left renal hilum. *B,* Sagittal ultrasound image of the left testicle of the same patient demonstrates multifocal seminoma *(arrows).*

30. **Which germ cell tumor has a tendency for early hematogenous metastases?**
Choriocarcinoma, which often metastasizes to the lung. It is known for its tendency to produce hemorrhagic metastases.

KEY POINTS: TESTICULAR CANCER

1. Testicular cancer is the most common soild neoplasm in men 20–40 years old.

2. Germ cell tumors are most the common tumor type overall.

3. The most common testicular neoplasm is seminoma in young men and lymphoma in the elderly.

4. Seminoma has the best prognosis of germ cell tumors and is radiosensitive.

5. Lymphatic spread of testicular cancer is first to retroperitoneal lymph nodes, unless there is invasion of the scrotal skin or prior surgery, in which case pelvic nodes may be involved early.

31. **What types of testicular tumors are hormonally active? Which of these is most common?**
Stromal tumors (Leydig and Sertoli). Leydig tumor is the most common and can produce androgens. Sertoli tumors may produce estrogens. Ten percent of Leydig tumors are malignant.

32. **What is the differential diagnosis for multiple intratesticular masses?**
   - Lymphoma (generally older patients; bilateral in 10–20% of cases; involvement of epididymis and spermatic cord favor lymphoma over seminoma, which can otherwise be very similar in appearance)
   - Leukemia (testes commonly involved, similar in appearance to lymphoma, bilateral or unilateral)
   - Bilateral seminomas
   - Metastases, other than leukemia/lymphoma
   - Adrenal rests (benign, bilateral, seen in 8% of people with congenital adrenal hyperplasia, may regress with therapy)
   - Leydig cell hyperplasia (often bilateral, commonly seen in Klinefelter's syndrome)

33. **What is an epidermoid inclusion cyst? Is it malignant? What does it look like?**
The epidermoid inclusion cyst is (along with the simple testicular cyst) one of the few intratesticular entities that is benign. It is a nonvascular, well-circumscribed solid tumor of germ cell origin that consists only of ectodermal elements (in contrast to teratoma, which contains all tissue elements). Classic epidermoid lesions have a lamellated "onion skin" appearance on both ultrasound and MRI (Fig. 26-8). They can also

Figure 26-8. Ultrasound image demonstrates characteristic "onion skin" appearance of epidermoid inclusion cyst.

appear as a target lesion with a hyperechoic center and a hypoechoic rim, or as a rim calcified hypoechoic lesion.

34. **Name several structures that may herniate through the inguinal canal into the scrotal sac.**
Bowel (which can be identified by the presence of gas and peristalsis), mesenteric fat, the peritoneum with ascites, and the urinary bladder can all herniate into the scrotal sac.

35. **What is a varicocele? How is it diagnosed? Is it more common on the left or the right? What are complications of a varicocele?**
A varicocele is a dilated, tortuous vein of the pampiniform plexus, or a vein that is more than 2 mm in diameter located posteriorly near the upper pole of the testes. A varicocele will show little flow on color Doppler at rest and demonstrate increased distention and flow when the patient is upright or performs the Valsalva maneuver. Approximately 85% of these veins are on the left due to compression of the left renal vein by the superior mesenteric artery as it crosses the aorta. Varicoceles present in 15% of the population and are bilateral 10% of the time. Complications include infertility (up to 50% of men presenting with infertility have varicoceles) and pain.

36. **Under what circumstances is a varicocele concerning? Why?**
Varicoceles are more concerning if they are nondecompressible or right-sided or if the patient presents with one after age 40. In these cases, cross-sectional imaging is indicated to evaluate for a possible ipsilateral mass obstructing gonadal venous return.

37. **What is a hydrocele? Name the common causes of a hydrocele.**
A hydrocele is excess fluid within the tunica vaginalis. On ultrasound, a hydrocele typically is hypoechoic with good sound transmission. If complicated by blood (hematocele) or pus (pyocele), it may contain septations or echogenic material. Causes are diverse and include congenital patent processus vaginalis, trauma, surgery, diabetes, neoplasm, epididymo-orchitis, and torsion.

38. **What is the clinical differential diagnosis for an acutely painful scrotum? How is this usually evaluated with imaging?**
Ultrasound is used to evaluate the painful scrotum. Epididymitis/orchitis accounts for 75–80% of cases of acute scrotal pain. Testicular torsion, or torsion of the testicular appendage, is also an important cause. Strangulated hernia, testicular neoplasm, and trauma can also cause scrotal pain.

39. **What are the most common types of testicular torsion? Why does it occur?**
Intravaginal torsion is more common and is due to the "bell clapper" deformity. It is present in 10% of men in autopsy series and refers to the complete investment of the testes and epididymis by the tunica vaginalis, which results in incomplete fixation of the testis. The testicle can then freely rotate around its vascular pedicle, causing torsion. Intravaginal torsion presents during the teenage years.
    Extravaginal torsion, in which the tunica and testes twist at the external ring, occurs in neonates. It is not associated will the bell clapper deformity.

40. **What is the key criterion in diagnosing testicular torsion?**
Absent or decreased blood flow. It is often stated that compromise of venous flow is more sensitive for detection of torsion than is abnormal arterial flow.

41. **Why is the sensitivity of ultrasound for torsion only about 90%?**
At the time of imaging, a testicle may have detorsed or be incompletely torsed (<360 degrees) and therefore may have blood flow (Fig. 26-9).

KEY POINTS: TESTICULAR TORSION

1. A testicular torsion is usually due to the bell clapper deformity in teenagers.

2. The diagnosis of a testicular torsion is based on the identification of abnormal blood flow, not the gray scale appearance

3. A normal gray scale appearance (<6 hours) suggests viability.

4. Venous flow becomes abnormal before arterial flow.

5. False-negative results may be due to detorsion or partial torsion.

6. A testicle may be hyperemic after detorsion, simulating orchitis.

Figure 26-9. Transverse images of both testes demonstrate little color flow in the left testis in the presence of torsion *(A)* and hyperemia after detorsion *(B)*.

42. **What is the imaging appearance of acute epididymitis?**
    The epididymis will be enlarged and have increased blood flow. Epididymitis most commonly involves the epididymal head and is often diffuse but also can commonly only involve the epididymal body and tail, which therefore *must* be examined. In subtle cases, asymmetry can be a helpful clue to the presence of epididymitis. Accessory findings include hydrocele (simple), pyocele (echogenic), and skin thickening.

43. **What are the complications of epididymitis?**
    Orchitis (diffuse or focal hyperemia and enlargement of the testicle, which may also be relatively hypoechoic, occurs in 20–40% of cases), pyocele, scrotal abscess, infarction, chronic epididymitis, and infertility (Fig. 26-10).

44. **What is a cause of isolated diffuse hyperemia of the testicle (orchitis without epididymitis)?**
    Viral causes of orchitis (e.g., mumps) or syphilis.

45. **What else may cause hyperemia of the testicle and epididymis?**
    Post-torsion luxury perfusion (increased blood flow may result after a time of hypoperfusion) and trauma. The clinical history may help differentiate among possibilities.

Figure 26-10. *A–B,* Sagittal images of the right testis in a patient with epididymo-orchitis. An enlarged, inflamed epididymis is represented by the *short arrow,* and a complex hydrocele with septations by the *long arrow.* Note the enlargement, heterogeneity, and hypervascularity of the epididymis and testis.

46. **What are the possible ultrasound findings after testicular trauma?**
    Nonsurgical findings include extratesticular hematoma/hematocele (simple to complex extratesticular fluid collection or cystic mass) or traumatic epididymitis.
    Findings that indicate a need for surgery include testicular fracture or rupture (look for fracture line in testicle), devascularization, intratesticular hematoma, and disruption of normal contour/tunica albuginea. Ninety percent of fractured testicles can be restored if surgery is performed within 72 hours of injury, so this is a surgical emergency.

47. **Describe the normal appearance of the penis on MRI.**
    The penis is composed of three vascular cylinders. There are two dorsally located corpora cavernosa and the single ventral midline corpus spongiosum. Each cylinder is surrounded by a T2-hypointense fibrous band, the tunica albuginea (Figs. 26-11 and 26-12). All three cylinders tend to be T2 hyperintense to surrounding structures. The cavernosal bodies communicate with one another through holes in the intercavernosal septum and therefore should always be isointense to one another. The spongiosum also tends to be relatively T2 hyperintense but may have different signal from the cavernosa since it is functionally a separate space and may have a different rate of vascular flow within its channels than do the cavernosa. When viewed in cross section, the cavernosa each have a small, medially located T2-hyperintense "dot," which is the cavernosal artery. The flattened T2 dark band seen in the spongiosum is the urethra.

48. **Describe the physiologic factors behind erection.**
    After an appropriate stimulus, vascular resistance decreases and blood flow through the cavernous arteries increases, resulting in expansion of blood sinusoids in the cavernosa. Expansion of the corpora compresses the draining veins in the nonexpendable tunica albuginea, and penile erection is sustained.

49. **What congenital abnormality of the penis is associated with bladder exstrophy?**
    Epispadias, the absence of the dorsal covering of the penis and ectopic dorsal location of the meatus, is associated with bladder exstrophy. Epispadias also may be associated with a foreshortened penis.

50. **The penile meatus is located more ventrally and proximally than expected. What is this congenital malformation called? What is an associated finding?**
    Hypospadias. A dilated utricle, which is a midline cystic structure typically within the prostate, is an associated finding.

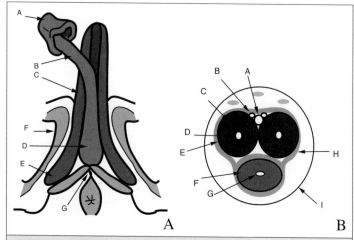

Figure 26-11. *A,* Axial line drawing of the penis (A = glans penis, B = corpora spongiosum, C = right corpus cavernosum, D = cavernosal artery, E = crus, F = ischiopubic ramus, G = perineal body). *B,* Coronal line drawing of the penis (A = dorsal artery of the penis, B = deep dorsal vein [note also the superficial dorsal veins], C = right corpus cavernosum, E = tunica albuginea, F = corpora cavernosa, G = urethra, H = Buck's fascia, I = epidermis).

Figure 26-12. Normal penile anatomy. *A,* Coronal T2-weighted image. *B,* T2-weighted image (a = spermatic cord, b = Buck's fascia and tunica albuginea, c = corpus cavernosum, d = central cavernosal artery, e = testis, f = corpus spongiosum, g = symphysis pubis, h = corpora cavernosum [again], i = urethra, j = prostate, k = seminal vesicles).

51. **What is the most common cancer of the penis in an adult? What are the risk factors? Where is the cancer most commonly located?**

Squamous cell cancer is the most common cancer of the penis but still accounts for less than 1% of all genitourinary malignancies in men. Risk factors include infection with human papilloma virus 16 or 18, lack of circumcision (due to the chronic irritative effect of smegma), and patient age (the sixth and seventh decades are the most common). Carcinoma of the penis is much more common in Asia and Africa than in Europe and the Americas. Carcinoma of the penis, which is most commonly found in the glans penis, is hypointense to the corpora on both T1 and T2 images.

52. **A patient with known prostate or bladder cancer presents with priapism. What must be considered?**
A metastasis to the penis may result in abnormal vascular shunting, a high-flow state called *malignant priapism.*

53. **What is Cowper's duct syringocele? What does it look like on MRI?**
It is cystic dilation of the main duct of the bulbourethral glands. It appears as a T2-hyperintense midline structure ventral to the proximal bulbous urethra (in the expected region of the Cowper's ducts). It may present with vague clinical symptoms, including postvoid dribbling, weak stream, frequency, and hematuria.

54. **A patient has a clinical history of painful deviated erections. What disease does the clinician suspect? What should one look for on MRI or ultrasound?**
Peyronie's disease, which represents inflammation that causes fibrosis of the connective tissue/tunica albuginea surrounding the corpora cavernosa (Fig. 26-13). It may be painful in its inflammatory form but is often painless in more chronic cases.
On MRI, the fibrosis is identified as T1- and T2-hypointense areas, which may enhance peripherally in association with the tunica albuginea.
On ultrasound, hyperechoic plaques are identified, which may shadow if calcium is present.

Figure 26-13. Peyronie's disease. *A,* Axial T1-weighted and, *B,* axial T2-weighted images demonstrate hypointense, densely calcified plaque *(arrows)* along the intercavernosal septum.

55. **Describe the characteristic clinical history or physical examination findings associated with penile fracture. What are the findings on MRI?**
Penile fracture occurs due to trauma to an erect penis, usually as a consequence of vigorous intercourse. The patient may describe acute onset of pain, rapid detumescence, and purple discoloration/deformity of the penis. Penile fracture is a surgical emergency. On MRI, look for discontinuity of T1- and T2-hypointense tunica albuginea and associated hematoma.

56. **A patient presents with a history of impotence. What can one look for on ultrasound to evaluate for potential causes?**
Doppler ultrasound can measure arterial flow in cavernosal arteries after administration of a vasodilator (normal peak systolic velocity is >30 cm/sec; if velocity is <25 cm/sec, arterial disease may be the cause).

BIBLIOGRAPHY

1. Cornud F, Flam T, Chauveinc L, et al: Extraprostatic spread of clinically localized prostate cancer: Factors predictive of pT3 tumor and of positive endorectal MR imaging examination results. Radiology 224:203–210, 2002.

2. Dambro TJ, Stewart RR, Carroll BA: The scrotum. In Rumack CM, Wilson SR, Charboneau JW (eds): Diagnostic Ultrasound, vol. 1, 2nd ed. St. Louis, Mosby, 1998, pp 791–821.

3. Dogra VS, Gottlieb RH, Oka M, et al: Sonography of the scrotum. Radiology 227:18–36, 2003.

4. Dunnick NR, Sandler CM, Newhouse JH, Amis ES Jr: Textbook of Uroradiology, 3rd ed. Philadelphia, Lippincott Williams and Wilkins, 2001, pp 394–450.

5. Noone TC, Semelka RC, Kubik-Huch RA, et al: Male pelvis. In Semelka RC (ed): Abdominal-Pelvic MRI. New York, Wiley-Liss, 2002, pp 981–1019.

6. Pretorius ES, Siegelman ES, Ramchandani P, et al: MR imaging of the penis. Radiographics 21:S283–299, 2001.

PATIENT SEDATION AND PAIN MANAGEMENT

Charles T. Lau, MD, and S. William Stavropoulos, MD

CHAPTER 27

1. **What is the purpose of sedation and pain management during an interventional radiology procedure?**
   The purpose is to enable a patient to tolerate a potentially painful procedure yet still maintain satisfactory cardiopulmonary function and the ability to cooperate with verbal commands and tactile stimuli.

2. **What is the difference between analgesia and anesthesia?**
   Analgesia is the relief of pain without alteration of a patient's state of awareness. Anesthesia is the state of unconsciousness.

3. **What is the difference between anxiolysis and amnesia?**
   Anxiolysis is the relief of fear or anxiety without alteration of awareness. Amnesia is the loss of memory.

4. **What capabilities should the patient maintain during conscious sedation?**
   The patient should:
   - Remain responsive and cooperative
   - Maintain spontaneous ventilation
   - Be able to protect the airway
   - Maintain protective reflexes

5. **Describe the levels of patient sedation.**
   The levels of patient sedation exist along a continuum: light sedation, moderate sedation, deep sedation, and general anesthesia. A patient under light sedation can respond to stimuli and maintains intact airway reflexes. A patient under moderate sedation should maintain spontaneous ventilation and be able to protect the airway. A patient under deep sedation can respond to vigorous stimuli but may lack airway reflexes. A patient under general anesthesia has no response to stimuli and lacks all protective reflexes.

6. **What details should the presedation evaluation of a patient include?**
   - Patient medical history
   - Previous adverse experience to sedation or anesthesia
   - Current medication use and drug allergies
   - Time and nature of last oral intake
   - History of alcohol or substance abuse
   - Focused physical examination including heart, lungs, and airway
   - Pertinent clinical laboratory findings

7. **How long should a patient typically fast before undergoing conscious sedation?**
   A patient should not have solid foods for 6–8 hours and clear liquids for 2–3 hours before the undergoing sedation.

8. **The physical status of a patient is often quantitated on a 5-point scale, known as the American Society of Anesthesiologists Physical Assessment Status. Describe this scale.**
   - Class I: healthy patient
   - Class II: mild to moderate systemic disturbance, well controlled
   - Class III: severe systemic disturbance that limits normal activities
   - Class IV: severe life-threatening illness
   - Class V: moribund, poor chance for survival

9. **Commonly, conscious sedation is administered by the provider (e.g., interventional radiologist) with patient monitoring provided by a qualified nurse. What patient factors should influence a provider to consider consulting an anesthesiologist to administer conscious sedation?**
   - ASA classification of III, IV, or V
   - Obesity
   - Pregnancy
   - Mental incapacity
   - Extremes of age

10. **What patient factors must be monitored during conscious sedation?**
    Level of consciousness, ventilation, oxygenation, blood pressure, and continuous cardiac monitoring.

11. **What equipment must be present when administering conscious sedation to a patient?**
    A patient undergoing conscious sedation should be under direct observation until recovery is complete. Equipment needed to monitor oxygenation; blood pressure; and heart rate, rhythm, and waveform should be present. Pharmacologic antagonists and commonly used agents need to be at hand as well as supplemental oxygen, a defibrillator, and appropriate equipment to establish airway and provide positive pressure ventilation.

12. **What pharmacologic agents are commonly used for patients undergoing conscious sedation? What is their reversal agent?**
    Benzodiazepines are typically used to provide conscious sedation. Common benzodiazepines include midazolam, lorazepam, and diazepam. Flumazenil is used as a reversal agent for benzodiazepines. The effect of flumazenil is usually visible in 2 minutes, with peak effects at 10 minutes. The initial dose in adults may be as high as 1 mg.

13. **What are the usual effects of benzodiazepines?**
    Benzodiazepines produce sedation and amnesia but do not provide analgesia. Significant adverse effects of benzodiazepines include respiratory and cardiovascular depression. Paradoxical reactions can occur with benzodiazepines and are more common in the elderly.

14. **What pharmacologic agents are commonly used for pain control? What is their reversal agent?**
    Opiates are commonly used to provide pain control. Commonly used opiates include fentanyl, morphine, and meperidine. Naloxone is used as a reversal agent for opiates and is typically administered as 0.4-mg IV doses (in adults) to a total of 2 mg. The effect of naloxone is usually visible in 2–3 minutes; however, its duration of action may be substantially shorter than a number of long-acting opiates, and repeated dosing may be necessary.

15. **What are the typical effects of opiates?**
Opiates provide systemic analgesia, mild anxiolysis, and mild sedation. Opiates do not induce amnesia.

16. **What pharmacologic agent used for pain control is contraindicated in patients taking a monoamine oxidase (MAO) inhibitor?**
Meperidine administered to a patient taking an MAO inhibitor can cause a variety of undesirable and potentially lethal side effects such as agitation; fever; and seizures progressing in some instances to coma, apnea, and death. The narcotic analgesic of choice for patients taking an MAO inhibitor is morphine.

17. **What are the strategies for dealing with a patient who has a known hypersensitivity to iodinated contrast media?**
Adverse reactions to iodinated contrast range from nuisance side effects, such as hives and emesis, to potentially lethal reactions, such as anaphylaxis and laryngeal edema. Patients with a history of even a minor hypersensitivity reaction to contrast may be at increased risk for a severe reaction, and special precautions should be exercised when administering contrast to these patients. Premedicating the patient with oral steroids and the use of low-osmolar contrast agents may reduce the risk of minor reactions, but there is, however, no proof that this strategy will prevent or reduce the risk of lethal contrast reactions. Alternative contrast agents such as gadolinium and/or CO_2 may be used in patients with a history of severe contrast reactions. If iodinated contrast must be used in a patient with a history of bronchospasm, laryngeal edema, or anaphylaxis, it may be wise to have an anesthesiologist standing by.

18. **List possible options for the management of an acute vasovagal reaction.**
A rapid infusion of normal saline or atropine (0.6–1.0 mg) may be given intravenously.

19. **What are the *ABCs* of patient resuscitation?**
Advanced Cardiac Life Support (ACLS) guidelines provide a series of algorithms regarding distressed patients in a variety of clinical settings. A common theme is that of the *ABCs* of resuscitation. Intervention in a patient with an unstable condition should always begin with the establishment of an *a*irway, followed by assessment of *b*reathing (ventilation) and *c*irculation (heart rate and blood pressure).

20. **Describe the management of acute hypotension.**
Remember your *ABCs!* During conscious sedation, an overdose of either a benzodiazepine or an opiate may cause respiratory depression that manifests as acute hypotension. Vigorous stimulation (sternal rub) may remedy the situation. If not, pharmacologic reversal may be needed. If hypoxia is not the etiology of the hypotension, evaluation of a patient's heart rate provides a simple algorithm for treating acute hypotension. A vasovagal reaction should be suspected if the patient is bradycardic, and treatment should proceed accordingly. If the patient is tachycardic, one should immediately evaluate for a source of blood loss. A fluid challenge with normal saline may help determine whether a patient is suffering from intravascular volume depletion. Pharmacologic intervention with epinephrine, phenylephrine, or dopamine may be indicated if the patient fails to respond to the fluid challenge. A complete algorithm for treating hypotension can be found in the ACLS guidelines.

21. **List possible options for the management of an acute hypertensive crisis.**
During a procedure, pain and anxiety may precipitate hypertension. A benzodiazepine, such as midazolam (Versed), mixed with an opiate, such as fentanyl, will likely decrease the blood pressure of an uncomfortable or anxious patient. To treat a patient in true hypertensive crisis, further pharmacologic intervention may be needed. IV labetalol, given as a bolus or a constant infusion, will often normalize blood pressure. Hydralazine and nitroprusside are other intravenous agents that may also be useful in this setting.

KEY POINTS: PATIENT SEDATION AND PAIN MANAGEMENT

1. A patient under moderate sedation should maintain spontaneous ventilation and be able to protect the airway.

2. The following equipment should be present when administering conscious sedation: pharmacologic antagonists, appropriate equipment to establish airway and provide positive pressure ventilation, supplemental oxygen, and a defibrillator.

3. The medications used to treat an anaphylactic reaction include diphenhydramine, methylprednisolone, and epinephrine.

4. Naloxone is used as a reversal agent for opiates.

5. Flumazenil is used as a reversal agent for benzodiazepines.

6. ACLS guidelines provide complete recommendations for the distressed patient.

7. Evaluation of a patient with an unstable condition should always begin with the *ABCs*.

22. **How can acute pulmonary edema be managed?**
Pulmonary edema interferes with the ability to oxygenate blood. Therapy consists of securing an airway, providing supplemental oxygen, and administering IV furosemide or other agents to induce diuresis.

23. **Describe the immediate options for management of an anaphylactic reaction.**
An anaphylactic reaction can be rapidly fatal. An airway should be secured immediately and oxygen administered. The mainstay of therapy consists of epinephrine (1:1000) given 0.1–0.3 mL subcutaneously every 15 minutes up to 1 mL total. Additional therapy includes saline for pressure support, diphenhydramine (50 mg IV), methylprednisolone (50 mg IV), and dopamine (5–10 µg/kg/min IV). Cardiopulmonary resuscitation may be required.

24. **Describe the immediate options for management of acute laryngeal edema.**
Laryngeal edema may lead to airway obstruction and death. An airway should be established, and oxygen should be administered. Epinephrine (1:1000) 0.1–0.3 mL subcutaneously every 15 minutes up to 1 mL total should be administered immediately. Additional agents include diphenhydramine (50 mg IV) and cimetidine (300 mg by mouth).

25. **Describe the immediate options for management of bronchospasm.**
The patient should be monitored closely and oxygen administered by nasal cannula or face mask. In severe cases, intubation may be required. Pharmacologic treatment includes epinephrine (1:1000), 0.1–0.3 mL given subcutaneously every 15 minutes up to 1 mL total, and aminophylline (4–6 mg/kg IV loading dose, then 25 mg/min continuous infusion). These agents may be supplemented with inhaled albuterol or metaproterenol.

26. **What are possible options for the management of generalized urticaria?**
A patient suffering from generalized urticaria can be treated with either diphenhydramine (50 mg IV) or cimetidine (300 mg by mouth). Vital signs should be obtained, and the patient should be observed to ensure that a more severe reaction is not evolving. The reaction should be documented in the patient's medical record.

WEBSITE

http://www.emedicine.com/emerg/topic695.htm

BIBLIOGRAPHY

1. Ray CE, et al: 2004 SIR 29th Annual Scientific Meeting Syllabus, 2004.
2. Wojtowycz M: Handbook of Interventional Radiology and Angiography, 2nd ed. St. Louis, Mosby, 1995.

CHAPTER 28

EQUIPMENT, TERMS, AND TECHNIQUES IN INTERVENTIONAL RADIOLOGY

Jeffrey A. Solomon, MD, MBA, and S. William Stavropolous, MD

1. **What are the characteristics of a diagnostic catheter?**
   Catheters may be selected for a specific application based on a number of characteristics (Fig. 28-1). Although there are an almost countless array of catheters, experience and personal preference play a large role in the selection process.
   - *Length:* Catheters are available in a variety of lengths, the most common being 65 and 100 cm. The appropriate length is based on the access site and desired application. For example, from a femoral approach, a 100-cm-long catheter may be used for a cerebral arteriogram, whereas a 65-cm-long catheter would suffice for a renal arteriogram.
   - *Tip configuration:* Tip configuration describes the curve on the leading edge of the catheter. A variety of curves are available that are designed to select branch vessels that originate at different angles. Common catheter curves include Cobra, Simmons, and Berenstein (see Fig. 28-1).
   - *Outer diameter:* Most diagnostic catheters used today are 4 or 5 Fr, meaning that they are less than 2 mm in diameter.
   - *Inner diameter:* This describes the inner channel of the catheter. Most catheters are designed to accommodate guidewires that are either 0.035 or 0.038 inch in diameter. It is important to match the inner diameter of the catheter with the devices (wire or coil) that are placed through it.
   - *Coating:* Some catheters have a hydrophilic coating that becomes very slippery when wet. This may facilitate crossing a stenosis.
   - *Stiffness:* Some catheters may contain braided fibers within the shaft. Braiding of polymers increases the stiffness of the catheter. Some clinical applications are better suited to stiffer catheters, whereas others are better served by floppier ones.

Figure 28-1. Types of catheters. *A*, Berenstein, *B*, Cobra, *C*, H1H, *D*, multipurpose-A, *E*, pigtail, *F*, Simmons, *G*, straight, *H*, tennis racket, *I*, = SOS.

2. **What is the difference between a Cobra 1 and a Cobra 2 catheter?**
   A Cobra 1 catheter and a Cobra 2 catheter have the same general shape except that the radius of the secondary curve of the catheter is greater for the Cobra 2 (Fig. 28-2). A Cobra 3 catheter again has the same general "Cobra" shape, but the secondary curve is even greater still. The same nomenclature applies to Simmons catheters and others as well.

3. **What is a French? What is a gauge?**
   A French (Fr) is a unit of measure of diameter and is often applied to catheters. One Fr is equal to one third of 1 mm. Therefore, a 6-Fr catheter will be 2 mm in diameter.
   A gauge (G) is also a unit used to measure diameter. A gauge (often applied to measurements of needles) describes the number of objects that have to be lined up side by side to make 1 inch.

Therefore, if 21 needles must be lined up to equal 1 each, the diameter of each needle is 21 G. One could convert gauge to French, but this has no clinical application and would be a tremendous waste of time.

4. **What are the two general categories of stents? How do they differ?**
    Improvements in biomedical engineering and metallurgy have helped expand the clinical applications for noncoronary stents. Although there are a variety of commercially available stents, they can be classified as either balloon-expandable or self-expanding. The characteristics of each type vary, making one type more suitable for certain clinical applications than the other. There is significant overlap for uses of both types of stent, and user preference plays a role in selection.

Figure 28-2. The difference between a Cobra 1 and a Cobra 2 catheter: The radius of the secondary curve on, *A,* the Cobra 1 catheter is smaller than, *B,* the Cobra 2 although the overall configuration of the catheters is similar.

5. **How is a balloon-expandable stent deployed?**
    The Palmaz stent is the prototypical balloon-expandable stent. Such stents come packaged either individually or premounted on a balloon. When the balloon is inflated, the stent expands to the diameter of the balloon. As the stent expands, it changes very little in length. The relatively constant size and method of delivery/deployment of this type of stent makes for precise and predictable placement. Balloon-expandable stents are the stent of choice for treating renal artery stenosis. Because they are made of laser-cut stainless steel, these stents may cause significant artifact on magnetic resonance imaging examinations. Balloon-expandable stents may be permanently deformed by extrinsic compression and therefore should not be used in situations in which they could be subject to these forces.

6. **What two materials are used to make self-expanding stents?**
    There are two broad categories of self-expanding stents: those made from woven elgiloy wires and those laser-cut from nitinol tubes. Self-expanding stents exert a continuous outward force and resist deformation and therefore are preferable to balloon-expandable stents in regions potentially subject to external compressive forces. To ensure full expansion, self-expanding stents are dilated with a balloon of appropriate diameter after deployment.

7. **How do woven elgiloy and nitinol self-expanding stents differ?**
    - *Woven stents,* such as Boston Scientific's Wallstent, have several unique characteristics. They are very radiopaque and can be easily seen on fluoroscopy, even in obese patients. The stents are reconstrainable, meaning that they can be almost entirely deployed, recaptured, moved, and then deployed in a different location. The trade-off, however, is that the length of the stent depends on its fully expanded diameter. These stents may shorten significantly as they expand over time, uncovering a region of pathology. Alternatively, if the stent does not expand to the degree expected, the stent may remain too long. Wall stents are available in large sizes (up to 24 mm in diameter) and are often used to create transjugular intrahepatic portosystemic shunts (TIPS) or to stent large central veins.
    - *Laser-cut stents,* such as the S.M.A.R.T stent, are not reconstrainable. However, because the stents are constructed of rings linked together, they are not subject to foreshortening and remain at a relatively stable length regardless of diameter. Nitinol is less radiopaque than elgiloy, and these stents may be difficult to see, especially in obese patients.

KEY POINTS: CHOICE OF STENT TYPE

1. Balloon-expandable stents are the stent of choice for renal arteries because they can be placed with greater accuracy.

2. Self-expanding stents are indicated when there may be an extrinsic compressive force acting on the stent.

8. **What is nitinol?**
Nitinol was developed by the U.S. Navy and stands for nickel titanium alloy. The metal is particularly useful for medical applications because it has thermal memory. This property allows stents to be made at a certain diameter, cooled, and then compressed onto a delivery system. When the stent is deployed at body temperature, the stent attempts to regain its original configuration and diameter. Therefore, a nitinol stent that is slightly oversized (by approximately 20%) with regard to the vessel will exert an outward force to keep the vessel open as the stent attempts to regain its original diameter.

9. **What do the terms *hoop strength* and *radial force* mean?**
   - *Hoop strength* is a measure of a stent's ability to avoid collapse and withstand the radial compressive forces of a vessel after dilatation.
   - Chronic outward *radial force* is the force a self-expanding stent exerts on a vessel as it tries to expand to its original diameter. The *radial resistive force* is the force a self-expanding stent exerts as it resists squeezing by a vessel.

10. **What is a sheath?**
A sheath is a device that may be placed into a vessel at the site of percutaneous access. Sheaths permit rapid exchanges of guidewires and catheters while maintaining access. Sheaths are sized based on the diameter of the catheter or device that they will allow to pass. For example, a 7-Fr sheath will accept devices up to 7 Fr in outer diameter. A 7-Fr sheath is in fact closer to 8 or 9 Fr in diameter.

11. **What is a guiding catheter?**
A guiding catheter is a special type of catheter that does not taper at its tip to the diameter of the guidewire. This configuration allows the passage of devices of large diameter through the catheter. When used in this manner, a guiding catheter functions similar to a long sheath. Unlike sheaths, guiding catheters lack a side port and hemostatic valve. Guiding catheters are sized based on the outer diameter. A 7-Fr guiding catheter will fit through a 7-Fr sheath, but a 7-Fr device will not fit through a 7-Fr guiding catheter. Guiding catheters are available with a variety of tip configurations.

12. **What is an up-and-over sheath?**
Sometimes called a Balkin sheath, an up-and-over sheath is a U-shaped sheath (Fig. 28-3). It is designed to facilitate interventions in which the arterial access is in one femoral artery and the lesion to be treated is in the contralateral extremity. A catheter and guidewire are placed into the aorta, and the contralateral iliac artery is selected. The sheath is then placed over the wire. The preshaped U curve assists passage over the aortic bifurcation. After angioplasty or stenting, arteriography can be performed by injecting contrast through the side arm of the sheath.

13. **What is the Trojan horse technique?**
The original balloon-expandable stents came from the manufacturer packaged in a small box. To use the stent, an appropriate balloon was selected, and the stent was hand-crimped onto the

balloon by the operator. If not mounted properly, stents had the tendency to slip on the balloon when being advanced across a tight stenosis. The Trojan horse technique minimizes this risk. Instead of pushing the stent across the lesion, the lesion is crossed with a sheath or guiding catheter (Fig. 28-4). The balloon-mounted stent is advanced through the catheter or sheath to the desired location, and then the sheath or catheter is withdrawn to expose the stent in the proper location. In this way, complications related to stent slippage are minimized. This is just one example of how the technique is used. The term applies to the technique in general and can be used to deliver any device in this manner, not just a balloon-expandable stent.

14. **What are the defining characteristics of guidewires?**
   Guidewires are available in a wide array of configurations. The selection of wire type depends on the intended application. Defining characteristics include:
   - *Length:* Wires are available in lengths from 70 to more than 300 cm. Short wires may be used for obtaining vascular access or placing drains. Longer, 300-cm wires are used in catheter exchanges or to perform procedures at a great distance from the access site.
   - *Diameter:* The most commonly used wires are 0.035, 0.038, or 0.018 inch in diameter. Wires as thin as 0.010 inch are available for special applications, such as cerebral interventions. The size of the wires should be selected based on the catheter used and the intended application.
   - *Stiffness:* Wires vary from very floppy to extremely stiff.
   - *Coating:* Some wires may have a hydrophilic coating. When wet, these wires become very slippery, and the coating may therefore facilitate the crossing of tight stenoses.
   - *Tip configuration:* Wires have specialized tips that have been engineered for specific applications. Some wires have preformed angles to assist the selection of vessels. Other wires have floppy or atraumatic tips to prevent vascular injury. Some specialized wires have shapeable tips that can be formed during a procedure to accomplish a specific task.

15. **What is an "exchange-length wire"? How long does it have to be?**
   An exchange-length wire is long enough to perform a catheter exchange without having to withdraw the wire. Most wires are 150 cm long and are paired with catheters that are either 65 or 100 cm long.

Figure 28-3. A Balkin sheath is commonly used when performing interventions in the contralateral lower extremity. The "up-and-over" design allows diagnostic angiography and interventional procedures to be performed via an access site in the contralateral leg.

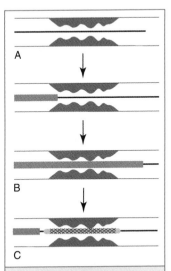

Figure 28-4. The Trojan horse technique. *A,* The lesion is crossed with a wire. *B,* A sheath or guiding catheter with a stent inside is used to cross the lesion. *C,* The sheath or guiding catheter is withdrawn, exposing the stent.

If a catheter needs to be exchanged over a wire, the wire needs to be at least twice as long as the catheter to make the exchange without having to pull the wire back and risk losing access. This is easy to remember: If a 100-cm-long catheter is advanced all the way into a vessel, a 200-cm wire will be needed to exchange the catheter; 100 cm of the wire will be used before the tip of the wire comes out of the catheter, and another 100 cm of wire is needed so that the catheter can be pulled out without moving the wire.

16. **What is a Cope loop?**
Dr. Constantine Cope is one of the pioneers of interventional radiology and is credited with some of the field's most ingenious inventions. One of these is the Cope loop, which is a pigtail catheter with a locking mechanism to prevent accidental displacement. A small string runs through the center of the catheter and is fixed to the distal curved end. The other end of the string exits the hub of the catheter. The curl on the catheter is straightened out as it is advanced over a guidewire. After the wire is removed, the string is pulled and tied, which causes the end of the catheter to curl and lock. The fixed diameter of the locked coil prevents migration. To remove the catheter, the hub and string are cut, releasing the distal lock.

17. **Who is the "stent" named after?**
The word *stent* derives from the surname of 19th century English dentist Charles Stent. He developed gums and resins used to make models of jaws, and the verb "to stent" came to mean "to hold tissue in place." The term *stent* was later adopted by surgeons to describe a device or material used to prop open a space.

18. **What does it mean to "Dotter" a lesion?**
Charles Dotter was an early pioneer in interventional radiology. Before the availability of angioplasty balloons, he described a technique in which stenoses were treated by passing dilators of successively larger diameter through them.

19. **What is a micropuncture set?**
A micropuncture set is used to obtain vascular access. It contains a 21-G, single-wall needle; an 0.018-inch wire, and a dilator. The dilator is tapered to the 0.018-inch wire to allow easy placement. The inner portion of the dilator can then be removed along with the wire to allow the dilator to accept a standard 0.035-inch wire. This set can be used as an alternative to double-wall needles. Some prefer this set for gaining access for thrombolysis because it uses the single-wall technique.

20. **What is the difference between the single-wall and the double-wall technique?**
To perform a single-wall technique, only the ventral wall of the vessel is punctured to gain entry to the vessel. A double-wall puncture (Seldinger technique) is performed by puncturing both the dorsal and ventral walls of the vessel and subsequently withdrawing the needle. When pulsatile blood is encountered, the tip of the needle will be in an intraluminal position, and a guidewire can be placed safely.

21. **What are the advantages and disadvantages of a single-wall puncture?**
Single-wall technique is preferred for bypass grafts and for patients at risk for puncture site hemorrhage, such as those undergoing thrombolysis. The disadvantage is an increased risk for access site dissection.

22. **What is a snare?**
A snare is a device that may be used to remove intravascular foreign bodies such as wires or coils (Fig. 28-5). A snare consists of a wire with a nitinol loop at the end. The plane of the loop is oriented perpendicular to the long axis of the wire. The snare is advanced through a catheter. Under fluoroscopic guidance, the loop is used to engage a free edge of the foreign body.

Figure 28-5. Steps used to retrieve a catheter fragment. *A,* A gooseneck snare is deployed in the vessel adjacent to the free end of the fragment. *B,* The free end of the catheter is engaged by the loop of the snare. *C,* The snare is pulled back into its outer catheter to tightly grasp the catheter. *D,* The snare, outer catheter, and catheter fragment are withdrawn in unison.

The wire and loop are then retracted into the catheter. This locks the foreign body between the snare loop and catheter. The snare, loop, and foreign body are then removed in unison.

23. What is a reverse curve catheter?

A reverse curve catheter is one in which the tip of the catheter doubles back on itself to form a partial loop (Fig. 28-6). Because of the loop at the end, special maneuvers must often be performed to form the loop once the catheter is inside the patient. After the loop is formed, the catheter is then pulled down to select a branch vessel. Once the tip of the catheter engages the orifice of the vessel, the use of the catheter may be slightly counterintuitive. The presence of the loop at the end of the catheter will cause the tip of the catheter to advance distally in the selected vessel if the catheter is pulled out. This is exactly opposite of what happens with a conventional catheter. One must push a reverse curve catheter inward to deselect a branch vessel. Reverse curve catheters may often provide very stable access to vessels because of the way they behave. The Simmons catheter is the prototypical reverse curve catheter.

Figure 28-6. The steps in using a reverse curve catheter. *A,* The catheter is formed in the aorta. *B,* The vessel is selected. *C,* As the catheter is pulled out, its tip moves further into the vessel.

24. What are the different ways to form a Simmons catheter?

There are a variety of ways to form a Simmons catheter. One way is first to place a wire over the aortic bifurcation and then form the catheter by placing the tip over the bifurcation and pushing up. The catheter may also be formed in the thoracic aorta where the diameter is sufficiently large. A technique commonly used at the Hospital of the University of Pennsylvania involves anchoring a suture with a wire in the tip of the catheter. The loop is formed by gently pulling on the string while advancing the catheter.

25. What is a Waltman loop?

The distal tip of any catheter can be looped back to form a reverse curve catheter. A Waltman loop is the configuration of a standard catheter once the distal end has been formed into a reverse curve loop. The simplest technique to do this involves selection of an aortic branch vessel. The tip is maintained in a constant position as wire and catheter are advanced in unison. This creates a large reverse curve that can stabilize access and facilitate difficult catheterizations.

26. **What is a "road map"?**
"Road-mapping" is an imaging technique present on many modern fluoroscopy units. An arteriogram is performed first. When the road map function is selected, the fluoroscopy monitor will display a static subtracted angiographic image from the prior run. When fluoroscopy is performed, a live subtracted fluoroscopic image is superimposed on the static angiogram. In effect, the vessels are highlighted with everything but the motion of the catheter and guidewire subtracted out. This technique facilitates selection of small or tortuous vessels.

27. **How do you select the proper injection rate for an arteriogram?**
The easiest way to select the proper rate is to give a test injection of contrast by hand to estimate the rate of flow. The injection rate should approximate the intrinsic rate of flow of the vessel. Giving a test injection is always wise to ensure that the catheter is in the appropriate location. Accidental power injection into the subintimal space or a tiny branch vessel may occur if this recommendation is not followed.

KEY POINT: INJECTION RATE

1. The best way to determine the appropriate injection rate for a given vessel is to give a test injection by hand and then to approximate the native rate of flow.

28. **What is meant by an injection of "20 for 40"?**
One must dictate the rate and volume for a power injected run. The term "20 for 40" means that the injection rate is 20 mL/sec for a total volume of 40 mL. This, therefore, will be a 2-second injection.

29. **What is a rate rise?**
A rate rise is another way that a power injection can be modified and describes the time in seconds that it takes from the beginning of the injection to reach the desired injection rate. For example, for an injection of "20 for 40" with no rate rise, the velocity of contrast in the catheter will immediately jump from 0 to 20 mL/sec. No rate rise implies a step function. If a rate rise of 0.6 second is used, it will take 0.6 second for the injection to reach maximum velocity. Rate rises are used to minimize the recoil of the catheter during rapid injections.

30. **What is a Hickman catheter?**
A Hickman catheter is a device used for chronic IV access, most commonly for chemotherapy or total parenteral nutrition. The line is available in single-, double-, or triple-lumen models. It is ideally placed in the internal jugular vein, with the exit site tunneled several centimeters away. The catheter has an antimicrobial cuff on its surface.

31. **What is a Permacath?**
Permacath is a brand name and therefore should not be used to describe the device in general terms. It is a type of tunneled dialysis catheter.

32. **What is a Medcomp?**
Medcomp is also a brand name and should not be used as a generic reference. It is a brand of nontunneled dialysis catheter.

BIBLIOGRAPHY

1. Duda SH, Wiskirchen J, Tepe G, et al: Physical properties of endovascular stents: An experimental comparison. J Vasc Interv Radiol 11:645–654, 2000.

CHAPTER 29

INFERIOR VENA CAVA FILTERS

S. William Stavropoulos, MD, and Jeffrey A. Solomon, MD, MBA

1. **What is an inferior vena cava (IVC) filter?**
   An IVC filter is a device inserted percutaneously into the IVC designed to prevent pulmonary emboli (PE) originating from lower extremity deep vein thrombosis (DVT) and to maintain caval patency.

2. **What are some common indications for IVC filter placement?**
   For patients with lower extremity DVT, accepted indications include:
   - A contraindication to anticoagulation
   - Recurrent thromboembolic disease despite adequate anticoagulation
   - Significant bleeding complication while undergoing anticoagulation
   - Inability to achieve anticoagulation

3. **What are the relative indications for IVC filter placement?**
   - Thromboembolic disease with limited cardiopulmonary reserve
   - Poor compliance with anticoagulation therapy
   - Chronic PE with pulmonary hypertension
   - Prophylaxis in the setting of prolonged immobilization
   - Large clot burden or free-floating pelvic/IVC thrombus

4. **What is a prophylactic IVC filter?**
   A prophylactic IVC filter is placed in patients who are at an increased risk for, but do not currently have, DVT or PE. These filters are most commonly placed in patients who will face prolonged immobilization. This population primarily consists of trauma patients with long bone or pelvic fractures and neurosurgical patients with transient or permanent motor deficits. Prophylactic filters may also be placed in patients with DVT risk factors before having surgery.

5. **What is Virchow's triad?**
   Virchow's triad is a basis for understanding the factors that contribute to thrombosis, including:
   - A hypercoagulable state caused, for example, by malignancy, nephrotic syndrome, or oral contraceptives
   - Vascular stasis due to shock, heart failure, venous obstruction, extrinsic compression, or other causes
   - Vascular injury due to a variety of causes, such as trauma, inflammation, surgery, or central lines

6. **What are the absolute contraindications to IVC filter placement?**
   Although rare, a lack of venous access; complete thrombosis of the IVC; or a severe, uncorrectable coagulopathy are each individually an absolute contraindication to IVC filter placement.

7. **What are the relative contraindications to IVC filter placement?**
   The decision to place a permanent medical device should be made on a case-by-case basis, and only after careful deliberation of the patient's history. One relative contraindication to filter placement is septic emboli or active bacteremia due to the theoretical risk of infectious seeding of the filter. IVC filters are not routinely placed in adolescents or pregnant women. A severe hypercoag-

ulable state or a history of IVC thrombus may preclude filter placement due to the risk of complete IVC thrombosis.

8. **What percentage of PE originates from the lower extremities?**
    Between 75% and 90% of PE originates from the lower extremities. The remainder of PE originates from the right atrium and upper extremities and likely account for some of the cases of recurrent PE after IVC filter placement.

9. **When would a superior vena cava (SVC) filter be placed?**
    Filters are rarely placed in the SVC because the small clot burden in the upper extremities is rarely thought to lead to clinically significant PE. SVC filters are indicated in the unique setting of symptomatic PE that can be traced with a high degree of certainty to upper extremity clot.

10. **Why is a venacavogram performed before IVC filter placement?**
    A venacavogram is performed to evaluate the size, anatomy, and patency of the IVC. It is important to know the diameter of the IVC because each filter can be safely placed in vessels up to a certain size. For instance, a Greenfield filter can be placed in a cava up to 28 mm in diameter, whereas a Bird's nest filter can be used in an IVC up to 40 mm. Filters can migrate into the heart or pulmonary artery if they are not sized appropriately. Ideally, the tip of the filter should rest in the infrarenal IVC. The venacavogram is helpful in identifying the location of the renal veins as well as variant anatomy that may affect filter placement. The presence of a nonocclusive clot in the cava may change the approach used to place the filter or its location. A jugular approach may be used when there is a large clot low in the IVC to help prevent pushing the clot centrally. To be effective, a filter needs to be placed above any clot in the IVC. This may warrant suprarenal placement.

11. **How is a venacavogram performed before IVC filter placement?**
    The venacavogram can be performed via access from a jugular or femoral vein or an arm vein. A 5-Fr pigtail catheter with radiopaque markers is recommended so that accurate measurements of the IVC can be taken. The tip of the catheter is placed just above the confluence of the iliac veins, and an injection rate is chosen that will cause contrast to flow down both the left and right common iliac veins. Identifying both iliac veins excludes the existence of a duplicated IVC, a normal anatomic variant that alters filter placement. Patients should perform a Valsalva maneuver to maximally distend the IVC during the contrast injection so that the caval diameter can be accurately measured, thus preventing caval migration. A radiopaque ruler can be placed underneath the patient to be used as a landmark to facilitate accurate filter placement.

12. **What do the renal veins look like on a cavogram?**
    Usually, the renal veins are not opacified by contrast injected into the IVC because the opacified blood in the cava flows preferentially back to the right atrium. The location of the renal veins, however, can be determined because unopacified blood from the renal veins mixes with and dilutes opacified blood in the cava. The location of the renal veins can be inferred from inflow defects in the stream of contrast in the IVC. If there is doubt about their location, a selective injection of the renal veins may be performed.

13. **Can a cavogram be performed if the patient is allergic to iodinated contrast or has an elevated creatinine level?**
    If iodinated contrast cannot be used due to an elevated creatinine level or a severe contrast allergy, a cavogram can be performed using intravenous carbon dioxide or gadolinium as an alternative contrast agent. If available, intravascular ultrasound (IVUS) can also be used.

14. **What are the common venous anomalies seen on a cavogram?**
    In interpreting a cavogram, one should be familiar with the common venous anomalies, including circumaortic renal vein, retroaortic left renal vein, caval duplication, and left-sided IVC.

15. **How common is IVC duplication? What does it look like on a cavogram?**
IVC duplication occurs in 0.2–0.3% of patients. In a patient with a duplicated IVC, the left common iliac vein does not join with the right common iliac vein but instead extends cranially to join the left renal vein. Simultaneous injections of the right and left femoral veins reveal two IVCs. The one on the right extends from the right common iliac vein into the right atrium. The one on the left extends from the left common iliac vein and joins with the left renal vein, which then empties into the right-sided IVC. If one understands this anatomy, one can understand why refluxing contrast down both common iliac veins during the cavogram excludes the presence of a duplicated IVC.

16. **What should be done in a patient with duplicated IVC who needs an IVC filter?**
Failure to recognize the presence of a duplicated IVC may lead to the placement of a single filter in the right-sided cava. A filter in this position would leave the entire left leg and left pelvis "unprotected" since a clot could bypass the filter by traveling from the leg, up the left-sided cava to the left renal vein, and then to the heart and lung. If the left-sided cava is recognized, a filter could be placed in each cava, or a single suprarenal filter could be placed.

17. **What are the characteristics of a left-sided IVC?**
Left-sided IVC occurs in 0.2–0.5% of patients. This vessel usually crosses to the right side of the abdomen at the level of the left renal vein and suprarenally continues in the position of the normal right-sided cava.

18. **What are characteristics of a circumaortic left renal vein? How common are they?**
A circumaortic left renal vein is an anatomic variant in which the left renal vein forms a ring around the aorta. It has a prevalence of between 1.5% and 8.7%. The anterior segment of the ring connects with the IVC at the expected level of the left renal vein, and the posterior segment connects with the IVC below the insertion of the anterior segment.

19. **Where should a filter be placed in a patient with a circumaortic left renal vein?**
If unrecognized, a circumaortic left renal vein may provide a collateral pathway for a clot to circumnavigate a filter and embolize to the lungs. If the filter is placed above the posterior segment, a clot may travel up the posterior segment to the anterior segment that is above the filter and then pass on to the lungs. Therefore, the filter should be placed below the lowest renal vein. This will ensure that a clot would encounter the filter as it travels centrally.

20. **List the IVC filters that are currently approved by the U.S. Food and Drug Administration (FDA).**
The following are FDA-approved caval filters: Bird's nest filter, titanium Greenfield filter, stainless steel over-the-wire Greenfield filter, Simon Nitinol Filter, Vena Tech LGM filter, Vena Tech LP filter, TrapEase filter, Optease filter, Gunther Tulip filter, and Recovery filter (Fig. 29-1).

KEY POINTS: IVC FILTERS

1. IVC filters prevent approximately 97% of symptomatic PE that originates from the lower extremities.

2. A cavogram before IVC filter placement is essential.

3. Retrievable IVC filters may be removed once they are no longer needed.

4. In most cases, IVC filters should be placed below the lowest renal vein when possible.

5. When fishing with a wire in a patient with a filter—be careful! You might actually "catch" something.

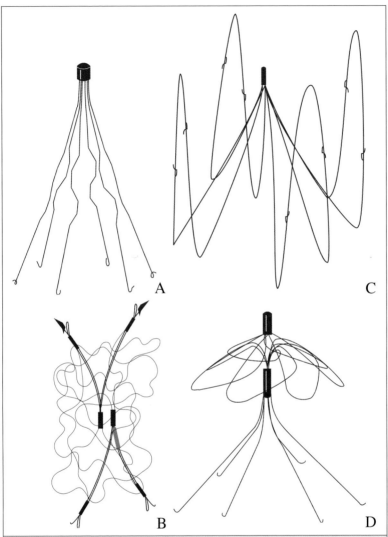

Figure 29-1. Examples of permanent IVC filters. *A*, Stainless steel over-the-wire Greenfield filter. *B*, Bird's nest filter. *C*, Vena Tech LP filter. *D*, Simon Nitinol Filter.

(Continued)

21. **What is a nonpermanent IVC filter?**
    Nonpermanent IVC filters can be removed. There are two categories of nonpermanent IVC filters: temporary and retrievable filters. A retrievable filter can be left in place permanently or can be removed if it is no longer needed. Currently, three FDA-approved retrievable IVC filters are available in the United States (Fig. 29-2). A temporary IVC filter must be removed at some point and is usually tethered to the skin by a wire or a catheter. There are no FDA-approved temporary IVC filters available in the United States at this time.

22. **What patients could benefit from a nonpermanent IVC filter?**
These patients include young trauma patients who are expected to recover, preoperative patients who only need short-term protection from PE, pregnant patients, young patients, and patients with a temporary contraindication to anticoagulation.

23. **Which of the currently FDA-approved filters can be used as a retrievable filter?**
The Gunther Tulip filter, the Recovery filter, and the Optease filter are currently FDA approved as both permanent and retrievable IVC filters.

24. **Can a patient with an IVC filter still get a PE?**
Yes! There are several ways for a patient with a filter to still get a PE. A patient may have had an anatomic variant that was not recognized during filter placement that permitted a clot to bypass the filter. Even in the absence of such variants, a filter will not protect a patient from PE originating in every part of the body. A filter will not offer protection from a clot

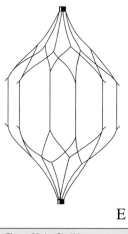

E

Figure 29-1, *Cont'd.*
E, TrapEase filter.

originating in the upper extremities or right atrium. Similarly, a clot from an ovarian vein that embolizes to the renal vein and then centrally will not be stopped by an infrarenal filter. Small clots may pass through a filter and large clots may propagate through a filter as pieces break off and embolize centrally. Overall, the rate of recurrent PE in patients with caval filters ranges from 3% to 5%. These rates are based on clinical findings and imaging studies performed in patients to detect symptomatic PE. The rates of asymptomatic PE after IVC filter placement are largely unknown.

25. **Where in the IVC should the filter be placed? Why?**
It is preferable that the filter be placed immediately below the lowest renal vein. With the apex of the filter sitting just below the renal veins, any clot caught by the filter is subject to high blood

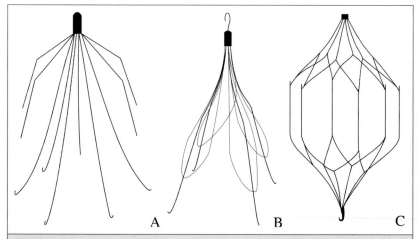

A   B   C

Figure 29-2. Examples of retrievable IVC filters. *A,* Recovery filter. *B,* Gunther Tulip filter. *C,* Optease filter.

flow from the renal veins and may be more likely to lyse. In theory, this may help maintain caval patency over the lifetime of the patient. Placement below the renal veins also decreases the risk of renal vein thrombosis if the filter is subject to a large clot burden. Suprarenal IVC filters are relatively safe but have a theoretical increased risk of renal vein thrombosis and therefore should be reserved for instances in which there is thrombus in the infrarenal IVC.

26. What complications are related to IVC filter placement?

Complications of filter placement can be related to the access site and include hematoma, venous thrombosis, and accidental arterial puncture. Complications related to the device include filter migration, malposition, fracture, infection, IVC perforation, failed deployment, and caval inclusion. IVC filter migration into the right atrium and pulmonary artery has been reported and can be fatal. IVC filters can be dislodged by wires or catheters placed during venous access performed at a later time. A potential complication for house staff may occur during central line placement. If the wire is inserted too far down the IVC in a patient with a filter, it may become entrapped. Attempts to pull the wire out may pull the filter with it and lacerate the cava. If you are placing a central line and the wire feels like it is "stuck," check the patient's record to see whether he or she has a filter. If the patient has a filter, you may want to call the interventional radiologist who can help remove the wire using fluoroscopic guidance.

27. How often does IVC occlusion occur after IVC filter placement?

IVC occlusion after filter placement can be due to either trapped thrombus in the filter or primary IVC thrombosis. Reports in the literature place the rate of symptomatic IVC occlusion between 2% and 10%.

BIBLIOGRAPHY

1. Asch MR: Initial experience in humans with a new retrievable inferior vena cava filter. Radiology 225:835–844, 2002.
2. Becker DM, Philbrick JT, Selby JB: Inferior vena cava filters: Indications, safety, effectiveness. Arch Intern Med 152:1985, 1992.
3. Cho KJ, Greenfield LJ, Proctor MC, et al: Evaluation of a new percutaneous stainless steel Greenfield filter. J Vasc Interv Radiol 8:181–187, 1997.
4. Crochet DP, Stora O, Ferry D, et al: Vena Tech-LGM filter: Long-term results of a prospective study. Radiology 216:857–860, 1993.
5. Dorfman GS, Cronan JJ, Tupper TB, et al: Occult pulmonary embolism: A common occurrence in deep venous thrombosis. Am J Roentgenol 148:263–266, 1987.
6. Ferris EJ, McCowan TC, Carver DK, et al: Percutaneous inferior vena cava filters: Follow-up of seven designs in 320 patients. Radiology 216:851–856, 1993.
7. Friedell ML, Goldenkranz RJ, Parsonnet V, et al: Migration of a Greenfield filter to the pulmonary artery: A case report. J Vasc Surg 3:929, 1986.
8. Golueke PJ, Garrett WV, Thompson JE, et al: Interruption of the inferior vena cava by means of the Greenfield filter: Expanding the indications. Surgery 103:111–117, 1988.
9. Grassi CJ: Inferior vena caval filters: Analysis of five currently available devices. Am J Roentgenol 156:813–821, 1991.
10. Huisman MV, Buller HR, ten Cate JW, et al: Unexpected high prevalence of silent pulmonary embolism in patients with deep venous thrombosis. Chest 95:498–502, 1989.
11. Katsamouris AA, Waltman AC, Delichatsios MA, et al: Inferior vena cava filters: In vitro comparison of clot trapping and flow dynamics. Radiology 166:361–366, 1988.
12. Kinney TB: Update on inferior vena cava filters. J Vasc Interv Radiol 14:425–440, 2003.
13. Millward SF, Marsh JI, Peterson RA, et al: LGM (Vena Tech) vena cava filter: Clinical experience in 64 patients. J Vasc Interv Radiol 2:429, 1991.
14. Molgaard CP, Yucel EK, Geller SC, et al: Access-site thrombosis after placement of inferior vena cava filters with 12-14 F delivery sheaths. Radiology 185:257–261, 1992.

15. Neuerburg JM, Gunther RW, Vorwerk D, et al: Results of a multicenter study of the retrievable Tulip vena cava filter: Early clinical experience. Cardiovasc Intervent Radiol 20:10–16, 1997.

16. Rogers FB, Shackford SR, Wilson J, et al: Prophylactic vena cava filter insertion in severely injured trauma patients: Indications and preliminary results. J Trauma 35:637, 1993.

17. Rousseau H, Perreault P, Otal P, et al: The 6-F Nitinol TrapEase inferior vena cava filter: Results of a prospective multicenter trial. J Vasc Interv Radiol 12:299–304. 2001.

18. Schutzer R, Ascher F, Hingorani A, et al: Preliminary results of the new 6F TrapEase inferior vena cava filter. Ann Vasc Surg 17:103–106, 2003.

19. Stavropoulos SW, Itkin M, Trerotola SO: In vitro study of guide wire entrapment in currently available inferior vena cava filters. J Vasc Interv Radiol 14:905–910, 2003.

20. Streiff MB: Vena caval filters: A comprehensive review. Blood 95:3669–3677, 2000.

21. Tobin KB, Pais SO, Austin CB: Femoral vein thrombosis following percutaneous placement of the Greenfield filter. Invest Radiol 24:442–445, 1989.

22. Winchell RJ, Hoyt DB, Walsh JC, et al: Risk factors associated with pulmonary embolism despite routine prophylaxis: Implications for improved protection. J Trauma 37:600, 1994.

23. Wojtowycz MM, Stoehr T, Crummy AB, et al: The bird's nest inferior vena cava filter: Review of a single-center experience. J Vasc Interv Radiol 8:171, 1997.

CHAPTER 30

PERIPHERAL VASCULAR DISEASE

Jeffrey A. Solomon, MD, MBA, and Jeffrey I. Mondschein, MD

1. What is the appropriate landmark for a femoral artery puncture?

Some of the risks of arteriography can be minimized by properly selecting the puncture site. Above the inguinal canal, the femoral artery (or more correctly, the external iliac artery) dives posteriorly. Punctures above the inguinal canal may be problematic for several reasons. Because the artery is so deep to the puncture site, manual compression may be difficult, leading to a hematoma or pseudoaneurysm formation. Furthermore, in the event of an access site complication that requires surgical intervention, the surgical approach for puncture above the inguinal ligament is more involved. A puncture that is too low may result in an arteriovenous fistula. A landmark that is commonly used for femoral artery puncture is the inguinal crease. This is a very inaccurate estimate for the location of the inguinal ligament, especially in obese patients. The best landmark is the middle of the medial third of the femoral head identified fluoroscopically (Fig. 30-1).

Figure 30-1. Leg arterial vascular anatomy. The *arrow* and *gray circle* indicate the preferred site for percutaneous access to the common femoral artery, over the middle third of the femoral head (A = external iliac artery, B = femoral bifurcation, C = deep femoral artery, D = superficial femoral artery, E = popliteal artery, F = anterior tibial artery, G = peroneal artery, H = posterior tibial artery).

2. What is Cope's law of vascular access?

"You can't stick a vessel where it isn't." In essence, this law suggests that the puncture site should be chosen carefully. The puncture should not necessarily be where you think the artery might be, but instead, where it actually is as determined with palpation or ultrasound.

3. If the femoral artery cannot be accessed, what are other options for obtaining access for an arteriogram?

Multiple options for access may exist in any given patient. The appropriate access site depends on the patient's symptoms, intended procedure, prior surgical history, and clinical setting. A brachial approach may be used if a femoral approach is not possible. Other access options include direct puncture of bypass grafts, direct translumbar aortic puncture, and retrograde popliteal access.

4. If a brachial approach must be used, is the right or left arm used?

A left brachial approach is preferred. A catheter placed from the left arm will traverse the left vertebral artery orifice, but not that of the left common carotid artery. This may reduce the risk of stroke.

5. **What are some complications unique to brachial access?**
    There is a small risk of stroke associated with brachial access. The arm cannot tolerate large hematomas, and bleeding after removal of a catheter or sheath may result in compartment syndrome. If a hematoma does develop, it must be followed up carefully to ensure that neurovascular compromise does not occur. Surgical evacuation of the hematoma may be required to prevent a neurologic deficit.

6. **What is claudication?**
    Claudication is derived from the Latin verb *claudicare*, which means "to limp." Claudication describes exercise-induced leg pain due to peripheral vascular disease (PVD). Patients with claudication typically complain of a burning or aching sensation in the thigh or calf, which starts after a predictable distance and remits with rest. With advanced disease, there may be progression to rest pain, skin ulceration, and tissue loss.

7. **What are the risk factors for PVD?**
    Risk factors for claudication and PVD include hypertension, diabetes, high cholesterol, cigarette smoking, and older age. Claudication is also more likely in people who already have atherosclerosis in other arteries, such as the coronary or carotid arteries.

8. **Does the location of leg pain suggest the location of arterial stenosis?**
    Leg pain usually occurs downstream to hemodynamically significant stenoses. Calf pain may result from disease of the superficial femoral artery, whereas thigh or buttock pain may be caused by iliac disease.

9. **What is Legs For Life?**
    Legs For Life is a national screening program initiated by the Society of Interventional Radiology (http://www.sirweb.org/) that is dedicated to improving the cardiovascular health of the community. It is a public education/community wellness program that screens people who may be at risk for PVD and helps them take the next step in resolving the pain they are experiencing. The primary goals of the Legs For Life program are to educate the public, primary care physicians, and medical community; identify patients at risk; and strengthen collaborative relationships among health care professionals who treat this condition.

10. **Why is it important to identify patients with claudication?**
    PVD affects more than 10 million Americans, and its prevalence is increasing. PVD is an important marker for many other serious conditions, including coronary artery disease, cerebrovascular disease, aneurysms, diabetes, and hypertension. Patients with PVD have a four- to six-fold increase in cardiovascular mortality compared with age-matched controls. The mortality rate for patients with claudication may be as high as 75% 15 years after being diagnosed with PVD. Early diagnosis of claudication affords patients the chance to modify their atherosclerotic risk factors and reduce their risk of coronary and carotid artery disease.

KEY POINTS: PVD

1. Asymptomatic arterial lesions rarely require treatment.

2. Patients rarely die from PVD, but this disease serves as a marker for other processes such as cerebrovascular disease and coronary artery disease, which can be life-threatening.

3. PVD is underdiagnosed in women.

11. **What is the Fontaine classification?**
    The Fontaine classification is a widely used classification system for lower extremity ischemia. It describes four stages based on signs and symptoms.
    - *Stage 1* is asymptomatic disease
    - *Stage 2a* is intermittent claudication when walking more than 200 meters
    - *Stage 2b* is intermittent claudication when walking less than 200 meters
    - *Stage 3* is rest pain
    - *Stage 4* is tissue necrosis or gangrene

12. **What is the Rutherford-Becker classification system?**
    This is another classification system for chronic lower extremity ischemia. It is popular in the United States and is based on clinical and objective criteria (Table 30-1).

TABLE 30-1.	RUTHERFORD BECKER CLASSIFICATION SYSTEM		
Grade	Category	Clinical Description	Objective Criteria
0	0	Asymptomatic	Normal treadmill/stress test
1	1	Mild claudication	Complete treadmill test, ankle pressure after exercise <50 but >25 mmHg less than blood pressure
	2	Moderate claudication	Between categories 1 and 3
	3	Severe claudication	Cannot complete treadmill test, ankle pressure after exercise <50 mmHg
2	4	Rest pain	Resting ankle pressure <40 mmHg, flat or barely pulsatile ankle or metatarsal pulse volume recording
3	5	Minor tissue loss, nonhealing	Resting ankle pressure <60 mmHg
	6	Major tissue loss, functional foot no longer salvageable	Same as category 5

13. **What are the clinical categories of leg ischemia?**
    See Table 30-2.

14. **What is the ankle-brachial index (ABI)?**
    The ABI is an essential component used for risk stratification for PVD. The ABI is used to screen for hemodynamically significant disease and to help define its severity. With the patient in the supine position, bilateral brachial blood pressures are obtained. A blood pressure cuff is placed on the calf of each leg, and an ankle systolic pressure is obtained. Determining ankle systolic pressure may require the use of Doppler. The ABI is calculated by dividing the ankle systolic pressure by the highest systolic pressure from either arm.

15. **How is the ABI interpreted?**
    A normal ABI is slightly greater than 1. A significant obstruction to blood flow to the lower extremities will lower the ankle pressure and the ABI. The risk of PVD and symptoms increases as the ABI decreases (Tables 30-3 and 30-4).

TABLE 30-2.   CLINICAL CATEGORIES OF ACUTE LEG ISCHEMIA

Category	Description	Capillary Return	Muscle Weakness	Sensory Loss	Arterial Doppler	Venous Doppler
Viable	Not immediately threatened	Intact	None	None	Audible (ankle pressure >30 mmHg	Audible
Threatened	Salvageable if treated promptly	Intact, but slow	Mild, partial	Mild, incomplete	Inaudible	Audible
Irreversible	Major tissue loss, amputation indicated regardless of treatment	Absent (marbling)	Profound paralysis, rigor	Profound, anesthetic	Inaudible	Inaudible

TABLE 30-3.   ABI BY SYMPTOMS

ABI	Symptoms
1.0–1.10	Normal
0.3–0.9	Claudication
≤0.5	Rest pain
≤0.2	Tissue loss

TABLE 30-4.   ABI BY RISK

ABI	Category
≥1.0	Normal (no/low risk)
0.90–0.99	Borderline (probably normal; no/low risk)
0.70–0.89	Mildly abnormal (low/moderate risk)
0.50–0.69	Abnormal (moderate/high risk)
<0.49	

16. **What can cause a falsely elevated ABI?**
    The ability to accurately determine the systolic blood pressure is predicated by the ability to compress the artery and obstruct blood flow. Diabetes may cause significant calcification of peripheral vessels, making them difficult to compress. This will factiously elevate the observed cuff pressure and the calculated ABI.

17. **What is meant by the terms *inflow* and *outflow*?**
At least two criteria must be met for an artery to remain patent. There must be sufficient flow of blood *into* the vessel. With respect to the femoral artery, "inflow" vessels include the aorta, common iliac artery, and external iliac artery. A stenosis of any of these vessels constitutes an "inflow" lesion. Even with perfect inflow, there also must be flow *out* of a vessel for it to remain patent. With respect to the femoral artery, the popliteal, peroneal, anterior, and posterior tibial arteries constitute "outflow" vessels.

18. **What are the basic steps in performing an angioplasty?**
A thorough diagnostic arteriogram is performed first. This is important so that the lesion can be sized and an appropriate balloon selected. The patient is then given heparin. It is important to give heparin before crossing the lesion to prevent thrombosis. The next step involves crossing the lesion with a catheter and guidewire. The lesion is then dilated. After the balloon is removed, an arteriogram is performed with the wire across the lesion to evaluate the result of the angioplasty. It is important to leave the wire in place until the follow-up arteriogram is performed in case a complication, such as a flow-limiting dissection or arterial rupture, occurs.

KEY POINT: ANGIOPLASTY

Outflow is a key determinant for the long-term patency of angioplasty.

19. **What constitutes a technically successful angioplasty?**
   - Restoration of luminal diameter with less than 30% residual stenosis
   - A pressure gradient less than 5 mmHg across the lesion
   - Absence of a flow-limiting dissection or vessel rupture
   - Relative reduction in the number and caliber of collateral vessels after a venous angioplasty

20. **What are the complications of angioplasty?**
The type and incidence of complications vary with the lesion's location and morphology. Complications include spasm, flow-limited dissection, plaque embolization, vessel rupture, access site trauma, renal dysfunction, contrast allergy, and death.

21. **What are the indications for stenting?**
Primary indications for stenting include failed angioplasty caused by a flow-limiting dissection or elastic recoil.

22. **What constitutes a hemodynamically significant arterial stenosis?**
A stenosis is generally considered significant if the luminal diameter is reduced by 50% and the systolic pressure gradient is in excess of 10 mmHg across the lesion. A lumen that is diminished by 50% will have a corresponding 75% reduction in cross-sectional area, which will likely reduce flow to a clinically significant level. In patients with claudication and lesions that are equivocal based on the aforementioned criteria, provocative testing may be performed. Tolazoline (Priscoline), a potent arterial dilator, is no longer commercially available. One may stimulate arterial dilatation with a prolonged inflation of a blood pressure cuff above the systolic pressure. A gradient greater than 20 mmHg after dilatation is considered significant. One should remember to treat the patient and not the arteriographic or pressure findings. The clinical history is also important in deciding whether a lesion is significant. There are few reasons to treat a patient with an entirely asymptomatic lesion.

23. **What is the kissing balloon technique?**
    This technique is most commonly used to perform angioplasty of the common iliac arteries (Fig. 30-2). Often, stenoses of the proximal common iliac arteries are associated with large, eccentric, calcified plaques. Sequential—as opposed to simultaneous—angioplasty may displace the plaque and lead to compromise of the contralateral iliac artery. The kissing technique mitigates this risk through the use of simultaneous angioplasty. This requires bilateral retrograde femoral artery access. The kissing technique may be used for the dilation of complex bifurcation stenosis in other locations as well.

Figure 30-2. The kissing balloon technique. *A,* Bifurcation lesion. *B,* Sequential angioplasty risks occlusion of the unprotected vessel. *C,* Simultaneous angioplasty prevents plaque displacement. *D,* Desired result.

24. **What are the basic principles in performing a thrombolysis procedure?**
    Thrombolysis therapy consists of the delivery of a lytic agent directly into a thrombosed vessel or graft. The catheter is, in large part, responsible for the specificity of the lysis. The immediate goal of the procedure is to lyse an unwanted clot while preventing a systemically lytic state to minimize bleeding complications. The secondary goal of a thrombolysis procedure is to uncover the cause of the thrombosis. Commonly, bypass grafts and native vessels thrombose due to stenoses in inflow vessels, anastomoses, or outflow vessels. Unless the underlying cause for the thrombosis is treated, thrombosis is likely to recur. Less commonly, there are instances in which grafts or vessel thrombose without underlying stenoses. Embolic disease, diminished cardiac output, and noncompliance with anticoagulation therapy are some causes of thrombosis in the absence of an underlying stenosis.

25. **In general, how is a thrombolysis procedure performed?**
    A thorough history and physical examination of the patient are performed. Particular attention should be given to any prior surgeries described in the history. Understanding the patient's vascular anatomy is key for planning access and intervention. Prior arteriograms, if available, should be reviewed. These may also help in the planning of the access site and in determining an appropriate endpoint to the procedure. A baseline physical examination is essential to monitoring the patient's progress or deterioration during the procedure. After laboratory findings are reviewed and consent has been obtained, a thorough diagnostic arteriogram is performed. The patient is given heparin and a sheath is placed. The thrombosis is crossed with a wire, and an infusion catheter is placed across the clot. Lytics are infused through the catheter, and the patient is sent to the intensive care unit for monitoring. Every 12–24 hours, the patient is brought back to the interventional suite for a follow-up arteriogram. Once the clot has resolved, the underlying lesion is treated.

26. **What is the guidewire traversal test?**
    This is an attempt to pass a guidewire across a thrombosed vessel before lysis. If the wire can be successfully passed across the occlusion, the clot is more likely to be fresh and lyse. If the guidewire traversal test fails, the occlusion is more likely to be chronic and less responsive to lytics. An end-hole catheter, positioned proximal to the clot, may be used to deliver lytics and

soften the clot to facilitate wire traversal. Once a wire has been passed, an infusion catheter can be placed. Placement of an infusion catheter within the bulk of the clot will help lend specificity to the lysis procedure and may reduce the overall time required for lysis.

27. **What are the contraindications to thrombolysis?**
    - *Absolute:* active internal bleeding, known intracranial pathology, stroke within the past 6 months, craniotomy in the past 2 months, irreversible limb ischemia, and infected bypass graft.
    - *Relative:* uncontrollable hypertension, history of gastrointestinal bleeding, bacterial endocarditis, diabetic retinopathy, coagulopathy, pregnancy, recent major surgery, recent major trauma, and recent cardiopulmonary resuscitation. In these patients, it is imperative to carefully analyze the potential risk-benefit ratio in each case.

28. **What is a PVR examination?**
    PVR stands for *pulse volume recording,* and it is a noninvasive method to evaluate arteries of the lower extremity. A brachial pressure and arterial waveform are obtained as reference standards. The process is then repeated at different stations, including the high thigh, low thigh, calf, ankle, and foot. The segmental pressures and waveforms are then analyzed to identify the level and severity of possible stenoses. Arterial waveforms provide especially useful information in the setting of calcified vessel. This test is one way that surveillance may be performed after a vascular intervention. It can also be used to plan an intervention in a symptomatic patient.

29. **What is Leriche's syndrome?**
    Leriche's syndrome describes chronic, lower extremity ischemia due to aortoiliac obstruction that is characterized by intermittent buttock claudication, absent femoral pulses, and sexual impotence (Fig. 30-3).

30. **What is an ACT measurement?**
    ACT stands for *activated clotting time.* It is a clotting test that may be performed in the interventional suite and is commonly used to monitor the effect of heparin. A small sample of whole blood is placed in the testing machine, and a result is available in less than 5 minutes. The reference range varies considerably, but it usually falls somewhere within 70–180 seconds. Although it can be obtained quickly, the ACT is less precise than partial thromboplastin time and can be affected by a host of factors, including ambient temperature, platelet count, and hemodilution.

31. **How are groin pseudoaneurysms managed?**
    Pseudoaneurysms resulting from femoral artery puncture can be managed in several ways, based on the patient's clinical status and the anatomy of the lesion. The first step is recognizing that the complication has occurred. A postprocedure groin check may reveal a pulsatile mass or ecchymosis. The patient may complain of groin pain. Ultrasound can be used to diagnose or

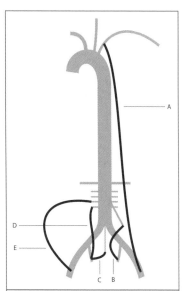

Figure 30-3. Collateral vascular pathways in aortic occlusion. Anterior supply: (A) Left subclavian artery to the left external iliac artery, via internal mammary and inferior epigastric arteries. Middle supply: (B) Inferior mesenteric artery to the internal iliac artery. Posterior supply: (C) Median sacral artery to the internal iliac artery. (D) Lumbar artery to the internal iliac artery. (E) Lumbar artery to the external iliac artery.

exclude the injury. If a pseudoaneurysm is found, several options exist. Manual or ultrasound-guided compression may cause the pseudoaneurysm to thrombose. Direct thrombin injection can also be performed if the anatomy of the lesion is suitable. Surgical intervention is also an option if other techniques fail.

32. **What are the major pathways of collateral circulation to supply the lower extremities in a patient with known aortic occlusion?**
    A simple way to help remember the collateral supply is to divide it into anterior, middle, and posterior pathways:
    - *Anterior:* subclavian artery through the internal mammary to the superior epigastric artery to the inferior epigastric artery and then into the external iliac artery
    - *Middle:* superior mesenteric to the inferior mesenteric artery via the arc of Riolan and the marginal artery of Drummond to the superior and inferior hemorrhoidal arteries to the internal iliac arteries and then to the external iliac arteries
    - *Posterior:* lumbar arteries to the internal iliac arteries via the retroperitoneal collaterals and then to the external iliac arteries by way of the iliolumbar and circumflex iliac arteries

WEBSITE

http://www.legsforlife.org

BIBLIOGRAPHY

1. Pentecost MJ, Michael H, Criqui GD, Goldstone J, et al: Guidelines for peripheral percutaneous transluminal angioplasty of the abdominal aorta and lower extremity vessels: A statement for health professionals from a special writing group of the Councils on Cardiovascular Radiology, Arteriosclerosis, Cardio-Thoracic and Vascular Surgery, Clinical Cardiology, and Epidemiology and Prevention, the American Heart Association. J Vasc Interv Radiol 14:495S–515S, 2003.

2. Sacks D, Bakal CW, Beatty PT, et al: Position statement on the use of the ankle brachial index in the evaluation of patients with peripheral vascular disease: A consensus statement developed by the Standards Division of the Society of Interventional Radiology. J Vasc Interv Radiol 14:389S, 2003.

EMBOLIZATION TECHNIQUES AND APPLICATIONS

Sara C. Chen, MD, and S. William Stavropoulos, MD

CHAPTER 31

1. Describe embolotherapy and some of its indications.

Embolotherapy is temporary or permanent vascular occlusion induced by the intravascular administration of materials via a percutaneous route. Embolization has a variety of clinical applications, including control of bleeding; treatment of vascular malformations; and tumor or organ ablation for curative, palliative, or preoperative purposes.

2. What materials are most commonly used for embolization?

There are a variety of embolic materials commercially available. Gelfoam, a temporary agent; metallic coils; and polyvinyl alcohol (PVA) particles are the most widely used embolics. Specific clinical situations may warrant the use of other agents, such as absolute ethanol, synthetic microspheres, or liquid "glues."

3. What is gelfoam, and how is it used?

Gelfoam is a reabsorbable gelatin that is most widely used in its sheet form. Wedges (1–2 mm) of gelfoam are divided from the larger sheets. The gelfoam can then be injected as "torpedoes" through a catheter placed in a blood vessel, or the gelfoam can be suspended in a contrast/saline slurry, which can then be injected.

4. How does gelfoam work? When is it used?

Gelfoam causes vascular occlusion by mechanically obstructing vessels, serving as a matrix for thrombus formation, and by causing endothelial inflammation that incites further thrombus formation. Gelfoam is reabsorbed in 5–6 weeks, during which time vessel recanalization is anticipated. Clinical situations in which temporary vascular occlusion is preferred include pelvic arterial hemorrhage after trauma, priapism, peripartum hemorrhage, and some cases of upper gastrointestinal (GI) bleeding. The rationale for using gelfoam in these situations is based on the belief that the use of a temporary agent will minimize the long-term ischemic effect on the end-organ.

5. What are metallic coils?

Metallic coils are made of either stainless steel or platinum. Dacron fibers are woven into some coils to promote thrombosis. Coils are available in a wide variety of shapes, sizes, and configurations. Special wires are used to push the coils through catheters that have been placed into the vessel intended to be embolized. Coils occlude vessels by causing mechanical obstruction, inducing clot formation, and provoking an inflammatory reaction.

6. When are coils preferred?

One way to classify embolics is based on whether they cause permanent or temporary occlusion. Another way is based on the size (diameter) of the vessel where the occlusion occurs. Coils cause vascular occlusion in vessels that are 1–2 mm in diameter and larger. Coils are preferred in clinical situations in which permanent occlusion is intended in vessels of this size. This includes the treatment of arteriovenous fistulas, GI bleeding, aneurysms, endoleaks after endovascular repair of abdominal aortic aneurysms, and traumatic vascular injuries in the proper clinical settings. Coils should not be used if occlusion is desired in vessels smaller than

1 mm. This includes situations in which the target of the embolization is an organ. For instance, when embolizing the uterus or performing chemoembolization of the liver, coils are not used. PVA particles or ethanol can be used to cause microvascular thrombosis, depending on the specific clinical situation.

7. **What happens when coils are the wrong size?**

   Although there is no TV show called "When Coil Embolization Goes Bad," any experienced interventional radiologist can tell a good tale about inappropriately sized coils. When coils are undersized, they can remain mobile after they are pushed out of the catheter and continue to travel with the flow of blood until they embolize to a vessel that is smaller than the diameter of the coil. If this happens while a venous embolization is being performed, the coils travel back toward the right heart and often out the pulmonary artery before lodging in a small vessel. The lungs are also a most likely final destination for coils that inadvertently pass through an arteriovenous fistula. When deployed in an artery, coils that are too small can migrate into distal branches or into another vascular distribution. This may result in nontarget embolization and decreased efficacy of the intended embolization. Coils that are too large can partially recoil into the parent vessel or cause the catheter to back out of the proper vessel. Retrievable coils are now available and allow optimization of positioning, configuration, and sizing before full deployment.

8. **When are PVA particles used?**

   PVA particles range in size from 50–2000 μm. Their mechanism of action is to physically obstruct vessels and incite extensive granulation tissue formation. PVA particles result in permanent occlusion. The size of the particle used is based on the location of desired thrombosis. The smaller the particles are, the more distal the embolization. Particle selection is often based on the experience of the operator. If the particles selected are too small, end-organ ischemia and necrosis may occur. On the other hand, if the particles are too large, collateral vessels may quickly reconstitute blood flow to the target organ, significantly decreasing the efficacy of the procedure. The smallest particles are reserved for tumor embolization or preoperative devascularization of other tissues because they can cause significant tissue ischemia via occlusion down to the capillary level.

9. **When performing an embolization procedure, why is it recommended to always place a vascular sheath at the access site?**

   A vascular sheath will assist in catheter exchanges during the procedure. More importantly, the sheath will maintain vascular access in the event the embolic agent clogs the delivery catheter and the catheter needs to be removed.

10. **What is postembolization syndrome?**

    Postembolization syndrome is an expected set of symptoms, including pain, fever, nausea, vomiting, and leukocytosis, that patients may experience after an embolization. The cause is likely secondary to organ ischemia/infarction. Prophylactic antibiotics to prevent superinfection of the ischemic tissue as well as pain control and antiemetic agents are helpful in treating postembolization syndrome. The syndrome is transient and should resolve within 3–5 days after the procedure.

11. **How can nontarget embolization be minimized?**

    Meticulous preembolization diagnostic angiography can ensure proper selective catheterization of the desired vessel.

12. **When performing an embolization procedure for an upper GI bleed, what information from the endoscopy report is essential?**

    Because clinically significant upper GI bleeding may be intermittent or too slow to be identified angiographically, arteriograms performed in this setting often display normal results. Empiric embolizations are commonly performed even when arteriograms have normal results.

Embolization of an arteriographically "normal" vessel can be performed safely because of the redundant collateral supply to the stomach and duodenum. Ischemic complications of such embolizations are rare unless the patient has a compromised network of collaterals from previous surgery. Before the procedure, it is therefore necessary to know exactly where the patient is bleeding. If the source is duodenal, the gastroduodenal artery is embolized. If the source is gastric, the left gastric artery is embolized.

13. **Can a lower GI bleed be treated with empiric embolization?**
     The colon and small bowel lack the extensive collateral network present in the stomach and duodenum. Empiric embolization of a vascular distribution will cause extensive ischemia and bowel necrosis. The approach to lower GI bleeds is therefore much different. To perform an embolization, the site of bleeding must be identified on the angiogram. Nuclear medicine bleeding scans are often performed before an arteriogram. These scans are noninvasive and can detect intermittent bleeding and hemorrhage that is much slower than that needed to be seen on an arteriogram. If the bleeding scan shows negative results, it is of virtually no value to perform an arteriogram. If the bleeding scan shows positive results and the site of hemorrhage can be identified on the arteriogram, embolization can be attempted.

14. **In the setting of pelvic trauma or peripartum hemorrhage in a patient with an unstable condition, is superselective embolization always indicated?**
     In emergent settings, with a patient with an unstable condition, the goal is efficient hemostasis and stabilization of the patient's condition. As such, embolization of the entire internal iliac artery, if necessary, can be performed, usually with gelfoam. The time saved by avoiding further catheterization may be life-saving. If the patient's condition is stable, selective embolization may be performed to reduce ischemic complications (Fig. 31-1).

Figure 31-1. *A*, Digital subtraction angiography (DSA) after a gunshot wound reveals acute hemorrhage from a branch of the left deep femoral artery. *B*, Delayed image from DSA prominently demonstrates the hemorrhage.

(Continued)

Figure 31-1, *Cont'd.* *C,* DSA after successful coil embolization of the injured artery demonstrates cessation of bleeding.

15. **Name some clinical indications for angiography in pelvic trauma patients.**
    The human pelvis represents a very large potential space, often able to accommodate 4–5 L of blood. Traumatic diastasis of the symphysis pubis can double the effective potential space of the pelvis. Pelvic bleeding can be difficult to control surgically. Splinting and external fixation are usually performed first to help reduce bleeding. Indications for arteriography include open pelvic fracture, expanding pelvic hematoma, and transfusion requirement greater than 4 units over 24 hours.

16. **Is empirical embolization indicated in pelvic trauma?**
    In the setting of a pelvic fracture, bleeding may be from a number of sources. Venous bleeding is by far the most common etiology. Bleeding from the periosteal surface of fractured bones is the next most common, followed by arterial hemorrhage. Therefore, in the setting of an arteriogram with normal results, arterial embolization is not usually performed.

17. **In bronchial artery embolization for hemoptysis, vigilance for which vessels is imperative?**
    Anterior spinal arteries arising from bronchial arteries must be identified to prevent nontarget embolization and subsequent paraplegia. Anterior spinal artery branches that arise from bronchial arteries have a classic "hairpin" appearance, traveling cranially for 1 cm or so before forming a loop and doubling back to travel caudally over the midline of the spine.

18. **Why should coils not be used in the bronchial arteries?**
    Life-threatening hemoptysis is often caused by chronic lung disease, such as sarcoidosis or cystic fibrosis. Because of the chronic nature of the lung disease, hemoptysis is likely to recur. Embolizing with coils makes future access to the embolized vascular territory difficult, if not impossible. Thus, particulate agents such as PVA are preferred.

19. **Why is it necessary to embolize both sides of a pseudoaneurysm, aneurysm, or arteriovenous fistula?**

Significant reconstitution of flow via collaterals can occur and cause recurrence of the lesion. For example, if only the proximal feeding vessel to a pseudoaneurysm is embolized, flow may then reverse in the outflow vessel and feed the pseudoaneurysm. Embolizing both sides of a pseudoaneurysm, aneurysm, or AV fistula is called "embolizing the front and back door of a lesion" and is also sometimes needed when embolizing bleeding vessels.

20. **What should always be placed when absolute ethanol is being used for renal artery sclerosis?**

An occlusion balloon must always be placed to prevent reflux of absolute ethanol into the aorta. The balloon should also be distal to the origin of the adrenal and gonadal arteries because catecholamine release or gonadal ischemia can result if ethanol is instilled into the respective arteries.

21. **How is chemoembolization theorized to work?**

Embolization of tumor vessels causes ischemia. This disables tumor cell membrane ion pumps and exocytosis functions and increases capillary permeability. As a result, there is increased intracellular accumulation and dwell time of the concomitantly delivered chemotherapeutic agent, leading to increased tumor cell apoptosis.

KEY POINTS: EMBOLIZATION TECHNIQUES AND APPLICATIONS

1. Embolotherapy has a variety of clinical applications, including control of bleeding; elimination of vascular malformations; and tumor or organ ablation for curative, palliative, or preoperative purposes.

2. Postembolization syndrome is a transient and expected set of symptoms, including pain, fever, nausea, vomiting, and leukocytosis, probably secondary to organ ischemia/infarction.

3. Meticulous pre-embolization diagnostic angiography to ensure appropriate selective catheterization of the desired vessel is required to minimize nontarget embolization.

4. Embolization on both sides of a pseudoaneurysm, aneurysm, or arteriovenous fistula is necessary to prevent reconstitution of flow via collaterals, which causes recurrence of the lesion.

5. Gas in the target organ within 3–5 days postembolization is thought to arise from tissue necrosis and does not automatically equal infection.

22. **What happens when the cystic artery is embolized during hepatic lesion embolization/chemoembolization?**

A transient chemical cholecystitis may result. This can be self-limited and may resolve with conservative management. Incidental embolization of the cystic artery is believed to contribute to postembolization pain in patients undergoing hepatic chemoembolization.

23. **What happens if the left or right gastric artery is embolized during hepatic chemoembolization?**

Injecting chemotherapeutic agents directly into the bowel can cause irreversible gastric ischemia and eventual necrosis. Thus, meticulous attention to possible variants in gastric/bowel vascular supply is necessary when performing pre-embolization diagnostic arteriograms.

24. **What is the significance of gas in the target organ postembolization?**
    There is little significance. Gas is often present in the target organ postembolization and is thought to arise from tissue necrosis. The presence of gas does not always indicate infection. Resorption of the gas may take weeks.

25. **What findings suggest that postembolization gas is due to infection?**
    Beyond 5 days postprocedure, when postembolization syndrome is expected to resolve, persistent fever, elevated serum markers of inflammation (erythrocyte sedimentation rate, C-reactive protein), and/or a fluid level in the embolized area suggest superinfection of the embolized tissue.

26. **When is uterine artery embolization (UAE) used in a nonemergent setting?**
    Uterine fibroids causing menorrhagia or pelvic pain can be treated effectively with bilateral UAE. UAE can be performed with permanent particles.

BIBLIOGRAPHY

1. Coldwell DM, Stokes KR, Yakes WF: Embolotherapy: Agents, clinical applications, and techniques. Radiographics 14(3):623–643, 1994.
2. Gee M, Soulen MC: Chemoembolization for hepatic metastases. Tech Vasc Interv Radiol 5(3):132–140, 2002.
3. Murphy KD: Embolotherapy. In Katz DS, Math KR, Groskin SA (eds): Radiology Secrets. Philadelphia, Hanley & Belfus, 1998, pp 502–510.
4. Pelage JP, Le Dref O, Mateo J, et al: Life-threatening primary postpartum hemorrhage: Treatment with emergency selective arterial embolization. Radiology 208(2):359–362, 1998.
5. Salem RS, Borsa JJ, Lewandowski RJ, et al: Arterial embolotherapy. Proceedings of the Society of Interventional Radiology Workshop, 29th Annual Meeting, 2004, pp 237–249.
6. Wells I: Internal iliac artery embolization in the management of pelvic bleeding. Clin Radiol 51(12):825–827, 1996.
7. Wojtowycz M: Handbook of Interventional Radiology and Angiography, 2nd ed. St. Louis, Mosby, 1995, pp 229–251.

CHAPTER 32

HEPATOBILIARY AND PORTAL VENOUS INTERVENTIONS

Jeffrey I. Mondschein, MD

1. **What are the indications for percutaneous transhepatic biliary drainage?**
   Percutaneous biliary drainage is indicated for the treatment of cholangitis or pruritus related to hyperbilirubinemia in the setting of benign or malignant obstructive biliary disease. Biliary drainage may also be performed in the setting of a traumatic bile leak to help divert bile and promote healing of the injured duct. In general, percutaneous drainage is only indicated if access of the ducts via endoscopic retrograde cholangiopancreatography is not possible.

KEY POINTS: BILIARY DRAINAGE

1. An obstructed, infected biliary system constitutes a medical emergency.

2. Complications from percutaneous biliary drainage can be life-threatening. An endoscopic approach is preferred when possible.

2. **What are the causes of benign and malignant biliary obstruction?**
   Common benign causes include bile duct calculi (Fig. 32-1), benign strictures, pancreatitis, and sclerosing cholangitis (Fig. 32-2). Less common benign causes include Caroli's disease, Mirizzi syndrome, and parasites. Malignant causes include pancreatic cancer (Fig. 32-3); metastatic disease; cholangiocarcinoma; and, less commonly, gallbladder carcinoma and ampullary tumors.

Figure 32-1. Percutaneous transhepatic cholangiogram performed to relieve biliary obstruction demonstrates multiple common bile duct stones, seen as filling defects among the injected intrabiliary contrast.

Figure 32-2. Percutaneous transhepatic cholangiogram demonstrates "beading" of the intrahepatic biliary ducts, with segments of duct dilation proximal to regions of duct stricture. This stricture-dilation pattern is common in sclerosing cholangitis.

Figure 32-3. Percutaneous transhepatic cholangiogram demonstrates intrahepatic biliary dilation due to malignant stricture of the common bile duct. This was due to carcinoma of the pancreatic head.

3. **What is the most commonly encountered biliary ductal anatomy?**
The main left bile duct is formed by the union of two horizontally oriented superior and inferior segmental ducts. Right lobe ductal anatomy is somewhat more complex and variable. The posterior-inferior and posterior-superior portions of the right hepatic lobe are drained by the right posterior ducts (also known as the "right dorsal caudal ducts"). The anterior-inferior and anterior-superior portions of the right hepatic lobe are drained by the right anterior ducts (also known as the "right ventral cranial ducts"). The main right hepatic duct is formed by the union of the right posterior and anterior ducts. The confluence of right and left ducts forms the common hepatic duct, which is joined by the cystic duct (from the gallbladder) to form the common bile duct. The most common biliary ductal anatomy (approximately 60% of the population) consists of a right posterior segment duct (RPSD) that joins the right anterior segment duct (RASD) to form the main right duct (Fig. 32-4).

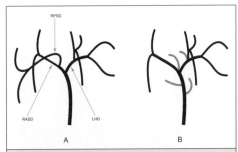

Figure 32-4. *A,* The most common biliary ductal anatomy consists of a right posterior segment duct (RPSD) that joins the right anterior segment duct (RASD) to form the main right duct. LHD = left hepatic duct. *B,* Variant insertions of the RPSD.

4. **What are the basic steps required to perform diagnostic percutaneous transhepatic cholangiography?**

Under fluoroscopic guidance, a 21- or 22-G needle is passed into the liver through an inferior intercostal or subcostal space at the level of the right midaxillary line. It is important to verify that the needle does not pass through the pleural space. The needle is withdrawn during injection of contrast in an effort to opacify a bile duct that may have been traversed as a result of the needle pass. When a bile duct is identified, contrast injection is continued, and the biliary tree is opacified. A diagnostic cholangiogram is performed with spot images obtained in anteroposterior and multiple bilateral oblique projections.

5. **What are the basic steps required to perform percutaneous transhepatic biliary drainage?**

If indicated by the diagnostic percutaneous transhepatic cholangiogram and clinical symptoms, a wire can be placed via the accessing needle into the biliary tree, followed by tract dilation and biliary drainage catheter placement. This is called the "one-stick" method. However, if the initial puncture was directed into a central duct, a "two-stick" technique may be used. Central duct punctures are less than ideal because the risk of injuring a major hepatic vessel is significant. Therefore, a second needle may be placed into an appropriate duct that will subsequently be dilated and used for access. The ideal access site will be an opacified peripheral duct that can be easily accessed under fluoroscopic guidance. Aside from a peripheral location, the duct's path should course through an angle that is gentle enough to allow a catheter to be advanced into the small bowel without extreme angulation. After the second access is obtained, the first needle can be removed. If left-sided biliary drainage is being performed, the needle is passed into the liver from a left subxiphoid approach.

6. **What is the difference between an external biliary drainage catheter and an internal/external biliary drainage catheter?**

External drains end internally within the bile ducts above the site of obstruction. The obstructed biliary tree is decompressed by draining the bile externally into a drainage bag. Internal/external drains cross the site of obstruction and end within the small bowel. Bile may drain internally from the biliary tree through side holes in the catheter into the small bowel, and the catheter may be capped externally. Internal/external drainage catheters are placed whenever it is possible to cross the site of obstruction, since this type of drainage is more physiologic. Internal drainage prevents loss of bile salts and electrolytes and allows the bile to aid in fat metabolism within the bowel. It is very important to monitor the volume status and electrolytes of patients draining bile externally. Such patients can lose a large volume of fluids rich in electrolytes.

7. **When should an internal/external drain be capped? When should it be uncapped?**

After a de novo biliary drainage, catheters are almost always placed to a bag for gravity drainage for a period of time. External drainage helps to decompress the biliary system. A pressurized system may promote bacterial translocation into the hepatic vasculature, resulting in sepsis. Obstructed systems are likely to be pressurized, and this is exacerbated by the contrast injected into the ducts during the procedure. Pruritus will often resolve faster if drainage is maximized. In the setting of a malignant obstruction, administration of chemotherapeutic agents may be delayed if the serum bilirubin level is excessively elevated. In certain situations, internal and external drainage may accelerate normalization of the serum bilirubin level and allow for the subsequent administration of chemotherapeutic agents.

Patients with drains placed for external drainage can lose a significant amount of fluids and electrolytes. Tubes are commonly capped when possible to allow more physiologic drainage of bile. Usually this occurs when concerns over infection have subsided and pruritus has resolved. If chemotherapy is planned, tube capping may be delayed until the serum bilirubin level is within an acceptable range.

After a tube has been capped, it should be uncapped for infectious concerns (fever, bacteremia, sepsis, elevated white blood count), leakage of bile around the catheter, pain, and rising bilirubin or other liver enzyme levels. After the tube is uncapped, additional tests may be indicated, such as a tube check to determine whether the tube is clogged or malpositioned.

8. **A patient begins to leak bile around an indwelling biliary drain. Why does this happen? What can be done?**
   Biliary drains are far from perfect and require considerable maintenance after they are placed. This is unfortunate for patients, and the maintenance often adversely affects their quality of life. Tubes leak for a variety of reasons. Standard biliary tubes consist of a catheter with side holes and a distal locking loop. For the tube to work properly, the side holes must be patent and properly positioned. The key to proper positioning is the proper location of the most peripheral side hole. This hole should be located just inside the biliary duct where access was obtained. If the most peripheral side hole of the catheter is malpositioned, leakage will also occur. Migration or malposition of the tube so that the hole is outside of the duct and in the parenchymal tract will result in bile leaking back along the catheter onto the skin. If the hole is too far in, the bile duct peripheral to the catheter may become obstructed and leak along the course of the catheter. A careful cholangiogram and meticulous tube placement will solve these problems. Another common cause of leaking is clogging of the side holes of the catheter with viscous bile. This can be managed with catheter exchange with consideration given to upsizing the tube if the complication occurs with frequency.

9. **What are the potential complications associated with percutaneous transhepatic biliary drainage?**
   Even in the absence of clinical signs of cholangitis, bile in an obstructed system is often colonized with bacteria. Biliary sepsis, a potentially lethal complication, may occur during or after a cholangiogram or biliary drainage. Antibiotics should be given during a biliary drainage, and patients should be monitored closely for signs of sepsis. Injury to blood vessels adjacent to the bile ducts within the hepatic parenchyma may be associated with pseudoaneurysms, hemorrhage, and hemobilia. Bile leakage and bile peritonitis may occur, as well as complications related to intraprocedural sedation (respiratory failure and aspiration). Pneumothorax and reactive or bilious pleural effusions are uncommon complications if care is taken during initial needle placement.

10. **After an initial drainage procedure, what additional management measures may be performed for the treatment of benign biliary obstruction?**
    Biliary drainage provides access to the bile ducts that may allow for retrieval of biliary calculi. Balloon dilation of benign ductal strictures with gradual upsizing of drainage catheter diameter may allow for remodeling of the bile duct with eventual relief of obstruction and removal of the drainage catheter. This therapy, when successful, usually takes several months. If unsuccessful, surgical intervention may still be possible, or catheters may be left in place for the long term.

11. **What can be done to manage the treatment of malignant biliary obstruction after initial drainage?**
    With some tumor types, access to the bile ducts will allow for the placement of radioactive isotopes for ductal brachytherapy. If the patient is not a candidate for surgical resection, the drainage catheters may be left in long term. Sometimes, internal metal stents may be placed across malignant strictures to allow for catheter removal for patient comfort. The decision to place a metallic stent depends on patient prognosis and life expectancy, since internal metal stents have limited long-term patency.

12. **What does the term *isolated ducts* mean? What is its significance?**
    In the case of a low obstruction of the common bile duct, the right and left systems will still communicate. Therefore, a right-sided biliary drain can be used to drain both the right and left

sides. If however, the level of obstruction is higher, as might occur with cholangiocarcinoma, this might not be the case and some ducts may not communicate with others—they will be "isolated." This is one reason why it is important to obtain cross-sectional imaging before biliary drainage. If only one ductal system is dilated, this information will help determine the access site (left-sided vs. right-sided drainage). By definition, patients with isolated ducts will have a portion of the biliary system that remains undrained if only a single catheter is placed. These patients may require more than one tube to treat infection, pruritus, or hyperbilirubinemia.

13. **How does stricture morphology help us to differentiate between benign and malignant disease?**
Benign strictures tend to taper smoothly, with gradual narrowing across their length. Malignant strictures, by contrast, are points of obstruction that end abruptly, sometimes with irregular borders or an appearance of "shouldering."

14. **If a histologic diagnosis is required, what methods may be used to biopsy the bile ducts?**
Once access to the bile ducts has been achieved, biopsy of a stricture site may be performed under fluoroscopic guidance. A variety of devices may be used to obtain tissue samples, including biopsy brushes, forceps, and needles. Often, several samples obtained on different days will be required to obtain a diagnosis.

15. **When is percutaneous cholecystostomy indicated?**
Although cholecystectomy is the preferred therapy for acute cholecystitis, some patients may not be surgical candidates due to their overall clinical status, sepsis, or other co-morbid conditions. Percutaneous cholecystostomy in combination with broad-spectrum antibiotic coverage is a temporizing measure until the patient's clinical status may be optimized for surgery.

16. **What are the basic steps involved in performing percutaneous cholecystostomy?**
With ultrasound guidance, the gallbladder is accessed with a needle. A wire is placed, and after tract dilation, a drainage catheter is placed into the gallbladder and allowed to drain externally. A subcostal, transhepatic path to the gallbladder is generally preferred because it may guard against bile leakage into the peritoneal space if the catheter is inadvertently dislodged.

17. **What are potential complications associated with percutaneous cholecystostomy?**
Complications include hemorrhage, infection, bile peritonitis, and respiratory failure or aspiration related to intraprocedural sedation. Pneumothorax is possible but relatively rare if a subcostal approach can be used.

18. **How long must a percutaneous cholecystostomy catheter remain within the gallbladder before it can be removed?**
Although some investigators have shown that catheters may sometimes be safely removed in less time, most believe that the cholecystostomy catheter should stay within the gallbladder for at least 4–6 weeks. This allows time for a mature tract to form between the gallbladder and skin surface in an effort to prevent bile leakage into the peritoneal space once the catheter is removed.

19. **Should the cholecystostomy catheter be placed to external drainage indefinitely?**
In the acute phase, even though there is evidence of active inflammation, the catheter should be maintained on external drainage. In the setting of cholecystitis due to obstructing biliary calculi,

the catheter should be maintained on external drainage. However, in the setting of acalculous cholecystitis, the catheter may be capped to allow for internal drainage after a cholangiogram is performed to document that there is no evidence of cystic duct obstruction.

20. **When is transjugular liver biopsy indicated and preferred over percutaneous liver biopsy?**
Because transjugular liver biopsy is a biopsy that is obtained from within a hepatic vein, bleeding complications resulting from transgression of the liver capsule may be avoided. Therefore, the trans-jugular procedure is indicated for patients with coagulopathies or platelet deficiency. Platelet dysfunction due to renal failure may also be an indication. In addition, any other issue that may make percutaneous biopsy difficult or risky (e.g., ascites) would be a potential indication for transjugular liver biopsy. Since transjugular biopsy cannot generally be used to obtain tissue from a specific liver lesion, it is used only to obtain a tissue diagnosis for medical (diffuse) liver disease such as viral hepatitis or transplant rejection.

21. **How is transjugular liver biopsy performed?**
A hepatic vein (most commonly, the right hepatic vein) is accessed using a transjugular approach (jugular vein to superior vena cava, through the right atrium to the inferior vena cava, and then into the right hepatic vein), and a stiff wire is placed. A stiff metal cannula is placed over the wire into the hepatic vein. An 18- or 19-G core biopsy needle is placed through the cannula and used to obtain multiple samples of liver tissue. Since the right hepatic vein courses posteriorly through the right lobe, the needle is directed anteriorly to avoid transgression of the liver capsule. However, since the middle hepatic vein courses more anteriorly, lateral or posterior sampling may be safer with this approach.

22. **What are the clinical signs and symptoms associated with portal hypertension?**
Esophageal, gastric, mesenteric, and rectal varices may bleed in response to elevated portal pressures, and mortality from the initial bleeding episode may be as high as 20–60%. Increased intrasinusoidal pressure may result in ascites and hepatic hydrothorax. Hepatic encephalopathy, hepatorenal syndrome with renal dysfunction, and hepatopulmonary syndrome with hypoxemia may also be encountered.

23. **How can we indirectly estimate portal venous pressure to confirm the diagnosis of portal hypertension?**
Catheterization of a hepatic vein is performed via jugular or femoral vein access. The catheter is advanced until it obstructs a small hepatic vein branch, or a balloon occlusion catheter is inflated within the hepatic vein to obstruct its outflow. The wedged hepatic vein pressure is actually a measure of sinusoidal pressure but allows for a reasonable indirect estimate of portal pressure. A corrected sinusoidal pressure measurement is obtained by subtracting the measured free hepatic venous pressure from the wedged hepatic venous pressure. Corrected sinusoidal pressure measurements less than or equal to 5 mmHg are considered normal. Measurements of 6–10 mmHg are compatible with mild portal hypertension, and those greater than 10 mmHg are compatible with more severe portal hypertension.

24. **What are the indications for creating a transjugular intrahepatic portosystemic shunt (TIPS)?**
The most common indication for TIPS placement is variceal bleeding related to portal hypertension that is refractory to endoscopic therapy (Fig. 32-5). Other indications include refractory ascites or hepatic hydrothorax, Budd-Chiari syndrome, portal hypertensive gastropathy, and hepatorenal or hepatopulmonary syndrome. TIPS placement may act as an effective bridge to liver transplantation for patients with end-stage liver disease and the manifestations of portal hypertension.

Figure 32-5. TIPS with a stent from the right hepatic vein to the right portal vein.

25. **What are the contraindications to TIPS creation?**
    A pre-TIPS total bilirubin level greater than 3 mg/dL, refractory coagulopathy with an interna-tional normalized ratio greater than 1.8, a Child-Pugh score greater than 12, and a serum creati-nine level greater than 1.9 mg/dL have all been found to be associated with poor outcomes. TIPS creation that is performed on an emergent basis is also associated with high mortality, and therefore, hemodynamic stabilization with transfusions, other medical interventions, and bal-loon tamponade of gastroesophageal varices are preferred before the TIPS procedure.

26. **What are the steps of the TIPS procedure?**
    - A hepatic vein, most commonly the right hepatic vein, is accessed via a right internal jugular vein approach. A wedged hepatic venogram may be obtained to opacify the portal vein and map its location.
    - A stiff metal cannula is placed, and a needle is passed from the right hepatic vein into the right portal vein under fluoroscopic guidance. Often, several needle passes are required to obtain portal access. The portosystemic pressure gradient measurement is obtained.
    - A stiff wire is placed into the portal vein, and dilation of the intrahepatic parenchymal tract is performed with an angioplasty balloon.
    - A flexible, self-expanding stent (usually 8 or 10 mm in diameter) is placed from the portal vein to the confluence of the hepatic vein with the inferior vena cava.
    - A venogram and repeat portosystemic pressure gradient measurements are obtained.

27. **What are the potential complications of TIPS creation?**
    Complications include hemorrhage, infection, contrast allergic reaction, and respiratory failure or aspiration due to intraprocedural sedation. In addition, since the TIPS causes shunting of por-tal venous blood away from the liver, the procedure may be complicated by decline in liver func-tion and hepatic encephalopathy.

28. **What are the short- and long-term goals of TIPS creation?**
    Successful TIPS creation will be associated with a final portosystemic pressure gradient meas-urement of <12 mmHg to prevent variceal bleeding. If the TIPS has been placed to treat refrac-tory ascites, lower pressures may be necessary for success (≤8 mmHg). If the patient becomes significantly encephalopathic and treatment with lactulose is insufficient to control symptoms, a reducing stent may be placed into the TIPS to intentionally raise the portosystemic pressure gra-dient. TIPS patency should be monitored at intervals using duplex Doppler ultrasound, which

will allow velocity measurements within the TIPS to be obtained noninvasively. Significant velocity increases from baseline may indicate the presence of TIPS stenosis, which may prompt TIPS venography and revision by balloon dilation or additional stent placement.

BIBLIOGRAPHY

1. LaBerge JM, Venbrux AC (eds): SCVIR syllabus: Biliary interventions. Fairfax, VA, SCVIR, 1995.
2. Patel NH, Haskal ZJ, Kerlan RK (eds): SCVIR syllabus: Portal hypertension: Diagnosis and interventions, 2nd ed. Fairfax, VA, SCVIR, 2001.

GENITOURINARY AND GASTROINTESTINAL INTERVENTIONAL RADIOLOGY

Charles T. Lau, MD, and S. William Stavropoulos, MD

CHAPTER 33

1. What are indications for a percutaneous nephrostomy (PCN)?

A PCN may be performed for a variety of indications, including (Fig. 33-1):

- To relieve obstruction in the setting of infection or to preserve renal function
- To assist in the removal of a stone or foreign body
- To divert urine to permit healing of a leak or fistula
- To provide access for ureteral intervention

2. What is the indication for an emergent PCN?

Pyonephrosis (infected urinary obstruction) may rapidly lead to urosepsis and death. It is, therefore, a urologic emergency, and emergent drainage is indicated.

Figure 33-1. PCN tube.

3. What are important technical factors to consider when performing a PCN?

A PCN is a relatively safe, minimally invasive technique that can be used to efficiently treat a variety of conditions. The safety and efficacy of the procedure, however, are predicated on the following well-established guidelines to help prevent complications. The skin puncture should be sufficiently lateral to the midline. This will ensure a relatively straight tract that avoids kinking of the catheter. The needle entry into the kidney should traverse the least vascular plane, and the access obtained should provide a path to all portions of the collecting system. It is also important that organs adjacent to the kidney, such as the colon, are not in the needle path.

4. What is the most common method of visualizing the collecting system for a PCN?

Fluoroscopy is the most common method, but this requires opacification of the collecting system. This can be accomplished by IV contrast injection with anterograde excretion, if the patient has satisfactory renal function. If the patient has impaired renal function or has a completely obstructed renal collecting system, fluoroscopy may not be a viable option. In these situations, an anterograde pyelogram can be performed via a 22- or 25-G needle. The anterograde pyelogram can be performed with iodinated contrast or carbon dioxide gas (Fig. 33-2).

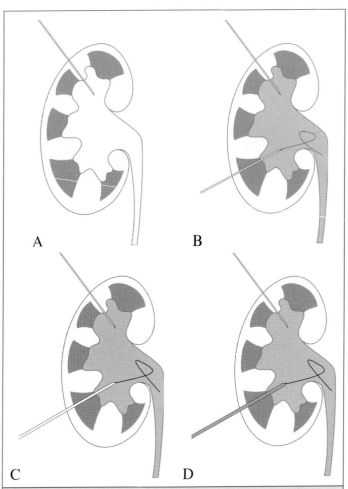

Figure 33-2. Schematic illustration of a PCN using the Seldinger technique. *A,* A posterior calyx is punctured with a 22-G needle under ultrasound guidance. *B,* After performing an anterograde pyelogram through this access point, a second 22-G needle is inserted into the opacified collecting system along the expected tract of the nephrostomy catheter. A 0.018-inch wire is then advanced through this needle. *C,* Exchange is made for a catheter that allows conversion to a 0.035-inch wire. *D,* The nephrostomy tract is dilated by exchanging successive dilators over the wire.

(Continued)

5. **What are alternative means of visualizing the collection system for a PCN other than fluoroscopy?**
   Ultrasound imaging can be used, which eliminates the need for contrast opacification of the collecting system. Ultrasound imaging also can be used to ensure that adjacent organs do not lie along a proposed nephrostomy tract. However, if the collecting system is not dilated, it may be difficult to visualize it with ultrasound. Computed tomography (CT) imaging is another option, particularly if the kidney is in an anomalous position.

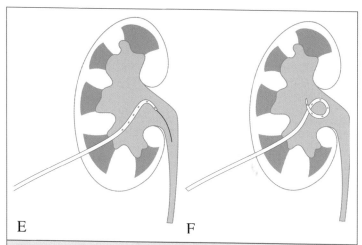

Figure 33-2, *Cont'd.* *E,* A 7- or 10-Fr locking loop nephrostomy catheter is finally advanced over the wire. *F,* The wire is removed, and the locking loop of the nephrostomy catheter is secured.

6. **Should access for a PCN be obtained through the renal parenchyma or directly into the renal pelvis?**
   Puncture of the collecting system should occur through the renal parenchyma because this is the least vascular plane. Direct access to the pelvis has a higher rate of vascular complications. Puncture through the renal parenchyma also helps to provide support for the catheter, minimize urine leakage, and decrease the chance of catheter displacement.

7. **From what approach should a PCN be performed?**
   A PCN tract should pass through the least vascular region of the kidney to minimize bleeding complications. Renal calyces are arranged in an anterior and posterior row. Between these two rows, in the interpolar kidney, is a relatively avascular plane of renal parenchyma called *Brödel's line*. This plane usually lies at 30–45 degrees, and the PCN tract should be made along this line.

8. **Aside from decreasing the chance of bleeding, what are the other benefits of performing a PCN through Brödel's line?**
   Such an approach also results in a PCN catheter exiting through skin near the posterior axillary line, so the catheter will not kink and the patient will not be uncomfortable lying on it when supine.

9. **What imaging modalities can be used to perform a percutaneous drainage of renal or perinephric abscesses?**
   Percutaneous drainage of renal and perinephric abscesses can be performed with ultrasound, CT, or even fluoroscopic guidance. Ultrasound is usually preferred because it provides real-time imaging, which allows for an accurate, safe, and fast procedure. It is important to place the drainage catheter in the most dependent portion of a large abscess cavity to ensure complete drainage of infected material.

10. **What are possible complications resulting from percutaneous drainage of renal or perinephric abscesses?**
    Percutaneous drainage is a safe and effective technique that can be used in the management of an abscess. Complications, however, may still occur. When collections adjacent to or within the

kidney are being drained, some infected material may intravasate into the vascular system, resulting in bacteremia or sepsis. It is important, therefore, to administer IV antibiotics both before and after drain placement. Drains placed within the kidney may accidentally traverse a blood vessel. Bleeding can be inconsequential and resolve spontaneously; may result in hematuria, if bleeding tracts into the collecting system; or may lead to a perinephric hematoma, if the hemorrhage tracts around the kidney. Rarely, adjacent organs may be inadvertently punctured during catheter placement.

11. **When is percutaneous management of urinary tract calculi preferred over extracorporeal shock wave lithotripsy (ESWL)?**
ESWL is the sole therapy used in approximately 90% of patients with symptomatic urinary tract calculi. However, percutaneous management is preferred in patients with a large stone burden. Percutaneous management may be also be used as an adjunct to ESWL if large stone fragments remain or if obstruction occurs after ESWL.

12. **What is the role of PCN in percutaneous treatment of urinary tract calculi?**
PCN is used to obtain a tract through which the endoscope may access the collecting system. It is important in this situation to create a tract that is straight and will permit the endoscope access to all portions of the collecting system.

13. **How are calculi removed during percutaneous treatment of the urinary tract?**
Different devices can be used through the endoscope once access to the collecting system has been obtained. These include a variety of stone baskets, which are three to eight wires arranged in a helical pattern. Forceps may be used to grab individual stones. Ultrasound and electrohydraulic lithotripters can also be used to pulverize calculi within the collecting system to facilitate removal.

14. **What are indications for ureteral stenting?**
Common indications include urinary tract calculi and benign ureteral stricture. Ureteral stenting is also indicated in patients with extrinsic ureteral obstruction, ureteral trauma, and retroperitoneal fibrosis. In the setting of malignant ureteral obstruction, stenting may be performed if the patient does not have bladder outlet obstruction. Stenting will allow the affected kidney to drain, and the patient will be able to void. The most commonly used ureteral stents are the double-J stent and nephroureteral stent.

15. **Describe the difference between a double-J ureteral stent and a nephroureteral stent.**
All ureteral stents are made of polyurethane or silicone; metallic stents are not used in ureters. A double-J ureteral stent is completely internal and has a "pigtail" at each end (Fig. 33-3, *A*). Its proximal coil is situated in the renal pelvis, and its distal coil is situated in the urinary bladder. A nephroureteral stent has a "pigtail" at its distal end that is placed in the bladder and another one that is looped in the renal pelvis (Fig. 33-3, *B*). The catheter exits through the skin at the percutaneous access site.

16. **How does a ureteral stent work?**
A ureteral stent is hollow and has multiple side holes. It drains urine past obstructions from the collecting system into the urinary bladder. Some believe that an element of capillary action augments this process. A ureteral stent also causes passive dilation of the ureter, which may or may not persist once the stent is removed.

17. **What are indications for esophageal stenting?**
Esophageal stenting is most commonly performed in the treatment of dysphagia due to cancer ingrowth and bronchoesophageal fistula (Fig. 33-4).

Figure 33-3. *A,* Double-J ureteral stent. *B,* Nephroureteral stent.

18. **What are technical complications associated with esophageal stenting?**
Even with the most experienced operators, stents may be malpositioned or migrate. Because esophageal malignancies may be friable, stenting may occasionally result in esophageal perforation, a potentially life-threatening complication.

19. **What factors should be considered when selecting the puncture site for a percutaneous gastrostomy?**
The site of the percutaneous gastrostomy should be subcostal and to the left of the midline (Fig. 33-5). The outer third of the rectus abdominis muscle should be avoided because the inferior epigastric artery courses in this region. Fluoroscopy should be performed so that the puncture avoids the colon and small bowel.

20. **G tube, G-J tube, J tube: What is the difference?**
A simple rule to follow in selecting an enteral access site is to use the stomach whenever possible. Direct gastrostomy (G) tubes are safe and easy to use. The stomach performs important digestive functions, and gastric access allows patients to receive bolus feeds. Jejunal access necessitates continuous feeds, which are not as well tolerated. The needs of the majority of patients can be met with G tubes.

Figure 33-4. Esophageal stent.

- A *G tube* is placed directly into the stomach and can be used for feeding or gastric decompression.
- *Gastrojejunostomy tubes (G-J tubes)* enter the stomach like a G tube but pass through the stomach and duodenum and terminate in the proximal jejunum (Fig. 33-6). G-J tubes are technically simpler to place than jejunostomy (J) tubes and are associated with a lower procedural risk (again, use the stomach, even for access, whenever possible). G-J tubes may have

Figure 33-5. Gastrostomy tube.

a single port that enters the small bowel. In patients with gastric outlet obstruction, G-J tubes with two ports may be used. One port is used to vent the stomach, and the other is used to administer feeds. In addition, a previously placed G tube can be converted to a G-J tube.

- *J tubes* enter the small bowel directly (Fig. 33-7). They may be used for feedings or for palliative decompression when placed above an obstruction.

KEY POINTS: GENITOURINARY AND GASTROINTESTINAL INTERVENTIONAL RADIOLOGY ✓

1. Urosepsis is an indication for emergent PCN.

2. A PCN tract should pass through the skin near the posterior axillary line, pass through the renal parenchyma in the relatively avascular plane denoted by Brödel's line, and enter the collecting system.

3. Although ureteral stents successfully drain the collecting system into the bladder and cause passive dilation of the ureter, they are considered a temporary measure and are not necessarily curative.

4. Patients with ascites should receive large-volume paracentesis before percutaneous gastrostomy.

5. J tubes and G-J tubes are reserved for patients with known gastroesophageal reflux disease and/or documented aspiration.

---

21. **When are feeding G tubes not the tube of choice?**
    Patients may not be candidates for *feeding* G tubes because of anatomic or functional reasons. Anatomic contraindications include prior gastrectomy or gastric pull-through, colon adhered to the stomach, and ascites. Patients with ascites are at high risk for constantly leaking fluid through the puncture site. Functional reasons include severe reflux with aspiration, gastroparesis, and gastric outlet obstruction. On the other hand, *decompressive* G tubes may be indicated in patients with gastric outlet obstruction.

Figure 33-6. Gastrojejunostomy tube.

Figure 33-7. Jejunostomy tube.

22. **When are small bowel feeding tubes indicated?**
J tubes and G-J tubes are usually reserved for patients with known severe gastroesophageal reflux disease with the risk of aspiration.

WEBSITES

1. http://www.emedicine.com/radio/topic796.htm.

2. http://www.medscape.com/viewarticle/423508_1.

3. http://www.emedicine.com/radio/topic798.htm.

BIBLIOGRAPHY

1. Dunnick NR, Sandler CM, Newhouse JH, Amis Jr ES: Textbook of Uroradiology, 2nd ed. Baltimore, Williams & Wilkins, 1997.
2. Wojtowycz M: Handbook of Interventional Radiology and Angiography, 2nd ed. St. Louis, Mosby, 1995.

EXTREMITY PLAIN FILMS AND TRAUMA

Woojin Kim, MD, and Neil Roach, MD

CHAPTER 34

1. How are fractures evaluated with plain films?
At least two views of the fracture site, taken at 90 degrees to each other, must be obtained. Remember, "one view equals no view." The radiographs obtained should include joints immediately above and below the fractured area for evaluation of associated dislocations.

2. Define the following terms: dislocation, subluxation, closed fracture, open fracture, intra-articular fracture, pathologic fracture, and occult fracture.
- *Dislocation* is complete loss of contact between the articular surfaces of a joint. A partial loss of congruity between articular surfaces defines *subluxation.*
- *Closed fracture* has intact skin over the fracture site. If there is communication between the fracture site and the outside environment, it is considered an *open fracture,* regardless of how small the overlying skin defect is.
- *Intra-articular fracture* involves the articular surface of a joint.
- *Pathologic fracture* is a fracture in abnormal bone weakened by a disease process.
- *Occult fracture* is a fracture that is not visible on a plain radiograph.

KEY POINTS: BASIC TERMINOLOGY

1. Dislocation is complete loss of contact between the bones of a joint.

2. Subluxation is partial loss of contact between the bones of a joint.

3. Open fracture has an open wound that allows communication between the outside environment and the fracture site.

4. Intra-articular fracture involves the articular surface.

5. Pathologic fracture is a fracture in an abnormal, diseased bone.

3. What is an avulsion fracture?
Avulsion fracture occurs when a fragment of bone is pulled off at the site of insertion of muscles, ligaments, and tendons.

4. What is a comminuted fracture?
A fracture with more than two fracture fragments.

5. What is an os acromiale?
Os acromiale is an accessory ossification center of the acromion. Although the os acromiale is normally fused by the age of 25, it remains unfused in a certain percentage of the population. It is an important entity to be aware of because it may be misinterpreted as an acromial fracture.

6. **Describe types I, II, and III acromioclavicular (AC) separation.**

As the term suggests, AC separation is widening of the AC joint space due to ligamentous injury.

- *Type I* AC separation is stretching or partial tear of the AC ligament with no displacement seen on a radiograph. One can radiographically assess this condition by obtaining and comparing weight-bearing views of both the uninjured and injured shoulders. This is a stable injury and has excellent prognosis of healing.

- *Type II* AC separation is complete tear of the AC ligament with widening of the AC joint. The majority of these injuries will heal without surgery.

- *Type III* AC separation is complete disruption of the AC and coracoclavicular ligaments. There is abnormal widening of the AC and coracoclavicular joints as a result. This type of injury requires internal fixation (Fig. 34-1).

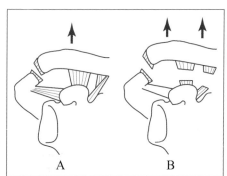

Figure 34-1. *A,* Type II AC separation. Note that only the AC ligament is ruptured. *B,* Type III AC separation. There is complete tear of both the AC and coracoclavicular ligaments.

7. **What is a "Y" view?**

It is a special radiographic view of the shoulder that shows the head of the humerus sitting between the two projections off the scapula, namely the acromion and the coracoid process, forming a Y. This view is helpful in determining the relative position of the humeral head and the glenoid fossa and aids in the diagnosis of shoulder (glenohumeral) dislocation.

8. **What are the radiographic features of anterior shoulder dislocation on an anteroposterior view?**

Anterior-inferior is the most common type of shoulder dislocation. The humeral head is displaced anteromedially and typically rests slightly inferior to the coracoid process. Hence, it is also known as "infracoracoid dislocation" or "subcoracoid dislocation."

9. **What are Hill-Sachs fractures and Bankart fractures?**

The Hill-Sachs fracture and Bankart fracture are complications of anterior shoulder dislocation. The Hill-Sachs fracture is a defect in the posterolateral aspect of the humeral head. It occurs when there is contact between this region of the humeral head and the anterior-inferior glenoid rim during anterior dislocation. The Bankart fracture is a fracture of the anterior-inferior glenoid rim secondary to this trauma.

10. **What is pseudosubluxation of the humerus?**

With this entity, there is inferior displacement of the humeral head with widening of the glenohumeral space. This is usually caused by hemarthrosis or lipohemarthrosis after trauma to the shoulder. As the term suggests, this is not true dislocation of the glenohumeral joint.

11. **What are the "posterior fat pad sign" and the "sail sign" in the elbow?**

The posterior fat pad and sail signs indicate the presence of an intra-articular elbow fracture. Fat is normally present between the synovium and capsule of the elbow joint, which is normally not radiographically visible, with the exception of occasional normal anterior fat pad that may be seen as a small lucency immediately adjacent to the anterior cortex of the distal humerus. With intra-articular fracture, however, subsequent hemarthrosis distends the synovium and causes displacement of this fat. The posterior fat pad becomes visible as a radiolucency and the anterior fat pad is lifted away from the bone as a triangular radiolucency, causing it to resemble a sail.

12. **Describe Monteggia's fracture and its associated finding.**
Monteggia's fracture is a fracture of the proximal ulna with radial head subluxation or dislocation. This fracture-dislocation was originally described by Giovanni Battista Monteggia in 1814. It is important to remember to look for the associated radial head dislocation or subluxation when you see a proximal ulnar fracture because failure to do so will result in radial head necrosis.

13. **Describe Galeazzi's fracture and its associated finding.**
Galeazzi's fracture is a fracture of the distal radius with associated distal radioulnar dislocation/subluxation. Ricardo Galeazzi described this fracture in 1935.

14. **Name all eight carpal bones. Which carpal bone gets fractured the most often?**
A well-known mnemonic used for memorizing all the carpal bones is the following (proximal row from radial to ulnar direction and then distal row from radial to ulnar direction): *some lovers try positions that they cannot handle*, which stands for *s*caphoid, *l*unate, *t*riquetrum, *p*isiform, *t*rapezium, *t*rapezoid, *c*apitate, and *h*amate. The following tip can help you remember the respective positions of trapezium and trapezoid: trapezi*um* is associated with the th*um*b.
The scaphoid is the carpal bone that is fractured the most often. Fracture of the scaphoid should be suspected when there is tenderness of the anatomic snuff box. Scaphoid fractures can be difficult to visualize on plain radiographs. The blood supply to the scaphoid enters from the waist (middle third) and distal pole by the scaphoid branches of the radial artery. As result, blood flows proximally from the distal pole. When this is disrupted by a fracture, avascular necrosis of the proximal fracture fragment occurs and can be seen as sclerosis.

15. **What is the "Terry-Thomas sign"?**
Scapholunate dissociation results from ligamentous disruption between the scaphoid and lunate. This is manifested by widening of the space between the scaphoid and lunate on the AP view of the wrist and is known as the Terry-Thomas sign. Terry Thomas (1911-1990) was a gap-toothed British comic actor.

16. **What are dorsal intercalated segmental instability (DISI) and volar intercalated segmental instability (VISI)?**
DISI and *VISI* are terms used to describe carpal instability based on the tilt of lunate on the lateral radiograph of the wrist. With DISI, the lunate tilts dorsally. With VISI, the lunate tilts in a volar direction (Fig. 34-2).

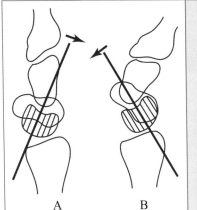

A   B

Figure 34-2. *A,* DISI. Note the dorsal tilt of the lunate (indicated by the vertical lines). *B,* VISI. Conversely, there is volar tilt of the lunate.

17. **Match the following fractures with the radiographic images in Figure 34-3: Barton's, baseball (mallet) finger, Bennett's, boxer's, Colles', Smith's, and triquetral.**
See Figure 34-3.

Figure 34-3. *A,* Triquetral fracture. Dorsal avulsion fracture *(arrow)* seen best on the lateral view. *B,* Colles' fracture. Nonarticular distal radial fracture with dorsal displacement of the distal fracture fragment. *C,* Mallet finger. Avulsion fracture of the base of the distal phalanx at the extensor digitorum tendon insertion site. *D,* Bennett's fracture. Intra-articular fracture-dislocation of the base of the first metacarpal. *E,* Smith's fracture. Nonarticular distal radial fracture with volar displacement of the distal fracture fragment.

(Continued)

Figure 34-3, *Cont'd*. *F,* Barton's fracture. Intra-articular oblique fracture of the dorsal aspect of the distal radius. *G,* Boxer's fracture. Transverse fracture of the distal fifth metacarpal.

18. **What is more common, anterior or posterior dislocation of the hip?**
    Posterior hip dislocation is more common. It is manifested by superior displacement of the femoral head. In anterior hip dislocation, the femoral head is displaced anteriorly and medially.

19. **What is a bipartite patella?**
    It is another normal anatomic variant that one should not misinterpret as being a fracture of the patella. It is a secondary ossification center that is seen in the upper outer quadrant of the patella. It is usually bilateral and has a smooth and sclerotic cortical border.

20. **What is a Segond fracture and its clinical implication?**
    It is an avulsion fracture of the proximal lateral tibia at the site of attachment of the lateral ligament. The fracture fragment may be very small. Even though it may not look so terrible on a radiograph, it is commonly associated with anterior cruciate ligament tear and meniscal injury.

21. **What is a tibial plafond fracture?**
    It is an intra-articular fracture of the distal tibia caused by impaction of the talus and is often comminuted.

22. **Match the following fractures with their radiographic images in Figure 34-4: Freiberg, Jones, Maisonneuve, and Segond fractures.**
    See Figure 34-4.

Figure 34-4. *A,* Jones fracture. Transverse fracture of the base of the fifth metatarsal. *B–C,* Maisonneuve fracture. Tear of interosseous membrane and fracture of the upper third of fibula *(B)* with associated medial malleolus fracture *(C) D,* Segond fracture. A small cortical avulsion fracture *(arrow)* of the proximal lateral tibia. *E,* Freiberg's infraction is osteonecrosis of the second or third metatarsal head from a subchondral fatigue fracture.

BIBLIOGRAPHY

1. Harris JH, Harris WH: The Radiology of Emergency Medicine. Philadelphia, Lippincott Williams & Wilkins, 2000.
2. Hunter TB, Peltier LF, Lund PJ: Radiologic history exhibit. Musculoskeletal eponyms: Who are those guys? Radiographics 20:819-836, 2000.
3. Schultz RJ: The Language of Fractures, 2nd ed. Baltimore, Williams & Wilkins, 1990.

CHAPTER 35

PLAIN FILM EXAMINATION OF SPINAL TRAUMA

Woojin Kim, MD, and Neil Roach, MD

1. **Describe a standard cervical spine examination.**
   A standard cervical spine examination includes anteroposterior (AP), lateral, and open-mouth odontoid views. Occasionally, bilateral oblique radiography may be obtained for evaluation of the neural foramina and facet joints.

2. **Describe how to interpret a lateral cervical spine film.**
   - Count the vertebral bodies. All seven cervical vertebral bodies should be visualized, as well as C7–T1. If not, then either a swimmer's view or limited lower cervical spine computed tomography scan can be obtained.
   - Evaluate the thickness of prevertebral soft tissue. It should be less than 5 mm anterior to C1–C3. From C4–C7, its thickness should not exceed 20 mm.
   - Assess four parallel lines for alignment. From anterior to posterior, these lines are anterior vertebral, posterior vertebral, spinolaminar, and posterior spinous (Fig. 35-1).
   - Examine the atlantoaxial interval, which is the distance between the posterior aspect of the anterior arch of C1 and the anterior aspect of the odontoid process of C2 (axis). This space should not exceed 3 mm in adults and 5 mm in children. This interval should remain constant with flexion and extension in adults. Widening of this space is indicative of disruption of the transverse atlantal ligament.
   - Compare the intervertebral disc spaces for widening or narrowing.

3. **What is a swimmer's view?**
   A swimmer's view is obtained when the lower cervical vertebrae cannot be seen on the lateral view, usually due to a patient's inability to cooperate or a large shoulder girdle obscuring the view. This view is obtained by having the patient, in the supine position, raise his or her arm over the head while lowering the other arm.

4. **Describe Jefferson's fracture and its mechanism of injury.**
   It is an unstable burst fracture involving the ring of C1 with lateral displacement of lateral masses and disruption of the transverse ligament. This fracture is associated with axial load injuries.

Figure 35-1. Normal lateral view of the cervical spine. Cervical vertebrae to C7–T1 can be visualized. Four parallel lines used for assessment of alignment are drawn: A, anterior vertebral; B, posterior vertebral; C, spinolaminar; and; D, posterior spinous process.

5. **Describe three different types of odontoid process (also known as "dens") fractures.**
   - *Type I* fracture involves the superior tip of the odontoid process. It is extremely rare, and some authorities even argue over its existence.
   - *Type II* is the most common and is characterized by a fracture through the base of the odontoid process. Unlike the other two types, this fracture is considered mechanically unstable.
   - *Type III* fracture involves the body of C2.

6. **What is os odontoideum?**
   Os odontoideum describes separation of the dens from the body of C2. It appears as a well-circumscribed ossicle with a smooth, thin cortex that is separated from the adjacent dens by a radiolucent gap. It was originally thought that this represented failure of fusion of the secondary ossification center with the remaining dens. Such a congenital anomaly, however, is now known as "persistent ossiculum terminale" and appears as a small ossicle at the tip of the dens. Most authorities now agree that os odontoideum is more likely an acquired posttraumatic abnormality. Regardless, this entity can be differentiated from an acute odontoid fracture by the presence of a sclerotic cortical margin and occasional hypertrophy of the anterior arch of axis. Os odontoideum can cause atlantoaxial instability. Some studies have demonstrated increased frequency of this entity in patients with Down syndrome.

7. **What is a hangman's fracture?**
   As the name suggests, hangman's fracture can be seen after a motor vehicle accident in which the chin strikes the dashboard. It is a hyperextension injury. There is bilateral fracture of the pars interarticularis. This type of fracture can be subtle on radiography and be easily overlooked (Fig. 35-2).

8. **What is a flexion teardrop fracture? What is its prognostic significance?**
   It is a severe hyperflexion injury of the cervical spine that results in anterior compression fracture of the vertebral body and disruption of the posterior ligament. Due to severe kyphotic angulation of the cervical spinal cord at this level,

Figure 35-2. Lateral plain film radiograph of a hangman's fracture. Note the disruption of the spinolaminar line *(arrow)*.

there is usually associated anterior cervical cord syndrome. The teardrop component is seen as a fracture fragment off the anterior-inferior corner of the involved vertebral body (Fig. 35-3). Remember that flexion teardrop fractures are the most severe and unstable spinal fractures. Schneider in 1956 described this fracture as a "teardrop" fracture-dislocation because it reminded him of the tear from a patient after he conveyed the seriousness of the injury.

9. **What is a clay shoveler's fracture?**
   It is a fracture of the spinous process, often seen in the lower cervical spine (Fig. 35-4). In the 1930s, there were a large number of men who worked as clay shovelers in Australia. This injury occurred as result of hyperflexion when the worker attempted to throw a shovel full of clay with the shovel stuck in the clay. In modern days, this fracture occurs as result of football and power-lifting injuries.

10. **What is the difference between unilateral and bilateral interfacetal dislocations?**
    Unilateral interfacetal dislocation (also known as "unilateral locked facet injury") is a rotational injury of the cervical spine that results in unilateral facet joint dislocation with associated posterior ligamentous tear. Bilateral interfacetal dislocation (also known as "bilateral locked facet injury") results from extreme hyperflexion, causing anterior dislocation of both facet joints. This is a serious injury that is commonly associated with spinal cord damage.

11. **What is the difference between compression and burst fractures?**
    Compression fractures are caused by anterior flexion. There is anterior wedging of the affected vertebral body, with the middle vertebral column remaining intact. Since only the anterior vertebral column is affected, this fracture is usually stable. Burst fractures are caused by axial loading injuries. The fracture lines extend through both the anterior and posterior cortices of the vertebral body. The posterior displacement of fracture fragments can cause spinal cord injury, and hence these fractures are considered unstable.

12. **What is a Chance fracture?**
    There is horizontal splitting of the posterior elements extending anteriorly to involve the vertebral body and/or intervertebral disc space. It is often associated with tearing of the posterior ligament complex. It is also

Figure 35-3. Flexion teardrop fracture. There is focal kyphosis at C5 with posterior displacement of the vertebral body and a teardrop fracture fragment *(arrow)*.

Figure 35-4. Clay shoveler's fracture. There is a minimally displaced fracture of the posterior spinous process of C7 *(arrow)*.

called a "seat belt fracture" after acute hyperflexion. Presence of this fracture should alert the clinician to the existence of significant intra-abdominal injury.

13. **What is a "Scotty dog"?**
On the oblique view of the lumbar spine, an outline of what looks like a dog can be seen. The parts of the dog are as follows: the transverse process makes up the nose, the pedicle makes up the eye, the superior articular facet makes up the ear, the pars interarticularis makes up the neck, the inferior articular facet makes up the front leg, the lamina makes up the body, the contralateral superior articular facet makes up the tail, and finally, the contralateral inferior articular facet makes up the hind leg (Fig. 35-5).

Figure 35-5. *A,* "Scotty dog" (see question 13). *B,* Fracture of pars interarticularis, the "neck" of the "Scotty dog."

14. **What is spondylolysis? Describe spondylolisthesis and its grading method.**
Spondylolysis is a defect or fracture of the pars interarticularis. On the "Scotty dog" view, it is seen as a band of radiolucency through the "neck," like a collar. L5 is most commonly involved. When this condition involves bilateral pars interarticularis, it is commonly associated with a condition called *spondylolisthesis,* which is anterior translation of the involved vertebral body with respect to its inferior adjacent vertebral body. It is graded I through IV, based on the degree of anterior displacement. If it is displaced anteriorly <25% of the vertebral body's AP dimension, it is considered to be grade I. Displacements of 25–50%, 50–75%, and >75% constitute grades II, III, and IV, respectively. Its etiology can be congenital, traumatic, degenerative, or pathologic, such as from Paget's disease or osteogenesis imperfecta.

BIBLIOGRAPHY

1. Harris JH, Harris WH: The Radiology of Emergency Medicine. Philadelphia, Lippincott Williams & Wilkins, 2000.
2. Hunter TB, Peltier LF, Lund PJ: Radiologic history exhibit. Musculoskeletal eponyms: Who are those guys? Radiographics 20:819-836, 2000.
3. Schultz RJ: The Language of Fractures, 2nd ed. Baltimore, Williams & Wilkins, 1990.

NONTRAUMATIC SPINE PLAIN FILMS AND DEGENERATIVE DISEASE

Christopher J. Yoo, MD, and Neil Roach, MD

CHAPTER 36

1. **Define scoliosis, and name the most common cause.**
   Scoliosis is defined as lateral curvature of the spine in the coronal plane, whereas *kyphosis* and *lordosis* refer to anterior and posterior curvature in the sagittal plane. In the majority of cases of scoliosis, the cause is idiopathic.

2. **Describe the three subgroups of idiopathic scoliosis.**
   - *Infantile idiopathic scoliosis* is typically detected before 4 years of age and is more common in boys. When diagnosed in the first year of life, 92% of cases resolve spontaneously.
   - *Juvenile idiopathic scoliosis* is diagnosed between 4 and 10 years of age and is seen predominantly in boys before the age of 6 and predominantly in girls between ages 7 and 10. Only 7% of cases resolve spontaneously.
   - *Adolescent idiopathic scoliosis* is diagnosed between age 10 and skeletal maturity and is the most common type of idiopathic scoliosis. There is a heavy predominance in girls.

3. **Although idiopathic scoliosis is the most common type of scoliosis, what other etiologic factors should be considered before making this diagnosis?**
   Other etiologic factors can be grouped as in Table 36-1.

TABLE 36-1. OTHER ETIOLOGIC FACTORS TO CONSIDER BEFORE MAKING THE DIAGNOSIS OF IDIOPATHIC SCOLIOSIS

Category	Examples
Congenital*	Block vertebra, hemivertebra, vertebral bar
Neuromuscular	Cerebral palsy, muscular dystrophy, spinal cord injury
Developmental	Skeletal dysplasia, neurofibromatosis
Neoplasm*	Osteoid osteoma, osteoblastoma
Trauma and other	Trauma, postradiation

*Particularly in otherwise healthy patients, effort should be focused on excluding congenital vertebral segmentation, fusion anomalies, and neoplasm.

4. **What is a limbus vertebra?**
   An abnormality of the anterior-inferior or anterior-superior corner of a vertebral body secondary to an unfused ring apophysis of the end plate. It appears as a corticated ossicle, usually triangular in shape and separated from the rest of the vertebral body by herniated disc material. It is not definitively known whether this is congenital or traumatic in nature (Fig. 36-1).

287

Figure 36-1. Lateral plain film examination of the neck demonstrates a triangular-shaped, well-corticated ossicle at the superior endplate of C5 *(arrow)*. This is a limbus vertebra.

5. **What is a butterfly vertebra? Hemivertebra? Block vertebra?**

These are all congenital vertebral anomalies. The vertebral bodies form initially from two chondral centers, side by side, which eventually fuse to form a single body. If one chondral center fails to form, a hemivertebra results. If the chondral centers fail to fuse in the midline and there is hypoplasia centrally, a butterfly vertebra results (Fig. 36-2, *A*). If there is nonsegmentation of these centers from the chondral centers above or below, a block vertebra may result (Fig. 36-2, *B*). These congenital anomalies can result in premature degenerative disease or structural abnormalities such as congenital scoliosis and kyphosis. They should also alert the radiologist to the possibility of other anomalies in the VACTERL complex (*v*ertebral, *a*norectal, *c*ardiac, *tr*acheal, *e*sophageal, *r*ectal, and *l*imb anomalies).

Figure 36-2. *A*, Frontal radiograph of the lumbar spine demonstrates a butterfly vertebral body segment at L4. *B*, Lateral radiograph of the thoracolumbar junction demonstrates nonsegmented block vertebrae.

6. **What descriptors are important when reporting scoliosis?**
Location and direction of the curvature, Cobb angle, rotational component, whether it is fixed (structural) versus not fixed (nonstructural), presence of congenital anomaly or neoplasm, and Risser stage.

7. **How do you measure the Cobb angle?**
One of two methods is used, depending on the severity of the scoliosis. Visually determine the highest vertebra at the beginning and the lowest vertebra at the end of the curvature. Draw a line parallel to the superior end plate of the top vertebral body and a line parallel to the inferior end plate of the lower vertebral body. The angle at the intersection of these two lines is the Cobb angle. If the scoliosis is mild, the intersection of the two lines will obviously be far away. Therefore, draw lines perpendicular to the previously described lines and measure the Cobb angle at their intersection. Use whichever method is convenient, because they will result in the same angle measurement (Fig. 36-3).

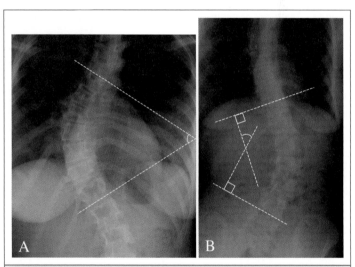

Figure 36-3. Frontal radiographs of patients with scoliosis demonstrate methods for measuring the Cobb angle in moderate *(A)* and mild *(B)* scoliosis.

8. **What is the Risser classification? Why is it significant in scoliosis?**
It is a gross measure of skeletal maturity as determined by the amount of ossification of the iliac apophysis. The apophyseal ossification begins laterally and progresses medially with increasing skeletal maturity. The Risser classification is significant in scoliosis because the likelihood of progression is high in low Risser stages (e.g., skeletal immaturity) and decreases once the patient reaches skeletal maturity (Fig. 36-4).

Figure 36-4. Risser stages for determining skeletal maturity through evaluation of degree of ossification of the iliac apophysis.

9. **What are the radiographic signs of degenerative disc disease?**
Disc space narrowing; osteophyte formation; end-plate sclerosis; Schmorl's nodes; vacuum disc phenomenon; facet osteoarthritis; neural foraminal narrowing; and in the cervical spine, uncovertebral joint hypertrophy.

10. **What is a Schmorl's node?**
A Schmorl's node is a herniation of intervertebral disc material through the vertebral end plate, resulting in a lucent area at the end plate with surrounding sclerosis on radiographs and computed tomography (CT) and possibly surrounding edema on magnetic resonance imaging (MRI) (Fig. 36-5).

11. **What is the best way to image degenerative disc disease?**
MRI is now the modality of choice for anatomic accuracy in imaging degenerative disc disease and its effects on the spinal canal and neural foramina.

12. **What are Modic changes of the vertebral end plates?**
These are MRI findings of the marrow adjacent to the vertebral end plates associated with degenerative disc disease in the lumbar spine.
   - *Modic type I* change refers to a marrow edema-like pattern that histopathologically correlates with subchondral vascularized fibrous tissue with end-plate fissures and is seen as low signal on T1-weighted images and high signal on T2-weighted images relative to normal marrow signal.
   - *Modic type II* change refers to a fatty marrow change seen as increased signal on T1-weighted images and as isointense or increased signal on T2-weighted images relative to normal marrow signal.
   - *Modic type III* change refers to subchondral sclerosis, which is seen as low signal on both T1- and T2-weighted images.

Figure 36-5. Lateral radiograph of the lumbar spine demonstrates multiple degenerative end-plate Schmorl's nodes *(arrows)*.

13. **What terms are used to describe the different types of disc extension beyond the vertebral body margin?**
The spectrum includes disc bulge, protrusion, extrusion, and sequestration (Fig. 36-6).
   - *Disc bulge* is diffuse enlargement of the intervertebral disc, which is usually symmetric or slightly eccentric to one side and results from laxity or stretching of the annulus fibrosus.
   - *Disc protrusion* is an area of more focal disc extension beyond the boundaries of the remainder of the disc but is still contained within the annulus fibrosus. The neck of the protrusion is the widest portion of the abnormality.
   - *Disc extrusion* is a focal disc extension in which the neck is narrower than the extruded portion of the disc and indicates extrusion through an annular fissure. Extrusions will often extend superiorly or inferiorly, along the long axis of the spinal canal.
   - *Disc sequestrum* is a free fragment of the intervertebral disc, which has extruded through the annulus and separated from the remainder of the disc to lie within the extradural space.

14. **Other than degenerative disc pathology, what other factors commonly contribute to neural foraminal narrowing and central canal stenosis?**
Facet osteoarthritis, which can result in sclerosis and subsequent enlargement of the facet joint complex, and ligamentum flavum hypertrophy both contribute to narrowing. Spondylolisthesis can also contribute, particularly if it is secondary to degenerative disease rather than spondylolysis. In

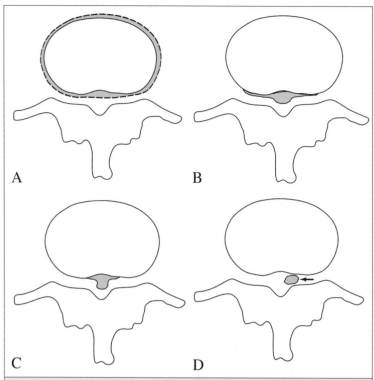

Figure 36-6. Illustrations of terms used to describe extension of the intervertebral disc beyond the margin of the vertebral body. *A,* A disc bulge is diffuse and symmetric. *B,* A disc protrusion (in this case, a central disc protrusion) has focality, and the neck is the widest part of the abnormality. *C,* An extrusion also has focality, but the neck is the narrowest part. *D,* A disc sequestrum has lost all connection to the disc and lies in the epidural space.

the cervical spine, osteophytes along the posterior margins of the vertebral end plates and uncovertebral hypertrophy, in addition to the previously mentioned factors, can contribute to narrowing.

KEY POINTS: TERMINOLOGY OF DEGENERATIVE DISC PATHOLOGY

1. Disc bulge: diffuse, symmetric extension of the disc beyond the end plate.

2. Disc protrusion: more focal extension of the disc. It may be central, left/right paracentral, or left/right lateral. The "neck" is wider than the more distal portion.

3. Disc extrusion: herniation of a portion of the disc. The "neck" is the narrowest part. The extrusion often extends superiorly or inferiorly along the long axis of the spinal canal.

4. Disc sequestrum: free disc fragment in the epidural space that has lost its connection to the disc.

15. **What nerve root exits the C3–C4 neural foramen? C7–T1? T3–T4? L3–L4?**
    In the cervical spine, C1 exits between the occiput and C1, whereas C8 exits at C7–T1.
    Therefore, the cervical nerve roots exit above the pedicles of the same-numbered vertebral body

(i.e., the C4 nerve root exits through the C3–C4 foramen). Because there are eight cervical roots, the relationship switches at the cervicothoracic junction, and in the thoracic and lumbar spine, the nerve root exits below the pedicle of the same-numbered vertebral body (i.e., T3 exits though the T3–T4 foramen, and L3 exits through the L3–L4 foramen).

KEY POINTS: THE PROBLEM OF THE C8 NERVE ROOT

1. C8 is a nerve root without a vertebral body. It exits between C7 and T1.

2. As a result of C8 exiting between C7 and T1, cervical nerve roots exit *above* the pedicles of the same-numbered body.

3. As a result of C8 exiting between C7 and T1, thoracic and lumbar nerve roots exit *below* the pedicles of the same-numbered body.

16. **What nerve root may be compressed by a right posterior disc protrusion at L3–L4?**
    If one looks at a sagittal T1-weighted MRI of the lumbar spine, one will notice that the nerve root exits the foramen just below the pedicle of the upper vertebral body (i.e., L3 root exits just below the L3 pedicle, which happens to be above the level of the intervertebral disc space). Therefore, a posterior disc bulge at L3–L4 will not impinge the L3 root since it has already exited unless the disc protrusion is large and/or extends craniad in the neural foramen. Instead, the right L4 nerve root is descending slightly lateral to the cauda equina, in the lateral recess, toward the L4–L5 neural foramen and can be impinged by a right posterior disc protrusion.

17. **What is failed back syndrome? What is the best way to evaluate affected patients?**
    Between 5% and 40% of patients have persistent symptoms after spine surgery, and this is referred to as *failed back syndrome*. Approximately 10% undergo another operation. Causes of failed back syndrome include residual or recurrent disc herniation; residual central canal, foraminal, or lateral recess stenosis; formation of scar tissue in the surgical bed; instability; arachnoiditis; surgical misadventure (operating on the wrong level); and surgical complications (infection, hematoma, and cerebrospinal fluid leak). The best method for evaluating these patients is with MRI, with and without IV gadolinium enhancement, which can help distinguish recurrent disc pathology versus postoperative fibrosis, which are two common causes of the syndrome.

18. **What is spondylolisthesis? Name the two major causes.**
    Spondylolisthesis is displacement of one vertebral body with respect to the vertebral body below. Anterolisthesis is more common than retrolisthesis. The most common causes are spondylolysis and degenerative facet arthrosis.

19. **What is the inverted Napoleon hat sign?**
    This is a radiographic sign seen on the anteroposterior view of the L-spine or pelvis and can be due to spondylolisthesis of L5 on S1. The anterior-inferior vertebral margin and transverse processes have the appearance of Napoleon's hat turned upside down (Fig. 36-7).

20. **What is OPLL?**
    OPLL stands for *o*ssification of the *p*osterior *l*ongitudinal *l*igament and typically involves the cervical spine. This appears as a longitudinal bony ridge parallel and adjacent to the posterior vertebral margins. It is more common among people of Japanese descent and occurs in up to 50% of patients with DISH (*see* question 21).

21. **What is DISH?**

    DISH stands for *d*iffuse *i*diopathic *s*keletal *h*yperostosis (also known as "Forestier disease"). DISH has many manifestations throughout the body, including calcification and ossification of ligamentous and tendinous insertion sites, particularly involving the pelvis and patella (known as "whiskering"); enthesophyte formation on the calcaneus and olecranon processes; and para-articular osteophyte formation, particularly around the hip joints. However, its most common manifestation is in the spine, where it is associated with calcification and ossification of the anterior longitudinal ligament and large bridging osteophytes anteriorly and laterally, sometimes interrupted by linear lucencies due to herniation of intervertebral disc material. OPLL can occur in DISH as well (Fig. 36-8).

Figure 36-7. The inverted Napoleon hat sign, which can indicate anterolisthesis of L5 on S1 as depicted on an anteroposterior view of the lumbar spine.

Figure 36-8. *A,* Lateral view of the cervical spine. The patient has OPLL *(arrows)* as well as DISH *(arrowheads). B,* DISH of the thoracic spine *(arrows).*

22. **What are three radiographic criteria for the diagnosis of DISH?**

    Flowing ossification over at least four contiguous vertebrae, minimal loss of disc height relative to ossification formation, and the absence of bony ankylosis and sacroiliac joint disease.

23. **What is the difference between an osteophyte and a syndesmophyte?**
    - *Osteophyte* formation begins at the site of Sharpey's fibers attachment between the annulus fibrosus and the anterior margin of the vertebral body just above or below the end-plate margin. Osteophytes typically begin by growing outward. An osteophyte eventually grows and meets an osteophyte on the other side of the disc space and may be called a "bridging osteophyte."
    - *Syndesmophytes* are ossifications of the annulus fibrosus and are more vertically oriented, attaching right at the end-plate margin. DISH in the spine is ossification of the anterior longitudinal ligament and, like an osteophyte, is also seen originating away from the end-plate margin.

24. **What is Scheurmann's disease?**
    This is an osteochondrosis of the thoracic spine, which occurs in adolescents typically between the ages of 13 and 17 years. It is characterized by vertebral end-plate sclerosis, multiple Schmorl's nodes, anterior wedging, and resultant kyphosis. Radiographic criteria for diagnosis require three contiguous abnormal vertebrae with at least 5 degrees of anterior wedge deformity.

25. **What is the radiographic appearance of Kümmell's disease?**
    Compression fracture of the vertebral body with intraosseous vacuum phenomenon. This is believed to represent osteonecrosis of the vertebral body with secondary fracture.

BIBLIOGRAPHY

1. Resnick D: Degenerative disease of the spine. In Resnick D (ed): Bone and Joint Imaging, 2nd ed. Philadelphia, W.B. Saunders, 1996, pp 355–377.
2. Resnick D: Diffuse idiopathic skeletal hyperostosis (DISH). In Resnick D (ed): Bone and Joint Imaging, 2nd ed. Philadelphia, W.B. Saunders, 1996, pp 378–387.
3. Stoller DW, Hu SS, Kaiser JA: The spine. In Stoller DW (ed): Magnetic Resonance Imaging in Orthopaedics and Sports Medicine, 2nd ed. Philadelphia, Lippincott Williams & Wilkins, 1997, pp 1059–1162.

CHAPTER 37

OSTEOPOROSIS

Neil Roach, MD

1. What is osteoporosis? How does it differ from osteomalacia and osteopenia?
- *Osteoporosis* is characterized by low bone mass and microarchitectural deterioration of bone tissue, leading to increased bone fragility and an increased risk of fracture. The bone has normal mineralization and histologic characteristics.
- *Osteomalacia* is characterized by incomplete mineralization of normal osteoid tissue. Osteomalacia in the growing child is also known as "rickets."
- *Osteopenia* is a descriptive term for decreased calcification or density of bone. Osteopenia if not due to from a particular cause, pathophysiology, or disease.

2. What are potential causes for generalized osteoporosis?
Arthritis may be either primary or secondary. Any patient who presents with osteoporosis should be evaluated for secondary causes before being diagnosed with primary osteoporosis. Causes of *primary osteoporosis* include involutional osteoporosis, juvenile osteoporosis, and idiopathic osteoporosis (premenopausal women or middle-aged men). *Secondary osteoporosis* has a wide differential diagnosis. Causes include endocrine diseases (such as hypogonadism, ovarian agenesis, hyperadrenocorticism, hyperthyroidism, hyperparathyroidism, diabetes mellitus, and acromegaly); gastrointestinal diseases (such as subtotal gastrectomy, malabsorption syndromes, chronic obstructive jaundice, primary biliary cirrhosis, severe malnutrition, and anorexia nervosa); bone marrow disorders (such as multiple myeloma, systemic mastocytosis, and disseminated carcinoma); connective tissue diseases (such as osteogenesis imperfecta, homocystinuria, Ehlers-Danlos syndrome, and Marfan syndrome); and miscellaneous causes (such as immobilization, chronic obstructive pulmonary disease, chronic alcoholism, chronic heparin administration, and rheumatoid arthritis).

3. What are some causes for regional or localized osteoporosis?
A focal area of bone loss can be highly localized (also known as a "lytic lesion"). Metastasis, multiple myeloma, and osteomyelitis are the most common causes of lytic lesions. Larger areas of bone loss, usually without violation of cortical bone, may be caused by a stroke or immobility of an extremity. Another cause for regional osteoporosis is reflex sympathetic dystrophy syndrome (RSD), or Sudeck's atrophy. RSD is a multifactorial disorder. The underlying cause is typically trauma, followed by regional or localized osteoporosis.

4. In what demographic groups is generalized osteoporosis most prevalent?
Bone loss starts to occur in men and women around 35 years old. Women have a greater rate of bone loss. White and Asian people are more likely to develop osteoporosis than are black people. Therefore, a white or Asian woman has the greatest risk of developing osteoporosis.

5. Are conventional radiographs sensitive enough to diagnose osteoporosis?
No. A large percentage (30–40%) of bone must be lost to appreciate a change on radiographic examination. There is also marked intra-reader and inter-reader variability for this diagnosis on radiographs.

6. **What radiographic features are useful in diagnosing osteoporosis?**
Decreased bone density, prominence of vertebral body end plates, and cortical thinning can be seen with osteoporosis but are subjective. Accentuation of trabecular stress lines from resorption of secondary trabecula is another radiographic sign of osteoporosis, and this is best appreciated around the femoral neck.

7. **Is computed tomography (CT) more sensitive than conventional radiographs for evaluating bone mineral density (BMD)?**
Yes. Quantitative CT (QCT) can be performed using software that is added to a standard CT scanner. This allows BMD to be measured. Other methods of assessment based on relative absorption of x-rays using a less expensive scanner are preferred.

KEY POINTS: OSTEOPOROSIS

1. Osteoporosis is the most common skeletal disorder worldwide.

2. Osteoporosis can start at any age.

3. Osteoporosis progresses silently over a long period.

4. Osteoporosis is preventable with therapy.

8. **What are the other quantitative methods of measuring BMD?**
Single-photon absorptiometry (SPA) and dual-photon absorptiometry (DPA) were the early techniques for measuring BMD. Both used radioactive sources to produce photons. These units have essentially been replaced with dual x-ray absorptiometry (DXA) units. This technique uses the same principles as DPA, except that the radionuclide source is replaced with an x-ray tube. Two distinct energy x-ray beams are used (usually 70 and 140 kVp). DXA is the examination of choice for the diagnosis and follow-up of osteoporosis.

9. **What are the units of measurement of BMD?**
BMD is measured in grams divided by area: gm/cm^2. Therefore, it is technically not a density (weight/volume) being measured but a weight divided by area.

10. **What sites of the skeleton are routinely assessed on a DXA scan?**
The lumbar spine, from L1 or L2 to L4, and the proximal femur (regions of interest are the femoral neck, trochanteric region, and Ward's triangle). Ward's triangle is a site at the proximal femur where bone mineral loss is thought to occur first (Figs. 37-1 and 37-2).

11. **How can large osteophytes and sclerotic changes in a patient with lumbar degenerative disease affect bone densitometry assessment?**
On an anteroposterior evaluation of the lumbar spine, the osteophytes and other degenerative changes in the vertebrae and posterior elements can cause pseudoelevation of the BMD. This can result in the BMD of an osteoporotic patient appearing falsely normal. This is one reason that BMD measurements are routinely obtained in two separate locations.

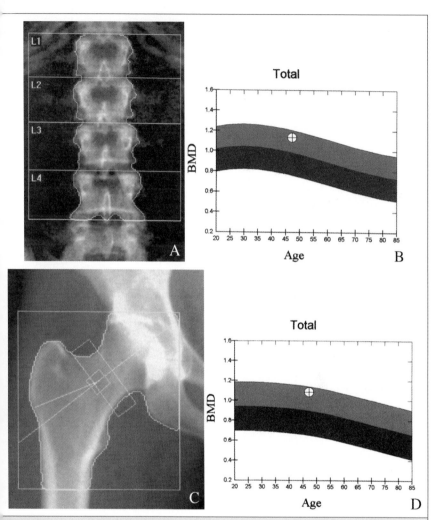

Figure 37-1. *A–B*, Normal lumbar spine DXA scan in a 47-year-old woman. *C–D*, Normal right hip DXA scan in the same patient.

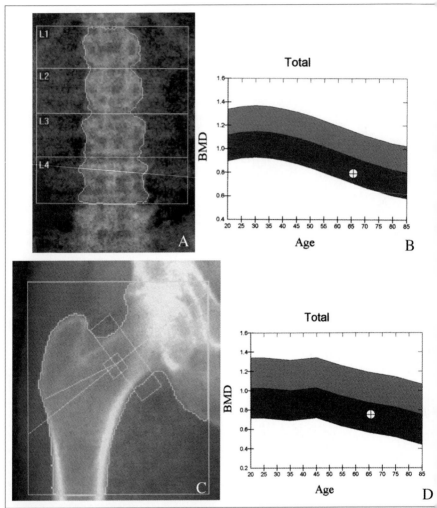

Figure 37-2. *A–B,* Osteoporosis in a 65-year-old woman. The T-score is –2.9. *C–D,* Osteopenia of the right hip with a T-score of –1.8 in the same patient.

12. **What are the World Health Organization criteria for the diagnoses of normal BMD, osteopenia, and osteoporosis?**
    - *Normal* is a BMD is within 1 SD of the young adult reference mean.
    - *Osteopenia* is a BMD between 1.0 and 2.5 SD below the young adult reference mean.
    - *Osteoporosis* is a BMD more than 2.5 SD below the young adult reference mean.

13. **What are T- and Z-scores?**
    - The *T-score* is the number of standard deviations above or below the young adult mean. The young adult mean is the expected normal value for the patient compared with others of the same sex and ethnicity in a reference population the manufacturer builds into the DXA soft-

ware. It is approximately what the patient should have had at his or her peak bone density at about age 20.

- The *Z-score* is the number of standard deviations of the patient's bone density above or below the values expected for the patient's age. By comparing the patient's BMD with the expected BMD for his or her age, the Z-score can help classify the type of osteoporosis. Primary osteoporosis is age-related and in which no secondary causes are found.

BIBLIOGRAPHY

1. National Osteoporosis Foundation: Physicians Resource Manual on Osteoporosis: A Decision-making Guide, 2nd ed. Washington, DC, National Osteoporosis Foundation, 1991.
2. World Health Organization: Assessment of fracture risk and its application to screening for postmenopausal osteoporosis. Report of a WHO study group. WHO Technical Report Series 843:1–129, 1994.

CHAPTER 38

OSTEOARTHRITIS AND INFLAMMATORY ARTHRITIS

Daniel Saurborn, MD, and Neil Roach, MD

1. **What imaging modality is best for diagnosis and follow-up of arthritic diseases?**
   Plain films are the mainstay for arthritis imaging. They are easy to obtain and give high-resolution information about cortical bone changes such as erosions and osteophytes. However, if plain radiographs are normal, magnetic resonance imaging (MRI) may be useful to evaluate for early changes such as cartilage thinning, early marrow edema, or synovial inflammation.

2. **What is the difference between an inflammatory arthritis and a degenerative arthritis?**
   Inflammatory arthritides are diseases of the synovium, which subsequently produce erosive changes of the adjacent bones. Examples of inflammatory arthritis include rheumatoid arthritis (RA) and psoriatic arthritis. Degenerative arthritis (osteoarthritis) occurs because the cartilage becomes thinned, either by a single traumatic event or repetitive events, which then allows bone cortex to rub against cortex, causing the bone to proliferate and produce an osteophyte reaction.

3. **Which joints are most often affected in RA?**
   RA has a predilection for the carpal/tarsal, carpometacarpal/tarsometatarsal, metacarpophalangeal/metatarsophalangeal, and proximal interphalangeal joints (Fig. 38-1). In adults it would be rare for the distal interphalangeal joints to be affected. Joint involvement tends to be bilateral but not necessarily symmetric. Generally, the metacarpophalangeal and the metatarsophalangeal joints are affected first.

Figure 38-1. Note the ulnar deviation of the metacarpals in this patient with RA. There is a typical marginal erosion of the metacarpal head *(arrow)*.

4. **What portion of the spine does RA most commonly affect?**
   In the cervical spine, RA commonly causes atlantoaxial (C1–C2) subluxation due to laxity of the transverse ligament and pannus formation.

5. **Can RA affect nonarticular structures?**
   Yes. Retrocalcaneal bursitis is common and is detected when the retrocalcaneal fat at the posterior-superior aspect of the calcaneus is obscured by edema. It is often accompanied by bone erosion.

6. **How do the inflammatory arthritides affect cartilage?**
   Inflammatory arthritides are a chronic synovitis, eroding bone that is "unprotected" by cartilage. These changes are noted first at the margins of joints, where cartilage is thinnest. Cartilage is also eroded by the joint inflammation, but tends to do so in an even and uniform manner.

7. **What finding, which is common in osteoarthritis (OA), is virtually never seen with RA?**
   The presence of significant osteophytes (productive bone changes) is not consistent with the diagnosis of RA. However, a joint that has been destroyed by RA may then develop OA due to cartilage loss.

8. **What additional joint findings are seen with RA?**
   Subluxations and malalignments at the metacarpophalangeal and metatarsophalangeal joints are typical. The subluxations tend to deviate the phalanges in the ulnar direction (*see* Fig. 38-1).

9. **Where are the "swan-neck" and "boutonniere" deformities located?**
   The chronic inflammatory changes of RA in the joints of the fingers produce retraction of the tendons. The swan-neck deformity is caused by hyperextension of the proximal interphalangeal joint with simultaneous flexion of the distal interphalangeal joint. If you try this manipulation on yourself, you will clearly recognize the etiology of the name. The boutonniere (or buttonhole) deformity is caused by hyperextension of the distal interphalangeal joint with simultaneous flexion of the proximal interphalangeal joint.

10. **When can RA be confused with other arthritides?**
    Severe erosions of the subchondral bone may develop late in the disease after the cartilage is destroyed and may give an appearance similar to erosive OA.

11. **What joints are typically affected by OA?**
    OA most often affects the proximal and distal interphalangeal joints of the hands as well as the major weight-bearing joints—the hips and the knees. In addition, the carpal joints at the base of the thumb are very commonly affected (the trapeziometacarpal and scapho-trapezio-trapezoidal joints). The most commonly affected joint in the foot is the first metatarsophalangeal joint. It is important to remember, however, that any joint damaged by trauma that results in an irregular articular surface can become prematurely arthritic.

12. **Where are Heberden's and Bouchard's nodes located?**
    - *Heberden's nodes* are osseous outcroppings involving the distal interphalangeal joints.
    - *Bouchard's nodes* involve the proximal interphalangeal joints. Both Bouchard's and Heberden's nodes are physical examination signs of hand OA.

13. **Which joints are rarely involved in primary OA?**
    Involvement of the radiocarpal, pan-carpal, and metacarpophalangeal joints is rare in OA but is common in RA and psoriatic arthritis.

14. **What are the hallmarks of osteoarthritic change in a joint?**
    Whereas erosive arthritides have uniform cartilage loss, degenerative OA results in segmental cartilage loss. In small joints, such as those in the fingers, the loss may appear to be uniform. The layer of bone just beneath the cartilage is called the *subchondral bone*. When exposed to increased stress, this layer becomes sclerotic. As this process continues, both the cartilage and the underlying bone can become eroded, producing cystlike pockets in the bone, called "geodes." At the edge of a joint where the cartilage is thinnest, exposed bone will become hypertrophic, resulting in irregular or pointed outcroppings of bone, called "osteophytes."

15. **What is erosive OA?**
    Erosive OA is a form of OA that is some-
    times called "inflammatory osteoarthritis"
    (Fig. 38-2). Although the joint distribution is
    the same as in typical OA, the erosive
    changes are more severe and there is soft
    tissue swelling, which may give a similar
    appearance to RA or psoriatic arthritis.
    These changes, however, involve the sub-
    chondral cortex in the main portion of the
    joint rather than the peripheral "bare areas."
    Ultimately, the phalangeal joints may
    become fused.

16. **Name the seronegative
    spondyloarthropathies.**
    Seronegativity refers to the absence of
    rheumatoid factor in blood tests of patients
    who present with inflammatory arthritis.
    This group of diseases includes psoriatic
    arthritis, Reiter's syndrome, ankylosing
    spondylitis, and enteropathic arthritis (asso-
    ciated with inflammatory bowel diseases
    such as Crohn's and ulcerative colitis).

Figure 38-2. Erosive OA involving the distal
interphalangeal joints, with a combination of
productive and erosive changes. Note the classic
"gull-wing deformity" of the distal interphalangeal
joint *(arrow)*.

17. **What mnemonic can be used to remember the triad of symptoms seen with
    Reiter's syndrome?**
    "Can't see (uveitis), can't pee (urethritis), can't climb a tree (arthritis)."

18. **What are the different presentations of psoriatic arthritis?**
    Psoriatic arthritis tends to involve the terminal interphalangeal joints of both hands. This is in
    contrast to RA, which more commonly involves more proximal joints in the hands and wrists.
    A second presentation pattern of psoriatic arthritis may involve multiple joints of a single hand.
    The third pattern involves only the joints of a single ray. The appearance is a combination of ero-
    sive and productive bony changes. The erosive changes occur at the peripheral bare areas, simi-
    lar to that with RA. However, psoriatic arthritis also produces productive bone formation
    adjacent to the joint, typically in an exuberant and irregular manner.

19. **What is the "pencil-in-cup" deformity?**
    The advanced erosive changes seen in psoriatic arthritis can produce a pointed appearance of
    the proximal phalanx that then pushes into the base of the more distal phalanx and deforms it
    like a cup.

20. **Does ankylosing spondylitis (AS) have a specific pattern of joint involvement?**
    AS preferentially involves the sacroiliac joints and lumbar spine and then may advance craniad to
    involve the thoracic and cervical spine. *Ankylosis* refers to the bony fusion of the opposing sur-
    faces, which results in sclerosis and loss of the normal sacroiliac joint cartilage space (Fig. 38-3).

21. **What is the term *bamboo spine* used to describe?**
    AS produces syndesmophytes, which are osseous bridges of the intervertebral disc spaces
    along Sharpey's fibers in the annulus fibrosus. Combined with fusion of the facet joints and ossi-
    fication of the longitudinal spinal ligaments, the appearance is likened to that of a stick of
    bamboo.

KEY POINTS: DIFFERENTIATING ARTHRITIS ON HAND X-RAY

1. Symmetric erosive change of the metacarpophalangeal and proximal interphalangeal joints of both hands suggests RA.

2. Extensive productive osteophyte changes of the distal interphalangeal joints, with less severe changes of the proximal interphalangeal and metacarpophalangeal joints, or a thickened "sausage-digit," suggests psoriatic arthritis.

3. Osteophyte production and joint-space narrowing without marginal erosions of the distal interphalangeal and proximal interphalangeal joints, with little or no involvement of the metacarpophalangeal joints, suggests degenerative joint disease.

4. A soft tissue mass with an overhanging rim of bone, adjacent to a joint space, suggests gout.

5. Calcifications within the soft tissues of the fingertips and/or resorption of the cortex of the finger tufts suggest scleroderma or polymyositis.

Figure 38-3. AS causes fusion of the sacroiliac joint. When this joint fuses, the normally dark-appearing cartilage becomes replaced by bone matrix *(double arrows)*.

22. **What is the radiologic appearance of gout?**
    Gout classically involves the first metatarsophalangeal joint. Be aware, though, that other joints of the hand and foot can also be affected. Although more than one joint may be involved, it does not tend to be symmetric as other inflammatory arthritides can be. The classic appearance of a gout erosion is termed the "overhanging margin," with a rim of eroded cortex hanging over a soft tissue density called a "tophus." Tophi are soft tissue deposits of monosodium urate crystals that may occur anywhere, particularly in the dorsal aspect of the foot and the extensor aspect of the elbow.

23. **What is pseudogout?**
    Calcium pyrophosphate deposition disease (CPDD) has a similar presentation as gout, with episodic and acute joint inflammation, leading to the term *pseudogout* based on clinical symptoms. CPDD is caused by calcium pyrophosphate crystals, whereas gout is caused by urate crystals.

24. **What are the unique features of CPDD?**
    CPDD resembles OA at first glance, with cartilage narrowing and subchondral sclerosis with osteophyte formation (Fig. 38-4). However, CPDD tends to involve the metacarpophalangeal

joints, particularly the second and third, but spares the interphalangeal joints. Other joints that may be involved include the elbow, carpal, radiocarpal, tibiotalar, and tarsal. The subchondral bone becomes involved by multiple cystlike lucencies that can eventually lead to collapse of the articular surface. Calcium pyrophosphate crystals tend to deposit within the fibrocartilage and are best seen in the triangular fibrocartilage (TFC) of the wrist and the meniscal cartilage of the knee. These cartilage calcifications are termed *chondrocalcinosis*. These deposits may also affect the hyaline cartilage, which becomes a more specific radiologic marker for the disease. Soft tissue calcification is also common in tendons, bursae, and synovium.

Figure 38-4. CPDD with calcium crystal deposition in the meniscus *(double arrows)*. This is called chondrocalcinosis.

BIBLIOGRAPHY

1. Brower A: Arthritis in Black and White. Philadelphia, W.B. Saunders, 1988.

2. Helms CA: Fundamentals of Skeletal Radiology, 2nd ed. Philadelphia, W.B. Saunders, 1995.

3. Taveras JM, Ferrucci JT: Radiology: Diagnosis, Imaging, Intervention, 2002 ed. on CD-ROM. Philadelphia, Lippincott Williams & Wilkins, 2002.

CHAPTER 39

OSTEOMYELITIS

Andrew Gordon, MD, and Neil Roach, MD

1. **What are the initial plain film findings in osteomyelitis?**
   Soft tissue swelling and blurred fascial planes.

2. **How long does it take before the initial skeletal findings of osteomyelitis are seen on a plain film?**
   Radiographically evident bone changes often take at least 7–10 days to develop.
   Skeletal lesions appear as enlarging ill-defined radiolucencies in the infected bone. Periosteal reaction is common (Fig. 39-1).

3. **Define sequestrum, involucrum, cloaca, and sinus tract.**
   - A *sequestrum* is a fragment of necrotic bone that is separate from the living parent bone. A sequestrum may be resorbed, be discharged through a sinus tract, or persist as a focus of infection (Fig. 39-2).
   - An *involucrum* is a layer of healthy bone that has formed around the dead bone. It may merge with the parent bone or become perforated with tracts through which pus can escape.
   - A *cloaca* is an opening in the involucrum through which granulation tissue and the sequestra may be discharged.
   - A *sinus tract* is a channel extending from the bone to the skin surface that is lined with granulation tissue.

Figure 39-1. Acute osteomyelitis of the distal tibia in a teenager bitten by a dog approximately 1 week earlier. *A,* Lateral radiograph of the ankle demonstrates an ill-defined lucency in the metaphysis of the distal tibia. *B,* On the sagittal short tau inversion recovery (STIR) image of the ankle, there is increased signal intensity in the marrow of the distal tibia, most focal at the site corresponding to the abnormality seen on the plain film. High-signal edema is also noted in the anterior soft tissues due to associated cellulitis. STIR images can be thought of as equivalent to fat-saturated T2-weighted images.

Figure 39-2. Sequestrum. Lateral radiograph of the tibia and fibula in a child with chronic osteomyelitis demonstrates a long segment of bone in the medullary canal of the tibia, separate from the parent bone. This finding is in keeping with a devascularized sequestrum. There has been marked resorption and cortical destruction of the tibia, indicated by radiolucency surrounding the sequestrum.

4. **What is Brodie's abscess?**

Brodie's abscess is a bone abscess found characteristically in subacute pyogenic osteomyelitis, but which also may be identified in chronic osteomyelitis. Brodie's abscess typically occurs near the ends of tubular bones, is especially common in children, and may be single or multiple. The wall of the abscess is lined by granulation tissue surrounded by dense bone. On radiographs, Brodie's abscess appears as a well-defined circular or elliptical radiolucency with adjacent sclerosis. When located in the metaphysis of children, it may connect with the growth plate through an identifiable channel (Fig. 39-3).

Figure 39-3. Brodie's abscess. Lateral radiograph of the knee of a child demonstrates a well-defined circular lucency with a sclerotic border in the proximal metaphysis of the tibia. This is the typical appearance of a Brodie's abscess of subacute osteomyelitis.

5. **Name the two imaging modalities that may be used to diagnose acute osteomyelitis if plain films show negative or equivocal results.**

Magnetic resonance imaging (MRI) and three-phase bone scan.

6. **What is the appearance of acute osteomyelitis on MRI?**

Because inflammation causes edema to replace marrow fat, a focus of osteomyelitis demonstrates low to intermediate signal intensity on T1-weighted images and high signal intensity on fat-saturated T2-weighted and short tau inversion recovery (STIR) images (*see* Fig. 39-1).

IV gadolinium may be administered when performing an MRI for the purpose of diagnosing osteomyelitis. Gadolinium is useful in differentiating an abscess from bone marrow edema in the marrow space or in differentiating a soft tissue abscess from surrounding cellulitis or phlegmon. An abscess demonstrates a thick, enhancing wall without central enhancement. The detection of sinus tracts and sequestra is also improved after gadolinium administration. However, bone marrow enhancement is nonspecific; it may be seen in infected bone and in noninfected regions of reactive marrow hyperemia.

7. **Are the MR findings of osteomyelitis specific? If not, what other processes may appear similar?**

No. Bone contusion, occult fracture, neuropathic joint, and neoplastic processes may also demonstrate marrow signal intensity changes similar to those seen in osteomyelitis. Clinical history, therefore, is important for proper image interpretation.

8. **List the three classes of radiotracers used predominantly to diagnose osteomyelitis.**

   - *Technetium (Tc)-99m diphosphonates* (most commonly methylene disphosphonate [MDP]). Tc-99m MDP is the radiotracer used in three-phase bone scans and is typically all that is required for diagnosing uncomplicated osteomyelitis.
   - *Gallium 67 citrate.* Gallium may be used in combination with Tc-99m MDP bone scans in more complicated cases. Gallium activity greater than Tc-99m MDP suggests infection.
   - *Autologous leukocytes* labeled with indium 111 or Tc-99m hexamethylpropyleneamine oxime (HMPAO). Radiolabeled autologous leukocytes are also used in combination with Tc-99m MDP bone scans in a similar fashion to gallium.

9. **Name the three phases of a three-phase bone scan, and describe the timing of each.**

Angiographic (blood flow) phase, blood pool phase, and delayed phase. During the angiographic phase, serial images are obtained every 5 seconds for the first minute after injection of the radio-tracer. During the blood pool phase, an image is obtained approximately 5 minutes after injection. Images are then obtained 2–3 hours later for the delayed phase.

10. **How can the diagnosis of osteomyelitis be differentiated from cellulitis on a three-phase bone scan?**

Both cellulitis and osteomyelitis demonstrate high soft tissue uptake of the radiotracer in the blood flow and blood pool phases. Differentiation between the two types of infection occurs in the delayed phase. In cellulitis, there is mild, diffuse bone uptake on delayed images. In osteomyelitis, there is focal, intense radiotracer uptake of the infected bone.

11. **List the four main routes through which osteomyelitis (and septic arthritis) may be acquired.**

   - Hematogenous spread of infection from the blood stream
   - Spread of infection from adjacent soft tissues
   - Direct inoculation (e.g., penetrating trauma)
   - Postoperative infection (a postoperative infection may result from hematogenous spread, spread from contiguous tissues, or direct implantation)

12. **Which organism is accountable for most cases of hematogenous osteomyelitis and septic arthritis?**
Staphylococcus aureus.

13. **Which disease is associated with an increased incidence of *Salmonella* osteomyelitis?**
Sickle cell disease.

14. **How does the vascular anatomy of tubular bones affect the location of infection in infants, children, and adults?**
Up to about 1 year of age, a fetal vascular pattern may be present in tubular bones. Some vessels at the surface of the metaphysis penetrate the preexisting physeal plate and extend into the epiphysis. These transphyseal vessels allow a pathway for the spread of infection. Therefore, in addition to infection at the metaphysis, epiphyseal and articular infection may occur in infants.

After about 1 year of age, there is obliteration of the transphyseal vessels. The physeal plate serves as a barrier such that the metaphyseal and epiphyseal blood supplies are completely separate; therefore, hematogenous osteomyelitis arising in the metaphysis cannot extend into the epiphysis. The terminal metaphyseal vessels turn acutely at the growth plate to join large sinusoidal veins, where the blood flow is slow and turbulent. The frequency of metaphyseal osteomyelitis in children is due to this combination of venous stasis and the barrier formed by the growth plate.

Once the growth plate closes in the mature skeleton, vascular communications between the metaphysis and epiphysis reestablish, and infection may localize from the metaphysis to the epiphyseal subchondral bone. Involvement of the joint may complicate epiphyseal infection.

15. **What are the plain film findings of chronic sclerosing osteomyelitis?**
The chronic phase of osteomyelitis, termed *chronic sclerosing osteomyelitis,* is characterized by thickened trabecula and thick, wavy periosteal new bone with resultant radiodensity and contour abnormalities of the affected bone (Fig. 39-4).

16. **Is malignancy a potential complication of osteomyelitis?**
Yes. Epidermoid carcinoma arises in 0.5% of patients with chronic osteomyelitis and draining sinus tracts. The latent period is usually 20–30 years. Radiographically, progressive destruction of the bone may suggest the diagnosis. Other secondary neoplasms arising in chronic osteomyelitis have also been described.

17. **Describe the plain film and MRI findings in septic arthritis.**
Septic arthritis is the infection of a joint and should always be considered when there is monoarticular inflammatory arthritis. Widening of the joint space is initially seen secondary to joint effusion. There may also be regional soft tissue swelling and periarticular osteopenia due to hyperemia. Later, cartilage destruction results in concentric joint space narrowing, and an inflamed

Figure 39-4. Chronic sclerosing osteomyelitis of the femur. The femoral shaft is markedly sclerotic (dense). Thick, wavy periosteal reaction on the medial and lateral aspects of the femur cause the bone to have an abnormal contour. The thick periosteal new bone is the involucrum.

pannus results in osseous erosions. Bone ankylosis and destruction can occur in the late stages of disease. It is the poorly defined osseous destruction that is most characteristic (Fig. 39-5).

MRI may be used as an adjunct to joint aspiration in the diagnosis of septic arthritis. However, the MR findings of septic arthritis are not specific and are the same as in any inflammatory arthritis. Initially, the joint effusion and synovitis are characterized by low intra-articular signal intensity on T1-weighted images and high signal intensity on T2-weighted and STIR images. After gadolinium is administered, the synovium enhances but the joint fluid does not. There may be low to intermediate T1 signal and high T2 signal in the adjacent soft tissues and bone marrow due to sympathetic hyperemia with edema or spread of infection outside of the joint. Later, bone erosions will appear as marginal subchondral defects that are low signal on T1-weighted images and high signal on T2-weighted images (Fig. 39-6).

Figure 39-5. Septic arthritis and osteomyelitis involving the fourth finger. Extensive intra-articular and periarticular erosions are seen to involve the proximal and distal interphalangeal joints of the fourth digit. There is marked concentric narrowing of the proximal interphalangeal joint due to cartilage destruction. Soft tissue swelling is evident overlying both joints. Ill-defined radiolucency of the head of the middle phalanx is suggestive of a component of osteomyelitis.

18. **Name the joints most commonly infected in infants and children, adults, and IV drug abusers.**
    - Infants and children: knee and hip
    - Adults: knee
    - IV drug abusers: sacroiliac, sternoclavicular, and acromioclavicular (also, even though it is not a joint, the spine is commonly involved in cases of osteomyelitis in IV drug abusers)

KEY POINTS: OSTEOMYELITIS

1. Plain film radiography, MRI, and nuclear medicine studies have roles in the imaging diagnosis of osteomyelitis.

2. The knee and hip are the most commonly infected joints of infants and children. The knee is the most common joint infected in adults.

Figure 39-6. Septic arthritis of the right hip on MRI. Coronal T1-weighted *(A)* and coronal STIR *(B)* images of the hips demonstrate decreased T1 and increased STIR signal within a distended right hip joint, indicative of joint effusion and synovitis. There is abnormal signal in the proximal right femur and in the regional hip musculature due to reactive edema. The left hip is normal.

19. **How is a definitive diagnosis of septic arthritis made in a child?**
    Radiographic findings of septic arthritis are nonspecific. However, plain films should be obtained first to exclude other potential causes for an irritable hip in a child, such as Perthes' disease or occult fracture. Although MRI has a role in the evaluation of suspected septic arthritis, aspiration of the joint is mandatory in establishing the diagnosis so that the appropriate antibiotic therapy may be started in a timely manner. The joint may be aspirated under ultrasound or fluoroscopic guidance.

20. **What is the differential diagnosis for unilateral sacroiliac joint disease?**
    - Infection
    - Psoriatic arthritis
    - Reiter's syndrome
    - Degenerative joint disease
    - Gout
    See Figure 39-7.

21. **Describe the radiographic findings of infectious spondylitis (infection of the spine).**
    Hematogenous spread of infection to the spine initially results in involvement of the anterior subchondral vertebral body and quickly spreads to the adjacent intervertebral disc. The initial findings on radiography are a decrease in the height of the vertebral body with loss of the normal definition of the end plate. Destruction of the vertebral body ensues. Spread of infection through the intervertebral disc results in involvement of the adjacent vertebra. Involvement of two contiguous vertebral bodies and the intervening disc is seen in the majority of patients.

    After many weeks, reactive sclerosis occurs in the involved vertebra. Soft tissue extension may occur and appears as a displaced psoas shadow in the lumbar spine, a paraspinal mass in the thoracic spine, or prevertebral soft tissue swelling in the cervical spine.

Figure 39-7. Unilateral sacroiliitis. Plain film *(A)* and computed tomography (CT) scan *(B)* of the pelvis demonstrate erosions with reactive sclerosis at the right sacroiliac joint. The left sacroiliac joint is normal. Although a few processes can present as unilateral sacroiliitis, in the appropriate clinical setting, these findings are suggestive of septic arthritis. CT is often helpful in evaluating complicated joints such as those at the pelvis.

22. **Can infection of the intervertebral disc (discitis) occur without involvement of the adjacent vertebral bodies?**

    Yes. In children and young adults up to the age of about 20–30 years, the intervertebral discs remain significantly vascular, and therefore, hematogenous spread of infection may occur directly to the disc tissue. The clinical manifestations of discitis are usually mild, and an organism cannot always be identified. Infection of an intervertebral disc may also occur via direct contamination during invasive diagnostic or therapeutic procedures.

23. **How does infectious spondylitis appear on MRI?**

    Patients are usually first imaged with MRI after the infection has spread through a disc and involves two contiguous vertebral bodies. The MR findings consist of a triad of (1) low signal intensity of the involved vertebral body marrow on T1-weighted images; (2) enhancement of the marrow after the administration of gadolinium, as well as possible intervertebral disc enhancement; and (3) high signal of the disc on T2-weighted and STIR images. A decreased disc height and destruction of the cortical end plate may also be seen.

    An epidural, subligamentous, or paraspinal abscess or phlegmon may be present. Differentiation of abscess from phlegmon requires IV gadolinium; a phlegmon enhances diffusely, whereas an abscess demonstrates low signal intensity on T1-weighted images with peripheral rim enhancement. Both exhibit high signal intensity on T2-weighted images (Fig. 39-8).

24. **What is Phemister's triad?**

    Phemister's triad refers to the classic radiographic findings of tuberculous arthritis:
    - Periarticular osteoporosis
    - Peripherally located osseous erosions
    - Gradual narrowing of the joint space

    Preservation of the joint space is the hallmark of tuberculous arthritis and helps to distinguish it from the rapid joint destruction of pyogenic (bacterial) arthritis.

    Monoarticular disease is the rule in tuberculous arthritis. The majority of joint infections arise secondary to contiguous spread of tuberculous osteomyelitis. Diagnosis of tuberculous arthritis is often delayed and requires synovial fluid and tissue for culture and histopathology.

Figure 39-8. Infectious spondylitis. *A*, Sagittal T2-weighted image of the lumbar spine demonstrates marked disc space narrowing at L5–S1. High signal is present in what is remaining of the intervertebral disc. There are erosions of the end plates of L5 and S1 and abnormal signal in both vertebral bodies. A paraspinal mass is noted anteriorly at this level. *B*, Sagittal T1-weighted image after the administration of IV gadolinium demonstrates enhancement of the involved vertebral bodies. The paraspinal mass remains low in signal intensity with mild peripheral rim enhancement, indicative of a paraspinal abscess (as opposed to phlegmon).

25. **What is Pott's disease?**
    The eponym of tuberculous spondylitis. The vertebra is affected in 25–60% of osseous tuberculosis cases. The first lumbar vertebral body is most commonly infected, although involvement of more than one vertebral body is typical. Infection may spread to contiguous vertebral bodies or skip multiple levels; it commonly spreads beneath the anterior longitudinal ligament (and less commonly the posterior longitudinal ligament). Tuberculous spondylitis characteristically involves the anterior portion of the vertebral body. Destruction and anterior collapse of the vertebral body may result in deformity and an angular kyphosis (gibbus deformity).
    Epidural or paraspinal abscesses are common and often travel long distances from their site of origin before perforating into a viscus or the body surface. Paraspinal masses out of proportion to the spondylitis may be seen on radiographs. A calcified psoas abscess favors tuberculous over pyogenic spondylitis. Another differentiation point is that tuberculous spondylitis is not as rapidly progressive as pyogenic disease.

26. **What plain film findings suggest an infection of a metallic prosthesis?**
    It is typically not possible to differentiate an infected prosthesis from a loosened, uninfected prosthesis with plain radiographs alone. Both demonstrate prominent lucency at the bone-cement interface. A radiolucent zone of 2 mm should suggest loosening or infection, especially if it has increased in size from a prior radiograph.

27.   What is a ring sequestrum?
A ring sequestrum indicates infection about a pin tract. A central radiolucent region created by the pin is surrounded by a ring of bone, which in turn is surrounded by an area of osteolysis due to infection. Pin tract infections are particularly common after percutaneous placement.

BIBLIOGRAPHY

1. Kaplan PA, Helms CA, Dussault R, et al: Musculoskeletal infections. In Kaplan PA, Helms CA, Dussault R, et al (eds): Musculoskeletal MRI. Philadelphia, W.B. Saunders, 2001, pp 101–116.
2. Leach TJ: Imaging of infectious arthritis. Semin Musculoskelet Radiol 7:137–142, 2003.
3. Resnick D, Niwayama G: Osteomyelitis, septic arthritis, and soft tissue infection: Mechanisms and situations. In Resnick D (ed): Diagnosis of Bone and Joint Disorders, 3rd ed. Philadelphia, W.B. Saunders, 1995.
4. Sammak B, Abd El Bagi M, Al Shahed M, et al: Osteomyelitis: A review of currently used imaging techniques. Eur Radiol 9:894–900, 1999.
5. Stabler A, Reiser MF: Imaging of spinal infection. Radiol Clin North Am 39:115–135, 2001.
6. Tehranzadeh J, Wong E, Wang F, Sadighpour M: Imaging of osteomyelitis in the mature skeleton. Radiol Clin North Am 39:223–250, 2001.

CHAPTER 40

BONE TUMORS

Judy S. Blebea, MD

1. **What radiographic features should be considered when evaluating a suspected bone tumor?**
   Morphologic features, periosteal reaction, location in a bone (epiphysis, metaphysis, diaphysis), distribution within the skeleton (axial vs. appendicular), presence of tumor matrix, and soft tissue mass.

   Morphologic features to consider are the pattern of bone destruction and the size, shape, margins, and zone of transition of the lesion. A lesion with a sharp border suggests a nonaggressive or benign lesion, whereas a poorly defined margin, especially one associated with cortical destruction, favors malignancy.

   Periosteal reaction reflects the rate of growth of the underlying lesion. Slow-growing lesions may produce a laminated periosteal reaction with uniform, wavy layers. Malignant lesions that grow in spurts can produce an onion-skin pattern, whereas aggressive lesions with rapid growth are associated with the sunburst or hair-on-end periosteal reaction. A Codman's triangle is the uplifting of the periosteum in a triangular configuration and can be seen with both benign and malignant lesions.

2. **How do cartilage tumor matrix and neoplastic bone matrix differ?**
   Cartilage matrix is typically ringlike, flocculent, or flecklike—in the shape of rings and arcs—whereas neoplastic bone matrix is typically cloudlike, amorphous, or ivory-like. The detection of tumor matrix can be helpful in recognizing the etiologic factor of the underlying lesion, that is, whether it is of osseous or cartilaginous origin.

KEY POINTS: PLAIN RADIOGRAPHIC FEATURES TO ASSESS FOR BONE TUMORS

1. Morphologic features/pattern of bone destruction, zone of transition

2. Periosteal reaction

3. Location in the bone/distribution in the skeleton

4. Presence of tumor matrix

5. Presence of a soft tissue mass

3. **Which imaging study is most useful in arriving at an accurate differential diagnosis for a bone tumor?**
   Plain radiography is the first step in detecting and diagnosing a bone tumor. Plain films should also be obtained initially, even with suspected soft tissue tumors, to identify possible underlying bone involvement or the presence of calcifications.

4. **What is the role of magnetic resonance imaging (MRI) and computed tomography (CT) in the evaluation of musculoskeletal tumors?**
   MRI is the most important diagnostic test for local staging and preoperative planning of primary bone and soft tissue tumors. It is also useful for monitoring the response to chemotherapy or radiation therapy as well as detecting postoperative tumor recurrence. CT may be helpful in the detection of tumor matrix and the location of the nidus in a suspected osteoid osteoma. CT is also used for percutaneous image-guided biopsy of bone tumors.

5. **What are some of the tumor features evaluated with MRI? Can MRI be used to distinguish between benign and malignant tumors?**
   The tumor location, extent, and relationship to the neurovascular bundle and the presence of skip lesions and joint involvement are important features that are assessed with MRI and help to determine the stage of the tumor and to plan a surgical approach. Even though MRI may help in the assessment of the aggressiveness of a lesion and in the recognition of certain "Aunt Minnie" lesions, it cannot be used to reliably distinguish between benign and malignant tumors and is generally nonspecific in determining tumor cell type. Biopsy of the lesion is often required.

6. **What is the role of IV gadolinium contrast in MRI of musculoskeletal tumors?**
   There is some controversy about the need for IV contrast during pretherapy MRI for a patient with a suspected musculoskeletal tumor. Contrast may be used to help distinguish tumor margins and assess tumor vascularity. Its use may also help distinguish malignant viable tissue from inflammatory changes and necrosis for preoperative biopsy planning. For a follow-up or post-therapy MRI evaluation, contrast can be helpful to assess the patient's response to chemotherapy, to determine the presence of a fluid collection postoperatively, and to detect tumor recurrence.

7. **What is the staging system adopted by the Musculoskeletal Tumor Society, and what three features form the basis of this staging system?**
   The Musculoskeletal Tumor Society has adopted the Enneking staging system. The grade, local extent, and presence of metastases are the three features assessed with this system.

8. **Which primary bone tumors tend to involve the epiphysis most commonly?**
   Chondroblastoma and giant cell tumors. Chondroblastoma is a benign lesion that is typically well defined and located in the epiphysis. Although benign, chondroblastomas can be locally invasive and metastasize to the lungs. A giant cell tumor usually arises in the metaphyseal region and extends to involve the epiphysis. Giant cell tumors are eccentrically located lesions with a nonsclerotic zone of transition that typically occurs after closure of the growth plate (Fig. 40-1). A clear cell chondrosarcoma may also occur in the epiphyseal region.

Figure 40-1. Plain film anteroposterior radiograph of the ankle demonstrates a geographic lesion that extends to the epiphyseal region in the distal tibia. In this patient with closed growth plates, the most likely diagnosis is giant cell tumor.

9. **What is the difference between a nonossifying fibroma (NOF) and a fibrous cortical defect?**
    Both are benign, usually asymptomatic, well-defined cortical-based lesions with sclerotic borders seen in the metaphysis or diametaphysis of long bones and are identical in their histology. They differ only in their size. Fibrous cortical defects are smaller (<2 cm), whereas NOFs are larger (>2 cm) and are usually detected incidentally on radiographs in children and often subsequently heal with sclerosis.

KEY POINTS: PRIMARY BONE TUMORS IN THE EPIPHYSEAL REGION

1. Chondroblastoma
2. Giant cell tumor
3. Clear cell chondrosarcoma

10. **What is the most common malignant tumor involving the skeleton?**
    Metastases.

11. **What is the most common *primary* malignant bone tumor in adults?**
    Multiple myeloma, which represents approximately 1% of all malignant diseases and about 10–15% of hematologic malignancies. The excessive proliferation of abnormal plasma cells can result in the formation of a single lesion (plasmacytoma) or multiple lesions (multiple myeloma).

12. **If the diagnosis of multiple myeloma is suspected, what radiographic evaluation should be performed?**
    A skeletal survey is usually obtained, and approximately 75% of patients with multiple myeloma will have positive radiographic findings with "punched-out" osteolytic lesions that demonstrate discrete margins and uniform size. Multiple compression fractures can also be seen. MRI is very sensitive for detecting the presence of marrow lesions and may help in determining tumor extent.

13. **What are the most common primary neoplasms that metastasize to bone?**
    A small number of primary tumors account for the majority of all metastatic bone lesions. Cancers most likely to metastasize to bone include *p*rostate, *b*reast, *k*idney, *t*hyroid, and *l*ung and are remembered by the mnemonic *PB* (lead) *KetTLe*. Other primary tumors that can metastasize to bone include colon, rectum, stomach, and bladder. The axial skeleton is seeded more than the appendicular skeleton due to the presence of red bone marrow. It is rare to have bone metastases below the elbow or knee. Lytic bone metastases must have destroyed 30–50% of the bone to be seen on x-rays. Nuclear medicine bone scans are more sensitive than radiographs for the detection of metastatic bone disease.

14. **Which tumors can give rise to lytic, expansile, "blown-out" metastases of bone?**
    Bone metastases from renal cell carcinoma and thyroid cancer can demonstrate this pattern. Bone metastases from malignant melanoma may be expansile as well.

15. **What is the second most common primary bone tumor after multiple myeloma?**
    Osteosarcoma (Fig. 40-2). About 75% of osteosarcoma lesions occur around the knee and typically arise in the metaphyseal region. The peak incidence is in the second and third decades, and there is a smaller second peak in patients older than 50 years; this later peak has more pelvic and craniofacial involvement. Osteosarcoma can develop after radiation exposure, with an average latent period of 11 years.

Figure 40-2. Plain film radiograph demonstrates exuberant bone formation in this osteosarcoma.

16. **Which type of tumor can present with bone pain, swelling, tenderness, fever, and increased sedimentation rate, mimicking an infection?**
    Ewing sarcoma, a malignant round cell tumor with a predilection for the long bones and pelvis. Plain films may demonstrate a permeative or moth-eaten pattern of bone destruction with an onion-skin type of periosteal reaction and an associated soft tissue mass.

17. **Where do sarcomas most commonly metastasize?**
    Sarcomas tend to undergo hematogenous spread, with pulmonary metastases being the most common.

18. **What is the most common benign skeletal neoplasm?**
    Osteochondroma (Fig. 40-3). This lesion accounts for 20–50% of benign bone tumors and 10–15% of all bone tumors. Osteochondromas occur most commonly in the first two decades of life, arise from the metaphysis pointing away from the joint, and can be either flattened (sessile) or stalklike. There is usually cessation of growth of the osteochondroma after closure of the growth plate. Osteochondromas can occur after radiation therapy in children and may present with pain due to mechanical irritation or fracture.

Figure 40-3. A sessile bony protuberance is noted arising from the femur; this represents an osteochondroma. Osteochondromas are the most common benign skeletal neoplasm.

19. **Which clinical and radiographic features suggest malignant degeneration of an osteochondroma?**
    Features suggesting malignant degeneration include pain, growth after closure of the growth plate, bony destruction, thickened cartilage cap, and soft tissue mass.

The risk of malignant transformation of a solitary osteochondroma is approximately 1%, whereas that of hereditary multiple osteochondromatosis is much higher and may be on the order of 25–30%. A sessile lesion is more likely to degenerate, usually undergoing malignant transformation to a chondrosarcoma (Fig. 40-4).

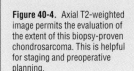
Figure 40-4. Axial T2-weighted image permits the evaluation of the extent of this biopsy-proven chondrosarcoma. This is helpful for staging and preoperative planning.

20. **What is the most common benign bone tumor of the hand? Where else may these lesions occur, and what are the features of malignant transformation?**
An enchondroma is the most common benign bone tumor of the hand. Small, peripheral enchondromas of the hand are usually well-defined lytic lesions that are typically benign, but may be detected as a result of pathologic fracture. Solitary enchondromas can also occur in the long bones and are usually oval in shape with central calcifications (Fig. 40-5). Features suggestive of malignant degeneration include an enlarging painful lesion with progressive destruction of the chondroid matrix and an expansile soft tissue mass.

Figure 40-5. An anteroposterior view of the femur demonstrates the presence of cartilage matrix, which is typically ringlike, flocculent, or flecklike, in this patient with an enchondroma.

21. **Which primary bone tumor has the characteristic history of pain at night that is relieved by aspirin?**
Osteoid osteoma. The classic radiographic appearance of this lesion is a round or oval lucent lesion, which represents the nidus, that typically measures less than 1 cm and is surrounded by a zone of bone sclerosis with cortical thickening.

22. **What is fibrous dysplasia?**

Fibrous dysplasia is a developmental anomaly of bone usually presenting as a solitary lesion with focal bone expansion, cortical thinning or thickening, and a "ground-glass" appearance. Patients with these lesions may be asymptomatic or present with pathologic fracture. Polyostotic fibrous dysplasia with associated endocrine dysfunction that is usually manifested as precocious female sexual development is known as *McCune-Albright syndrome*.

KEY POINTS: IMAGING OF BONE TUMORS

1. Order a plain film first.

2. Use MRI for staging and preoperative planning.

3. Use CT for image-guided biopsy and detection of the nidus of an osteoid osteoma or pulmonary metastases.

4. Use MRI for follow-up to detect response to therapy and/or tumor recurrence.

23. **Which of the following has an increased incidence of skeletal malignancy: high-dose radiation therapy, bone infarction, Paget's disease, or chronic osteomyelitis?**

All of the above, with osteosarcoma and fibrosarcoma being the most common forms of malignant degeneration.

24. **What is a bone island?**

A bone island, or enostosis, is a benign lesion that appears radiographically as an oval or round sclerotic focus that may have radiating bone spicules from the center of the lesion. Bone islands are typically asymptomatic, incidentally discovered, and usually do not show increased radiotracer uptake on a nuclear medicine bone scan.

25. **What is the most common location for a skeletal hemangioma?**

The most common site of involvement is the spine, particularly the thoracic segment. Most vertebral hemangiomas are small and asymptomatic, demonstrating a coarse, vertical trabecular pattern or corduroy appearance in the vertebral body on plain films or CT.

BIBLIOGRAPHY

1. Greenspan A: Differential Diagnosis of Tumors and Tumor-Like Lesions of Bones and Joints. Philadelphia, Lippincott Williams & Wilkins, 1998.

2. Rand T, Ritschl P, Trattnig S, et al: Imaging of Bone and Soft Tissue Tumors. New York, Springer Verlag, 2001.

3. Resnick D: Diagnosis of Bone and Joint Disorders, 4th ed. Philadelphia, W.B. Saunders, 2002.

CHAPTER 41

SHOULDER MRI

Neil Roach, MD

1. **What MRI planes are used for evaluating the shoulder?**
   Because the scapula is attached to the chest wall at approximately 45 degrees, oblique sagittal and oblique coronal planes are used for the evaluation of the shoulder. Axial images are also obtained.

2. **Name the four muscles of the rotator cuff.**
   The supraspinatus, infraspinatus, and teres minor attach to the greater tuberosity of the humeral head. The subscapularis tendon attaches to the lesser tuberosity.

3. **What is impingement syndrome?**
   This is caused by entrapment of the supraspinatus tendon, biceps tendon, and subacromial-subdeltoid bursa between the humeral head and coracoacromial arch. It is thought that 95% of rotator cuff tears are related to chronic impingement. The diagnosis of impingement is made clinically.

4. **In what age group of patients do rotator cuff tears most commonly occur?**
   Rotator cuff tears are rare in the normal population younger than 40 years old. Impingement syndrome is a chronic process, beginning at about age 25 years, that causes degeneration of the rotator cuff tendons. Rotator cuff tears can be seen in pitchers and weightlifters before the age of 40 years.

5. **What is the typical magnetic resonance (MR) appearance of a rotator cuff tear?**
   Increased T2 signal (fluid) is seen within the tendon (Fig. 41-1). Normal tendons have low signal intensity on all pulse sequences.

Figure 41-1. Oblique coronal proton density *(A)* and fat-suppressed T2-weighted *(B)* images of the right shoulder at the anterior leading edge of the supraspinatus tendon. A small focal tear *(arrow)* is seen where the supraspinatus tendon (which should be dark) inserts on the greater tuberosity. On T2, fluid is seen in the region of the tear.

6. Which tendon of the rotator cuff is most commonly torn?
The supraspinatus. Most tears occur in the critical zone of the tendon, which is a relatively hypo-vascular area of the tendon that is approximately 1–2 cm proximal to the insertion of the supraspinatus tendon on the greater tuberosity.

7. What MR features indicate that a rotator cuff tear is chronic?
A high-riding humeral head in close proximity to the undersurface of the acromion indicates a chronic rotator cuff tear. This can be seen on radiographs or MR imaging (MRI). Atrophy of muscles can be seen on MRI. This is appreciated by fatty infiltration on T1-weighted images and decreased muscle bulk.

8. What are Hill-Sachs and Bankart deformities?
Both are secondary to anterior dislocations. The Hill-Sachs lesion is an impaction fracture of the posterolateral aspect of the humeral head and is seen best on axial images above the coracoid process. The Bankart lesion is defined as an injury to the anterior-inferior glenoid and can be an osseous or nonosseous abnormality. Bankart lesions are also best appreciated on axial images (Fig. 41-2).

Figure 41-2. *A,* Axial fat-suppressed T2-weighted image demonstrates an osseous defect of the anterior-inferior aspect of the glenoid, a Bankart lesion. *B,* Axial proton density image demonstrates a defect is seen in the posterior-lateral aspect of the humeral head *(arrow),* representing a Hill-Sachs deformity resulting from prior anterior-inferior humeral dislocation.

9. What other shoulder abnormalities can be diagnosed on routine shoulder MR?
Fractures, biceps tendon tears or dislocations, glenohumeral and acromioclavicular osteoarthritis, glenoid labral tears, joint effusion, osteonecrosis, and osteomyelitis.

KEY POINTS: SHOULDER MRI

1. There are three primary diseases that can be seen on MRI of the shoulder: osteoarthritis, rotator cuff tears, and abnormal structures related to the clinical diagnosis of instability.

2. Radiographs should be obtained before MR images. Many times, rotator cuff tears can be diagnosed by the narrowing of the distance between the undersurface of the acromion and humeral head.

10. **What is a SLAP lesion?**

SLAP is a type of glenoid labral tear that extends anteriorly and posteriorly. SLAP is an acronym that stands for superior labrum anterior and posterior. It is usually seen in athletes who throw or after shoulder trauma. Subtle SLAP lesions may be difficult to diagnose on routine MRI. MR arthrography increases the sensitivity for detecting these abnormalities.

11. **Which is better for the detection of calcific tendinitis: radiographs or MRI?**

Calcific tendinitis is a type of tendon pathology seen about the shoulder. It is formally known as *calcium hydroxyapatite* (HA) *deposition disease*. The shoulder is the most common site of involvement. On MRI, the nodular calcium deposits show low signal intensity on all pulse sequences. The involved rotator cuff tendons may show focal thickening related to the calcified nodules. It can be difficult to appreciate calcific tendonitis on MRI, but this diagnosis can be clearly seen on radiographs.

12. **What is meant by glenohumeral instability?**

Patients in whom the humeral head slips or subluxates out of the glenoid are said to have instability during activities. Orthopedic surgeons like to describe instability by direction: anterior, posterior, or multidirectional. Instability can also be characterized as traumatic or atraumatic. *Anatomic instability* refers to subluxation or dislocation of the humeral head. Functional instability refers to pain, clicking, or locking of the shoulder. The most common glenohumeral instability is anterior instability from a previous dislocation.

BIBLIOGRAPHY

1. Beltran J, Kim DH: MR imaging of shoulder instability injuries in the athlete. Magn Reson Imag Clin North Am 11(2):221–238, 2003.
2. Feller JF, et al: Magnetic resonance imaging of the shoulder: Review. Semin Roentgenol 30(3):224–240, 1995.
3. Kaplan PA, Dussault R, Anderson MW, Major NM: Musculoskeletal MRI. Philadelphia, W.B. Saunders, 2001, pp 175–176.
4. Rafii M, et al: Rotator cuff lesions: Signal patterns at MR imaging. Radiology 177(3):817–823, 1990.

CHAPTER 42

MRI OF THE ELBOW AND WRIST

Christopher J. Yoo, MD, and Neil Roach, MD

1. **Name the bones and articulations of the elbow.**
   The elbow joint involves the radius and ulna of the forearm and the humerus of the upper arm. There are three articulations: the radiocapitellar, ulnotrochlear, and proximal radioulnar.

2. **Name the muscles that cross or surround the elbow joint.**
   Biceps, brachialis, triceps, brachioradialis, extensor tendons, flexor tendons, anconeus, pronator teres, and supinator.

3. **Name the labeled structures on the magnetic resonance (MR) images in Figure 42-1.**

4. **Describe the anatomy of the medial and lateral collateral ligament complexes.**
   The medial collateral ligament (MCL) complex consists of three bundles: anterior, posterior, and transverse. The anterior is the most important stabilizer against valgus strain. The lateral collateral ligament (LCL) complex consists of three components as well: the radial collateral ligament (RCL), annular ligament, and lateral ulnar collateral ligament (LUCL). The annular ligament encircles the radial head and attaches to the anterior and posterior margins of the

Figure 42-1. Anatomy of the elbow shown on MR images. *A,* Coronal proton density image through the posterior aspect of the radial head (1 = humerus, 2 = radial head, 3 = ulna, 4 = common flexor tendon, 5 = common extensor tendon, 6 = medial collateral ligament, 7 = lateral ulnar collateral ligament, 8 = radial collateral ligament). *B,* Sagittal proton density image through the ulnotrochlear articulation (1 = trochlea, 2 = ulna, 3 = olecranon, 4 = coronoid process, 5 = anterior fat pad in the coronoid fossa, 6 = posterior fat pad in the olecranon fossa, 7 = triceps, 8 = biceps tendon, 9 = brachialis).

Continued

Figure 42-1, *Cont'd.* *C,* Axial T1-weighted image at the level of the distal humeral epiphysis (1 = trochlea, 2 = capitellum, 3 = ulna, 4 = cubital tunnel retinaculum, 5 = flexor carpi ulnaris, 6 = ulnar nerve, artery, and vein in the cubital tunnel, 7 = brachialis, 8 = biceps tendon).

radial notch of the ulna. The LUCL arises from the lateral epicondyle, courses posterior to the radial head, and inserts on the lateral aspect of the ulna onto the supinator crest (Table 42-1).

TABLE 42-1. ANATOMY OF THE MCL AND LCL COMPLEXES

	Origin	Insertion
MCL complex		
Anterior bundle	Medial epicondyle	Medial aspect of coronoid
Posterior bundle	Medial epicondyle	Medial aspect of olecranon
Transverse bundle	Medial aspect of coronoid	Medial aspect of olecranon
LCL complex		
RCL	Lateral epicondyle	Annular ligament
Annular ligament	Anterior margin of radial notch	Posterior margin of radial notch
LUCL	Lateral epicondyle	Supinator crest of lateral ulna

5. **What pattern of injury is seen with a valgus injury? Whom does it most commonly affect?**
   Athletes who throw develop these injuries, which arise from repeated valgus stress and injury. Valgus-type injuries can include the following, even though not all components will be seen because there is a spectrum of severity of injury: MCL strain/tear, common flexor tendon/muscle strain/tear, medial epicondyle edema, medial heterotopic ossification, lateral bony impaction injury of the radius and capitellum, and ulnar neuropathy.

6. **What is the LUCL? Explain its significance in instability of the elbow joint.**
   The LUCL is a component of the LCL complex, as previously described, originating from the lateral epicondyle and coursing posterior to the radial head to insert on the lateral aspect of the

KEY POINTS: MR SIGNS OF TENDON INJURY ✓

1. Tendon enlargement

2. Increased intrinsic signal intensity on T1-weighted, proton density–weighted, and T2-weighted images

3. Fluid/edema surrounding the tendon

4. Disruption of the tendon fibers

ulna at the supinator crest. Disruption or laxity of the LUCL results in an entity called *posterolateral rotatory instability,* which is the most common form of chronic elbow instability.

7. **What are golfer's elbow and tennis elbow? Which is more common? What muscle groups do they involve?**
    Golfer's elbow and *tennis elbow* are lay terms for medial and lateral epicondylitis, respectively. They do not represent inflammation of the epicondyle itself, but rather are injuries of the tendons and muscles, including tendonopathy; partial and complete tendon tears; muscle strain; muscle tear; and, in young patients, perhaps bony avulsion or delayed physeal closure. Lateral epicondylitis is more common (tennis elbow). The common flexor tendon and associated muscles are involved in medial epicondylitis, and the common extensor tendon and associated muscles are involved in lateral epicondylitis (Fig. 42-2).

Figure 42-2. Common extensor tendonopathy/tennis elbow. *A,* Coronal T1-weighted image shows thickening and increased intermediate signal in the common extensor tendon insertion *(arrow). B,* Coronal T2-weighted image with fat saturation shows increased high signal intensity in the common extensor tendon insertion *(arrow).* The tendon is intact, and no full-thickness tear is seen. Compare with Figure 41-1, *A.*

8. **What causes the anterior and posterior fat pad signs in conventional radiographs? What is the significance of these signs? What role does MRI play in the evaluation of patients?**
    The anterior fat pad in the coronoid fossa and the posterior fat pad in the olecranon fossa can be displaced by a joint effusion. Elevation of the anterior fat pad has been called the *anterior sail sign.*

Visualization of either a posterior fat pad sign or an anterior sail sign may indicate the presence of a joint effusion or hemarthrosis. In the setting of elbow trauma, these signs are higly suggestive for the presence of a fracture, whether or not a fracture is visualized radiographically. MR can be used to diagnose fractures when the sail sign or posterior fat pad sign is present but the fracture is radiographically occult and can also detect associated tendon or ligament injury.

Figure 42-3. *A,* Lateral plain radiograph of the elbow shows elevation of the anterior fat pad, "the anterior sail sign," and elevation of the posterior fat pad. *B,* Sagittal T1-weighted image through the ulnotrochlear articulation shows high signal intensity anterior *(arrow)* and posterior *(arrowhead)* fat pads displaced by intermediate signal intensity joint fluid *(asterisks). C,* Sagittal T2-weighted image with fat saturation in the same plane shows the high signal intensity joint fluid *(asterisks)* displacing the anterior *(arrow)* and posterior *(arrowhead)* fat pads, which now appear dark as a result of fat saturation.

9. **Which patients most commonly present with biceps tendon rupture? Describe the MR appearance of complete rupture.**
   Biceps rupture usually involves the dominant arm and is most commonly seen in men, especially weightlifters or workers who perform heavy lifting. The MR appearance of complete rupture is easily recognized since there is complete disruption of the biceps tendon near the insertion with proximal retraction of the tendon, which often has a wavy appearance (Fig. 42-4). Fluid/hemorrhage usually fills the cubital fossa and surrounds the ruptured tendon.

Figure 42-4. Biceps tendon rupture. *A*, Sagittal T2-weighted image with fat saturation shows the wavy appearance of the retracted biceps tendon *(arrow)*, with extensive edema around the tendon and in the cubital fossa. *B*, Axial T2-weighted image through the distal humeral metaphysis shows the retracted tendon *(asterisk)* with surrounding edema.

10. **What are the boundaries and contents of the cubital tunnel? The presence of which anomalous muscle is a rare cause of symptoms related to the cubital tunnel?**

    The cubital tunnel contains the ulnar nerve and the recurrent ulnar artery and vein. The floor of the tunnel is the elbow capsule and MCL, and the roof consists of the cubital tunnel retinaculum proximally and the flexor carpi ulnaris distally *(see* Fig. 42-2, *C)*. The anconeus epitrochlearis, when present, can cause static compression of the ulnar nerve within the confines of the cubital tunnel, resulting in ulnar neuropathy. The anconeus epitrochlearis sits just deep to the cubital retinaculum.

KEY POINTS: TUNNEL NEUROPATHIES ✓

1. Cubital tunnel: medial elbow, ulnar neuropathy

2. Carpal tunnel: volar wrist, median neuropathy

3. Guyon's canal: volar wrist, ulnar neuropathy

11. **What is Panner's disease?**

    This is an osteochondrosis/avascular necrosis of the capitellum, similar to Legg-Calvé-Perthes disease of the femoral epiphysis. On plain radiographs, one may see sclerosis and deformity of the capitellum. On MR, Panner's disease manifests as low marrow signal on T1-weighted images and variable signal on T2-weighted or short tau inversion recovery (STIR) images, progressing from high to low with more advanced disease.

12. **Where does the pseudodefect of the capitellum occur compared with osteochondritis dissecans (OCD) in the capitellum?**

    OCD typically occurs anteriorly, whereas the pseudodefect is seen posterolaterally. The pseudodefect is actually the normal appearance of the capitellum on sagittal images (Fig. 42-5).

Figure 42-5. OCD of the capitellum. *A,* Sagittal T1-weighted image through the radiocapitellar articulation shows a large osteochondral defect and adjacent low-signal-intensity marrow that represents marrow edema. *B,* Sagittal T2-weighted image with fat saturation at the same level shows the same osteochondral defect with surrounding marrow edema and edema within the osteochondral fragment.

13. **What is the differential diagnosis for olecranon bursitis? Describe its appearance on MRI.**

    The differential diagnosis includes acute or repetitive trauma, gout, rheumatoid arthritis, calcium pyrophosphate deposition disease, hydroxyapatite deposition disease, dialysis, and infection. On MRI, olecranon bursitis typically appears as simple or complex fluid enlarging the bursa, often with surrounding edema in the soft tissues and/or bone, depending on the etiologic factors.

14. **Name the labeled structures in Figure 42-6.**

Figure 42-6. *A,* Axial T1-weighted image through the wrist at the level of the pisiform (1 = APL, EPB; 2 = ECRB, ECRL; 3 = EPL; 4 = ED, EI; 5 = EDM; 6 = ECU; 7 = flexor digitorum superficialis and profundus tendons; 8 = flexor pollicis longus tendon; 9 = flexor carpi radialis longus tendon outside the carpal tunnel; 10 = median nerve; 11 = flexor retinaculum; 12 = pisiform; 13 = scaphoid; 14 = ulnar artery and veins in Guyon's canal; 15 = ulnar nerve in Guyon's canal).

(Continued)

Figure 42-6, *Cont'd.* *B,* Axial T2-weighted image with fat saturation at the same level as in *(A)* (1 = ulnar artery, 2 = ulnar veins, 3 = ulnar nerve, 4 = median nerve). *C,* Coronal gradient-echo image (1 = scaphoid, 2 = lunate, 3 = triquetrum, 4 = trapezium, 5 = trapezoid, 6 = capitate, 7 = hamate, 8 = triangular fibrocartilage, 9 = scapholunate ligament, 10 = lunatotriquetral ligament).

15. What is the role of MRI in evaluation of scaphoid fractures? What is the appearance of avascular necrosis (AVN) of the proximal pole?

MR has much higher sensitivity for scaphoid fractures and, more importantly, can be used to diagnose early AVN of the proximal fracture fragment. MR is useful to assess the viability and probability of successful union of the fracture fragments, thus helping direct treatment options. In radiographically occult fractures, a low T1- and T2-signal intensity fracture line may be seen with surrounding edema on MR. In the presence of AVN, the proximal fracture fragment appears as low signal intensity on T1-weighted images and heterogeneously high to low signal intensity on T2-weighted images. Uniformly low T2-signal intensity and lack of enhancement of the proximal fracture fragment on postgadolinium MRI suggest the lack of blood supply and, therefore, poor prognosis for healing (Fig. 42-7).

16. Define negative, neutral, and positive variance. Which of these is related to Kienböck's malacia?

Ulnar variance refers to the length of the ulna in relationship to the radius at the distal radioulnar joint. If the ulna is longer than the radius as determined by straight lines drawn along the distal articular surfaces, this is termed *positive ulnar variance*. If the ulna is more than 2 mm shorter than the radius, this is termed *negative ulnar variance*. All other cases are termed *neutral ulnar variance*. Negative ulnar variance is associated with increased incidence of Kienböck's disease (AVN of the lunate), which is thought to be due to altered compressive forces at the radiolunate articulation secondary to decreased load bearing at the triquetral-triangular fibrocartilage-ulnar axis.

17. Name the contents of the carpal tunnel. What are classic signs and symptoms of carpal tunnel syndrome (CTS)?

The carpal tunnel contains the median nerve and tendons of the flexor digitorum superficialis and profundus as well as the tendon of the flexor pollicis longus. Classic signs and symptoms of CTS include paresthesia in the median nerve sensory distribution (the first three digits and

Figure 42-7. AVN of the scaphoid after fracture. *A,* Coronal proton density weighted image shows irregular shape and abnormal low signal intensity of the scaphoid. *B,* Anteroposterior radiograph of the wrist shows irregular shape and abnormal sclerosis of the scaphoid *(arrow).*

the radial aspect of the fourth digit) that may be worse at night, thenar atrophy, and positive Phalen's and Tinel's tests.

18. **Describe the MR appearance of CTS.**
    The MR appearance of CTS includes flattening and edema of the median nerve in the carpal tunnel, enlargement of the nerve proximal to the tunnel, and volar bowing of the retinaculum. The etiologic factor can sometimes be seen on MR, including flexor tenosynovitis, trauma, infection, and mass (ganglion cyst, lipoma, neuroma, fibrolipomatous hamartoma).

19. **What is the role of MRI in CTS?**
    Currently MRI is not commonly used as a primary diagnostic tool for CTS because it is costly and neither sensitive nor specific enough. It may be helpful when electromyography is equivocal or when an atypical etiologic factor is being considered. MRI is useful in evaluating for a cause of recurrent symptoms in postoperative patients who have undergone surgical release (Fig. 42-8, *A–B*).

20. **What are the two most common causes of recurrent symptoms in patients who have had surgical release of the carpal tunnel?**
    The two most common causes are an incomplete release, meaning failure to completely divide the flexor retinaculum, and scar formation joining the surgically divided retinaculum, resulting in a closed canal (Fig. 42-8, *C–D*).

21. **What are the boundaries and contents of Guyon's canal? What situations can cause neuropathy related to Guyon's canal?**
    Guyon's canal is a triangular space on axial images located superficial to the carpal tunnel on the ulnar aspect of the wrist and contains the ulnar nerve, artery, and vein. The flexor retinaculum is the floor. The radial surface of the pisiform is the ulnar margin. A superficial fascial layer is the roof (*see* Fig. 42-6, *A*). Acute or chronic trauma, mass, anomalous muscle, or inflammation related to infection or arthritis can cause ulnar nerve entrapment within the canal.

Figure 42-8. *A,* Axial T1-weighted image through the carpal tunnel demonstrating marked enlargement of the median nerve *(asterisk)* within the carpal tunnel secondary to a fibrolipomatous hamartoma. *B,* Sagittal T1-weighted image through the carpal tunnel demonstrating a mixed soft tissue and fatty mass *(arrowheads)* enlarging the median nerve. *C,* Axial T1-weighted and, *D,* fat-saturated T2 images after carpal tunnel release in a patient with recurrent symptoms of CTS. Images show low T1 and T2 signal intensity fibrosis and scarring of the flexor retinaculum *(arrows)* with flattening and increased signal of the median nerve *(arrowheads).*

22. **What is de Quervain's tenosynovitis? Describe its MR appearance.**
    This is tenosynovitis of the first extensor compartment involving the abductor pollicis longus and extensor pollicis brevis. The tendons may be enlarged with increased intrinsic signal, and there should be fluid surrounding the tendons within the tendon sheaths (Fig. 42-9).

23. **What ligament is injured in gamekeeper's thumb or skier's thumb?**
    The ulnar collateral ligament of the first metacarpal joint is injured with forced adduction or hyperadduction of the first digit, often seen in skiers gripping ski poles during a fall but also seen in other contact sports. Historically this was seen in European gamekeepers who would grip a small animal's neck, much like a ski pole, and break the neck using an adduction motion, which would cause chronic repetitive strain on the ulnar collateral ligament (Fig. 42-10).

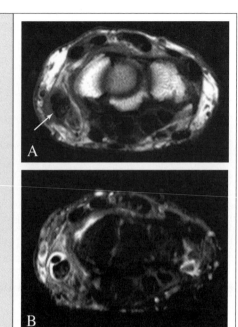

Figure 42-9. Axial T1-weighted *(A)* and fat-saturated T2-weighted *(B)* images in the proximal wrist show enlargement and increased T1 and T2 signal intensity within the first extensor compartment *(arrow)* involving the abductor pollicis longus and extensor pollicis brevis tendons with surrounding fluid within the tendon sheath, in keeping with de Quervain's tenosynovitis.

24. **What is a Stener lesion? Describe its significance.**
    A Stener lesion is characterized by displacement of the avulsed ulnar collateral ligament such that the adductor pollicis aponeurosis is interposed between the avulsed ligament and its insertion, effectively precluding healing. This requires surgical repair to prevent chronic instability.

KEY POINTS: OTHER IMPORTANT CLINICAL ENTITIES

1. Kienböck's malacia (negative ulnar variance)

2. Ulnar abutment syndrome (positive ulnar variance)

3. Medial epicondylitis (wrist flexors and common flexor tendon)

4. Lateral epicondylitis (wrist extensors and common extensor tendon)

25. **What is the most commonly injured intrinsic ligament of the wrist? With what form of instability is this injury associated?**
    The scapholunate ligament is injured more commonly than the lunatotriquetral ligament. Injury to the scapholunate predisposes the patient to dorsal intercalated segment instability (DISI), whereas injury to the lunatotriquetral ligament is associated with volar intercalated segment instability (VISI).

Figure 42-10. Gamekeeper's thumb. *A,* Plain radiograph of the first digit shows a small, bony, ossific density adjacent to the ulnar aspect of the base of the proximal phalanx *(arrow),* representing an avulsion fracture involving the ulnar collateral ligament of the first metacarpophalangeal joint. *B,* Stress image of the same patient reveals hyperabduction at the first metacarpophalangeal joint, indicating ligamentous laxity of the affected side *(arrow).* *C,* Coronal T1-weighted image shows thickening and disruption of the ulnar collateral ligament of the first metacarpophalangeal joint *(arrow).* The avulsed fracture fragment is not seen here.

26. **Describe the typical patient populations who experience traumatic versus degenerative tears of the triangular fibrocartilage (TFC).**
    Typically younger patients get traumatic tears of the TFC, whereas older patients and patients with positive ulnar variance and ulnar abutment syndrome more commonly develop degenerative tears.

27. **What mass in the wrist has been called the King James lesion? Where does it most commonly occur?**
    A ganglion cyst. This facetious term was derived from the sometimes used "treatment" for this lesion, which consisted of putting the hand on a hard flat surface and slamming it with a King James version of the Bible. Ganglion cysts most commonly occur on the dorsum of the wrist near the scapholunate ligament but can occur anywhere. The typical patient population is young adults, more commonly women.

BIBLIOGRAPHY

1. Berquist TH: Nerve compression syndromes. In Berquist TH (ed): MRI of the Hand and Wrist. Philadelphia, Lippincott Williams & Wilkins, 2003, pp 163–178.
2. Chung CB, Kim HJ: Sports injuries of the elbow. MRI Clin North Am 11(2):239–253, 2003.

3. Desharnais L, Kaplan PA, Dussault RG: MR imaging of ligamentous abnormalities of the elbow. MRI Clin North Am 5(3):515–528, 1997.

4. Fritz RC: MR imaging of osteochondral and articular lesions. MRI Clin North Am 5(3):579–602, 1997.

5. Fritz RC, Stoller DW: The elbow. In Stoller DW (ed): Magnetic Resonance Imaging in Orthopaedics and Sports Medicine, 2nd ed. Philadelphia, Lippincott Williams & Wilkins, 1997, pp 743–849.

6. Ho CP: Magnetic resonance imaging of tendon injuries in the elbow. MRI Clin North Am 5(3):529–543, 1997.

7. Rosenberg ZS, Bencardino J, Beltran J: MR features of nerve disorders at the elbow. MRI Clin North Am 5(3):545–565, 1997.

CHAPTER 43

MRI OF THE HIP

Gregory Goodworth, MD, and Neil Roach, MD

1. **What is the first radiologic examination for the evaluation of hip pain?**
   Plain radiographs. These are inexpensive, easy to obtain, and can often delineate the etiologic factor of hip pain.

2. **When should a magnetic resonance image (MRI) of the hip be performed?**
   Hip MRI is the modality of choice for symptomatic patients whose conditions cannot be resolved after evaluation of plain films. Common indications include osteonecrosis, trauma with radiographically occult fractures, stress and insufficiency fractures, labral tears, musculoskeletal neoplasms, septic arthritis and osteomyelitis of the hip, transient osteoporosis, and bone marrow edema.

3. **Which modality is best for the evaluation of suspected osteoarthritis (degenerative changes) of the hip?**
   Plain radiographs.

4. **Does an MRI examination of the hip usually include one or both hips?**
   Both hips. Even if a patient has a complaint of unilateral hip pain, both hips should be examined when a bilateral disease process is suspected, such as osteonecrosis in a patient receiving long-term steroid therapy. Since most hip MRI examinations are for fracture, tumor, or osteonecrosis, it is often useful to image the entire pelvis to search for other lesions. A unilateral protocol is used to evaluate patients with unilateral hip pain without suspicion of contralateral disease, such as a trauma patient with clinical suspicion of an occult fracture. If very high resolution images are required, the unilateral protocol allows for a smaller field of view and thus higher resolution.

5. **Is IV contrast helpful for an MRI evaluation of the hip?**
   Only very rarely. IV contrast may aid in the guidance of percutaneous biopsy by helping to distinguish viable tumor from cystic or necrotic tumor. Enhanced images may also help localize a soft tissue abscess and guide surgical drainage. Contrast may help assess tissue viability in tumors or osteonecrosis.

6. **What is avascular necrosis (AVN) of the hip?**
   Osteonecrosis, previously referred to as *AVN* or *aseptic necrosis,* is a process of subchondral bone necrosis secondary to diminished or disrupted blood supply. The pathologic condition is very similar to that of a bone infarct; however, the articular location of hip AVN makes it clinically more critical than most bone infarcts.

7. **What is the natural history of osteonecrosis? Why is the articular location so critical?**
   Compromised blood supply leads to infarct of the subchondral bone beneath the articular surface of the femoral head. Eventually the weight-bearing surface will collapse and fragment, disturbing joint mechanics and resulting in severe osteoarthritic changes of the hip. The risk of developing osteonecrosis is greatly influenced by the type of fracture. A nondisplaced fracture carries a relatively low risk, approximately 10%, of developing osteonecrosis. A displaced femoral neck fracture runs a risk as high as 80%, depending on vascular anatomy.

8. **What is the blood supply to the femoral head?**
   The femoral head is predominantly nourished by a variable combination of the medial femoral circumflex artery (MFCA) and the ligamentum teres artery, which travels with the round ligament. Thus, hip dislocations may tear the ligamentum teres artery, whereas femoral neck fractures may tear the MFCA and its branches (Fig. 43-1).

9. **Is osteonecrosis a unilateral or bilateral process?**
   It depends on the etiologic factor. Unilateral osteonecrosis is usually secondary to traumatic disruption of the blood supply to the femoral head and is often a sequela of hip dislocation or femoral neck fracture. Bilateral osteonecrosis is usually nontraumatic in etiology.

Figure 43-1. Arterial anatomy of femoral head and neck (A = deep femoral artery, B = MFCA, C = lateral circumflex femoral artery, D = anastomosis of medial and lateral circumflex femoral arteries, E = artery of round ligament of the femoral head).

10. **Which is more common: unilateral or bilateral osteonecrosis?**
    Bilateral disease accounts for approximately 50–80% of cases. The most common cause in the United States is steroid therapy.

11. **What is an idiopathic cause of osteonecrosis in children?**
    Perthes disease. Also known as *Legg-Calvé-Perthes disease* or *coxa plana,* Perthes disease usually affects children between the ages of 3 and 12 years and results from an inadequate blood supply to the femoral head. In most cases (87%), only one hip joint is affected. Most children with Perthes disease eventually recover, but it can take anywhere from 2 to 5 years for the femoral head to regenerate. Treatments are available to encourage the femoral head to grow into a functional shape.

12. **How is MRI useful in the treatment of osteonecrosis?**
    Early detection. MRI is the most sensitive modality for detection of early osteonecrosis, before femoral head cortical collapse. Early detection allows for possible joint-sparing therapies such as steroid reduction, supportive therapies such as non-weight-bearing, and core decompression. Small lesions that involve less than 25% of the weight-bearing portion of the femoral head have a better chance of responding to therapy without progression to femoral head collapse. Large areas of osteonecrosis will not respond to minimally invasive therapies such as core decompression. It is generally believed that if more than 50% of the articular surface is involved, then the prognosis is poor, with eventual collapse and fragmentation of the femoral head, requiring total hip arthroplasty.

13. **What are the MRI characteristics of osteonecrosis?**
    Variable with heterogeneous signal characteristics. However, on fat-saturated T2-weighted images or short tau inversion recovery (STIR) images, most patients (up to 80%) will demonstrate the characteristic "double line" within the femoral head marrow (Fig. 43-2). This sign is composed of concentric rings with an inner low signal intensity ring surrounded by a high signal intensity outer ring. The irregular, inner low signal intensity line demarcates the peripheral aspect, or reactive interface, of the necrotic segment. This is paralleled by a high-signal-intensity line of marrow edema.

14. **What are radiographically occult hip fractures?**
    Fractures that are not evident on plain radiographs. Examples include nondisplaced traumatic fractures, stress fractures, and insufficiency fractures. MRI is a very useful modality for detecting these fractures.

15. **Why is MRI a useful modality for the detection of radiographically occult hip fractures?**

    MRI has very high sensitivity. Traumatic fractures can sometimes be nondisplaced and often impossible to identify on plain films. However, as soon as a fracture occurs, there is associated edema, which produces an immediate change in the bone marrow signal intensity (increased on fat-saturated T2 or STIR) images that is easily seen on an MRI (Fig. 43-3). Fractures are hypointense to marrow on T1-weighted images. Additionally, subtle cortical fracture lines, which may not be evident on plain radiographs for days or weeks until there is visible evidence of healing, may be easily seen on MRI.

Figure 43-2. *A,* STIR and, *B,* T1-weighted images of AVN of both femoral heads.

16. **What are the MRI signal characteristics of an acute fracture?**

    Fracture lines are low signal intensity on all pulse sequences. The edema associated with a fracture demonstrates low signal intensity on T1-weighted images and high signal intensity on T2-weighted and STIR sequences. Traumatic fractures can sometimes be nondisplaced and are often impossible to identify on plain films. MRI is very sensitive for the identification of a nondisplaced fracture. Usually a fracture line will be visible, but occasionally only diffuse edema without a fracture line will be present.

17. **Suppose there is clinical suspicion of an occult fracture related to trauma, but the plain radiographs display normal results and the MRI reveals only diffuse edema without any sign of a dark fracture line. Does this scenario exclude a fracture?**

    No. These findings may represent a bone contusion, which is a microfracture of cancellous bone with associated edema and hemorrhage. On MRI, bone contusions often present as a speckled area in cancellous bone with low T1 signal and high T2 signal intensity. The absence of cortical involvement not only explains the lack of a visible pathologic condition on the plain radiograph, but also highlights why MRI is far superior to computed tomography (CT) for diagnosis of occult fractures. Unless there is cortical disruption, CT may not demonstrate the fracture, especially the microfractures of a bone contusion, whereas MRI will demonstrate these changes. Contusions within the subchondral portion of the femoral head may lead to subsequent bone resorption and rapid development of osteoarthritis.

18. **How many types of stress fractures are there?**
Two: fatigue and insufficiency. Fatigue fractures are commonly referred to simply as *stress fractures*. A fatigue stress fracture results from repeated stress on a normal bone. An insufficiency fracture occurs in abnormal bone that has been weakened by decreased mineralization and fractures under stress of routine or normal activity.

19. **In the hip, where do stress fractures usually occur?**
The transcervical neck. Rarely do stress fractures involve the intertrochanteric region. Stress fractures of the femoral neck are not often seen on plain film because as many as 67% may only involve cancellous bone rather than cortical bone. The fracture in the femoral neck usually can be classified into one of two types: tension or compression. Tension stress fractures are usually perpendicular to the line of force transmission in the femoral neck, usually originate at the superior surface of the neck, and have increased risk of displacement.

Figure 43-3. *A*, STIR and, *B*, T1-weighted images of an occult right hip fracture. The fracture line is hypointense to bone marrow on T1 and shows surrounding edema, which is hyperintense on STIR.

Compression stress fractures have radiologic changes of callus formation on the inferior femoral neck without apparent cortical disruption.

20. **How are stress fractures of the hip usually treated?**
Tension stress fractures are unstable and often require surgical stabilization. Treatment of compression stress fractures is usually nonsurgical with conservative rest and protective weight bearing.

KEY POINTS: MRI OF THE HIP

1. Plain films are the first modality for identification of hip fracture, but MRI demonstrates nondisplaced fractures and microfractures not visible on plain film.

2. The most common cause of hip osteonecrosis in the United States is steroid therapy.

21. **Once a stress fracture or other occult fracture of the hip is diagnosed, which modality is best for follow-up?**
Plain radiographs. Routine plain films may be used to detect any changes or displacement of the fracture. A displaced femoral neck stress fracture in a young adult is a surgical emergency that requires open reduction and internal fixation.

22. **Who are prone to fatigue stress fracture?**
Young, active persons such as endurance athletes, ballet dancers, and military recruits. Development of a stress fracture is often associated with initiation of a new activity or increased frequency/intensity of a routine athletic activity.

23. **Who is most prone to insufficiency stress fracture?**
Patients prone to osteoporosis, such as women and elderly patients, or patients with metabolic bone diseases. In the elderly, a fall is often thought to be the cause of an acute femoral fracture; however, the fall actually may have resulted from displacement of a long-standing insufficiency fracture. Interestingly, it is thought that the displacement of an insufficiency fracture of the femoral neck may lead to a fall as the hip loses its stability. There is no radiographic difference between a completed insufficiency fracture and an acute, traumatic femoral fracture.

24. **Does diffuse marrow edema without a fracture line always indicate a bone contusion or microfracture?**
No. Often, the extensive edema related to subchondral contusions or occult fractures, which do not exhibit a fracture line, may lead to their misdiagnosis as osteonecrosis or transient osteoporosis of the hip.

25. **What is transient osteoporosis of the hip?**
Transient osteoporosis of the hip is most common in women in the later stages of pregnancy, although it may also occur in older men (ages 50–70). It presents as sudden onset of pain that is increased with weight bearing. Its cause is unknown, but it generally resolves in 6–12 months with supportive therapy. On MRI, it is depicted as marked increase in marrow signal on STIR imaging and decrease of marrow signal on T1-weighted images, reflecting the presence of marrow edema (Fig. 43-4).

Figure 43-4. *A*, STIR and, *B*, T1-weighted images of transient osteoporosis of the left hip. The bone edema is hyperintense to normal marrow on STIR images and hypointense on T1-weighted images.

CHAPTER 44

MRI OF THE KNEE

Hanna M. Zafar, MD, MHS, and Neil Roach, MD

1. **What structures in the knee are best evaluated in the sagittal plane? How about the coronal and axial planes?**
   - *Sagittal:* anterior and posterior cruciate ligaments, medial and lateral menisci, patellar ligament, and quadriceps tendon
   - *Coronal:* medial and lateral collateral ligaments and medial and lateral menisci
   - *Axial:* patella, patellar retinacula, extensor mechanism, and popliteal cysts

2. **Identify the following labeled normal structures of the knee on Figures 44-1 through 44-4.**
   A. Anterior cruciate ligament (Fig. 44-1)
   B. Posterior cruciate ligament (Fig. 44-1)
   C. Medial collateral ligament (Fig. 44-1)
   D. Patellar retinacula (Fig. 44-2)
   E. Vastus medialis muscle (Fig. 44-2)
   F. Anterior cruciate ligament (Fig. 44-3)
   G. Posterior cruciate ligament (Fig. 44-3)
   H. Patellar tendon (Fig. 44-3)
   I. Quadriceps tendon (Fig. 44-3)
   J. Anterior horn of lateral meniscus (Fig. 44-4)
   K. Posterior horn of lateral meniscus (Fig. 44-4)
   L. Popliteal tendon (Fig. 44-4)

Figure 44-1.

Figure 44-2.

Figure 44-3.

Figure 44-4.

3. **What are the red and white zones of the menisci? Can MRI be used to differentiate between these zones?**
The red zone is the peripheral one third of the meniscus, which is vascular. The white zone is the central two thirds of the meniscus, which is avascular. Clinically, meniscal tears that involve the periphery are more likely to heal after repair, because of greater blood supply, than are tears that involve the central portion. Concordantly, the treatment of tears in these zones differs. MRI can be used to differentiate between these zones based on anatomy; however, MRI cannot help in the differentiation of these two zones based on enhancement.

4. **Describe the clinical presentation of meniscal injury. Which portions of the menisci are more likely to be involved in injury?**
The clinical presentation of a patient with a meniscal tear is pain and locking of the knee. The posterior horn of the medial meniscus is the primary weight-bearing surface and is more likely to be injured than the anterior horn of the medial meniscus. The lateral meniscus is not usually injured because it is smaller and attaches only at the lateral intercondylar tubercle, which procures greater mobility when compared with the medial meniscus.

5. **What is the appearance of normal and torn meniscus on MRI?**
The medial and lateral menisci are crescent-shaped structures that lie at the medial and lateral aspects of the superior articular surface of the tibia. They are composed mainly of fibrocartilage and demonstrate low signal intensity on all pulse sequences. On sagittal images, the menisci appear as bow-tie shaped structures. A meniscal tear is diagnosed by increased signal intensity within the meniscus that extends to the articular surface (Fig. 44-5).

6. **What is the grading system for meniscal tears on MRI?**
See Table 44-1.

Figure 44-5. Medial meniscus tear. Sagittal proton density image of the lateral aspect of the knee demonstrates linear high signal intensity within the posterior horn of the medial meniscus. This increased signal extends to both articular surfaces, and the vertical orientation is more consistent with a traumatic etiology.

TABLE 44-1.	GRADING OF MENISCAL TEARS ON MRI
Grade I	Focal, globular intrasubstance increase in signal intensity without extension to the articular surface
Grade II	Horizontal, linear intrasubstance increase in signal intensity without extension to the articular surface
Grade III	Increased signal intensity that extends to at least one articular surface
Grade IV	Complex tear with macerated meniscus.

Note that only grade III and IV injuries are true meniscal tears.

7. **What common meniscal variant is associated with tears of the lateral meniscus, and what is the appearance on MRI?**
    Discoid meniscus is a common variant occurring in 3% of the population that appears as morphologic enlargement of the meniscus (Fig. 44-6). Patients usually present with clicking of the knee on extension and flexion. This entity is diagnosed on MRI if more than three sagittal images demonstrate bridging of the posterior and anterior horns. On lateral images, this results in a rectangle appearance of the meniscus, compared with the usual rapid tapering that occurs from the periphery of the meniscus to the free edge, which has a bow tie appearance.

Figure 44-6. Discoid meniscus. Sagittal proton density image of the lateral aspect of the knee reveals bridging of the anterior and posterior horns of the lateral meniscus. Compare this rectangular morphology with the bow tie–shaped appearance of the normal meniscus illustrated in Figure 44-4.

8. **How can traumatic meniscal tears be differentiated from degenerative meniscal tears?**
    Traumatic tears are more likely to be oriented vertically, whereas degenerative tears are more likely to be oriented horizontally.

9. **What is a bucket handle tear? Describe the findings on MRI.**
    A bucket handle tear is a subtype of a traumatic, or vertical, tear that comprises 10% of all meniscal tears. This is usually seen on MRI through the following: (1) absence of the inner body segment, resembling a bow tie, known as the "absent bow tie sign" and (2) identification of a displaced meniscal fragment, which is usually located in the intercondylar notch on coronal images, simulating a third cruciate ligament.

10. **What are the sensitivity and specificity of MRI in the detection of medial and lateral meniscal tears?**
    MRI has approximately a 93% sensitivity and an 88% specificity for medial meniscal tears and a 79% sensitivity and a 96% specificity for lateral meniscal tears.

11. **What are meniscal cysts? How are they diagnosed on imaging?**
    Meniscal cysts are thought to be due to extrusion of meniscal fluid after a meniscal tear. Typically, they arise within the meniscus or in the parameniscal soft tissues at the meniscocapsular junction (more so in the medial compartment compared with the lateral compartment). MRI is more sensitive than either physical examination or arthroscopy in the diagnosis of meniscal cysts. On MRI, cysts usually appear as high-signal lesions within a swollen meniscus that is not as bright as fluid on T2-weighted images. When the fluid is expressed outside the meniscus in the parameniscal soft tissues, it demonstrates high signal intensity on T2-weighted images.

12. **What are the points of attachment for the cruciate ligaments?**
    The anterior cruciate ligament (ACL) arises on the medial surface of the lateral femoral condyle at the intercondylar notch and attaches on the anterior portion of the intercondylar eminence of the tibia. The posterior cruciate ligament (PCL) arises from the lateral surface of the medial

femoral condyle within the intercondylar notch and attaches at the posterior surface of the inter-condylar eminence.

13. **Which is more commonly injured: the ACL or the PCL?**
The ACL is much more commonly injured than the PCL.

14. **What is the MRI appearance of a torn ACL?**
The majority of ACL tears occur at the femoral origin. MRI signs of an ACL tear include (1) visible disruption of the ligament, (2) irregular or wavy contour, (3) focal signal abnormality within the ligamentous substance, (4) edema, and (5) "empty notch" sign on coronal images (absence of the ACL in its expected location) (Fig. 44-7).

15. **What are the classic bone contusions associated with ACL tears?**
Characteristically, ACL tears are associated with valgus force and are usually associated with contusions to the lateral femoral condyle and posterolateral tibial plateau. This is one of several indirect signs of ACL injury.

Figure 44-7. ACL tear. Sagittal proton density image of the midplane of the knee demonstrates an abnormal, wavy contour in the expected region of the ACL. Compare the signal intensity of the ACL with the normal-appearing PCL, which is seen posteriorly with low signal intensity and smooth borders.

KEY POINTS: MRI OF THE KNEE

1. Abnormal signal within a meniscus is not sufficient to diagnose meniscal tear on MRI. Abnormal meniscal signal intensity must extend to the meniscal surface to be called meniscal tear on MRI.

2. Diagnosis of an ACL tear should prompt a search for commonly associated injuries, including medial collateral ligament injury, medial meniscal tear, Segond fracture of the proximal lateral tibia, and bone contusions.

16. **What is the sensitivity and specificity of MRI for the detection of complete ACL and PCL tears?**
MRI has a 94% sensitivity and a 94% specificity for complete ACL tears and a 91% sensitivity and a 99% specificity for complete PCL tears.

17. **What are the components of the medial collateral ligament and lateral collateral ligament?**
The medial collateral ligament comprises the deep layer, which includes the medial meniscofemoral and meniscotibial ligaments, and the superficial layer, which is the tibial collateral ligament. The lateral collateral ligament comprises the fibular cartilage ligament, the biceps femoris tendon, and the iliotibial band.

18. What is O'Donoghue's unhappy triad?
This common football and skiing injury occurs as a result of valgus stress and twisting motion during weight bearing. Classically, this results in medial collateral ligament injury, ACL tear, and medial meniscus tear. Remember that the deep layer of the medial collateral ligament comprises deep fibrous attachments of the medial meniscus to the femur and the tibia (the medial meniscofemoral ligament and the meniscotibial ligaments, respectively). Therefore, injury to the medial collateral ligament is usually associated with medial meniscus injury.

19. What is the grading system for medial collateral ligament injury?
See Table 44-2.

TABLE 44-2. GRADING SYSTEM FOR MEDIAL COLLATERAL LIGAMENT INJURY	
Grade I (sprain)	The medial collateral ligament is intact, but edema is seen tracking along the ligament into the adjacent soft tissues.
Grade II (partial tear)	Abnormal signal is present within portions of the ligament, or there is complete disruption of the deep layer of the medial collateral ligament with an intact superficial layer.
Grade III (complete tear)	High signal is present in the medial collateral ligament with complete disruption of the ligament.

20. What is the difference between osteochondral fractures and osteochondritis dissecans?
Both osteochondral fractures and osteochondritis dissecans are associated with shearing, or tangential impaction, injury to the distal femur. This motion results in subchondral fragmentation or fracture along the lateral aspect of the medial femoral condyle, which is a non–weight-bearing surface. However, osteochondral fractures are acute, usually due to a sports-related injury, whereas osteochondritis dissecans is chronic. As a result, the fracture fragment in osteochondral fractures is usually associated with intact vasculature, whereas the fragment in osteochondritis dissecans is usually avascular (Fig. 44-8).

21. How are osteochondral fractures diagnosed?
Osteochondral fractures are fractures of cartilage and bone and can be seen on plain film as foreign bodies in the joint space with an effusion.

Figure 44-8. Osteochondritis dissecans. Coronal fat-saturated T2-weighted image in the midplane of the knee is significant for abnormal increase in signal intensity in the lateral aspect of the medial femoral condyle *(arrow)*. There is a rim of low signal intensity surrounding this lesion without displacement of bone into the joint space. This image illustrates osteochondritis dissecans with stable bone fragment.

22. Why and how is osteochondritis dissecans graded?
Management of osteochondritis dissecans is contingent on determining fragment stability. Once the fracture is identified, one must next attempt to determine whether the fracture is in situ,

attached to the cartilage by a flap, detached from the cartilage, or dislodged from the joint. MRI signs of an unstable fragment include one or more of the following findings on T2-weighted or Short tau inversion recovery (STIR) images: (1) linear high signal intensity between the fragment and the underlying bone, (2) cystic changes between the fragment and the underlying bone that are 5 mm or larger, (3) a high signal intensity linear defect in the overlying cartilage, or (4) a focal cartilage defect at the level of the lesion that is 5 mm or larger.

23. **Define SONK, and describe its appearance on MRI.**

SONK stands for *spontaneous osteonecrosis of the knee* and usually presents in the sixth or seventh decade of life as acute onset of pain without inciting trauma. Recently, SONK has been thought to be a result of subchondral insufficiency fracture, usually involving the lateral aspect of the medial femoral condyle, with resultant localized osteonecrosis. MRI demonstrates subchondral sclerosis, edema, and flattening of the medial femoral condyle with concomitant thinning of the articular cartilage. The appearance on T2-weighted images includes a central zone of low signal intensity with a periphery of high signal intensity.

24. **What is jumper's knee?**

Jumper's knee, also known as *patellar tendinitis,* is an overuse syndrome that classically occurs in young athletes who kick, jump, and run. These actions place stress on the patellofemoral joint with intrasubstance degeneration and partial tearing of the tendon. This injury is analogous to a rotator cuff tear clinically, pathologically, and radiologically.

25. **Describe the appearance of jumper's knee on MRI.**

Jumper's knee commonly occurs near the origin of the patellar ligament at the inferior pole of the patella. MRI of acute pathology reveals thickening of the posterior aspect of the proximal tendon, abnormally increased signal intensity on gradient recalled echo [SW1] within the tendon, and ill-defined margins on both T1 and T2.

BIBLIOGRAPHY

1. Campbell SE, Sanders TG, Morrison WB: MR imaging of meniscal cysts: Incidence, location, and clinical significance. Am J Roentgenol 177:409–413, 2001.

2. Greenspan A: Orthopedic Radiology: A Practical Approach, 3rd ed. Philadelphia, Lippincott, 2000, pp 227–271.

3. Hauger O, Frank LR, Boutin RD: Characterization of the "red zone" of knee meniscus: MR imaging and histologic correlation. Radiology 217:193–200, 2000.

4. Helms CA: The meniscus: Recent advances in MR imaging of the knee. Am J Roentgenol 179:1115–1122, 2002.

5. Oei EH, Verstijnean AC, Ginai AZ, et al: Diagnostic performance of magnetic resonance imaging of the knee differs according to the lesion. J Bone Joint Surg 85A:2258, 2003.

6. Yamamoto T, Bullough PG: Spontaneous osteonecrosis of the knee: The result of subchondral insufficiency fracture. J Bone Joint Surg 82A:858–866, 2000

CHAPTER 45

MRI OF THE FOOT AND ANKLE

Neil Roach, MD

1. **What are the four compartments about the ankle? What do they contain?**
   Medial, lateral, anterior, and posterior. The compartmental organization is helpful in thinking of tendon anatomy.

   The *medial compartment* contains (anterior to posterior) the posterior tibialis tendon (PTT), flexor digitorum longus tendon (FDL), and flexor hallucis longus tendon (FHL). "Tom, Dan, and Harry" (The *an* in Dan refers to the posterior tibial *a*rtery and *n*erve.)

   The *lateral compartment* contains the peroneal brevis and longus.

   The *anterior compartment* contains (medial to lateral) the extensor *T*ibials, extensor *H*allucis longus tendon, and extensor *D*igitorum longus tendons. "Tom, Harry, and Dick."

   The *posterior compartment* contains the Achilles tendon.

2. **What is the most commonly injured ankle tendon?**
   The Achilles tendon. It usually tears 3–5 cm superior to its calcaneal insertion, where the tendon's blood supply is poorest. Tears may also occur at the musculotendinous (usually the lateral gastrocnemius) junction, but this is much less common. The least common tears occur at the calcaneal insertion secondary to injury or ill-fitting shoes. Normal tendon signal is very low on both T1- and T2-weighted images. The tendon morphologic features should be evaluated on both sagittal and axial images, with the anterior surface of the normal tendon flat or concave on axial images.

3. **Describe the magnetic resonance (MR) appearance of Achilles tendon tears.**
   Achilles abnormalities tend to cover a progressive sequence of disorders:
   - *Peritendinitis:* The Achilles tendon does not have a sheath; therefore, only peritendinitis, not synovitis, can occur. Peritendinitis is seen as infiltrative changes in the fat surrounding the tendon.
   - *Tendonopathy:* Any internal tendon signal is indicative of tendonopathy.
   - *Chronic tendonopathy:* This is visualized on magnetic resonance imaging (MRI) as an enlarged and abnormally shaped tendon.
   - *Interstitial tears:* These are depicted on MRI as longitudinally oriented internal signal changes first seen on T1 scans. As these tears become more severe, T2 images will be abnormal also.
   - *Partial tears:* These are horizontally oriented signal abnormalities.
   - *Complete tears:* These are complete Achilles disruption with retraction of the torn ends. They are similar in appearance to the end of a mop.

4. **Which of the flexor or medial tendons is most commonly torn?**
   The PTT is the most common of the medial tendons to tear. These tears most often occur in middle-aged females. PTT disruption results in "adult onset" flat foot. PTT tears usually occur near the tendon insertion site and are associated with accessory navicular or a cornuate navicular bones. Normally, the PTT is twice the size as the FDL or FHL. One must suspect a PTT tear if there is tenosynovitis and/or if the tendon is greatly enlarged. Therefore, comparing the size of the PTT to the FDL or FHL can be useful.

5. **Name the three ligaments that form the lateral collateral ligament.**
   The anterior talofibular, calcaneofibular, and posterior talofibular.

6. **Which of these three ligaments tends to tear first?**
   The anterior talofibular is the most commonly injured ligament. The calcaneofibular is the next most commonly injured ligament. The posterior talofibular ligament is easily identified on coronal MRI images but is rarely injured.

7. **Which bones form the hindfoot, midfoot, and forefoot?**
   The hindfoot is composed of the calcaneus and talus. The midfoot has the navicular, the three cuneiform bones, and the cuboid. The forefoot is composed of the metatarsals and phalanges.

8. **What are the articulations of the subtalar joint?**
   The posterior facet is the largest and the "true" subtalar joint.
   The middle facet is formed by the sustentaculum tali (of the calcaneus) and the anterior talus. It has a flat joint surface.
   The anterior facet (vestigial) may be independent of or contiguous with the middle facet and has a rounded surface.

9. **Describe the tarsal canal and the sinus tarsi.**
   The tarsal canal and sinus tarsi form the boundary between the posterior subtalar joint and the anteriorly located talocalcaneal navicular joint. The tarsal canal and sinus extend from postero-medial to anterolateral. The tarsal canal extends to the medial aspect of the foot, posterior to the sustentaculum tali. The canal widens to form the sinus tarsi, which is cone-shaped and opens laterally. The sinus tarsi contain fat, blood vessels, and the interosseous and cervical ligaments and branches of the tibial nerve.

10. **Which ligament is least likely to tear about the ankle?**
   The medially located deltoid ligament is very strong and uncommonly torn. Eversion injuries rather than ligament tears usually cause avulsion fractures of the medial malleolus. The deltoid is composed of four ligaments, two of which are superficial and two of which are deeper.

11. **What are the three plantar compartments, and why are they important?**
   The plantar compartments of the foot are important for the evaluation of infection and tumor extent. The three plantar compartments are separated by fascial planes.
   The medial compartment (first ray) contains the abductor hallucis muscle, the flexor hallucis brevis muscle, the tendon of the flexor hallucis longus muscle, the medial plantar nerve and vessels, and the first metatarsal bone.
   The central compartment (second, third, and fourth rays) contains the flexor digitorum brevis muscle, the quadratus plantae, the four plantar lumbricales muscles, the tendon of the flexor digitorum longus muscle, a portion of the tendon of the flexor hallucis longus muscle, and the lateral plantar nerve and vessels. The central compartment also contains the second, third, and fourth metatarsals. The thick, longitudinally oriented plantar aponeurosis forms the floor of the central compartment. This compartment is important since it communicates with the calf and can serve as a pathway for spread of infection.
   The lateral compartment (fifth ray) contains the fifth metatarsal and the abductor digiti minimi and flexor digitorum minimi brevis muscles.

12. **What is tarsal coalition?**
   This is fusion of one or more intertarsal joints. The fusion can be osseous, fibrocartilaginous, or fibro-osseous. Patients usually present in adolescence with a spastic flat foot. It can be bilateral in 20–25% of cases. Hereditary forms exist. Calcaneonavicular fusion is the most common type based on plain film experience. Computed tomography (CT) and MRI are demonstrating that talocalcaneal fusion may be more common. Secondary signs of tarsal coalition include talar beaking and a ball-and-socket ankle joint. MRI diagnosis of an osseous coalition, demonstrated by continuity of the bone marrow, is straightforward (Fig. 45-1). Fibrocartilaginous or

fibro-osseous coalitions require evaluation of articular surfaces for irregularities and for low signal fibrous tissue bands that are more difficult to appreciate.

Figure 45-1. Coronal T1-weighted MR image of the ankle demonstrates an osseous calcaneal-talar coalition *(arrow)* at the level of the middle facet of the subtalar joint.

13. **What are the common sites for stress fractures of the foot?**
Calcaneal and metatarsal stress fractures are the most common stress fractures in the foot. On T1-weighted images, the edema and hemorrhage of the fracture appear as bands of low signal traversing the normally high-signal bone marrow. Fat-suppressed T2-weighted or short tau inversion recovery (STIR) images show areas of increased signal intensity in the region of the fracture (Fig. 45-2).

Figure 45-2. *A,* T1 axial scan of the forefoot shows a stress fracture of the second metatarsal. *B,* Coronal fat-suppressed T2-weighted image outlines the soft tissue and bone marrow edema from the stress fracture in *(A).*

14. **Which part of the dome of the talus is typically injured in repetitive trauma? What part of the talar dome is typically involved if there is a single bad traumatic event?**
Osteochondral injuries are most common in adolescents and in males. If the injury is caused by repetitive injury, the medial talar dome is usually affected. If the injury is caused by a single bad traumatic event, the lateral talar dome is usually involved.

15. **MRI and/or MR arthrography of the ankle may be useful in evaluating the different types of osteochondral injuries. How are osteochondral injuries classified?**
    - *Stable:* ill-defined rim of high T2 signal is present around the lesion, but the cartilage is intact
    - *Loose in situ:* the cartilage is injured
    - *Partially loose:* incomplete but well-defined ring of high T2 signal is present around the lesion
    - *Loose complete:* well-defined ring of signal surrounds the fragment and/or a cyst associated with the lesion
    - *Free:* intra-articular body with an empty crater

16. **What are some characteristics used to differentiate between osteomyelitis and neuropathic arthropathy?**
The distinction between neuropathic joint arthropathy and osteomyelitis is based on distribution of disease, the association with an ulcer, and the MRI signal characteristics of the bone marrow. Neuropathic arthropathy usually affects the Lisfranc, metatarsophalangeal, and subtalar joints. Osteomyelitis can affect any bone, but it is usually associated with contiguous spread from an ulcer and abnormal adjacent soft tissues. STIR sequences are very sensitive to edema in bones, whether this edema is due to osteomyelitis or to neuropathic/osteoarthritic changes. Because bone edema is not specific for bone infection, STIR images may lead to false-positive diagnoses of osteomyelitis and the finding of bone edema must be interpreted in light of other MRI findings. Postgadolinium images are also helpful in the evaluation of edema versus cellulitis.

17. **What MRI findings are related to plantar fasciitis?**
This is seen as increased T2 signal adjacent to the proximal insertion of the plantar fascia with or without a plantar enthesophyte. The fascia may be thickened. Refractory cases can demonstrate bone marrow edema adjacent to the plantar fascia insertion on the calcaneus (Fig. 45-3).

18. **What is plantar fibromatosis?**
Patients present with pain on weight bearing and have palpable nodular thickening along the course of the plantar fascia. Males are affected twice as often as females. Plantar fibromatosis can be bilateral in 10–40% of patients and may occur in any age group. On T1-weighted images, the lesion can be hypointense or isointense to muscle. On

Figure 45-3. Sagittal STIR image of the ankle shows soft tissue and bone marrow edema in a patient with plantar fasciitis *(arrows)*.

T2-weighted images, the lesion may be hypointense or slightly hyperintense. These lesions enhance intensely with gadolinium and are usually bright on STIR images.

19. **What are Morton's neuromas?**
They are small, focal masses of fibrosis and do not represent a true neuroma involving the plantar digital nerves. They occur most commonly between the third and fourth metatarsals and can

be bilateral in 25% of cases. Women ages 25–50 years are the most likely to be affected. T1- and T2-weighted MR images demonstrate low signal intensity secondary to fibrosis.

20. **What characterizes the tarsal tunnel? What is tarsal tunnel syndrome?**
   The tarsal tunnel is located on the medial side of the ankle. It begins superiorly at the medial malleolus and extends inferiorly to the navicular bone. The lateral side of the tunnel is formed by the calcaneus, including the sustentaculum tali, and the talus. The flexor retinaculum forms the medial wall, and the abductor hallucis muscle forms the floor of the tunnel. The posterior tibial nerve and its divisions—the posterior tibial artery and vein and the PTT, FDL, and FHL tendons—are within the tunnel.

   Patients with tarsal tunnel syndrome usually present with pain and paresthesia along the distribution of the posterior tibial nerve and its branches. They typically complain of pain and burning on the plantar aspect of the foot. Half of the cases are idiopathic, with the remainder secondary to scarring, osseous deformities, soft tissue masses, or varicose veins.

21. **What is sinus tarsi syndrome, and what does it look like on MRI?**
   There is loss of the normal fat within the sinus tarsi. In acute or subacute cases, there is low T1 signal and high T2 signal secondary to inflammation. In chronic cases, there is low T1 and T2 signal secondary to fibrosis. Patients complain of weakness and instability in the ankle with palpable tenderness over the sinus tarsi. Most cases are idiopathic, but some patients have a history of ankle inversion injury. Other causes of sinus tarsi include inflammatory conditions, such as rheumatoid arthritis or gout, and ganglion cysts.

22. **Of the bones of the foot/ankle, which is the most likely to develop avascular necrosis? What is the typical cause of this?**
   The talus. This is related to fracture of the neck of the talus and loss of the blood supply to the dome. This eventually leads to deformity and collapse of the dome.

KEY POINTS: MRI OF THE FOOT AND ANKLE

1. Tendon tears are generally related to a progressive sequence of disorders.

2. MRI can detect fractures that are not appreciated on radiographs or CT scans. This occurs commonly in the foot and ankle.

3. The deltoid ligament practically never tears. Avulsion fractures of the medial malleolus generally occur before deltoid ligament tears.

4. Tarsal coalitions are usually seen in children and adolescents.

BIBLIOGRAPHY

1. Beltran J, Campanini DS, Knight C, McCalla M: The diabetic foot: Magnetic resonance imaging evaluation. Skeletal Radiol 19(1):37–41, 1990.

2. Cheung Y, Rosenberg ZS, Magee T, Chinitz L: Normal anatomy and pathologic conditions of ankle tendons: Current imaging techniques. Radiographics 12(3):429–444, 1992.

3. Kaplan PA, Dussault R, Anderson MW, Major NM: Musculoskeletal MRI. Philadelphia, W.B. Saunders, 2001.

4. Klein MA, Spreitzer AM: MR imaging of the tarsal sinus and canal: Normal anatomy, pathologic findings, and features of the sinus tarsi syndrome. Radiology 186(1):233–240, 1993.

5. Wechsler RJ, Schweitzer ME, Deely DM, et al: Tarsal coalition: Depiction and characterization with CT and MR imaging. Radiology 193(2):447–452, 1994.

BRAIN: ANATOMY, TRAUMA, AND TUMORS

Gul Moonis, MD, and Laurie A. Loevner, MD

CHAPTER 46

1. **Identify the parts of the brain labeled 1 through 6 in Figure 46-1.**
   See figure legend for answers.

Figure 46-1. Axial T2-weighted image of the brain at the level of the basal ganglia (1 = putamen, 2 = caudate head, 3 = sylvian fissure, 4 = frontal horn of the lateral ventricle, 5 = occipital lobe, 6 = thalamus).

2. **What are the two primary imaging modalities used to image the brain?**
   The two major noninvasive cross-sectional imaging modalities used in neuroimaging are computed tomography (CT) and magnetic resonance imaging (MRI). Catheter angiography is reserved for the detection of intracranial vascular processes such as aneurysms and intracranial vasculitis. Myelography involves the injection of contrast material into the subarachnoid space by lumbar puncture, allowing visualization of the spinal cord and nerve roots, which are seen as "filling defects" within the contrast-opacified cerebral spinal fluid (CSF). Myelography (usually followed by postmyelography CT) is reserved for patients with contraindications to MR (patients with pacemakers, severe claustrophobia), patients with surgical hardware (pedicle screws), patients with equivocal MRI findings, and obese patients who exceed weight limits for MR scanners.

3. **What are the clinical indications for obtaining CT and MRI of the brain?**
   A CT scan is a good initial screening examination for evaluating the brain for the presence of abnormalities. It is the primary imaging modality for assessing for acute intracranial hemorrhage, subarachnoid hemorrhage, mass effect, hydrocephalus, and stroke. However, the greater tissue contrast of MR and its multiplanar capabilities make MR the imaging modality of choice for the assessment of a large spectrum of pathologic processes, including, but not limited to, metastatic disease, primary glial neoplasms, neurodegenerative disorders, and inflammatory

and infectious processes. MR is less sensitive than CT for the detection of subarachnoid hemorrhage and calcification. In many instances, CT and MRI play complementary roles in the evaluation of pathologic conditions (especially lesions at the skull base and those involving the calvarium).

4. **What are contraindications for performing MRI of the brain?**
Contraindications include implanted electronic devices, such as pacemakers, neurostimulator devices, non–MR-compatible vascular clips, ferromagnetic metallic implants, and foreign bodies in the eye. Severe claustrophobia is a relative contraindication and, if necessary, most patients with this condition can successfully undergo MRI with sedation. MRI cannot be performed on individuals who have a metallic intracranial aneurysm clip. Most aneurysm clips used after 1995 are made of titanium and are MR compatible.

5. **Define the terms *intra-axial* and *extra-axial*, which are commonly used to localize intracranial pathologic conditions.**
An *intra-axial* abnormality arises from the brain parenchyma. An *extra-axial* lesion is one that arises outside of the brain substance and may be pial, dural, subdural, epidural, or intraventricular in origin. The most common extra-axial mass is a meningioma. In adults, the most common solitary intra-axial masses are primary brain tumors and metastatic disease. An intra-axial mass lesion expands the brain, results in gyral swelling, and/or results in effacement of the cerebral sulci. Imaging features that identify a mass as extra-axial include inward buckling of the gray and white matter, the presence of a cleft (which may be CSF, dura, and/or small vessels) separating the extra-axial mass from the brain, and the presence of remodeling of the adjacent osseous calvarium (Fig. 46-2).

6. **Contrast agents are sometimes used in cranial CT (iodine-based materials) and are commonly used in brain MRI (gadolinium chelates) to detect areas of breakdown of the blood-brain barrier, which are identified as regions of enhancement (high density). What factors determine the degree of enhancement of a lesion?**
The volume of contrast delivered to the lesion, the vascularity of the lesion, the permeability of blood vessels in the lesion, and the size of the extravascular intralesional space determine the degree of enhancement.

7. **What is the imaging modality of choice for imaging acute head trauma?**
An unenhanced brain CT. CT is readily available and is a fast, accurate method for detecting acute intracranial hemorrhage. On CT, acute hemorrhage is hyperdense to brain and may display mass effect. Emergency physicians and neurosurgeons want to know the exact cause of a trauma patient's clinical symptoms. Specifically, the most significant concern is whether there is a treatable lesion. CT plays a primary role in evaluating the extent of trauma and in determining the appropriate management. It is sensitive in distinguishing brain contusions from extra-axial hematomas (subdural and epidural). CT is also excellent for detecting depressed facial and calvarial fractures. When diffuse axonal shear injury is suspected, MRI is more sensitive and can be obtained when the patient is clinically able to tolerate this examination.

8. **How does one differentiate a subdural hematoma from an epidural hematoma?**
An epidural hematoma is usually caused by an arterial injury (most commonly the middle meningeal artery is injured as a result of a fracture of the temporal bone through which it courses) (Fig. 46-3, *A*). An epidural hematoma is extra-axial, runs between the periosteum of the inner table of the skull and the dura, and is confined by the lateral sutures (especially the coronal sutures) where the dura inserts. As a result, an epidural hematoma is usually lenticular in shape. In contrast, a subdural hematoma is usually caused by injury to the bridging cor-

Figure 46-2. *A,* Intracranial meningioma. Axial T2-weighted image demonstrates a large meningioma in the right middle cranial fossa, which is isointense to gray matter. Note the CSF cleft surrounding this mass *(arrow),* indicating its extra-axial site of origin. *B,* Coronal contrast-enhanced MR image demonstrates homogeneous enhancement of this mass, characteristic of a meningioma. *C,* Axial unenhanced CT image of the same mass demonstrates that the meningioma is isodense to the brain parenchyma *(asterisk).*

tical veins (Fig. 46-3, *B*). A subdural hematoma runs between the dura and the pia-arachnoid meninges on the surface of the brain and is not confined by the lateral sutures. As a result, subdural hematomas are usually crescentic in shape. However, in the midline the dural reflection is attached to the falx cerebri. Therefore, subdural hematomas (unlike epidural hematomas) do not cross the midline, but rather track in the interhemispheric fissure. Subdural hematomas are commonly seen in closed head trauma, elderly patients with minor head trauma, and in the setting of rapid decompression of hydrocephalus and extra-axial hematomas where abrupt changes in intracranial pressure make the bridging cortical veins vulnerable.

Figure 46-3. *A,* Axial unenhanced CT scan shows a hyperdense, lenticular-shaped epidural hematoma in the left frontotemporal region. Note the mass effect on the adjacent left lateral ventricle that is effaced *(arrow)*. *B,* Axial unenhanced CT scan demonstrates a left hemispheric subdural hematoma *(arrow)* that crosses the coronal suture. The hematoma is confined by the falx anteriorly. *C,* Unenhanced CT demonstrates diffuse hyperdensity in the basilar cisterns (suprasellar and interpeduncular cisterns), compatible with subarachnoid hemorrhage *(arrow)*. Note the early dilation of the temporal horns *(white arrowhead)*, consistent with hydrocephalus.

KEY POINTS: EPIDURAL HEMORRHAGE

1. Arterial injury, usually middle meningeal artery

2. Associated with temporal bone or other skull fractures

3. Biconvex, lenticular shape; blood contained by dural sutures

4. Surgical emergency

9. **What is the CT appearance of traumatic subarachnoid hemorrhage (SAH)?**

   SAH appears as hyperdensity in the subarachnoid spaces. The subarachnoid spaces are identified by their serpentine appearance, dipping in between the gyri of the brain (Fig. 46-3, *C*). The
   presence of SAH in the setting of trauma usually indicates the presence of superficial cortical
   contusions.

10. **What is the Glasgow Coma Scale? How is it used?**

    The Glasgow Coma Scale was devised to provide a uniform approach to the clinical assessment
    of trauma patients with acute head trauma. To measure level of awareness and responsiveness,
    it assigns numeric values (1–5) to each of the following: eye opening, best motor response, and
    best verbal response. Scores of 13–15 correspond to mild closed head injury, 9–12 to moderate
    head injury, and 8 or less to severe brain injury. This scale does not correlate with survival out-
    come in cases of severe head trauma with coma.

KEY POINTS: SUBDURAL HEMORRHAGE

1. Venous injury to bridging cortical veins

2. Skull fracture may not be present

3. Usually crescentic, not contained by sutures; does not cross falx or tentorium

4. Trauma patients, older patients, child abuse victims

11. **What are the advantages and drawbacks of MRI in assessing the trauma
    patient?**

    It is important to remember that the availability and speed of CT, as well as its high sensitivity in
    detecting treatable lesions, makes it the imaging modality of choice for the initial assessment of
    trauma patients with head injury! MRI is more sensitive in distinguishing between the different
    ages of blood (hyperacute, acute, subacute, and chronic), in detecting shear injury (diffuse
    axonal injury), and in detecting injury in the posterior fossa and the undersurfaces of the frontal
    and temporal lobes. MRI is less sensitive than CT in detecting subarachnoid hemorrhage,
    intracranial air, and fractures. In addition, there are logistic difficulties in performing MRI on
    trauma patients. MRI times are significantly longer, performing MRI in patients on ventilators
    and other monitoring devices can be very cumbersome, and the location of most MRI scanners
    is outside of the emergency department.

KEY POINTS: SUBARACHNOID HEMORRHAGE

1. Blood in subarachnoid spaces; hyperdensity in CSF spaces

2. Aneurysm rupture or posttraumatic superficial cortical contusions

3. Vasospasm several days afterward may lead to secondary infarction

12. **Define *penetrating injury to the brain*, and identify common causes.**

    Penetrating injuries result in brain "lacerations," and they are most commonly associated with
    bullets, stab wounds, and depressed/dislodged bone fragments. There is risk of injury to all vital
    structures traversed by the penetrating object. The most important of these are the brain and
    vascular structures (arteries and veins/dural venous sinuses).

13. **What are the five patterns of brain herniation/herniation syndromes?**
    The brain lives in a confined compartment (the skull) and is further compartmentalized by inelastic dural attachments (the falx cerebri, falx cerebelli, and tentorium). Brain swelling, or mass lesions when large enough, forces brain from one compartment into another. If untreated, this can result in further brain damage and vascular injury. Five patterns of brain herniation are inferior tonsillar/cerebellar, superior vermian (upward), temporal lobe, subfalcine, and central transtentorial. Mass effect, especially in the posterior fossa, may also result in acute, obstructive hydrocephalus.

14. **What is the imaging manifestation of a brain contusion?**
    Contusions are parenchymal bruises of the brain with associated petechial hemorrhage usually related to direct trauma to the head. The most common locations are the inferior, anterior, and lateral surfaces of the frontal and temporal lobes. This is due to direct impact of the brain against the rough edges of the inner table of the skull along the floor of the anterior cranial fossa, the sphenoid wing, and the petrous ridges. On CT, hemorrhagic contusions appear as focal areas of hyperdensity (blood) with surrounding hypodensity (edema) in characteristic anatomic locations of the brain. On T2-weighted images, acute hemorrhagic contusions are hypointense (dark) with surrounding high-intensity (bright) edema. On gradient-echo susceptibility images, these lesions are detected with increased sensitivity as areas of signal drop-out (hypointensity, or "dark").

15. **What are the imaging manifestations of diffuse axonal injury?**
    Diffuse axonal injury (DAI) is commonly associated with coma, immediate cognitive decline, and poor outcome in patients with significant closed head injury. The stress induced by rotational acceleration/deceleration movement of the head causes differential motion to occur between the neuronal body and axon, which is the area of greatest density difference in the brain. This causes axon disruption and formation of retraction balls. The sites most commonly involved include the body and splenium of the corpus callosum, brain stem, superior cerebellar peduncle, internal capsule, and gray-white junction of the cerebrum. On CT, DAI may not be initially detected. On follow-up MRI, rounded or elliptical T2 hyperintense foci are seen in characteristic locations, and they are commonly hemorrhagic.

16. **Primary brain tumors in adults usually arise from what cell line?**
    Most primary intra-axial tumors of the brain arise from the supporting microglial cells. Gliomas account for 35–45% of all intracranial tumors. Glioblastoma multiforme (GBM) accounts for 35% of gliomas and has a very poor prognosis, with survival rates commonly less than 1 year. Astrocytomas, ependymomas, medulloblastomas, and oligodendrogliomas are other, more commonly encountered primary brain tumors.

17. **What is the most common benign extra-axial tumor in adults?**
    The prototypical extra-axial tumor in adults is the meningioma. This tumor commonly affects middle-aged women and arises from the arachnoid of the meninges. The most common locations are the parasagittal dura of the falx, the cerebral convexities, the sphenoid wing, and the olfactory groove and planum sphenoidale. Other locations include the tuberculum sella and orbit, the cerebellopontine angle, and the cavernous sinus. On unenhanced CT imaging, the majority of meningiomas are slightly hyperdense compared with normal brain tissue, with calcifications present in approximately 20% (Fig. 46-2, *C*). There may be associated osseous hyperostosis involving the adjacent bone. On MRI, meningiomas are isointense to slightly hyperintense relative to gray matter on T2-weighted images. Meningiomas enhance intensely and homogeneously (Fig. 46-2, *A* and *B*). There is often the presence of a CSF cleft between the mass and the brain, identifying its extra-axial location. Even though the presence of a dural tail is typical of a meningioma, it may not be seen in up to 30% of cases.

18. **What are the most common neoplasms arising in the corpus callosum?**
The corpus callosum is the largest white matter tract, and it connects the two cerebral hemispheres in the midline. The most common tumors that affect the corpus callosum are the GBM and lymphoma. The extension of a neoplasm from one hemisphere to the other via the corpus callosum produces the so-called "butterfly" pattern (Fig. 46-4). Other non-neoplastic white matter diseases that commonly involve the corpus callosum include demyelinating disease (especially multiple sclerosis) and trauma (diffuse axonal injury).

Figure 46-4. GBM. Axial contrast-enhanced T1-weighted MR image demonstrates a peripherally enhancing, expansile mass involving the splenium of the corpus callosum with extension into both occipital lobes in a pattern characteristic of a "butterfly" glioma.

19. **What are the most common systemic neoplasms to metastasize to the brain?**
Breast cancer, carcinoma of the lung, and melanoma most commonly spread hematogenously to the brain. Hemorrhagic brain metastases are common with melanoma, choriocarcinoma, thyroid cancer, and renal cell carcinoma; however, because breast and lung cancer are so much more common, it is more likely that a hemorrhagic metastasis will be related to one of these latter cancers. Calcified metastases may be seen with mucinous adenocarcinomas (lung, colon, stomach, ovary, and breast) and bone cancers (osteosarcoma and chondrosarcoma).

20. **What are the most common primary brain tumors that calcify?**
Oligodendroglioma, ependymoma, astrocytoma, craniopharyngioma, and ganglioglioma are among the primary central nervous system (CNS) tumors that most commonly calcify.

21. **What is the imaging appearance of leptomeningeal carcinomatosis/subarachnoid seeding (SAS)? What are the most common tumors producing it in adults?**
SAS/leptomeningeal tumor is characterized by tiny nodules of tumor implanted on the surface of the brain and/or spinal cord. There is "sugar-coating" of the subarachnoid spaces. T1-weighted MRI with contrast enhancement is best at demonstrating this nodular enhancement, particularly in the basilar cisterns, over the cerebral convexities, and along the cranial nerves (Fig. 46-5). Communicating hydrocephalus may result from obstruction of the arachnoid villi. Many primary CNS tumors seed the subarachnoid spaces (GBM, oligodendroglioma, ependymoma). Metastatic systemic tumors that commonly spread to the CSF/leptomeninges

Figure 46-5. Leptomeningeal spread of breast cancer. Axial contrast-enhanced T1-weighted MR image at the level of the cerebellum demonstrates numerous enhancing nodules studding the surface of the cerebellum/subarachnoid space along the cerebellar folia (*arrow*).

include breast and lung carcinoma, melanoma, and hematologic malignancies (lymphoma and leukemia).

22. **Why would a mass appear hyperdense on unenhanced CT of the head?**
Masses may be hyperdense due to the presence of acute blood, calcification, dense cellularity (lymphoma, meningioma, medulloblastoma, and germinoma), and/or the presence of proteinaceous material.

23. **What is the most common tumor in the cerebellopontine angle cistern (CPA)?**
The majority are vestibular schwannomas (75%), followed by meningiomas (10%) and epidermoid tumors (5%). Uncommon neoplasms that may involve the CPA include metastatic disease, facial nerve schwannoma, exophytic brain stem glioma, and hemangioma. Non-neoplastic lesions that may appear here include aneurysms arising from the vertebrobasilar arteries, arachnoid cysts, and lipomas. On imaging, small vestibular schwannomas are usually isolated to the internal auditory canal (IAC), isointense to brain parenchyma, and homogeneously enhanced. Contrast-enhanced MR is commonly necessary to detect them. However, larger tumors are usually heterogeneous due to the development of cystic and/or necrotic areas, and they cause expansion of the porous acusticus (the opening of the IAC) (Fig. 46-6). Eighty-five percent of vestibular schwannomas involve the IAC. In contrast, meningiomas rarely involve the IAC (5%), they usually enhance homogeneously, and there is usually associated dural enhancement. It is important for the radiologist to try to distinguish schwannoma from meningioma because this can affect the surgical approach in resecting these lesions.

Figure 46-6. Left IAC vestibular schwannoma. Axial contrast-enhanced T1-weighted MR image demonstrates the mass *(arrow)* in the left cerebellopontine angle cistern with a characteristic ice cream cone appearance, with enhancement extending into the left IAC.

24. **What is the most common clinical presentation of a vestibular schwannoma?**
Unilateral sensorineural hearing loss. Adult patients with unilateral sensorineural hearing loss should be evaluated with enhanced MRI. Conductive hearing loss is usually evaluated with temporal bone CT to assess for an abnormality of the ossicles and middle ear. In children, temporal bone CT is commonly the first imaging modality used to assess both sensorineural and conductive hearing loss, since the sensorineural hearing loss in pediatric patients is often related to congenital malformations easily detected on CT.

25. **Define transtentorial herniation.**
To understand this, one must appreciate important central anatomy. The medial temporal lobes (uncus, hippocampus) overhang the tentorium; the brain stem passes through the tentorial hiatus; the posterior cerebral arteries course around the brain stem and medial to the temporal lobes; and the third cranial nerves originate from the midbrain, crossing the interpeduncular cistern below the posterior cerebral arteries and medial to the medial lobes. Transtentorial herniation is caused by a mass effect with a vector force that is directed inferiorly and medially. The temporal lobe shifts over the tentorium, resulting in compression of the third nerve (leading to

ipsilateral papillary dilation), posterior cerebral arteries, and midbrain. Compression of the contralateral cerebral peduncle against the tentorium produces ipsilateral motor weakness, referred to as the "Kernohan-Woltman notch" phenomenon (false localizing sign).

26. **What is the most common posterior fossa/infratentorial mass in adults?**
    The most common infratentorial neoplasm in adults is a metastasis. A metastasis appears as a well-defined, enhancing mass at the gray-white junction and may have surrounding vasogenic edema. The most common primary posterior fossa tumor in adults is a hemangioblastoma. The typical imaging findings of hemangioblastoma are that of a cystic mass with an enhancing mural nodule (Fig. 46-7). The mural nodule is highly vascular. However, solidly enhancing hemangioblastomas can also be seen. Multiple hemangioblastomas are associated with von Hippel-Lindau disease.

Figure 46-7. *A,* Hemangioblastoma. Sagittal unenhanced T1-weighted MR image demonstrates a superficial mass in the superior cerebellar vermis *(arrow).* Note the multiple flow voids (black blood in vessels) within this lesion that are compatible with hypervascularity. Also note the cerebellar tonsils herniated into the foramen magnum due to mass effect. *B,* Axial gadolinium-enhanced T1-weighted MR image shows an enhancing cystic mass in the cerebellar vermis.

27. **What are the three parts of the anterior lobe of the pituitary gland?**
    The pituitary gland is composed of two physiologically and anatomically distinct lobes (anterior and posterior). The anterior lobe, or adenohypophysis, represents 75% of the volume of the gland and is divided into the pars tuberalis, pars intermedia, and the pars distalis. The posterior lobe, or neurohypophysis, is composed of the posterior pituitary lobe, the infundibular stalk, and median eminence of the hypothalamus. Microadenomas are the most common intrasellar neoplasm in adults. Microadenomas are defined as neoplasms that are 10 mm or smaller. They are hypointense relative to the pituitary gland on unenhanced and enhanced T1-weighted imaging (Fig. 46-8, *A*). Autopsy series indicate that small, incidental lesions of the pituitary gland are common. Therefore, clinical correlation is critical so insignificant lesions (e.g., cysts) are not treated. In about 75% of cases, microadenomas have associated hormonal abnormalities. Macroadenomas are larger than 10 mm, enlarge the sella turcica, and commonly spread outside of the sella into the suprasellar cistern or cavernous sinus. As a result, they often present with visual symptoms (classically, bitemporal hemianopsia) related to compression of the optic chiasm and prechiasmatic optic nerves (Fig. 46-8, *B*), headache, and other cranial nerve palsies.

Figure 46-8. *A,* Pituitary microadenoma. Enhanced T1-weighted coronal image through the sella turcica demonstrates a small, round lesion in the right lateral aspect of the pituitary gland *(arrow)* that demonstrates differential decreased enhancement compared with the normal gland. *B,* Pituitary macroadenoma. Coronal unenhanced T1-weighted MR image demonstrates a large mass emanating from the pituitary gland, with extension into the left cavernous sinus and encasement of the left cavernous internal carotid artery *(arrow)*. There is also a hemorrhagic component of the mass invading the left temporal lobe *(white arrow)*.

28. **What are the newer imaging techniques to help diagnose brain tumors?**
    These include MR spectroscopy, perfusion MRI, and diffusion MRI. Functional MRI is used for preoperative localization of eloquent brain cortex before surgery.

29. **Pineal region masses are associated with what visual disturbance?**
    The clinical manifestations of pineal region masses are dependent on their size and location near critical anatomic structures: the aqueduct of Sylvius, the tectal plate, and the vein of Galen/internal cerebral veins. Pineal region masses may cause paresis of upward gaze (Parinaud's syndrome) due to compression of the tectal plate or obstructive hydrocephalus due to compression of the aqueduct. Pineal region tumors are categorized into those arising from germ cell origin (60%) and those from pineal cell origin. The majority of these tumors arise from germ cells, are seen in males, and are germinomas. Intrinsic pineal cell tumors (pineocytoma and pineoblastomas) are seen in male and female patients equally. CSF seeding is

Figure 46-9. Pineoblastoma. Sagittal T2-weighted MR image demonstrates a rounded mass *(arrow)* in the region of the pineal gland with mild mass effect on the midbrain. The mass is only minimally hyperintense to gray matter.

not uncommon. Because pineal tumors are commonly hypercellular, they appear hyperdense on unenhanced CT, and they are intermediate in signal intensity on T1- and T2-weighted MR images (Fig. 46-9).

BIBLIOGRAPHY

1. Nelson SJ, McKnight TR, Henry RG: Characterization of untreated gliomas by magnetic resonance spectroscopic imaging. Neuroimaging Clin North Am 12(4):599–613, 2002.

2. Ricci PE: Imaging of adult brain tumors. Neuroimaging Clin North Am 9(4):651–669, 1999.

3. Smirniotopoulos JG: The new WHO classification of brain tumors. Neuroimaging Clin North Am 9(4):595–613, 1999.

CHAPTER 47

BRAIN: INFLAMMATORY, INFECTIOUS, AND VASCULAR DISEASES

Gul Moonis, MD, and Laurie A. Loevner, MD

1. **How is multiple sclerosis diagnosed?**

   Multiple sclerosis (MS) is the most common of the acquired demyelinating disorders. The disease has a characteristic relapsing-remitting course and usually presents between the third and fifth decades of life with a female predominance. On magnetic resonance imaging (MRI), the demyelinating lesions of MS are ovoid and hyperintense (bright) on T2-weighted images and occur predominantly in the white matter, especially in the periventricular location (usually perpendicular to the ventricular surface) (Fig. 47-1). The corpus callosum, white matter around the temporal horns of the lateral ventricles, and middle cerebellar peduncles are other favored locations of MS plaques. There may be enhancement of the plaques (ring-like or solid) that denotes active disease. Occasionally, MS plaques can be large and masslike (tumefactive MS), in which case differentiation from a tumor may be difficult.

   Figure 47-1. MS in a young patient. Axial flair image demonstrates numerous ovoid, periventricular lesions characteristic of MS plaques. These are oriented along the perivascular spaces, and the appearance has been referred to as "Dawson's fingers."

2. **What is the differential diagnosis of MS based on imaging findings?**

   It is important to recognize that the diagnosis of MS is a clinical one (neurologic symptoms spaced over time and in multiple distributions), with supporting radiologic findings. The diagnosis cannot be made on imaging findings alone because other inflammatory and vascular processes can present with similar imaging findings. White matter lesions similar to MS can be seen with a spectrum of inflammatory conditions, including Lyme disease, sarcoidosis, and vasculitis.

3. **What are the causes of intracranial abscesses?**

   Infectious agents gain access to the central nervous system (CNS) by direct spread from a contiguous focus of infection, such as sinusitis, otitis media, mastoiditis, orbital cellulitis, or dental infection. Infection from these locations may also spread to the intracranial compartment by retrograde venous reflux. Hematogenous spread of infection can also occur from a distant nidus of infection such as the lung. Polymicrobial infection is common with brain abscesses. Four stages have been described in abscess evolution: early cerebritis, late cerebritis, early capsule formation, and late capsule formation. A mature abscess is characterized by a "ring-enhancing" lesion on cross-sectional imaging.

4. **What is the imaging differential diagnosis of a ring-enhancing lesion in the brain?**

    The following disease processes can have an imaging presentation identical to brain abscess: metastatic disease, primary CNS glioma, resolving hematoma, and demyelinating disease. Interpreting the radiologic findings in conjunction with the clinical history is usually very helpful in differentiating among these possible etiologies.

5. **What advanced MRI techniques may be useful in distinguishing brain abscess from neoplasm?**

    Differentiating a subclinical brain abscess from cystic or necrotic tumor with conventional computed tomography (CT) or MRI can be difficult. [1]H-MR spectroscopy and diffusion-weighted MRI can be useful in this regard (Fig. 47-2). Typically, on diffusion-weighted MRI, an abscess is hyperintense (bright).

Figure 47-2. *A,* Frontal lobe abscess secondary to frontal sinusitis. Axial contrast-enhanced T1-weighted MR image demonstrates two ring-enhancing lesions in the left frontal lobe *(arrow)* and enhancing soft tissue within and anterior to the frontal sinus. *B,* On the corresponding diffusion-weighted image, there is restricted diffusion (high signal intensity) within these lesions that is compatible with abscesses.

6. **What anatomic location in the brain is preferentially involved by herpes simplex encephalitis?**

    In adults, the type 1 herpes simplex virus is responsible for fulminant, necrotizing encephalitis. The virus preferentially involves the temporal lobes, but involvement of the frontal lobes (especially the cingulate gyrus) is not uncommon. Often, there is bilateral temporal lobe involvement, though this is usually asymmetric. On MRI, there is T2-weighted hyperintensity in the temporal and frontal lobes with enhancement (Fig. 47-3). Clinically, the patient presents with acute confusion, disorientation, and/or seizures progressing to stupor and coma. The majority of cases are a result of reactivation of dormant virus in the trigeminal ganglion. There is commonly asymmetric temporal lobe involvement. Hemorrhage in the affected area is not uncommon.

Figure 47-3. *A,* Herpes simplex encephalitis. Axial flair MR image shows abnormal T2 hyperintensity in the left medial temporal lobe involving gray and white matter. *B,* Axial enhanced T1-weighted MR image shows mild patchy enhancement *(arrow)* that is consistent with cerebritis.

7. **What is the differential diagnosis of an intracranial mass in a patient with HIV infection?**

It is crucial to determine whether the cause of an HIV-related brain mass is neoplastic or infectious because these entities are managed in very different ways. Among infectious etiologies, toxoplasmosis and brain abscesses secondary to fungal or bacterial etiologies have to be considered. The major neoplastic consideration is primary CNS lymphoma. Toxoplasmosis is the leading cause of focal CNS disease in AIDS and results from infection by the intracellular parasite *Toxoplasma gondii.* It is usually caused by reactivation of old CNS lesions or by hematogenous spread of a previously acquired infection. On imaging, single or multiple ring-enhancing lesions in the white matter and/or basal ganglia with mass effect may be observed. A single lesion favors the diagnosis of lymphoma over that of toxoplasmosis (Fig. 47-4). Occasionally, progressive multifocal leukoencephalopathy (PML), a demyelinating disease caused by a viral infection, may result in ring-enhancing lesions. PML is caused by a virus that infects the oligodendrocytes in immunocompromised patients.

Figure 47-4. *A,* Toxoplasmosis in an HIV-positive patient. Axial flair MR image demonstrates extensive signal abnormality involving the left basal ganglia and adjacent frontal and temporal lobes with mass effect.

(Continued)

8. **What is a stroke?**
   A stroke occurs when the blood supply to a vascular territory of the brain is suddenly interrupted (ischemic stroke) or when a blood vessel in the brain ruptures, spilling blood into the spaces surrounding the brain cells (hemorrhagic stroke). Ischemic stroke is the most common form of stroke, responsible for approximately 80% of vascular accidents. In adults, these blockages are usually associated with two conditions: atherosclerosis-related occlusion of vessels (60%) and cardiac embolism (20%).

9. **What are the common causes of stroke that one must consider in children and young adults?**
   Only 3% of cerebral infarctions occur in patients younger than 40 years old. The most common causes of stroke in the young are cardiac disease, hematologic diseases (hypercoagulable states), and vascular dissection (from trauma or disease of the vessel wall). Other causes include CNS vasculitis, fibromuscular dysplasia, or venous sinus thrombosis.

10. **What are the imaging manifestations of ischemic stroke in the acute stage?**
    Commonly, in the acute setting, a CT of the head may be normal! The earliest signs (within 6 hours) of an acute infarct on CT are loss of the gray-white differentiation with obscuration of the lateral lentiform nucleus. There may be a high density noted in the proximal middle cerebral artery, representing acute thrombus or calcified embolus. This is referred to as the "hyperdense artery sign" (Fig. 47-5, *A*). Within 12–24 hours, there will be low density in the appropriate vascular distribution, with increasing mass effect. Mass effect peaks between 3–5 days. Findings of acute ischemia are detected earlier on MRI. With the use of diffusion-weighted imaging, acute ischemic changes can be seen within minutes of onset of the ictus. High signal intensity is noted within the involved vascular territory on T2-weighted images, with characteristic restricted diffusion (also hyperintense) on diffusion-weighted images (Fig. 47-5, *B* and *C*). Swelling of the involved cortex and arterial enhancement are noted early in the time course.

Figure 47-4, *Cont'd.* *B*, Axial enhanced T1-weighted MR image at the same axial level as Fig. 47-4, *A*, shows a rim-enhancing lesion in the center of the left basal ganglia *(arrow)* abnormality with extensive surrounding edema and midline shift from left to right.

Figure 47-5. Hyperdense middle cerebral artery consistent with acute thrombus or calcified embolus. Axial unenhanced CT of the head *(A)* demonstrates hyperdensity in the left middle cerebral artery *(arrow)* that is compatible with acute thrombus.

(Continued)

Figure 47-5, *Cont'd.* Corresponding axial flair *(B)* and diffusion-weighted *(C)* MR images demonstrate diffuse hyperintensity involving gray and white matter in the left middle cerebral artery territory, which is characteristic of stroke. The hyperintensity on the diffusion-weighted image represents restricted diffusion, which is compatible with acute ischemia.

11. **How can one differentiate acute from chronic stroke on imaging?**
Chronic stroke is manifested by encephalomalacic change in the involved vascular territory with accompanying dilation of the sulci and cisterns. There is also ex vacuo dilation of the ipsilateral ventricle. There is absence of mass effect. Again, if it is difficult to distinguish the age of a stroke on CT, MRI that includes a diffusion-weighted sequence can be invaluable.

12. **What are watershed infarctions?**
Also known as "border zone infarcts," these occur in the vascular watersheds (the most distal arterial territory with connection between the major arterial branches). In severe hypotension/shock the systemic blood pressure is not sufficient to pump arterial blood to the end arteries. In the cerebrum, not enough blood gets to the "watershed zones" between the anterior and middle cerebral arteries, or the middle and posterior cerebral artery territories, respectively, and in those areas infarcts are likely to develop. Some other causes of cerebral watershed infarcts include heart failure, decreased systemic perfusion pressure, and low blood pressure in the setting of a high-grade stenosis of a major artery (internal carotid) supplying the brain.

13. **What are lacunar infarctions?**
These are small infarcts caused by occlusion/disease of the perforating arteries (arteriolar lipohyalinosis). Initially these are slightly hypodense on CT. By 4 weeks, sharply circumscribed, cystic lesions develop. These are most commonly seen in the deep gray matter (basal ganglia, thalami), brain stem, internal capsule, and corona radiata. These small infarctions are usually 1 cm or smaller.

14. **What are the risk factors for venous sinus thrombosis and venous infarction?**
Venous sinus thrombosis is associated with many systemic conditions, including acute dehydration, hypercoagulable states, chemotherapeutic agents (L-asparaginase), sinusitis and mastoiditis, hematologic malignancies, pregnancy, and trauma. Unenhanced CT reveals the presence of high density and enlargement of the dural venous sinuses. The "empty delta sign," which refers to enhancement around the clot in a dural venous sinus, may also be present

(Fig. 47-6, *A*). The diagnosis of venous thrombosis is improved significantly with MRI. On unenhanced T1-weighted images, high signal intensity clot is noted within the venous sinuses (Fig. 47-6, *B*). There may be associated venous infarction. Venous infarctions have a high rate of hemorrhagic transformation compared with arterial infarctions.

Figure 47-6. *A,* Venous sinus thrombosis. Axial contrast-enhanced T1-weighted MR image demonstrates acute clot in the superior sagittal sinus *(arrow).* Note the characteristic "empty delta" sign *(arrow)* that represents nonenhancing clot within the superior sagittal sinus. *B,* Sagittal unenhanced T1-weighted MR image taken in the midline shows relative high signal intensity in the superior sagittal sinus *(arrows),* which is consistent with acute thrombosis.

15. **What is the most common cause for nontraumatic subarachnoid hemorrhage (SAH)?**
    An aneurysm rupture. An aneurysm is a focal dilation of an artery, most commonly encountered at branching points in the intracranial vasculature. Aneurysms are usually due to a congenital weakness in the media and elastica of the arterial wall but can be acquired in the setting of trauma or mycotic infections. The approximate relative frequency of aneurysm formation in the intracranial vasculature is as follows: anterior communicating artery (30%), distal internal carotid artery (ICA) and posterior communicating artery (30%), middle cerebral artery (25–30%), and the posterior vertebral-basilar circulation (10–15%). Multiple aneurysms are seen in approximately 15% of cases. There is increased incidence of intracranial aneurysms in patients with polycystic kidney disease, Marfan syndrome, and fibromuscular dysplasia (as well as other rarer entities, including moyamoya disease, Ehlers-Danlos syndrome, and Takayasu's arteritis).

16. **What is the work-up of a patient presenting with SAH?**
    If the patient presents with the classic history of "the worst headache of my life," a CT scan should be obtained to look for SAH. If the results of the CT scan are negative but there is high clinical suspicion for SAH, a spinal tap should be performed to look for red blood cells and/or xanthochromia in the cerebrospinal fluid (CSF). If CSF analysis is positive for subarachnoid blood, then a diagnostic conventional catheter angiogram is the next step to find the aneurysm, providing an anatomic road map for the neurosurgeon. Increasingly, CT angiography is being used rather than conventional catheter angiography for aneurysm detection.

17. **If there are multiple aneurysms seen on catheter angiography in a patient with SAH, which one most likely bled?**

If multiple aneurysms are identified, greater suspicion falls on the aneurysm that is the largest in size, on the aneurysm with a lobulated contour (nipple sign), or on the one closest to the largest clot on CT. Extravasation of contrast from the aneurysm is rarely seen but is diagnostic.

18. **What are common locations for hypertensive intraparenchymal hemorrhages?**

In adults who present with nontraumatic intraparenchymal hemorrhage in the brain, hypertension is the most common etiologic factor. The arteries in the brain injured by exposure to chronic hypertension typically are the perforating arteries, which supply the basal ganglia, thalami, and pons (Fig. 47-7). Other areas that may also be affected by hypertensive bleeds include the centrum semiovale and, occasionally, the cerebellum.

19. **What is amyloid angiopathy?**

Amyloid angiopathy results from deposition of amyloid in the media and adventitia of small and medium-sized vessels of the superficial layers of the cortex and leptomeninges. Amyloid deposition increases with age. Pathologically, there is loss of elasticity and increased fragility of the vessels that cause hemorrhages that are usually lobar and most often in the frontal and parietal lobes. These parenchymal hemorrhages may be associated with subdural and subarachnoid hemorrhage. The usual course is multiple hemorrhagic incidents spaced over time.

Figure 47-7. Left thalamic hypertensive hemorrhage. Axial unenhanced CT of the head demonstrates a large focus of hemorrhage centered in the left thalamus *(arrow)* with extension into the ventricular system and hydrocephalus.

20. **Review the MR signal characteristics of intracranial hemorrhage.**

See Table 47-1.

21. **What are the imaging features of cerebral hypoxia/anoxia?**

Hypoxia refers to a lack of oxygen supply to the cerebral hemispheres. This can have a multifactorial etiology, including drowning, asphyxiation from smoke inhalation, severe hypotension, strangulation, perinatal hypoxic insult, cardiac arrest, and carbon monoxide poisoning. On MRI, there is increased T2 signal in the perirolandic and occipital cortex as well as the basal ganglia (Fig. 47-8). Additionally, the watershed zones between major vascular territories and the hippocampi are also prone to hypoxic/ischemic damage. Layers three, four, and five of the cortex are sensitive to global ischemia/hypoxia and may become necrotic and hemorrhagic (laminar necrosis).

TABLE 47-1.   MR SIGNAL CHARACTERISTICS OF INTRACRANIAL HEMORRHAGE

	Age	T1-Weighted	T2-Weighted
Hyperacute	Hours old, mainly oxyhemoglobin with surrounding edema	Hypointense	Hyperintense
Acute	Days old, mainly deoxyhemoglobin with surrounding edema	Hypointense	Hypointense, surrounded by hyperintense margin
Subacute	Weeks old, mainly methemoglobin	Hyperintense	Hypointense, early subacute with predominantly intracellular methemoglobin Hyperintense, late subacute with predominantly extracellular methemoglobin
Chronic	Years old, hemosiderin slit or hemosiderin margin surrounding fluid cavity	Hypointense	Hypointense slit or hypointense margin surrounding hyperintense fluid cavity

Figure 47-8. Hypoxic injury in a patient who was found in respiratory arrest. Axial flair *(A)* and diffusion-weighted *(B)* MR images demonstrate abnormal hyperintensity in the bilateral caudate heads and the right putamen *(arrows)*. The diffusion hyperintensity is consistent with acute hypoxic/ischemic injury.

BIBLIOGRAPHY

1. Falcone S, Post MJ: Encephalitis, cerebritis, and brain abscess: Pathophysiology and imaging findings. Neuroimaging Clin North Am 10(2):333–353, 2000.

2. Gaskill-Shipley MF: Routine CT evaluation of acute stroke. Neuroimaging Clin North Am 9(3):411–422, 1999.

3. Lee SK, Brugge KG: Cerebral venous thrombosis in adults: The role of imaging evaluation and management. Neuroimaging Clin North Am 13(1):139–152, 2003.

4. Yoshiura T, Wu O, Sorensen AG: Advanced MR techniques: Diffusion MR imaging, perfusion MR imaging, and spectroscopy. Neuroimaging Clin North Am 9(3):439–453, 1999.

CHAPTER 48

ADVANCED IMAGING OF THE SPINE

Linda J. Bagley, MD, and Laurie A. Loevner, MD

1. **Identify parts of the spine labeled in Figure 48-1.**
   See the figure legend for the answers.

2. **What imaging modalities are most often used in the evaluation of spine pathology?**
   Plain films, computed tomography (CT), magnetic resonance imaging (MRI), myelography, discography, and angiography have roles in spinal imaging.

3. **Describe the strengths, weaknesses, and most appropriate uses of CT in spinal imaging.**
   Plain films are often the initial imaging study of the spine. Pathologic conditions of the osseous spine, including fractures, degenerative changes, tumors, infections and congenital anomalies (including transitional vertebrae), may be detected with plain films.

   However, multidetector CT provides superior evaluation of the bony anatomy and pathologic conditions. Images may be rapidly acquired and reconstructed at narrow intervals (1 mm) with edge enhancing algorithms. Multiplanar, three-dimensional images can subsequently be created. In the setting of acute spinal trauma, CT has been shown to be more time efficient and significantly more sensitive than plain films for fracture detection. CT, unlike plain films, also allows excellent evaluation of retropulsed

Figure 48-1. *A,* Axial T1-weighted MR image of a normal vertebra. *B,* Sagittal T2-weighted MR image of the spine. (A = Vertebral body, B = pedicle, C = lamina, D = facet joint, E = disc, F = spinal cord, G = conus medullaris, H = nerve root.)

bone into the spinal canal. As a result, CT is often used to image traumatic and nontraumatic osseous spinal pathologic conditions. The major drawback of CT is its limited contrast resolution of the soft tissues within the spinal canal, including the spinal cord, nerve roots, epidural compartment, and subdural compartment.

4. **Describe the strengths and drawbacks of MRI.**
   MRI provides the best and most direct evaluation of the contents within the spinal canal, including the spinal cord, nerve roots, and epidural, as well as the subdural compartments. Additionally, it provides the most detailed evaluation of the soft tissues, including the intervertebral discs, ligaments, and musculature. Optimal resolution is obtained at high-field strengths using phased array surface coils. A number of safety concerns arise, however, with the use of MRI. Many implantable devices, such as pacemakers, are not MR compatible, and patients must be appropriately screened. Ferromagnetic objects may become projectiles within the magnetic field and injure patients and/or health care providers. When MRI is performed in critically ill patients, MR-compatible ventilators and monitoring devices must be used. When patients with spinal cord injuries are imaged, spinal precautions must be maintained, and fixation devices must be MR compatible. MRI of patients with prior spinal surgery is often of limited diagnostic value due to artifacts arising from metallic hardware. MRI is also relatively time-consuming and requires patient cooperation (remaining motionless) to obtain high-quality studies.

5. **In patients with contraindications to MRI, what radiologic study may be used to assess the contents within the spinal canal?**
   In patients with suspected spinal cord or nerve root compression who cannot be evaluated with MRI, myelography is an alternative, but somewhat invasive, technique that may be used to evaluate the spinal canal contents. Myelography is most often performed in patients with contraindications to MRI or nondiagnostic MR studies. Nonionic contrast material is instilled into the subarachnoid space of the spinal canal, typically via lumbar puncture. Risks of this procedure are relatively low but include headache, allergic contrast reaction, infection, hematoma, neural damage, and seizure. The contrast material in the subarachnoid space will outline the spinal cord and nerve roots.

   Figure 48-2. Anteroposterior plain film from a lumbar myelogram demonstrates an extra-dural impression on the thecal sac at L4-L5 *(arrows)* with decreased opacification of the L4 nerve root sleeve.

   Impressions on the contrast column and/or displacement of neural structures are findings indicative of a pathologic condition (Fig. 48-2). Myelography is often complemented with cross-sectional CT scanning, performed after the myelogram is obtained to better distinguish the anatomy and pathologic condition in the spinal canal.

6. **What is discography? When is it used?**
   Discography involves the injection of contrast material into the nucleus of the intervertebral disc, usually followed by CT scanning of the injected disc. This test is usually performed in patients with multilevel disc disease and/or axial back pain in an attempt to reproduce the patient's symptoms and thereby identify the "culprit" disc. Patterns of contrast diffusion may suggest annular degeneration and/or frank tears, but imaging findings must be correlated with patient symptomatology.

7. **What is the primary role of catheter angiography of the spine?**
   Conventional spinal catheter angiography is primarily used for the detection, characterization, and possible endovascular treatment of spinal vascular malformations.

KEY POINTS: SPINE IMAGING MODALITIES ✔

1. Spine plain films are used to evaluate for fractures, degenerative changes, and alignment.

2. CT is used to evaluate for osseous pathologic conditions, especially fractures.

3. MR is the best modality for imaging the spinal cord, bone marrow, and epidural/subdural spaces.

4. Myelography is reserved largely for symptomatic patients who cannot undergo MR examination.

5. Spinal catheter angiography is used primarily for spinal vascular malformations.

8. **What is spinal dysraphia?**

Spinal anomalies with incomplete midline closure of mesenchymal, osseous, and neural structures are grouped under the term *spinal dysraphia*. Most defects occur in the lumbosacral region.

9. **Differentiate open and occult forms of spinal dysraphia.**

Myeloceles and myelomeningoceles are two types of open dysraphic anomalies. Neural tissue (the neural placode, with or without associated meninges) protrudes through the spinal canal and soft tissue defects. Associated abnormalities include Chiari II malformation, hydrocephalus, syringohydromyelia, spinal lipomas, dermoid and epidermoid inclusion cysts, agenesis of the corpus callosum, diastematomyelia, and abnormal spinal curvature. In the occult form of dysraphia, the defects are covered by skin, and no neural tissue is exposed. Occult dysraphias include meningoceles, dorsal dermal sinuses (epithelial lined tubes connecting the spinal cord and the skin), and fat-containing lesions (lipomyelomeningoceles, filum terminale lipomas, and intradural lipomas) (Fig. 48-3). Midline cutaneous stigmata (dimples, nevi, and hairy patches) are often present.

Figure 48-3. Sagittal T1-weighted *(A)* and axial T1-weighted *(B)* MR images demonstrate a large defect in the posterior elements of the sacrum. A lipomyelomeningocele protrudes through the defect *(arrows)*. The spinal cord is tethered to the predominantly fatty mass.

10. **What are the clinical findings and imaging features of a tethered spinal cord?**
    The conus medullaris normally terminates at approximately the L1–L2 level. With a tethered spinal cord/thick filum terminale syndrome, the conus medullaris is identified at L2 or below, and the filum terminale is greater than 2 mm in thickness. Associated anomalies (lipomas, diastematomyelia, and myelomeningocele) are common. Patients typically present in childhood or young adulthood with pain, dysthesias, bowel and/or bladder dysfunction, spasticity, and/or kyphoscoliosis.

11. **List and describe caudal spinal anomalies.**
    Caudal spinal anomalies are malformations of the distal spine, spinal cord, and meninges associated with disorders of the hindgut, kidneys, urinary bladder, and genitalia. Caudal spinal anomalies include:
    - *Caudal regression syndrome:* varying degrees of lumbosacral agenesis with renal and anogenital anomalies and possible fusion of the lower extremities
    - *Terminal myelocystocele:* cystic dilation of the distal spinal cord, which is tethered; associated with partial sacral agenesis or spina bifida
    - *Anterior sacral meningocele:* cerebrospinal fluid (CSF)–filled sac that protrudes into the pelvis anterior to the sacrum
    - *Occult intrasacral meningocele:* mild dural developmental anomaly with associated remodeling of the sacrum
    - *Sacrococcygeal teratoma:* most common presacral mass in children; contains tissue from all three germ layers (endoderm, mesoderm, and ectoderm) and is often cystic and solid

12. **What are the split notochord syndromes?**
    Persistent midline adhesions between endoderm and ectoderm can result in splitting of the notochord. With this split, paired hemicords (diastematomyelia) may result. Persistent endodermal-ectodermal adhesions/communications may produce dorsal enteric fistulas and neuroenteric cysts.
    - *Diastematomyelia* predominantly occurs in female patients. In 85% of cases, the split occurs between T9 and S1. The cord is split by a fibrous, osseous, or osteocartilaginous septum, and the hemicords may or may not share a dural sac. Associated neurologic and orthopedic anomalies are common (Fig. 48-4).
    - *Dorsal enteric fistulas* are very rare and extend from the mesenteric surface of the gut through the prevertebral tissues, vertebrae, and spinal cord to the dorsal skin surface.

Figure 48-4. Diastematomyelia. Coronal reformatted CT scan performed after myelography reveals two spinal cords *(arrows)* within the thecal sac.

    - *Neuroenteric cysts* are most often intradural, extramedullary cystic masses in the thoracic region. Vertebral anomalies are seen in fewer than half of the cases.

13. **What is the most common disorder of the spine affecting adults?**
    Degenerative changes in the spine generally begin to appear in adolescence and are often *asymptomatic*. Degenerative changes occur within the discs; vertebrae; joints; and soft tissues, including the ligaments. Although many degenerative changes are asymptomatic, more than

10 million adults seek medical care, and more than 200,000 operations are performed for back pain each year in the United States.

14. **What are the MRI findings of degenerative disease affecting the spine?**
Degenerative changes within the disc may initially manifest as decreased signal intensity within the disc on T2-weighted MR images, secondary to decreased water content and increased fibro-cartilaginous tissue. Discs may lose height. Annular fissures and frank tears may occur. Diffuse disc bulges, focal disc protrusions, and free disc fragments may be seen. The advantage of MRI over plain film radiographs is that the relationship between the degenerative disc and the contents (neural tissue) within the spinal canal can be seen.

Osseous degeneration may take the form of osteophytes, end-plate changes that include stages of edema, fatty replacement, and eventually sclerosis, which are readily distinguished with MRI. Facet and uncovertebral joint degenerative change may manifest with osteophytes, synovial proliferation, and/or synovial cyst formation. The ligamentum flavum may hypertrophy, and epidural lipomatosis may contribute to spinal stenosis.

Degenerative changes may combine to produce central canal, lateral recess, and/or foraminal stenosis with possible resultant spinal cord or nerve root compression.

15. **What are the most common lumbar and cervical spine levels to be affected by degenerative disease?**
Approximately 90% of lumbar disc extensions beyond the vertebral body end plate occur at L4–L5 or L5–S1, with approximately 7% occurring at L3–L4 and 3% at L1–L2 and L2–L3. The majority of cervical disc extensions beyond the end plate (90%) occur at C5–C6 or C6–C7. Even though spondylotic changes are quite common in the thoracic spine, thoracic disc extensions beyond the end plate are seen less commonly than cervical or lumbar disc abnormalities.

16. **What is the natural history of most disc extensions beyond the vertebral body end plate?**
Again, most discogenic disease is asymptomatic. In one study, 64% of normal volunteers demonstrated some abnormality of the lumbar spine on MRI. Furthermore, symptoms related to most disc abnormalities improve with conservative therapy (bed rest, anti-inflammatory and pain medication): 90% will decrease in size, and clinical symptoms will improve in 75% of cases.

17. **What is Baastrup's disease?**
Apparent enlargement and flattening of the spinous process, particularly in the lumbar spine, which may be secondary to excessive lordosis resulting in close contact of the spinous processes and subsequent sclerosis of the spinous processes and degeneration of the inter-spinous ligaments. This may cause pain and tenderness and is seen well on radiographs or MRI (Fig. 48-5).

18. **How can residual/recurrent disc abnormalities be differentiated from scar tissue?**
Scar/granulation tissue and residual/recurrent disc abnormalities often appear as soft tissue adjacent to the disc space, within the lateral recess, and/or within the neural foramen. This soft tissue may be inseparable from the nerve roots. Contrast-enhanced CT and unenhanced MRI are approximately 80% accurate in differentiating these entities. Contrast-enhanced MRI, however, is the most reliable modality for this task, with reported accuracy of approximately 95%. Disc abnormalities are typically of lower signal intensity than scar material on T2-weighted images. Scar and granulation tissue will enhance with gadolinium administration; disc material generally will not. At times, residual/recurrent disc abnormalities and scar tissue may coexist (Fig. 48-6). In the postoperative patient, enhancement may commonly be seen (and is not necessarily

Figure 48-5. Baastrup's disease. Sagittal T1-weighted *(A)* and sagittal fat-saturated T2-weighted *(B)* images demonstrate enlargement and flattening of the spinous processes. Because of the close contact of the spinous processes, there is bony sclerosis and marrow edema of the affected levels *(arrows).*

indicative of a pathologic condition) in the disc space, vertebral end plates, paraspinal soft tissues, joints, and within nerve roots that were previously compressed.

19. **What is arachnoiditis?**
   This term refers to inflammation of the nerve roots of the cauda equina with adhesion of the nerve roots to each other and/or to the thecal sac. Patients may present with nonspecific back pain and/or paresthesias. The key imaging features of this diagnosis are abnormal morphologic features and distribution of nerve roots, which may or may not enhance. Three imaging patterns have been described. The nerve roots may be centrally clumped, appearing as a "pseudocord" within the thecal sac. Alternatively, the nerve roots may be adherent to the periphery of the thecal sac—"the empty sac" appearance (Fig. 48-7). Uncommonly, the nerve roots may clump together to form a large, mildly enhancing mass, which fills the thecal sac.

20. **Review the epidemiologic factors of spinal trauma.**
   Approximately 30,000 injuries to the spinal column occur in the United States each year. Most injuries are secondary to blunt trauma, and penetrating trauma accounts for approximately 10–20% of cases.

Figure 48-6. *A,* Axial unenhanced T1-weighted MR image demonstrates a large amount of soft tissue contiguous with the disc space, extending to the left lateral recess and surrounding the S1 nerve root *(arrow).*

(Continued)

Roughly 2–3% of blunt trauma victims are affected, with a higher incidence of spinal injuries seen in those with significant craniofacial trauma. Approximately 40–50% of spinal injuries produce a neurologic deficit—often severe and sometimes fatal. Survival is inversely correlated with patient age. Mortality during initial hospitalization is about 10%. Because most spinal trauma patients are young, the costs of lifetime care and rehabilitation are extremely high, often exceeding $1 million per individual.

Figure 48-6, *Cont'd.* *B,* Gadolinium-enhanced T1-weighted MR image shows that the central tissue does not enhance *(single arrow)* (residual or recurrent disc herniation) but that the peripheral tissue extending into the lateral recess does *(double arrows)* (scar tissue).

21. **What are the appropriate indications for performing cross-sectional imaging of the spine in the setting of blunt trauma?**
    Pain, neurologic deficit, distracting injuries, altered consciousness (due to head injury, intoxication, or pharmaceutical intervention), and high-risk mechanism of injury have been shown to be appropriate clinical indications for spinal imaging.

Figure 48-7. Axial T1-weighted MR image is notable for the displacement of nerve roots along the periphery of the thecal sac—the "empty sac" appearance *(arrow).*

22. **What are the most common mechanisms of cervical spine injury?**
    Hyperflexion, hyperextension, and vertical compression (axial loading).

23. **Name the most common fractures associated with each of these mechanisms of injury.**
    - *Hyperflexion* may cause compression fractures, flexion-teardrop fractures, and spinous process fractures. When associated with posterior ligamentous injury, subluxations and bilateral facet dislocations may result. When hyperflexion occurs with rotation, this mechanism may result in unilateral facet dislocations.
    - *Hyperextension* injuries include extension-teardrop fractures, fractures of the atlas, "hangman's" fractures (through the pars interarticularis of C2) *(see* Fig. 35-2), laminar fractures, and fracture/dislocations. When hyperextension occurs with rotation, pillar fractures and pedicle-laminar separation may result.
    - *Vertical compression* or axial loading injuries (when force is transmitted through the top of the skull through the occipital condyles and vertebral column) result in burst fractures of the vertebral bodies. In the cervical spine, burst fracture of the atlas (C1) is most common.
    - *Lateral flexion* usually occurs in conjunction with vertical compression. Isolated lateral flexion is the typical mechanism of injury resulting in isolated fractures of the uncovertebral joint of the cervical spine.
    - Some injuries, such as odontoid fractures and atlanto-occipital dislocations, result from *complex, often combined* forces.

24. **What is the role of MRI in spinal trauma?**
    Fractures of the spine are best evaluated with thin-section CT with coronal and sagittal reformatted images. Spinal cord injuries and other traumatic sequelae within the spinal canal (e.g., subdural hematoma) are best evaluated with MRI and should be suspected when there are focal neurologic deficits or when neurologic symptoms are disproportionate to the findings detected on plain films and CT scans. Cord contusions are generally manifested as hyperintense, intramedullary lesions on T2-weighted MR images. The cord may be expanded (Fig. 48-8). The presence of hemorrhage within a contusion is associated with a worse prognosis and may alter the signal intensity characteristics of the lesion. MRI may also characterize many compressive lesions, such as epidural and subdural hematomas, disc abnormalities, and osteophytes.

Figure 48-8. Sagittal T2-weighted MR image of the cervical spine reveals abnormal signal intensity within the cord *(arrow)* (cord contusion) associated with kyphotic deformity. Also note increased signal intensity within the disc, suggestive of acute injury, and extensive signal abnormality within the interspinous ligaments and paraspinal soft tissues.

25. **What additional structures may be injured in association with cervical spinal trauma that may not be detected on plain films or CT scans?**
    It is always important to think about ligamentous and arterial (especially vertebral artery) injuries in patients with significant trauma to the cervical spine. If there is subluxation or dislocation involving the cervical spine on plain film radiographs or CT, ligamentous injury must be present. However, in the absence of subluxation/dislocation, ligamentous injuries can be missed. Special MRI sequences such as fat-saturated T2-weighted images usually detect ligamentous injury, including frank disruption and/or edema. MRI and MR angiography may be used to evaluate for associated vascular injuries (dissections, occlusions, pseudoaneurysms) that may accompany spinal trauma. In particular, cervical spine fractures involving a transverse process and/or the foramen transversarium (the osseous canal where the cervical portion of the vertebral artery lives) are at higher risk of vertebral artery injury.

26. **Name the most common sites of infection in the spine.**
    Infections may occur within the vertebra (most commonly the vertebral body [osteomyelitis]), within the disc space (discitis), within the epidural space (abscess), in the meninges (meningitis), and in the paraspinal soft tissues.

27. **What patient populations are particularly prone to the development of infectious spondylodiscitis?**
    Infectious spondylodiscitis most commonly occurs in elderly patients, diabetic patients, and in men more often than women. Other groups particularly susceptible to this disorder include IV drug abusers, dialysis patients, alcoholics, and the immunocompromised.

28. **What is the most common infectious agent responsible for spondylodiscitis?**
    The infecting organism may be bacterial, fungal, or parasitic. The most common cause of discitis is *Staphylococcus aureus*.

29. **What is the typical clinical presentation of discitis?**
    Patients may present with back pain, fever, focal neurologic deficits, an elevated white blood cell count, and/or an elevated erythrocyte sedimentation rate.

30. **What are the typical imaging findings of spondylodiscitis on plain film radiographs and CT?**

On radiographs and CT, disc space narrowing, endplate irregularity/destruction, and demineralization may be apparent (Fig. 48-9). However, these findings commonly occur in the later stages of infection. Spondylodiscitis may be detected earlier with MRI. The finding of increased signal intensity within the intervertebral disc on T2-weighted images in the appropriate clinical setting should raise suspicion. Loss of disc height with endplate irregularity/destruction and abnormal signal intensity in the vertebral bone consistent with edema and/or osteomyelitis can be late imaging findings. Paravertebral soft tissue swelling and/or fluid collections/abscesses may be present. Typically, enhancement is seen within the marrow and disc space. Epidural phlegmons may demonstrate solid enhancement, and the presence of peripheral or "rim-enhancement" is usually indicative of abscess formation.

Figure 48-9. Sagittal reformatted CT scan of the cervical spine demonstrates multilevel, severe endplate destruction and sclerosis; marked disc space narrowing; and prevertebral soft tissue swelling secondary to discitis and osteomyelitis. Changes are most pronounced at C5–C6 *(arrows)*.

31. **Describe the imaging appearance of spondylodiscitis caused by atypical organisms, such as tuberculosis.**

With granulomatous infections, such as tuberculosis, as well as fungal infections, there may be relative sparing of the disc space and endplates until late in the infection. Earlier involvement of the vertebral bodies is common. Tuberculosis is typically associated with anterior subligamentous involvement, resulting in infection of multiple, contiguous levels of the spine.

32. **Which noninfectious disorders can have imaging findings similar to those of infectious spondylodiscitis?**
   - Degenerative disease/instability
   - Neuropathic arthropathy
   - Dialysis-related arthropathy (amyloid deposition)
   - Postoperative changes
   - Richter's syndrome (lymphomatous transformation of chronic lymphocytic leukemia)

33. **What is the most common inflammatory disorder that affects the spinal cord?**

Multiple sclerosis. Patients typically have symptoms of numbness, weakness, and/or urinary incontinence that wax and wane. Other inflammatory conditions that involve the spinal cord include systemic lupus erythematosus (SLE), acute disseminated encephalomyelitis (ADEM) and other autoimmune disorders, sarcoidosis, and infections such as syphilis and HIV. A variety of other viral, bacterial, fungal, and parasitic organisms can infect the spinal cord.

34. **What are the classic imaging findings of multiple sclerosis that affect the spinal cord?**

The imaging findings of inflammatory disorders are often nonspecific. All of these processes produce intramedullary lesions that are hyperintense on T2-weighted images (Fig. 48-10). These lesions sometimes enhance and may be associated with cord expansion. More specific diagnoses are often made through correlation of imaging findings with clinical and laboratory data.

The spinal cord is commonly involved in patients with multiple sclerosis. The lesions of multiple sclerosis are often ill-defined, multiple, and located in the dorsolateral white matter of the cord (they are commonly small, but some lesions may extend over several spinal segments). In the active phase of demyelination, the plaques may expand the cord and typically enhance. Chronic lesions lead to focal or generalized cord atrophy.

The imaging findings of Behçet's syndrome are similar to those of multiple sclerosis. With autoimmune diseases—including SLE, viral infection, postviral and postvaccination syndromes (including ADEM), and paraneoplastic disorders—focal cord signal abnormality, sometimes associated with cord expansion and enhancement, is often present.

Figure 48-10. Sagittal T2-weighted MR image reveals a long segment of hyperintensity within the thoracic cord secondary to demyelinating disease *(arrow)*.

35. **What is the typical MRI appearance of sarcoidosis? How can its appearance, combined with the clinical history, distinguish it from other inflammatory disorders?**
Extensive leptomeningeal enhancement on the surface of the spinal cord. In sarcoidosis, a long segment of the cord may be expanded with abnormal signal intensity. With sarcoid, unlike many of the other inflammatory conditions, there typically is pronounced enhancement of the leptomeninges on the surface of the cord. Foci of intramedullary enhancement may also be present.

36. **What is the typical time course for the development of radiation myelitis after irradiation for treatment of tumor?**
Radiation myelitis generally presents within 6 months to 3 years after treatment. It will occur within the treatment portal, and the marrow of the vertebrae within the port will typically be fatty replaced. On MRI, the cord usually has T2-weighted hyperintensity, is expanded, and may enhance.

37. **What portion of the spinal cord is typically involved with syphilis?**
Syphilis has a predilection for the dorsal columns of the spinal cord. With syphilitic infection, enhancement may be seen along the pial surface of the cord and nerve roots. A vasculitis may accompany the infection and lead to cord infarctions. Vacuolar myelopathy occurs in approximately 15–30% of patients with AIDS and more commonly affects the posterolateral cord. Pathologically, vacuoles and lipid-laden macrophages are seen in the white matter.

38. **Name the two most common vascular disorders of the spinal cord.**
   - Spinal cord infarcts
   - Vascular malformations

39. **What is the arterial vascular supply to the spinal cord?**
The anterior spinal artery is the main arterial supply to the spinal cord. Additional supply is through paired posterior spinal arteries. The anterior spinal artery is located in the midline. In the cervical and upper thoracic cord, contributions to the anterior spinal artery are from the ver-

tebral, cervical, and superior intercostal arteries. A small component of supply to the mid-thoracic cord arises from the mid-thoracic intercostal arteries. The predominant contribution to the anterior spinal artery in the lower thoracic and lumbar regions (otherwise known as the artery of Adamkiewicz) is most often from thoracic intercostal or lumbar arteries, usually on the left (Fig. 48-11).

Figure 48-11. Anteroposterior plain film radiograph from a spinal angiogram demonstrates the anterior spinal artery *(arrow)* making its classic "hairpin" turn.

40. **What are the typical clinical characteristics and imaging findings of spinal cord infarcts?**
Spinal cord infarcts most often occur in elderly patients with atherosclerotic vascular disease. Patients undergoing thoracoabdominal aneurysm repair are particularly at risk. Lower thoracic intercostal or upper lumbar arteries are often sacrificed with aneurysm repair procedures, thereby jeopardizing the artery of Adamkiewicz. Patients experience sudden onset of paraplegia, often associated with pain. On MRI, signal abnormality is seen within the central gray matter (Fig. 48-12).

Figure 48-12. Axial T2-weighted MR image demonstrates central hyperintensity of the spinal cord due to infarct *(single arrow)* and also reveals aneurysmal dilation of the aorta *(double arrows)*.

41. **List the four types of spinal vascular malformations, and describe their clinical and imaging characteristics.**
   - *Dural arteriovenous malformations* are the most common of the spinal vascular anomalies seen in adults. They typically affect middle-aged and older men, who present with chronic,

progressive motor and sensory deficits, usually in the lower extremities. Bowel, bladder, and sexual dysfunction also often occur. These are acquired lesions, most often occurring in the lower thoracic and upper lumbar spine. Arterial supply is from the dural arteries. MRI is notable for diffuse enlargement and signal abnormality within the cord, generally involving the conus. Large vessels, representing dilated veins, are seen within the thecal sac. Enhancement may be present within the cord. The diagnosis is confirmed with spinal angiography. Treatment consists of embolization and/or surgery.

- *Arteriovenous malformations* are seen in younger patients (often teenagers) and often present acutely secondary to intramedullary and/or subarachnoid hemorrhage. The arteriovenous malformation nidus is located within or on the surface of the cord and is supplied by the anterior or posterior spinal arteries. In the juvenile variant, the nidus also involves the vertebral column.
- *Arteriovenous fistulas* are relatively uncommon. They are direct intradural fistulous connections from the anterior or posterior spinal arteries to the pial veins. These lesions typically occur in the thoracic and lumbar regions. Patients with these lesions may have a slowly progressive myelopathy or radiculopathy or may present with subarachnoid hemorrhage. These lesions usually present in the second to fourth decades.
- *Cavernomas* may occur anywhere in the spinal cord. They may present at any age, chronically or acutely (secondary to hemorrhage). Back pain is often reported. On imaging studies, they are often well-demarcated intramedullary lesions with a surrounding hemosiderin ring (hypointense on T2-weighted MR images). Surrounding signal abnormality due to edema or gliosis may be present, and these lesions may be calcified. Symptomatic lesions are treated with surgical excision.

42. **How are spinal tumors classified anatomically?**
    - Extradural
    - Intradural-extramedullary
    - Intramedullary

KEY POINTS: CLASSIFICATION OF TUMORS AND OTHER LESIONS WITHIN THE SPINAL CANAL

1. Extradural (outside the thecal sac): disc pathology, metastasis, epidural abscess, hematoma, bone abnormality

2. Intradural-extramedullary (inside the thecal sac but outside the cord): nerve sheath tumor (neurofibroma, schwannoma), meningioma, metastases, lipoma, arachnoid cyst

3. Intramedullary (inside the cord): tumors (astrocytoma, ependymoma, hemangioblastoma), multiple sclerosis, cord infarct, arteriovenous malformation, syrinx

43. **What is the most common epidural spinal tumor in adults?**
    Metastases are the most common neoplasms involving the epidural space. Epidural involvement is usually related to direct extension from an adjacent vertebral bone metastasis, though involvement of the epidural space in the absence of bone involvement on imaging can occur (lymphoma, leukemia, breast cancer, and lung carcinoma). On plain films and CT, metastases may appear as lytic or sclerotic lesions. Pathologic compression fractures may result. Typically, metastases will demonstrate increased uptake of radiotracer on bone scintigraphy. MRI is the most sensitive modality for the detection of osseous metastases, which appear as foci of signal abnormality within the marrow space, typically hypointense on T1-weighted images and hyper-

intense on fat-suppressed T2-weighted images with variable enhancement characteristics. MRI optimizes
detection of spinal cord and/or nerve root compression
(Fig. 48-13).

44. **What is the most common benign osseous lesion
    involving the spine?**
    Usually an incidental finding, hemangiomas are benign,
    present in approximately 11% of patients, and typically
    have a characteristic appearance on MRI. Because they
    contain internal fat, they are hyperintense on T1-weighted
    and fast spin-echo T2-weighted images.

45. **What is the differential diagnosis for an
    intradural-extramedullary tumor?**
    The most common intradural-extramedullary tumors are
    benign and include meningiomas and neural neoplasms
    (neurofibromas and schwannomas). Meningiomas most
    commonly occur in the mid-thoracic region and are much
    more common in women than in men. Nerve sheath tumors
    typically enhance avidly and extend along or envelop a
    nerve root. These tumors may have both intradural and
    extradural components. These tumors are often slow-
    growing, therefore bony remodeling, neural foraminal
    expansion, and/or vertebral body scalloping are common
    secondary imaging findings.

Figure 48-13. Sagittal T1-
weighted MR image of the
thoracic and lumbar spine
demonstrates markedly
decreased signal intensity
within multiple vertebrae with
multiple pathologic compression fractures and resultant
compromise of the spinal
canal *(arrow)*.

46. **What neoplasms are associated with
    leptomeningeal seeding of tumor?**
    Leptomeningeal metastatic disease may occur with
    both primary central nervous system (CNS) neo-
    plasms and with systemic malignancies.
    Medulloblastoma, ependymoma, glioblastoma mul-
    tiforme, and other high-grade astrocytomas are the
    primary CNS tumors that have been most often
    associated with leptomeningeal seeding. This phe-
    nomenon, however, may also occur with choroid
    plexus tumors, other glial tumors (including pilo-
    cytic astrocytomas), germ cell tumors, retinoblas-
    tomas, and primary spinal tumors.
       Systemic tumors, including lymphoma, may
    directly invade the subarachnoid space or may dis-
    seminate via lymphatic or hematogenous means. On
    MRI, leptomeningeal tumor often produces
    enhancement along the surface of the spinal cord
    that may be nodular and diffuse and is most promi-
    nent along the lumbar nerve roots/cauda equina.
    There may be associated edema (T2-weighted
    hyperintensity) within the spinal cord (Fig. 48-14).
    Imaging of the brain may be notable for communi-

Figure 48-14. Gadolinium-enhanced
T1-weighted MR image reveals pathologic, nodular enhancement along the
conus medullaris *(arrows)*.

cating hydrocephalus. Adequate CSF sampling (up to three high-volume spinal taps) remains
more sensitive than imaging for the detection of leptomeningeal disease.

47. **What are the most common intramedullary spinal tumors?**
    - Ependymoma
    - Astrocytoma
    - Hemangioblastoma
    - Metastasis

48. **What are the distinguishing clinical and imaging features of these intramedullary tumors?**

    - *Ependymomas* occur in all age groups and are slightly more common in men. Ependymoma is the most common primary tumor of the lower spinal cord, conus medullaris, and filum terminale. Imaging findings include bony remodeling (spinal canal expansion, vertebral body scalloping, and/or pedicle erosion), spinal cord expansion, a centrally located mass within the conus or filum, and heterogeneous signal intensity and enhancement—often with hemorrhage and/or hypercellularity (Fig. 48-15).

    Figure 48-15. Sagittal gadolinium-enhanced T1-weighted MR image of the thoracic spine demonstrates an irregularly enhancing ependymoma of the conus medullaris *(arrow)*.

    - *Astrocytomas* most often occur in the thoracic cord in young adults and children. On MRI, the spinal cord is typically expanded with decreased T1-weighted and increased T2-weighted signal intensity. These tumors are most often eccentric in location and enhance. Cysts may be seen within or adjacent to the lesions.

    - *Hemangioblastomas* are the third most common primary intramedullary tumor, but account for less than 5% of such tumors. These tumors are commonly seen in patients with von Hippel-Lindau disease. Hemangioblastomas are most often single, are located in the thoracic region, enhance avidly, and are commonly associated with cysts. Because these tumors are often vascular, enlarged vessels may be seen within the spinal canal. Whereas most are intramedullary, hemangioblastomas may also be intradural-extramedullary or extradural in location.

    - *Intramedullary metastases* are less common and are typically found in patients with widespread metastatic disease. The most common primary tumor to metastasize to the spinal cord is carcinoma of the lung. Cord metastases may also be seen with breast carcinoma, melanoma, lymphoma, colon carcinoma, and renal cell carcinoma.

BIBLIOGRAPHY

1. Czervionke LF, Haughton VM: Degenerative disease of the spine. In Atlas SW (ed): Magnetic Resonance Imaging of the Brain and Spine, 3rd ed. Philadelphia, Lippincott Williams & Wilkins, 2002, pp 1633–1714.

2. Flanders AE, Croul SE: Spinal trauma. In Atlas SW (ed): Magnetic Resonance Imaging of the Brain and Spine, 3rd ed. Philadelphia, Lippincott Williams & Wilkins, 2002, pp 1769–1824.

3. Harris JH, Mervis SE: Mechanistic classification of acute cervical spine injuries. In Harris JH, Mervis SE (eds): The Radiology of Acute Cervical Spine Trauma, 3rd ed. Philadelphia, Lippincott Williams & Wilkins, 1996, pp 213–244.

4. Hoffman JR, Mower WR, Wolfson AB, et al: Validity of a set of clinical criteria to rule out injury to the cervical spine in patients with blunt trauma. National Emergency X-Radiography Utilization Study Group. N Engl J Med 343(2):94–99, 2000.

5. Hurst RW: Vascular disorders of the spine and spinal cord. In Atlas SW (ed): Magnetic Resonance Imaging of the Brain and Spine, 3rd ed. Philadelphia, Lippincott Williams & Wilkins, 2002, pp 1825–1854.

6. Naidich TP, Blaser SI, Delman BN, et al: Congenital anomalies of the spine and spinal cord: Embryology and malformations. In Atlas SW (ed): Magnetic Resonance Imaging of the Brain and Spine, 3rd ed. Philadelphia, Lippincott Williams & Wilkins, 2002, pp 1527–1632.

7. Osborn AG: Nonneoplastic disorders of the spine and spinal cord. In Osborn AG (ed): Diagnostic Neuroradiology. St. Louis, Mosby, 1994, pp 820–875.

8. Osborn AG: Normal anatomy and congenital anomalies of the spine and spinal cord. In Osborn AG (ed): Diagnostic Neuroradiology. St. Louis, Mosby, 1994, pp 785–819.

9. Sze G: Neoplastic disease of the spine and spinal cord. In Atlas SW (ed): Magnetic Resonance Imaging of the Brain and Spine, 3rd ed. Philadelphia, Lippincott Williams & Wilkins, 2002, pp 1715–1768.

CHAPTER 49

HEAD AND NECK I

Mary Scanlon, MD, and Laurie A. Loevner, MD

1. **The hyoid bone divides the neck into two distinct regions. Name them.**
   The hyoid bone divides the neck into the suprahyoid neck (extending from the skull base to the hyoid bone) and the infrahyoid neck (extending from the hyoid to the cervicothoracic junction) (Fig. 49-1). The hyoid bone is a logical dividing point because its fascial attachments functionally cleave the neck into these two distinct anatomic regions. Magnetic resonance imaging (MRI) is the study of choice for the evaluation of lesions in the suprahyoid neck. MRI's superior soft tissue contrast and multiplanar capabilities enable excellent evaluation of the skull base, as well as evaluation for intracranial extent of disease from direct growth and from perineural and meningeal spread. In the infrahyoid neck, where there is abundance of fat and less complex anatomy, computed tomography (CT) is the imaging study of choice.

2. **What are the three subdivisions of the pharynx?**
   Nasopharynx, oropharynx, and hypopharynx. The nasopharynx extends from the base of the skull to the superior surface of the soft palate. The oropharynx extends from the soft palate to the hyoid bone. The hypopharynx extends from the hyoid bone to the inferior aspect of the cricoid cartilage. The oral cavity is a separate anatomic compartment distinct from the pharynx. It is located anterior to the oropharynx, from which it is anatomically demarcated by a ring of structures that include the circumvallate papillae of the tongue, anterior tonsillar pillars, and soft palate.

Figure 49-1. Enhanced axial CT scan of the neck shows the normal hyoid bone *(arrows)*. The hyoid bone divides the neck into the suprahyoid neck (extending from the skull base to the hyoid bone) and the infrahyoid neck (extending from the hyoid to the cervicothoracic junction).

3. **What are the boundaries of the nasopharynx?**
   The nasopharynx is divided into three subsites: the posterior-superior wall, lateral wall (also known as the *fossa of Rosenmüller*), and anterior-inferior wall (which is the superior surface of the soft palate). Laterally, the torus tubarius serves as the cartilaginous opening of the eustachian tube.

4. **What structures are part of the oropharynx?**
   The oropharynx includes the posterior third of the tongue (base of tongue), vallecula, palatine tonsils and tonsillar fossa, soft palate, and uvula.

5. **What structures are part of the hypopharynx?**
    The hypopharynx includes the piriform sinuses laterally, postcricoid region inferiorly (essentially the anterior wall of the hypopharynx), and posterior pharyngeal wall.

6. **What structures are part of the oral cavity?**
    The oral cavity includes the lips, anterior two thirds of the tongue, buccal mucosa, gingiva, hard palate, retromolar trigone, and floor of the mouth.

7. **Name the three anatomic subsites of the larynx.**
    The supraglottis, glottis, and subglottis. The soft tissues of the larynx are supported by a cartilaginous framework that includes the cricoid, thyroid, and arytenoid cartilages.

8. **What are the boundaries of the supraglottis?**
    The superior extent of the supraglottis is the tip of the epiglottis, and the supraglottis extends inferiorly to the laryngeal ventricle (which separates the false from the true vocal cords). The supraglottis includes the epiglottis, false vocal cords, aryepiglottic folds, and arytenoid cartilage. The laryngeal ventricle separates the false vocal cords of the supraglottis from the true vocal cords of the glottis. The aryepiglottic folds separate the supraglottic airway from the laterally situated piriform sinus of the hypopharynx.

9. **What structures compose the glottis?**
    The glottis is made up of the true vocal cords and the anterior and posterior commissures (Fig. 49-2).

Figure 49-2. Enhanced axial T1-weighted MR scan of the neck at the level of the glottis. The glottis is made up of the true vocal cords *(arrows)* and the anterior *(arrowhead)* and posterior commissures. Also, note the arytenoid cartilages (A), thyroid cartilage (T), and cricoid cartilage (C).

10. **Where is the subglottis?**
    The subglottis is the region of the larynx that extends from the undersurface of the true vocal cords through the inferior surface of the cricoid cartilage.

11. **Name and identify the extramucosal spaces of the head and neck in Figure 49-3.**
    Lateral to the pharyngeal airway are the parapharyngeal space (PPS), masticator space (MS), parotid space (PS), and carotid space (CS). Posterior to the pharyngeal airway are the retropharyngeal space (RPS) and the perivertebral space (PVS). The PPS is the central, primarily fat-containing space around which the other extramucosal spaces are located. The PPS contains fat, lymphatics, nerves, and minor salivary gland tissue. The MS contains the muscles of mastication (lateral and medial pterygoid and masseter and temporalis muscles), the ascending ramus of the mandible, and the V3 branch of the trigeminal nerve. The PS includes the parotid gland, facial nerve, retromandibular vein, external carotid branches, and intraparotid lymph nodes. The CS

includes the internal carotid artery, internal jugular vein, cranial nerves IX through XII, sympathetic plexus, and lymph nodes of the deep cervical chain. The RPS includes predominately fat and lymph nodes. The PVS includes the longus colli/capitis muscle complex, paraspinal musculature, vertebral body, posterior triangle of the neck, neurovascular structures within the spinal canal, and brachial plexus. The transverse process of the vertebral bodies further divide this space into the prevertebral portion anteriorly and the paraspinal portion posteriorly.

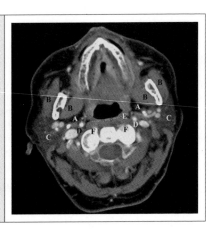

Figure 49-3. Enhanced axial CT scan of the suprahyoid neck, showing the extramucosal spaces (A = parapharyngeal space, B = masticator space, C = parotid space, D = carotid space, E = retropharyngeal space [dashed line], F = perivertebral space).

12. **Describe how displacement of the fat in the PPS helps to localize lesions/masses to their correct anatomic subsite in the extramucosal compartment.**

    The PPS is the central, primarily fat-containing space that is surrounded by the MS anteriorly, CS posteriorly, PS laterally, and pharyngeal mucosal space medially. Deviation of the fat in the PPS can help localize large masses to one of these four spaces. Large MS lesions will deviate the PPS fat posteromedially, a mass in the PS will deviate it medially, a CS mass will deviate the PPS fat anteriorly, and submucosal extension of a pharyngeal mucosal mass will deviate the fat medially.

13. **Displacement of the longus colli/longus capitis prevertebral muscle complex will help differentiate masses in what two extramucosal spaces?**

    The RPS and PVS. If these muscles are depressed posteriorly, the mass is arising either from the pharyngeal mucosal space or the RPS. If the muscle is elevated anteriorly off of the spine, then the lesion is arising from the PVS (usually the bone). If one can localize a mass to the correct extramucosal space and if the anatomic components of that space are known, then a differential diagnosis can be readily formulated.

14. **Displacement of the cervical internal carotid artery will help differentiate masses in what two extramucosal spaces?**

    The PPS (prestyloid) and CS (poststyloid). Masses in the PPS, when large enough, will displace the adjacent internal carotid artery posteriorly, whereas masses in the CS will elevate the adjacent internal carotid artery anteriorly.

15. **What are the imaging criteria for diagnosis of a pathologic lymph node?**

    Imaging criteria for pathologic nodes are based on nodal size and architecture. Any lymph node, regardless of size, that exhibits central low density (necrosis or cystic degeneration) is pathologic until proven otherwise (Fig. 49-4). The size criteria used depends on nodal location. The cervical nodes are anatomically classified by a grading system, from I to VII. Level I nodes are the submental and submandibular nodes. Levels II, III, and IV are the nodes in the internal jugular chain, with level II nodes located from the base of the skull to the hyoid bone, level III nodes located between the hyoid bone and cricoid cartilage, and level IV nodes located below the cricoid cartilage. Level V nodes are posterior to the sternocleidomastoid muscle. Level VI nodes are in the deep visceral chain, and level VII nodes are in the superior mediastinum. Level II–VII nodes are considered pathologic in size if they are greater than 1 cm. Level I and the jugulodigastric nodes (the only named level II node) are considered pathologic if they are greater than 1.5 cm.

Figure 49-4. Necrotic lymph nodes due to metastatic head and neck cancer. (A-B) Enhanced axial CT scan of the neck shows the characteristic appearance of a pathologic low-density (necrotic or cystic) cervical lymph node *(arrows)*. This node is a submental/submandibular node. Normal lymph nodes should be normal in size and enhance homogeneously. (C) Enhanced axial T1-weighted MR image shows a conglomerate nodal mass *(arrows)* at level II of the left anterior cervical lymph chain. Note the peripheral enhancement with central hypointense necrosis.

16. **What is the best cross-sectional imaging study to identify pathologic nodes?**
If the only clinical question is whether there is pathologic lymphadenopathy in the neck, then CT is the study of choice. It is more accurate than MRI in detecting nodal necrosis, especially in nodes of normal size.

KEY POINTS: NECK LESIONS

1. Neck lesions above the hyoid bone should be studied first with MRI. Pathologic conditions of the neck below the hyoid bone should be primarily imaged with CT scanning.
2. The most common cause of a cystic neck mass in an adult is metastatic adenopathy.

17. **What is the most common cause of a calcified cervical lymph node?**
In the adult, the most common cause is metastatic papillary thyroid carcinoma. In a child, metastatic neuroblastoma is the most common cause of calcified lymph nodes. Other less common causes of calcified lymph nodes include tuberculosis, other nontubercular granulomatous infections, sarcoid, and treated lymphoma.

18. **What is the most common cause of a cystic mass in the lateral neck of an adult?**
Metastatic nodal disease. Causes of such metastases include papillary thyroid cancer and squamous cell carcinoma. Carcinoma of the base of the tongue and tonsillar carcinoma are the most common primary head and neck carcinomas that result in cystic metastases. Metastatic cancer should always be the primary consideration of a cystic neck mass in adults. Branchial cleft cysts (BCC) are usually diagnosed in young patients. They most often are found at the angle of the jaw anterior to the sternocleidomastoid muscle and just touching the posterior aspect of the submandibular gland.

19. **What are the most common causes of cervical lymph node metastases in an adult?**
For a patient older than 40 years, if you say lymph node metastases from squamous cell carcinoma of the head and neck, you will be right 85% of the time. In patients between the ages of 20 and 40 years, the major differential diagnosis includes lymphoma, metastatic squamous cell carcinoma, metastatic thyroid cancer, and inflammatory adenitis.

20. **In patients with head and neck cancer, how does the presence of metastatic adenopathy affect prognosis?**
The presence of nodes dramatically reduces the 5-year survival of patients with squamous cell carcinoma. It follows the rule of 50%. The presence of a single lymph node reduces the 5-year survival by 50%. If the nodes are bilateral, 5-year survival is reduced by another 50%. If there is nodal fixation or extracapsular extension of tumor, expected survival goes down yet another 50%. Fixation of nodes (nonmobility) is probably best determined clinically. Extranodal spread can be suggested on CT by the demonstration of shaggy, irregular margins to the nodes, the presence of soft tissue stranding in the neck fat around the nodes, and enlarging nodal size. Seventy-five percent of nodes 3 cm or greater in dimension have extracapsular extension.

21. **What is the role of the radiologist in the evaluation and staging of head and neck cancer?**
The clinician and radiologist must work together as a team. The clinician/endoscopist can accurately assess the mucosa of the aerodigestive tract. The radiologist, with cross-sectional

imaging, sees the submucosa. When clinical and radiologic data are combined, there is 85% accuracy in staging patients. The radiologist is best at assessing submucosal spread of tumor, identifying necrosis in normal-sized nodes, and identifying retropharyngeal nodes (generally clinically occult).

22. List the most common neck masses in a child.

Inflammatory adenitis and congenital mass lesions are the two most common causes of neck masses in children. Malignancy is third. Lateral neck masses include cystic hygroma, BCC, inflammatory adenitis, and lymphoma. Midline masses include thyroglossal duct cysts (TGDCs), hemangiomas, and dermoids/epidermoids.

The most common congenital neck mass is a thyroglossal duct cyst. It can occur anywhere from the foramen cecum at the base of the tongue to the natural location of the thyroid gland. Most are located in the infrahyoid neck (65%), but they can occur at the hyoid (15%) or above (20%). Seventy-five percent are located in the midline. The more inferior the cyst, the more likely it is to be off-midline.

Thyroid carcinoma, usually papillary, arises in less than 1% of TGDCs. The presence of a nodule or calcification associated with the cyst should raise suspicion for the presence of carcinoma.

BIBLIOGRAPHY

1. Branstetter BF IV, Weissman JL: Infection of the facial area, oral cavity, oropharynx, and retropharynx. Neuroimaging Clin North Am 13(3):393–410, 2003.
2. Henrot P, Blum A, Toussaint B, et al: Dynamic maneuvers in local staging of head and neck malignancies with current imaging techniques: Principles and clinical applications. Radiographics 23(5):1201–1213, 2003.
3. Mack MG, Balzer JO, Herzog C, Vogl TJ: Multi-detector CT: Head and neck imaging. Eur Radiol 13(Suppl 5): M121–M126, 2003.
4. Som PM: Lymph nodes of the neck. Radiology 165:593–600, 1987.

CHAPTER 50

HEAD AND NECK II

Mary Scanlon, MD, and Laurie A. Loevner, MD

PARANASAL SINUSES

1. **Through what structure do the maxillary, frontal, and anterior ethmoid air cells drain?**

   The ostiomeatal complex (OMC) is the common drainage pathway for the paranasal sinuses. It refers to the uncinate process, a small bone around which mucus and secretions drain through the maxillary sinus ostium, infundibulum, hiatus semilunaris, and middle meatus (Fig. 50-1). The posterior ethmoid and sphenoid sinuses drain via the sphenoethmoidal recess into the superior meatus. Only the lacrimal duct drains into the inferior meatus. Acute bouts of sinusitis are typically treated medically, and diagnosis is made on clinical grounds. Imaging is reserved for patients who have chronic symptoms despite maximum medical therapy. Computed tomography (CT) is never performed during acute infection but rather after 4–6 weeks of maximum medical therapy. Delineation of OMC anatomy and the identification of any anatomic variants that narrow this common drainage pathway are key for the ear, nose, and throat (ENT) surgeon to plan possible surgical correction.

2. **Malignancy most commonly arises in which paranasal sinus?**

   The most common site involved is the maxillary sinus, followed by the nasal cavity and the ethmoid air cells. It is relatively rare to have a malignancy arise within the frontal or sphenoid sinus. The role of the radiologist is not, however, to be the histologist, but rather to map the extent of disease so that the surgeon can plan his or her surgical approach. Eighty percent of sinonasal malignancies are squamous cell carcinomas. Another 10% are adenocarcinomas and adenoid cystic carcinomas arising from minor salivary gland rests. Other cell types include melanoma and olfactory neuroblastomas (esthesioneuroblastoma). The hallmark of squamous cell carcinoma is bony destruction.

Figure 50-1. Coronal unenhanced CT scan of the paranasal sinuses at the level of the osteomeatal unit performed using a bone algorithm (A = uncinate process, B = maxillary sinus ostia, C = infundibulum *[dotted line]*, D = hiatus semilunaris, E = middle meatus).

3. **On an unenhanced CT scan, what are common causes of hyperdense tissue within the paranasal sinuses?**

   The big three are inspissated secretions, mycetoma (fungus ball), and blood.

   Inspissated secretions due to chronic sinusitis are the most common of these entities. These dense secretions may also be seen within chronic polyps of the sinonasal cavity. With polyposis there is expansion and bony remodeling. The dense appearance on CT is due to high protein content and viscosity. Blood within a paranasal sinus usually demonstrates an air-fluid-hemorrhage level(s).

4. **What classic radiologic finding supports the diagnosis of acute sinusitis in the appropriate clinical setting?**
   An air-fluid level in a paranasal sinus, in the absence of trauma or sinus irrigation, is the characteristic finding in acute sinusitis.

5. **Name the three major salivary glands and the ducts that drain them.**
   The parotid, submandibular, and sublingual. The parotid is drained by *Stensen's duct,* which courses from the parotid gland and passes over the masseter muscle to insert into the cheek at the level of the second maxillary molar. The submandibular gland is drained by *Wharton's duct,* which drains on either side of the frenulum in the floor of the mouth. The sublingual glands consist of 12–18 small, paired glands located in the sublingual space in the floor of the mouth. The sublingual glands have many draining ducts, known as the *ducts of Rivinus,* which drain into the floor of the mouth. If there is a dominant sublingual duct opening into Wharton's duct, it is called the *duct of Bartholin.*

6. **What salivary gland has the highest incident of calculi/stones? Why?**
   By 4:1, it is most common to have calculi/stones in the submandibular gland. The submandibular gland is more prone to stone formation due to its more alkaline and viscous secretions. In addition, its draining duct is wider, has a narrower orifice, and takes an upward course. On thin-cut unenhanced CT, more than 90% of these stones are radiopaque.

7. **Which salivary gland contains lymphoid tissue? What is the significance of this tissue?**
   The parotid gland is the first salivary gland to form and the last to encapsulate. As such, it is the only salivary gland to contain lymphoid tissue. For this reason, it is the only salivary gland that has the potential for lymphadenopathy from systemic diseases (e.g., rheumatoid arthritis, Sjögren's syndrome, HIV), metastases to intraglandular nodes (usually from skin cancer of the scalp), lymphoma, and Warthin's tumors. One of the major lymphatic drainage pathways of the scalp is to the lymph nodes in the parotid gland.

8. **What is the most common benign tumor of the salivary glands?**
   The pleomorphic adenoma (mixed benign tumor), which is seen most often in the parotid gland, where it represents approximately 80% of all parotid masses. Parotid gland masses follow the 80% rule. Eighty percent are benign, 80% are pleomorphic adenomas, 80% occur in the superficial lobe, and approximately 80% of untreated pleomorphic adenomas remain benign (up to 20% undergo malignant degeneration to squamous cell carcinoma).

9. **What are the most common malignancies of the salivary glands?**
   The most common malignant lesion of the parotid gland is mucoepidermoid carcinoma. In the submandibular, sublingual, and minor salivary glands, the most common malignancy is adenoid cystic carcinoma.

10. **How is the size of the salivary gland related to the likelihood of a mass in the gland being malignant?**
    In an adult, the rule is that the larger the salivary gland, the lower the incidence that a mass within it will be malignant. The reverse is true in the pediatric population. In an adult, a parotid mass has a rate of malignancy of about 15–20%; the submandibular gland, 40–50%; and the sublingual glands, greater than 50%.

11. **What imaging features distinguish a benign thyroid mass from a malignant thyroid mass?**

    None. There is nothing specific about the appearance of an intrathyroidal mass (such as calcification, low attenuation, or hemorrhage) that distinguishes a benign nodule from a malignant nodule (Fig. 50-2). Any thyroid mass that measures between 1.2 and 1.5 cm in two planes should be further studied with histologic analysis. Tissue for cytology is usually obtained by fine needle aspiration in the doctor's office for palpable lesions and under ultrasound guidance in the radiology department for lesions that are nonpalpable. Missed cancers that are 1.2 cm or larger in two planes tend to have a higher incidence of unfavorable biologic behavior (lymphatic spread and angioinvasion).

    Other findings on cross-sectional imaging that suggest that a thyroid mass is malignant include the presence of pathologic lymphadenopathy in the neck, extension of the thyroid mass outside of the thyroid capsule, and vascular invasion (spread into the adjacent internal jugular vein). Eighty percent to 90% of thyroid carcinomas are papillary carcinoma. Other malignant tumors of the thyroid gland include anaplastic carcinoma, follicular cancer, medullary carcinoma, and primary lymphoma. Rarely, metastatic disease to the thyroid gland occurs (from primary lung, breast, and renal cell carcinomas).

Figure 50-2. Normal thyroid gland and thyroid mass. *A*, Enhanced axial neck CT at the level of the thyroid gland. Note the normal right and left lobes of the thyroid gland (L) and the isthmus *(arrows)*. *B*, Enhanced axial neck CT in a different patient shows a 1.3-cm low-density mass in the left thyroid lobe *(arrows)*. This is nonspecific regarding benign (i.e., goiter or adenoma) versus malignant disease (cancer).

12. **What is the most common cause of proptosis in an adult?**

    Graves' disease is the most common cause of unilateral or bilateral proptosis. This is secondary to increased orbital fat and extraocular muscle enlargement. The extraocular muscle bellies are typically involved with characteristic sparing of the tendon insertions. This is in contrast to the pattern of involvement with orbital pseudotumor (the second most common cause of proptosis), in which the tendons are involved. Patients do not have to be hyperthyroid to have Graves' ophthalmopathy. It may occur before, during, or after treatment. The key clinical feature of orbital pseudotumor is eye pain associated with the proptosis. Ocular lymphoma and metastatic disease are other common causes of proptosis (Fig. 50-3).

13. **Which metastatic lesion to the orbit is classically associated with enophthalmos?**
Intraorbital, retrobulbar (behind the globe) metastatic breast carcinoma is commonly associated with enophthalmos. This is due to the frequent scirrhous reaction of breast carcinoma that results in retraction of adjacent tissues, similar to what is commonly seen in the breast (retraction and dimpling of skin).

14. **What is the most common primary ocular malignancy in a child? In an adult?**
In a child, retinoblastoma is the most common malignant tumor, and 95% of these masses are calcified. CT is best for detection of calcification (which can be difficult to see with magnetic resonance imaging [MRI]), whereas MRI is best for detecting intracranial extension. In an adult, the most common primary ocular malignancy is melanoma, although overall, the most common intraocular malignancy in an adult is a metastasis. The uveal track is involved with both. Melanomas may grow along the optic nerve and into the subarachnoid space, with resultant dissemination throughout the neural axis. In both the child and adult, malignant masses are commonly associated with a retinal detachment. Whenever a nontraumatic retinal detachment is identified, there must be careful evaluation for the presence of an associated intraocular mass.

Figure 50-3. Coronal enhanced T1-weighted MR image shows a large mass *(arrows)* in the right orbit along the superior muscle complex that represents metastatic prostate carcinoma.

15. **What key clinical and imaging features distinguish an optic nerve glioma from an optic nerve meningioma?**
The age of the patient and appearance of the optic nerve. Meningiomas occur in middle-aged adults, whereas optic nerve gliomas occur in children (mean age, 8–9 years). Meningiomas straighten the optic nerve because they arise from the surrounding dura of the optic nerve sheath complex, whereas gliomas kink the nerve as the tumor arises from the nerve itself. With meningiomas the mass can be separated from the optic nerve. Both can occur in children with neurofibromatosis, but optic nerve gliomas are the most common.

16. **Hearing loss is classified into what two major subtypes?**
Sensorineural and conductive. MR is the best imaging study to evaluate unilateral or asymmetric sensorineural hearing loss in an adult. The most common neoplasm associated with this is an acoustic (vestibular) schwannoma, and thin-section MRI with contrast enhancement should be obtained through the internal auditory canal and cerebellopontine angle. The remainder of the acoustic pathway, including the cochlear nuclear complex, medulla, and thalami, as well as the temporal lobes should also be evaluated. High-resolution, thin-section unenhanced CT of the temporal bones is the best imaging study for sensorineural hearing loss in patients younger than 15 years because congenital anomalies or atresias involving the otic capsule, semicircular

canals, and vestibular aqueduct are commonly the cause. CT is the study of choice in patients with conductive hearing loss at any age since it is best for demonstrating the sequela of chronic otitis media or cholesteatoma.

KEY POINTS: SINUSITIS AND HEARING LOSS

1. The best predictor of acute sinusitis in the appropriate clinical setting (facial pain, nasal drainage, fever) is the presence of an air-fluid level on a CT scan.

2. CT is the imaging modality of choice for conductive hearing loss.

3. MR is the imaging modality of choice in adult-onset sensorineural hearing loss.

17. **How is tinnitus clinically subcategorized?**
    Tinnitus is classified as pulsatile or nonpulsatile. Pulsatile tinnitus is further divided into subjective (patient hears beating) and objective (patient hears beating and so does the physician with a stethoscope). Pulsatile tinnitus is most often secondary to a vascular problem, including masses, malformations, or an anomaly. Causes include glomus tumor, dural arteriovenous fistula, aberrant internal carotid artery, or a high-riding jugular bulb. In subjective pulsatile tinnitus, CT is the first imaging study to perform. In objective pulsatile tinnitus, one may perform an MR study, although patients are often assessed with conventional catheter angiography because the most concerning potential diagnosis is dural fistula. The most common cause of pulsatile tinnitus reported in the neurologic literature is benign intracranial hypertension (pseudotumor cerebri). Tinnitus without a pulsatile quality may be an early symptom of an acoustic tumor or otosclerosis. Other causes include cholesteatomas, noise damage, and old age. Relatively rare causes include multiple sclerosis and Arnold-Chiari I malformation.

18. **Cholesteatoma is commonly noted to be a "pearly-white" mass seen in the middle ear on otoscopic examination. What is a cholesteatoma?**
    Cholesteatoma can be acquired or congenital. Acquired cholesteatomas are basically an ingrowth of skin through a perforation in the tympanic membrane (TM). Patients have a history of chronic otitis media with TM rupture and often have a history of myringotomy tube placements. The ingrowth of skin results in accumulation of squamous and keratin debris in the middle ear. The presence of associated osseous erosions on CT imaging is key to the diagnosis. Therefore, one must be familiar with the normal anatomy of this region (Fig. 50-4). In the absence of such erosions, a cholesteatoma can look exactly like chronic granulation tissue or chronic otitis media. Most commonly, cholesteatomas occur through a defect superiorly in the pars flaccida portion of the TM. Tissue first fills Prussak's space in the epitympanicum and erodes the scutum, then the ossicles, and may eventually progress to erode through the roof of the epitympanicum/tegmen tympani or undergo fistulization to the lateral semicircular canal or facial canal. Less commonly, cholesteatomas occur through a defect inferiorly in the pars tensa portion of the TM.

19. **What neoplasms occur in the jugular foramen?**
    Glomus tumors, neural neoplasms (schwannoma), meningioma, and metastatic disease. Glomus jugulare tumors are the most common. They arise from Arnold's nerve, a branch of cranial nerve X, which resides in the pars vascularis compartment of the jugular foramen. The jugular foramen is made up of two parts separated by a bony spur, the jugular spine. Anteriorly is the pars nervosa, which contains cranial nerve IX; posteriorly is the pars vascularis, which contains the internal jugular vein and cranial nerves X and XI. Glomus tumors, when large, erode the jugular spur and cause permeative bony changes (in contrast to the smooth osseous scalloping seen with schwannomas). In addition, unlike the other masses in this location that may compress the internal jugular vein, glomus tumors commonly grow directly into the jugular vein.

Figure 50-4. Normal temporal bone anatomy. *A-B,* Unenhanced axial CT images (A = head of malleus, B = body of incus, C = tympanic portion of the facial nerve, D = semicircular canals, G = vestibule, H = cochlea, IAC = internal auditory canal). *C,* Unenhanced coronal CT image (A = scutum, B = tegmen tympani, C = tympanic portion of the facial nerve, D = lateral semicircular canal, E = basal turn of the cochlea).

20. **Unilateral middle air fluid in an adult should trigger the search for what lesion?**
Nasopharyngeal carcinoma, which most often arises from the lateral wall of the nasopharynx (fossa of Rosenmüller). Infiltration of the levator veli palatini muscle leads to eustachian tube dysfunction and serous otitis media. Nasopharyngeal carcinomas can infiltrate widely in all directions. Superiorly, they can extend into the clivus, sphenoid sinus, as well as the neural foramina and osseous structures of the skull base.

BIBLIOGRAPHY

1. Moonis G: Imaging of sinonasal anatomy and inflammatory disorders. Crit Rev Comput Tomogr 44(4):187–228, 2003.
2. Okahara M, Kiyosue H, Hori Y, et al: Parotid tumors: MR imaging with pathological correlation. Eur Radiol 13(Suppl 4):L25–L33, 2003.
3. Shah GV, Fischbein NJ, Patel R, Mukherji SK: Newer MR imaging techniques for head and neck. Magn Reson Imaging Clin North Am 11(3):449–469, 2003.

POSITRON EMISSION TOMOGRAPHY

Andrew Newberg, MD

1. **What instructions do patients need to prepare for a fluorodeoxyglucose (FDG) positron emission tomography (PET) scan?**

   The most important issue regarding a PET scan is that the FDG will compete with nonradioactive glucose. Thus, if a person has recently eaten or has diabetes with a blood glucose level greater than 150 mg/dL, the sensitivity of the PET scan will be diminished. Typically, blood glucose levels greater than 200 mg/dL should exclude an individual from having a PET scan. Therefore, nondiabetic patients should have nothing by mouth (NPO) overnight or at least for 4–6 hours if their scan is later in the day. Diabetic patients should be managed carefully since some have difficulty forgoing eating. Also, insulin drives glucose, including FDG, into the muscles, so care should be taken regarding the administration of insulin too close to the scan time. It is preferred that the patient not inject insulin or eat before the PET scan, but if this is not possible, the referring physician must balance glucose levels, eating, and insulin in the diabetic patient. The scan itself takes place approximately 30 minutes after the IV injection of FDG, and performance of a whole body scan takes an additional 30–60 minutes, depending on the type of scanner.

2. **Is bowel activity normal on the FDG PET scan in Figure 51-1?**

   In general, bowel activity can be a normal finding on a PET scan, which sometimes makes the evaluation of cancer in the bowel more difficult. Some centers recommend a bowel preparation to minimize constipation, which might result in substantial smooth muscle uptake in the bowel. Bowel uptake that is very focal and intense should raise suspicion, but it is very important to correlate such findings with either anatomic imaging or endoscopy.

3. **What structures in the head and neck normally take up FDG? Is the neck uptake normal in Figure 51-2?**

   Normal uptake in the head and neck can be observed in the facial muscles, tongue (especially when patients are talking at the time of injection), neck muscles, brown fat, thyroid tissue, and vocal cords. The uptake of FDG can be very intense and can mimic or obscure cancer in these regions. Minimizing talking and patient movement as well as keeping the environment quiet and dimly lit both during injection and for approximately 15–20 minutes after injection may help to diminish uptake in these areas.

Figure 51-1. Normal FDG PET scan shows mild diffuse uptake throughout the bowel (a normal variant), mild uptake in the liver, significant uptake in the brain and heart, and marked uptake in the bladder.

401

Figure 51-2. The neck uptake in this patient is related to muscle uptake or brown fat. Other structures normally seen in the neck include salivary glands, oropharynx, tongue, vocal cords, and sometimes the thyroid. Uptake in the heart, brain, kidneys, and bladder is within normal limits. There are several small foci of mildly increased uptake in the lungs, which is suggestive of an active metabolic process, such as neoplasm.

4. **Is the lung nodule in the right upper lobe benign or malignant in Figure 51-3?**

   A lung nodule that has a moderate amount of uptake needs to be further evaluated for malignancy. Typically, a standardized uptake value (SUV, a quantity that incorporates the patient's size and the injected dose) that is more than 2.0 is considered to be suggestive of malignancy, whereas lesions with SUVs less than this value are considered to be benign. This nodule in the right upper lobe has an SUV of 4.0. Benign lesions include inflammatory or infectious etiologies. However, there are examples in which active infectious or inflammatory processes may result in SUVs comparable to those observed in malignant disease, so the clinical history and anatomic correlation are required for adequately assessing any finding on an FDG PET scan.

5. **Is the patient in Figure 51-3 a good surgical candidate?**

   One of the important uses of FDG PET imaging is presurgical evaluation of patients with known lung cancer. If the FDG PET scan demonstrates malignant lesions on the contralateral hilar regions or distant metastases, the patient no longer is a surgical candidate and would proceed to systemic therapy. In this particular patient, there are additional areas of uptake that are concerning for malignancy in the left supraclavicular region and the right inguinal region, which would require additional follow-up. If these areas are confirmed to be malignant, then the patient would no longer be a surgical candidate.

Figure 51-3. FDG PET scan of patient with lung cancer shows intense uptake in the right upper lobe with a standardized uptake value (SUV) of 4.0. There are additional areas of increased uptake that are also concerning for malignancy in the left supraclavicular region and the right inguinal region, which would require additional follow-up. Uptake in the heart, kidneys, and bladder is normal.

6. **How can FDG PET change the management of patients with lung cancer?**
   Studies have revealed that FDG PET changes the surgical management of patients in up to 40% of cases. In some cases, distant metastases or restaging indicates that the cancer is inoperable, thus preventing surgery that would have not been useful. In as many as 20% of patients, PET shows that enlarged nodes that may have prevented surgery from being considered are actually benign, so that surgery can be performed. This ability to change management has also contributed to the finding that FDG PET is cost-effective in the management of this patient population, since it can greatly alter the management and guide appropriate treatment.

KEY POINTS: INDICATIONS FOR PET SCANNING

1. Oncologic staging: Medicare approves PET for staging or restaging of non–small cell lung cancer, breast cancer, colorectal cancer, melanoma, lymphoma, head and neck cancer, and esophageal cancer

2. Brain tumors: differentiation of residual/recurrent brain tumor from radiation necrosis

3. Seizures: presurgical, interictal identification of refractory brain seizure foci

4. Cardiac imaging: metabolic assessment of myocardial viability

7. **What are potential confounding diseases that can mimic lung cancer?**
   There are several nonmalignant diseases that can mimic lung cancer by appearing as focally intense areas of increased uptake on an FDG PET scan. Most infectious processes such as pneumonia, active tuberculosis, or other abscesses can all appear as focal areas of increased activity. Sarcoidosis and other granulomatous diseases can also present as focally increased uptake (Fig. 51-4). Iatrogenic causes, such as postsurgical or postradiation therapy, can have increased activity, although radiation changes are usually more diffuse, involving most of the radiation field.

Figure 51-4. FDG PET scan of a patient with sarcoidosis shows multiple areas of intensely increased activity in the hilar regions; these findings appear similar to those found in lung cancer. This scan also demonstrates increased activity in other regions, such as the left axilla, abdominal, and pelvic lymph nodes.

8. **How is dual time point imaging used?**
   The physiology of glucose uptake is such that malignant cells continue to take up more and more glucose over time, whereas normal tissues establish an equilibrium. By taking FDG PET images at several time points, the later time point images should reveal malignant regions as increasing in intensity, especially compared with the background levels. Thus, dual time point imaging can contribute to making more accurate diagnoses, especially when the FDG uptake is borderline high on earlier images and increases on later images.

9. **How important prognostically is an FDG PET scan with negative results after treatment for lymphoma?**
   Studies evaluating the prognostic value of PET imaging for lymphoma after therapy have been quite dramatic. Patients with a PET scan with negative results have generally been shown to have greater than a 90% cure rate with excellent long-term survival. Patients with PET scans with positive results after therapy have less than a 10% chance of cure and most have a survival of less than 2–3 years. Thus, FDG PET after chemotherapy for patients with lymphoma has very important prognostic implications and may also suggest additional therapy for patients with scans with positive results (Fig. 51-5).

Figure 51-5. FDG PET scans in a patient with lymphoma before *(left)* and after *(right)* chemotherapy. The pretherapy scan shows multiple foci of increased activity in the neck and abdominal lymph node chains. The post-therapy scan reveals a complete resolution of these findings, suggesting a good response to therapy and good overall prognosis.

10. **What are the current indications for FDG PET in patients with lymphoma?**
    Currently, FDG PET scans are recommended for initial staging, especially to evaluate whether there is disease above and below the diaphragm. PET imaging can also be valuable in the early stages of therapy to assess whether the particular intervention is working. PET can be used to obtain prognostic information after therapy. Finally, PET can be used to evaluate the possibility of recurrence of disease and therefore can be a primary means of following up patients over the long term.

11. **How useful is PET in the evaluation of colon cancer?**
    A meta-analysis of studies evaluating almost 600 patients with colorectal cancer showed a sensitivity and specificity of whole body FDG PET of 97% and 75%, respectively. The specificity was found to be greater for local recurrence and hepatic metastases (>95%). FDG PET imaging was responsible for a change in patient management in almost 30% of cases.

12. **How does correlation with anatomic imaging help in detecting cancer accurately?**
    Fusing computed tomography (CT) and PET images has significant advantages over PET or CT alone. Studies have suggested that combining CT with PET may increase the diagnostic accuracy in up to 40% of patients compared with PET or CT alone. Specific advantages of fusing CT and PET images include discriminating metastases from physiologic foci of activity, improving lesion detection on both PET and CT, precisely localizing metastatic foci, differentiating bone from soft tissue, differentiating liver from adjacent bowel, and identifying specific structures of the neck. These advantages have led to a change in management in 10–20% of patients over that of PET alone.

13. **How does PET help with patient planning for radiation therapy?**
FDG PET can play several roles with respect to planning for radiation therapy. Since PET can detect distant metastatic disease, it may change the need for performing radiation therapy in the first place. PET can also be beneficial in helping to evaluate the area that requires radiation. A number of studies have shown that PET may show that the area of increased metabolism extends beyond the abnormal region on anatomic imaging, which would result in expanding the target volume for radiation treatment. Alternatively, PET may show that some areas believed to be involved with cancer on anatomic imaging are hypometabolic and are therefore not actively neoplastic. In this setting, the radiation volume can be reduced. Such changes in the plan for radiation therapy can occur in as many as 25% of patients.

14. **Is FDG PET useful for evaluating peritoneal seeding?**
FDG PET can detect peritoneal seeding, but the sensitivity and specificity of PET for making such a diagnosis are much less than for other more focal lesions. Peritoneal seeding can be difficult to detect on other imaging modalities as well; therefore, PET can still be useful when CT or magnetic resonance imaging (MRI) findings are equivocal since diffusely increased FDG uptake in various abdominal areas can be suggestive of peritoneal seeding. However, PET can often demonstrate negative results in patients with peritoneal seeding.

15. **How useful is FDG PET in the evaluation of osteomyelitis?**
FDG PET has been shown to be useful for evaluating infections both in bones and soft tissues. Studies have suggested that FDG PET has a high sensitivity (90–100%) and specificity (81–89%) in the detection of osteomyelitis in lower limb prostheses. Similar sensitivities and specificities have been reported in the detection of chronic osteomyelitis. Areas of osteomyelitis typically have intense uptake that is localized in the bone itself. More recently, PET has been used to evaluate soft tissue infectious or inflammatory disease, such as vascular graft infection, inflammatory bowel disease, and fever of unknown origin (Fig. 51-6).

Figure 51-6. FDG PET scan of a patient with suspected osteomyelitis of the spine reveals intense activity in two adjacent mid-thoracic vertebral bodies. This finding is consistent with osteomyelitis.

16. **How is PET used in the interictal evaluation of patients with seizure disorders?**
FDG PET scans are commonly used to evaluate seizure patients who are refractory to medications before surgery is performed to remove specific seizure foci. The FDG PET scan findings are also correlated with other clinical findings such as electroencephalography, Wada test, MRI findings, and neuropsychological tests. FDG PET has a sensitivity of more than 70% in the detection of seizure foci. The most common approach is to perform an interictal scan in which a seizure focus is expected to have reduced glucose metabolism. A clearly observed seizure focus on FDG PET can confirm the location of the seizure focus so that surgery can then be performed. In Figure 51-7, there is hypometabolism in the left temporal lobe, which is consistent with a seizure focus.

Figure 51-7. Interictal FDG PET brain scan in a patient with seizures reveals decreased metabolism in the left temporal lobe, consistent with a seizure focus.

17. **What are the most common areas for seizure foci, and what are the implications for finding multiple abnormal areas?**
    The temporal lobe is the most common focus of partial epilepsy and is also the region that can be most accurately evaluated with FDG PET imaging. The frontal lobes are the next most common area where seizure foci arise. This area is also relatively easy to observe on FDG PET, and the sensitivity and specificity for the detection of seizure foci in both regions are similar. On scans in which more than one area appears to be involved or when the regions of hypometabolism extend to other structures, the likelihood of resolution of seizures after surgery is typically diminished, sometimes substantially.

18. **How useful is FDG PET for the evaluation of primary brain tumors or new metastatic disease?**
    FDG PET has generally not been very useful for detecting primary brain or new metastatic tumors because the normal brain has such a high metabolism, and thus it is often difficult to find a tumor embedded in areas that already have high metabolism. However, some studies have suggested that the degree of hypermetabolism in tumors that have been detected may have prognostic implications since highly metabolic tumors tend to be the most aggressive and portend the worse prognosis. Low-grade tumors have lower metabolism and have an overall better prognosis.

19. **What are the sensitivity and specificity for differentiating tumor recurrence from radiation necrosis in patients with brain cancer?**
    Even though FDG PET appears to be useful in grading brain tumors and determining their prognosis, the major use of PET imaging is its ability to distinguish radiation necrosis from tumor recurrence. The ability to differentiate these two entities has critical clinical implications and is also often difficult with MRI or CT. In general, radiation necrosis should have virtually no metabolism, whereas recurrent tumor has increased metabolism. The ability to detect tumor recurrence is enhanced by the contrast of the tumor over the background hypometabolism induced by the radiation therapy (or surgery). Reports have generally scored the sensitivity and specificity of PET for detecting tumor recurrence as approximately 85% and 60%, respectively (Fig. 51-8).

20. **What are the characteristic features of Alzheimer's disease on the FDG PET scan in Figure 51-9?**
    The classic pattern of Alzheimer's disease on an FDG PET scan is hypometabolism in the temporoparietal regions. This may also involve the posterior cingulate gyrus. The subcortical areas, sensorimotor area, visual cortex, and cerebellum are generally less affected. However, more recent studies have shown that other areas may be hypometabolic, particularly when the patient

Figure 51-8. FDG PET brain scan in a patient after radiation therapy of a tumor in the left parietal region reveals decreased metabolism in the left parietal lobe with an intense region of activity centrally. These findings are consistent with recurrent brain tumor in the setting of radiation necrosis.

Figure 51-9. FDG PET brain scan in a patient with Alzheimer's disease shows bilateral temporoparietal hypometabolism. This is the most typical feature in Alzheimer's disease, although other structures, including the frontal lobes and visual cortex, can also be involved.

suffers specific neurocognitive deficits. Temporoparietal hypometabolism can also be observed in other conditions, including Parkinson's disease, bilateral parietal subdural hematomas, bilateral parietal stroke, and bilateral parietal radiation therapy ports.

21. **What is the typical metabolic pattern in the PET study of a patient with depression (Fig. 51-10)?**
    FDG PET studies of depressed patients usually demonstrate decreased metabolism, which can be global or affect more specific regions, such as the frontal lobes. More recent

Figure 51-10. FDG PET brain scan in a patient with moderate depression reveals globally decreased cerebral glucose metabolism compared with the subcortical structures of the basal ganglia and thalami.

studies have suggested that certain areas may actually have increased activity, such as the limbic regions. This more global pattern can usually be distinguished from specific neurodegenerative diseases, such as Alzheimer's or Pick's disease, which typically affect the temporoparietal and frontal lobes, respectively.

BIBLIOGRAPHY

1. Hustinx R, Benard F, Alavi A: Whole-body FDG-PET imaging in the management of patients with cancer. Semin Nucl Med 32(1):35–46, 2002.
2. Kostakoglu L, Goldsmith SJ: 18F-FDG PET evaluation of the response to therapy for lymphoma and for breast, lung, and colorectal carcinoma. J Nucl Med 44(2):224–239, 2003.
3. Newberg AB, Alavi A: Role of positron emission tomography in the investigation of neuropsychiatric disorders. In Sandler MP, Coleman RE, Patton JA, et al (eds): Diagnostic Nuclear Medicine, 4th ed. Philadelphia, Lippincott Williams & Wilkins, 2003, pp 783–819.
4. Valk PE, Bailey DL, Townsend DW, Maisey MN (eds): Positron Emission Tomography: Basic Science and Clinical Practice. London, Springer, 2003.
5. Zhuang H, Alavi A: 18-Fluorodeoxyglucose positron emission tomographic imaging in the detection and monitoring of infection and inflammation. Semin Nucl Med 32(1):47–59, 2002.

CHAPTER 52

BONE SCANS

Andrew Newberg, MD

1. What should a patient know about a bone scan?

A bone scan requires the IV injection of a small amount of a radioactive tracer that is absorbed into the bones. The tracer carries a relatively low dose of radioactivity and is extremely unlikely to result in any allergic or adverse reactions. The patient can eat and take medicines regularly and will be able to continue all daily activities before and after the scan. The scan itself occurs approximately 2 hours after injection of the tracer, and the scan time is approximately 45 minutes for a whole body scan. Three-phase bone scans require scanning for approximately 20 minutes at the time of the injection.

2. What are the normal structures observed on a bone scan? Describe the typical nonmalignant findings in asymptomatic patients.

Normally, all of the bones should be visible on a bone scan, including individual vertebrae and ribs. The kidneys and bladder are also seen in most patients. Normal soft tissue uptake can occur in the breasts and sometimes in vascular structures such as the uterus. Calcified cartilage is also commonly seen in the costochondral and thyroid cartilage. Common nonmalignant findings in asymptomatic patients include degenerative disease in the spine or joints, dental or sinus disease, calcification of atherosclerotic disease, and prior fractures (Fig. 52-1).

3. Why is a "superscan" associated with a negative prognosis in the patient with prostate cancer shown in Figure 52-2?

A "superscan" implies that so much of the methylene diphosphate (MDP) is taken up by the bones that there is no significant excretion in the kidneys and bladder or uptake in the soft tissues. The scan appears almost too good with high contrast between the bones and other tissues. The most common causes of a "superscan" are renal failure, hyperparathyroidism, metabolic bone disease, Paget's disease, or widespread metastatic disease. Thus, in a patient with cancer, a "superscan" implies widespread osseous metastases

Figure 52-1. Anterior and posterior projections of a normal bone scan using technetium (Tc)-99m–labeled methylene diphosphate show uniform activity throughout the bones, kidney, and bladder and mild degenerative changes.

that cannot be individually distinguished but rather occupy almost the entire skeleton.

4.   **Is there a way to successfully treat someone with bone pain associated with multiple osteoblastic metastases?**
Patients with bone pain from osteoblastic metastases can be treated primarily with four modalities: cancer-specific chemotherapy, radiation therapy, narcotic/pain management, or beta-emitting radiopharmaceutical agents that target bone. The latter option is often the best when multiple sites are involved that cannot be easily targeted by radiation therapy or would result in excessive radiation to uninvolved tissues or the whole body. Radiopharmaceutical agents, such as strontium-89 (Metastron) or samarium-153 (Quadramet), can be injected intravenously in patients with osteoblastic metastases for relief of pain. Studies suggest that up to 80% of patients experience some pain relief, with almost 50% having complete relief. The relief can last a mean of 6–8 months, and patients can be re-treated with similar pain relief. Although these treatments are not considered a cure, they can substantially improve a patient's quality of life and decrease reliance on narcotic medications.

Figure 52-2. The findings on this bone scan (anterior and posterior projections) are consistent with a "superscan," in which there is intense activity throughout virtually all of the bones with no significant excretion in the kidneys or bladder. Some areas, such as the proximal humeri and left femur, are particularly intense. This patient had widespread metastatic prostate cancer.

5.   **Figure 52-3 shows a scan of a patient complaining of swelling and pain in the distal arm after a recent traumatic event. What is the diagnosis?**
Patients with such symptoms after a traumatic event will typically either have osseous or soft tissue uptake characteristic of focal injury. In such patients, a three-phase bone scan will help make that determination. The first two phases—the blood flow, or vascular, phase and the blood pool, or tissue, phase—help to demonstrate whether there is soft tissue edema. If there is also focal uptake on the delayed bone images, then an osseous injury is suspected, which may be superimposed on soft tissue injury. However, the scan in Figure 52-3 shows diffusely increased uptake on all three phases, which is suggestive of reflex sympathetic dystrophy (RSD). RSD is a response to a traumatic event and results from autonomic dysfunction in the extremity, causing altered regulation of blood flow. On a bone scan, the typical result is increased flow and uptake on all three phases. However, other patterns have also been described. Regardless, the findings are almost always diffuse since they affect the entire extremity, including all of the fingers and distal arm.

6.   **What causes a bone scan that does not show the bones clearly?**
Usually a suboptimal bone scan is related to technical factors, such as not waiting at least 2 hours between the injection and the scan, poor preparation of the MDP, a significantly infiltrated injection dose, patient motion, and the camera being set to the incorrect energy window (e.g., for iodine-123 rather than Tc-99m). Physiologic reasons for suboptimal scans include large patient size, resulting in significant photon attenuation, or poor circulation states, such as congestive heart failure in which the tracer is not adequately delivered to the bones. Finally, patients with osteoporosis will simply not have enough bone for good visualization of osseous structures, and patients with iron overload will have inhibited uptake of the tracer.

7. **Is a bone scan an appropriate study for a 65-year-old patient with multiple myeloma?**
In general, bone scans are not sensitive for lytic bone lesions, and therefore, patients who demonstrate multiple myeloma or lytic abnormalities on computed tomography (CT) or x-ray should not be referred for a bone scan. Such patients should undergo a bone survey with multiple plain film x-rays. Patients with certain cancers that can have mixed lytic and blastic bone metastases may still benefit from a bone scan. Also, a patient with multiple myeloma with lytic disease in weight-bearing bones that might be susceptible to pathologic fracture may benefit since the fracture would show up as a focus of increased uptake. If a nuclear medicine scan is needed to better differentiate bone metastases, a fluorodeoxyglucose positron emission tomography (FDG PET) scan may be the most appropriate choice.

Figure 52-3. This bone scan shows diffusely increased activity throughout the entire right (left side of image) arm and hand on the blood pool images (top) and delayed images (bottom). These findings are consistent with reflex sympathetic dystrophy.

8. **Does a bone scan that shows a worsened condition after chemotherapy portend a bad prognosis?**
Even though a bone scan that shows apparent worsening abnormalities, characterized by increased activity in known lesions or the observation of new lesions, can be suggestive of progression of disease, the apparent worsening abnormalities may also be associated with the "flare" phenomenon. The flare phenomenon results from increased osteoblastic activity in lesions that is associated with the bone's healing response after chemotherapy. The flare response is therefore associated with a good prognosis, suggesting effective therapy. The flare response can occur 2–6 months after chemotherapy. Thus, a patient with a bone scan that demonstrates apparent worsening abnormalities in this time period should be followed up with another bone scan 4–6 months later to determine whether the lesions subsequently regress. If there is improvement on the latter scan, then the previous scan can be considered to be related to a flare response associated with effective treatment.

9. **What are the most common findings on a bone scan that suggest metastatic disease?**
Bone scan findings of metastatic disease most commonly have intensely increased activity and may either be a solitary focus or multiple foci (Fig. 52-4). Widespread disease may appear as a "superscan," in which all of the bones have diffusely intense uptake (*see* question 3). Cold, or photopenic, defects can be observed in patients with lytic bone metastases. Since the sensitivity of bone scans is not 100%, scans can have negative results in the face of metastatic disease. Finally, metastatic disease can be observed in the soft tissues, including organs such as the lungs or liver.

10. **What are the causes of "cold," or photopenic, defects on bone scans?**
There are a number of benign and malignant reasons for photopenic regions on a bone scan. Bones with avascular necrosis in the early stage will have photopenia. Lytic bone tumors or metastases can be cold since there is an absence of osteoblastic activity. Any metal objects, either external, such as jewelry, or internal, such as a pacemaker or joint prosthesis, can attenuate or block photons. Bone can also be affected by disuse or radiation therapy, in which there is an overall decrease in uptake in a focal area.

Figure 52-4. Anterior and posterior views of a bone scan show a patient with multiple foci of intense activity throughout the axial skeleton, consistent with prostate cancer. In particular, there are foci of intense uptake in multiple ribs, throughout the spine, the skull, the right scapula, and the pelvis.

KEY POINTS: COMMON FINDINGS OF METASTATIC DISEASE ON BONE SCANS

1. Solitary focal lesions

2. Multiple focal lesions

3. Superscan

4. Photon-deficient lesions

5. Normal findings (false-negative scan)

6. Soft tissue uptake

11. **Are three-phase bone scans alone useful for the diagnosis of osteomyelitis? What other scans can be used to improve diagnostic accuracy?**
Three-phase bone scans can be positive for osteomyelitis if there is a focal area of intense uptake. This is particularly true when a patient has a superficial area of infection, such as an ulcer or cellulitis. In such a case, the question to be answered is whether the underlying bone is affected, which can be readily detected on a three-phase bone scan. However, increased uptake on all three phases of a bone scan can also occur in acute fractures, surgical manipulation, metastatic disease, avascular necrosis, and Paget's disease. If any of these other conditions are potentially expected, a three-phase bone scan by itself is not likely to be useful due to poor specificity. Additional studies to consider are an indium-labeled white blood cell scan for the extremities; a gallium scan for the spine; or a PET scan, which can be used for any site of suspected osteomyelitis. Since these three studies evaluate infectious or inflammatory processes rather than the bone's response, they have higher specificity than a bone scan.

KEY POINTS: CAUSES OF COLD DEFECTS ON A BONE SCAN ✓

1. Avascular necrosis

2. Malignant bone tumors

3. Metastases

4. Prosthesis, pacemaker, jewelry, lead shield

5. Barium in colon

6. Disuse atrophy

7. External radiation therapy

8. Early osteomyelitis

12. **Is lung uptake normal on a bone scan?**
     Lung uptake is almost never normal on a bone scan and is usually associated with malignant pleural effusions, large tumors, inflammatory processes, or metastatic disease. Metastatic osteosarcoma has particularly intense uptake when involving the lungs. Lung uptake itself is usually detected by comparing the left and right hemithoraxes, observing for increased uptake in the intercostal spaces.

13. **Can Paget's disease be distinguished from cancer in the bones? What is the "Mickey Mouse sign"?**
     Paget's disease typically is associated with focal areas of intensely increased uptake in the flat bones and the ends of the long bones. The uptake is usually diffuse, although there can be focal areas of increased uptake. There is no definitive way of excluding metastatic disease or primary bone tumors from Paget's disease on the basis of uptake in the bones. However, the pattern of Paget's in terms of its distribution and appearance may help in the diagnosis. For example, it is less likely that an individual will have an entire hemipelvis as the only site of metastatic disease, but this can commonly be a presentation of Paget's. In the spine, the "Mickey Mouse sign" refers to foci in which there is uptake in both the entire vertebral body and the spinous process, which is almost always Paget's disease rather than metastatic disease (Fig. 52-5).

14. **Intense activity on a bone scan in multiple joints can be the result of which disorders?**
     Polyarticular uptake on a bone scan is typically associated with arthritic conditions such as osteoarthritis, rheumatoid arthritis, psoriatic arthritis, gout, or ankylosing spondylitis. The diagnosis of these different disorders can be suggested by the specific joints involved, such as the knees, acromioclavicular joints, and interphalangeal joints in osteoarthritis; the metacarpal-phalangeal joints in rheumatoid arthritis; and involvement of the great toe in gout.

15. **Can shin splints be differentiated from stress fractures on a bone scan?**
     In general, shin splints demonstrate linear increased activity primarily on the delayed bone images in the posterior tibia. Stress fractures should be more focally increased with intense uptake on delayed bone scans and are often more anterior in their location. Furthermore, stress fractures commonly demonstrate increased activity on the first two phases of the bone scan, so any patient being referred for stress fractures should have a three-phase bone scan.

Figure 52-5. Anterior and posterior views of a bone scan show a patient with Paget's disease associated with multiple areas of intense MDP uptake in the mandible, proximal humeri, femurs, right rib, and spine. The increased activity in the distal femurs can be distinguished from degenerative changes since Paget's involves much of the femur rather than only the joint area, which would be typical of osteoarthritis.

16. **Is a prostate-specific antigen (PSA) level relevant to bone scan findings in patients with prostate cancer?**

    Several studies have demonstrated that a low PSA level (<10 ng/dL) is associated with a very low chance of having bone metastases. In fact, some have suggested that for low-risk patients with a PSA of less than 10 ng/dL, bone scintigraphy may not be necessary. On the other hand, PSA levels greater than 20 ng/dL are associated with a significantly greater chance of bone metastases. However, most large trials have still revealed relatively low occurrence of abnormalities on bone scans in the early work-up of prostate cancer patients. Therefore, knowledge of the PSA level is beneficial since equivocal findings may be considered less likely to be metastases in a patient with a very low PSA level.

17. **What is the significance of a single rib lesion in a patient being evaluated for metastatic disease from a known primary cancer?**

    The traditional view is that a single rib lesion has approximately an 8–10% chance of being a metastasis. This can be modified somewhat by the characteristics of the finding. Typically, linear areas of increased activity that appear to extend along the rib are more suggestive of metastatic disease, whereas small, macular lesions are more likely the result of trauma. In addition, the patient's history might reveal a recent fall, which would also more likely suggest that the finding is the result of trauma.

18. **Which benign bone tumors have increased uptake on a bone scan?**

    Osteoid osteomas have increased uptake on delayed bone scan images and may even have an observable photopenic center. They commonly arise in the femur or spine. Uptake is also very intense for osteochondromas and chondroblastomas. Enchondromas do not typically have significantly increased uptake on a bone scan.

19. **Do bone scans have a role in the evaluation of child abuse?**

    A bone scan may be an important study in the evaluation of potential child abuse since it enables a ready evaluation of all of the bones in one scan and can often demonstrate old or occult fractures. Thus, even if the child does not complain of pain in a particular bone, the bone scan can reveal prior trauma. If there are multiple fracture sites that would not occur from a typical fall or disease process, then child abuse might be suspected as the cause.

20. **Are planar bone scans sufficient for the evaluation of spondylolysis?**
Patients with back pain and suspected spondylolysis can undergo bone scans for the evaluation of abnormalities in the spine. Planar imaging may be sufficient to demonstrate a focus of increased uptake in the region of the posterior elements of the vertebra. However, a tomographic image is often necessary for diagnosis if the planar scan has negative or equivocal results. Studies suggest that single photon emission computed tomography (SPECT) imaging enhances the sensitivity of planar bone scans. The usual findings are focal increased uptake in the posterior elements of the vertebra, which can be unilateral or bilateral. Interestingly, uptake can be seen on the affected side due to the remodeling or on the contralateral side due to altered biomechanics.

21. **Is increased uptake in the kidneys a clinically relevant finding on a bone scan?**
If one or both kidneys has increased uptake on a bone scan, this finding can be clinically relevant since such a finding can occur in the setting of hydronephrosis and obstruction. Increased uptake on a bone scan may also be the result of the effects of chemotherapy or from the involvement of tumor, nephrocalcinosis, radiation nephritis, or acute tubular necrosis. Thus, a patient with abnormally increased uptake in one or both kidneys should be followed up with additional imaging, including both anatomic and scintigraphic if clinically indicated.

22. **What are the causes of liver uptake on a bone scan?**
The most problematic cause of liver uptake on a bone scan is the presence of hepatic metastases, which most likely are associated with melanoma or cancers of the colon, breast, or lung. Sometimes there can be increased activity in the liver associated with overlying soft tissue activity, in which case the liver is not the actual source of the increased activity. Diffuse hepatic necrosis, although rare, can result in increased liver uptake on a bone scan. Finally, a colloid formation of the tracer due to poor preparation techniques can result in the equivalent of a sulfur colloid (liver/spleen) scan.

23. **What can cause uptake in the muscles on the scan in Fig 52-6?**
Increased uptake in the muscles on a bone scan usually implies some type of inflammatory process, such as myositis, which was the case in this patient. Other considerations include rhabdomyolysis, hypercalcemia, hematomas, and tumors. The latter two conditions are usually more focal. There are technical factors, such as poor preparation of the radiopharmaceutical agent, or possibly not waiting long enough after injection before imaging. However, the intensity and diffuseness of the uptake on this scan is indicative of myositis.

Figure 52-6. Anterior and posterior views of a bone scan show diffuse, intense uptake throughout most of the skeletal muscle groups. Such a finding is consistent with widespread myositis.

BIBLIOGRAPHY

1. Abdel-Dayem HM: The role of nuclear medicine in primary bone and soft tissue tumors. Semin Nucl Med 27(4):355–363, 1997.

2. Atkins RM, Tindale W, Bickerstaff D, Kanis JA: Quantitative bone scintigraphy in reflex sympathetic dystrophy. Br J Rheumatol 32(1):41–45, 1993.

3. Collier BD, Fogelman I, Rosenthal I (eds): Skeletal Nuclear Medicine. St. Louis, Mosby, 1996.

4. Haukaas S, Roervik J, Halvorsen OJ, Foelling M: Related articles, links, abstract: When is bone scintigraphy necessary in the assessment of newly diagnosed, untreated prostate cancer? Br J Urol 79(5):770–776, 1997.

5. Sarikaya I, Sarikaya A, Holder LE: The role of single photon emission computed tomography in bone imaging. Semin Nucl Med 31(1):3–16, 2001.

CHAPTER 53

V/Q SCANS

Andrew Newberg, MD

1. How would you prepare a patient for a ventilation-perfusion (V/Q) scan?

Patients should be informed that the test takes approximately 20–30 minutes and consists of two parts. During the ventilation part, the patient will have a face mask placed over the mouth and nose and will be asked to inhale an odorless radioactive gas. The mask will be left on for approximately 5–10 minutes, and images of the lungs will be acquired. Then, the patient will be asked to lie down to receive an IV injection of a radioactive material (macroaggregated albumin [MAA]) to measure the blood flow to the lungs. Images are acquired in multiple projections around the body over a period of approximately 20 minutes. There is no specific preparation for the patient. The patient does not need to be without food. Even though patients can receive oxygen, subjects who are dependent on significant amounts of oxygen (i.e., require O_2 by face mask) are unlikely to be able to successfully perform the ventilation component of the study.

2. In what order should radiographic studies be obtained in the work-up of a patient with acute shortness of breath?

The first radiologic study in any patient with shortness of breath should be a chest x-ray. This will exclude many causes and is also necessary for adequate evaluation of V/Q scans. The next study is dependent on a number of variables, which include the current protocols for an individual hospital, but more importantly, on whether the patient has normal or abnormal x-ray findings. Many hospitals now use helical contrast-enhanced, multidetector-row, computed tomography (MDCT) scanning to evaluate patients for pulmonary embolism (PE), whereas others use the V/Q scan. In patients with significant abnormalities on x-ray, it is more likely that the V/Q scan will result in an intermediate scan result that will not provide additional clinical information. Therefore, only patients with relatively unremarkable chest x-rays should proceed to V/Q scans in the current medical setting. If CT and/or V/Q scan are equivocal, the pulmonary angiogram is the "gold standard" for the detection of PE.

3. How do aerosols compare to Xenon (Xe)-133 for ventilation scans?

Xe-133 is a radioactive isotope of a noble gas. It can be inhaled into the lungs and will wash out quickly in a normal lung, although there will be persistent activity (gas trapping) in parts of the lung affected by airway disease such as asthma or chronic obstructive pulmonary disease (COPD). Xe-133 is the ventilatory agent used for the large PIOPED study of V/Q scanning, so there is more data supporting the use of Xe-133 in the evaluation of ventilation. Radioaerosols are typically technetium (Tc)-99m–labeled particles, such as diethylenetriaminepentaacetic acid (DTPA), suspended in air. Such aerosols are deposited on the lining of the alveolar spaces and therefore do not wash out. However, even though gas trapping cannot be assessed because the particles remain in the lungs, particles have the advantage of allowing for imaging in multiple projections, which can be more easily compared with the perfusion images.

4. What are normal findings on a V/Q scan?

Normal findings consist of uniform ventilation throughout both lung fields (Fig. 53-1). On an Xe-133 ventilation scan, there is usually good inflow of the gas; uniform activity during the equilibrium phase, which lasts approximately 3 minutes while the patient breathes into the closed system of the machine; and then rapid and uniform washout within about 1–2 minutes.

Perfusion should also be uniform throughout, with the exception of the cardiac silhouette. There should be no activity observed in the brain since this would suggest a right-to-left shunt.

5. **What findings are necessary to classify a V/Q scan as "high probability" for PE?**
   The PIOPED study, which prospectively evaluated patients with suspected PE, helped establish the criteria by which V/Q scans are currently read. A high probability for PE, requires that the scan have the equivalent of two or more large segmental perfusion defects (75–100% involvement of the segment) that are not matched by ventilatory abnormalities. Four or more moderately sized perfusion defects (25–75% involvement of the segment) would also represent a high probability for PE. The implication of a high probability scan is that the patient has a greater than 80% chance of having a PE (Fig. 53-2).

Figure 53-1. *(A)* Normal V/Q scan with ventilation that shows uniform activity on the initial first breath *(upper left),* followed by an equilibrium phase, and then a washout phase (each view represents 45 seconds). Just below the ventilation scan is the image of the brain that is used to observe whether there is any right-to-left shunt. *(B)* Perfusion images are shown in multiple projections (top row: anterior, posterior, right lateral, and left lateral projections; bottom row: left posterior oblique, right posterior oblique, right anterior oblique, and left anterior oblique projections) and also demonstrate uniform activity throughout both lungs.

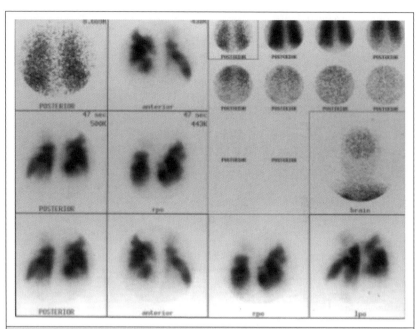

Figure 53-2. V/Q scan shows a high probability for PE. There is relatively uniform ventilation (upper right corner of scan) with only mild gas trapping in the upper lobes. There are multiple wedge-shaped perfusion defects throughout both lungs that are mismatched (i.e., no corresponding ventilation defect). Also note that there is mild uptake in the brain, consistent with a right-to-left shunt (*see* question 18).

6. **What are the causes of gas trapping on a V/Q scan?**
   Gas trapping refers to radioactive gas that persists in certain areas of the lungs during the washout phase of the ventilation scan. Potential causes for gas trapping are given in the following Key Points box. The implication of gas trapping is that there is an airway process that is contributing to the patient's symptoms. If the airway abnormality can be treated by medication or surgical interventions, then the gas trapping should also be resolved.

KEY POINTS: POTENTIAL CAUSES OF GAS TRAPPING ON A V/Q SCAN

1. Asthma
2. COPD
3. Chronic bronchitis
4. Mucous plug
5. Cystic fibrosis
6. Smoke inhalation
7. Tumors (e.g., carcinoma, adenoma)
8. Foreign body

7. **How does a quantitative V/Q scan assist in preparing patients for lung surgery?**
Quantitative V/Q scans help in the preoperative assessment of patients by demonstrating the areas of the lung that have the poorest overall function. This may help direct surgeons to preferentially resect areas that have the worst function. Perhaps, more importantly, the quantitative analysis provides a percentage of function for the various lobes and for the overall lung. When this percentage is multiplied by the forced expiratory volume in the first second (FEV_1), the surgeon can predict how much overall lung function will be left if certain parts of the lung are removed. For example, if a patient requires an upper and middle right lobectomy for lung cancer and the remaining lower lobe of the right lung and the whole left lung account for 70% of the lung function, then the surgeon can determine whether the patient will have adequate pulmonary function after surgery. In general, the remaining FEV_1 should be at least 700 mL/min. In the case described, the patient needs to have a preoperative FEV_1 of at least 1000 mL/min so that the remaining 70% will provide the necessary function for postoperative survival.

8. **What is the significance of a "triple match" on a V/Q scan and chest x-ray?**
A *triple match* refers to a ventilation defect and perfusion defect on a V/Q scan that match each other and are also matched to an opacification on the corresponding chest x-ray. The implication of such a finding is that it might represent a pulmonary infarct resulting from a PE. The revised PIOPED data indicate that a triple match defect in the upper or middle lung zones is still associated with a low probability for PE, but in the lower lung zone, it is associated with an intermediate probability.

9. **What can cause liver and splenic uptake on an Xe-133 ventilation scan?**
The primary cause of uptake in the liver and spleen on a ventilation scan is fatty infiltration of these organs since Xe-133 is lipid-soluble and a small percentage will cross the alveolar lining and enter into the blood stream. Uptake in the liver or spleen does not usually result in a poor prognosis and has no bearing on the diagnosis of PE. However, it is a relatively common finding on V/Q scans (Fig. 53-3).

10. **If the clinical suspicion for PE is high and the V/Q scan result is low probability, what is the patient's actual probability for having a PE?**
A high clinical suspicion for PE may occur in the setting of factors including predisposing conditions such as cancer or immobility, a sudden onset of shortness of breath, sudden requirement for O_2, or abnormalities on electrocardiogram or chest x-ray suggesting PE. In such a case, even a low probability result on the V/Q scan still carries as high as a 40% chance of a PE. Thus, a corroborative test, such as a pulmonary angiogram, would be necessary. On the other hand, a high-probability V/Q scan result would carry more than a 95% chance of a PE and would be enough to support the initiation of anticoagulant therapy.

11. **What are the causes of mismatched perfusion defects on a V/Q scan?**
Even though mismatched perfusion defects (a region with normal ventilation but no perfusion) are most likely to be associated with PE, there are other potential causes that should be excluded:
- Acute PE
- Chronic PE
- Other emboli (drug abuse, iatrogenic, fat)
- Vascular-obstructive tumor or obstructive adenopathy
- Hypoplasia of the pulmonary artery
- Swyer-James syndrome
- Vasculitis (post-external radiation therapy [post-XRT], collagen vascular)

12. **How can V/Q scans be used in the evaluation of chronic PE?**
Patients who have pulmonary hypertension or some other pulmonary process that might list chronic PE as a potential etiologic factor can undergo V/Q scans to assess for mismatched

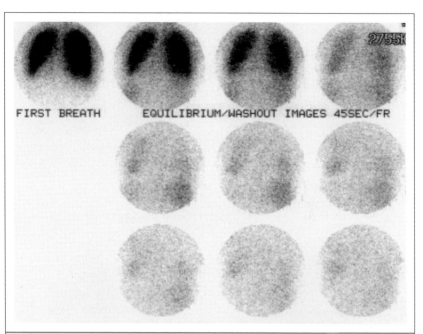

Figure 53-3. First breath, equilibrium, and washout phases of an Xe-133 ventilation scan showing increased uptake below the diaphragm in the liver and spleen.

perfusion defects. A V/Q scan cannot be easily used to determine the age of perfusion defects, and therefore, there is no way to definitively state whether a perfusion defect is attributable to chronic or acute PE. However, in the setting of a chronic disease process, such a finding would be consistent with chronic PE. If there is evidence for PE, then anticoagulant treatment can be started.

13. **Why is α_1-antitrypsin deficiency the most likely cause of the perfusion scan findings in Figure 53-4?**
In general, the upper lung zones in patients with airway disease related to COPD or asthma typically are more affected than the lower lobes. However, most of the lung becomes affected over time. On the V/Q scan, the result is a markedly heterogeneous perfusion pattern that shows the greatest decreases in the upper lung zones. In contrast, α_1-antitrypsin deficiency typically affects the lower lung zones first. Therefore, the V/Q scan findings usually show markedly decreased and heterogeneous perfusion in the lower lung zones, such as is the case in this patient with α_1-antitrypsin deficiency.

14. **Can idiopathic pulmonary fibrosis (IPF) be easily distinguished from PE?**
As shown in Figure 53-5, IPF can commonly result in perfusion defects that are often mismatched to the ventilation pattern. IPF usually results in multiple nonsegmental defects and therefore can be distinguished from PE. When such defects appear in a segmental pattern, PE cannot be excluded. Furthermore, since one of the criteria for an intermediate-probability V/Q scan is a scan that cannot be classified as high or low probability, many scans of patients with IPF will be considered to be of intermediate probability.

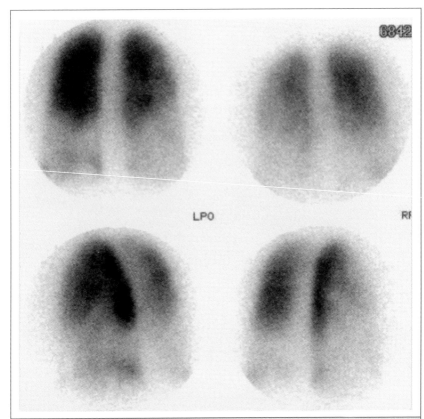

Figure 53-4. Perfusion scan (clockwise from top left: posterior, anterior, right posterior oblique, and left posterior oblique views) of a patient with α_1-antitrypsin deficiency shows characteristic abnormal flow in the lower lung zones compared with that in the upper lungs. The upper lungs have relatively uniform and preserved perfusion.

15. **Does the severe airway disease depicted in Figure 53-6 prevent adequate interpretation of V/Q scans?**
    This is a common problem since many patients with relatively severe COPD are referred for a V/Q scan because of worsening shortness of breath, and the question is whether the clinical symptoms are associated with a COPD flare or PE. Initial analysis of the PIOPED data suggested that severe airway disease usually associated with nonuniform matched perfusion and ventilation patterns made adequate assessment of PE too difficult. Therefore, such scans were read as intermediate or indeterminate. However, subsequent analysis has shown that if all of the perfusion abnormalities can be matched to the ventilatory findings, the scan can be interpreted as a low-probability scan. Thus, even though airway disease makes interpretation difficult, it is still possible to provide clinically relevant information using a V/Q scan.

16. **Could the V/Q scan in Figure 53-7 result from a lung tumor?**
    Lung tumors, if small, can elude detection, with no significant abnormality on the perfusion or ventilation scan observed. Larger tumors can appear as cold or photopenic defects on the V/Q scan since the tumor is a region that is not receiving blood in the same manner as the rest of the lung or is closed off from the other ventilatory areas. Large central or hilar tumors can preferen-

Figure 53-5. Perfusion scan (top row: first breath ventilation, posterior, left posterior oblique, and right posterior oblique views; bottom row: right lateral, right anterior oblique, anterior, and left anterior oblique views) of a patient with pulmonary fibrosis shows multiple areas of decreased perfusion. Most of these abnormal areas appear nonsegmental, and all of them are mismatched compared with the ventilation.

Figure 53-6. Perfusion scan (top row: first breath ventilation, posterior, left posterior oblique, and right posterior oblique views; bottom row: right lateral, right anterior oblique, anterior, and left anterior oblique views) of a patient with severe COPD primarily affecting the upper and mid-lung zones. The abnormal areas on the perfusion images appear to match the ventilation abnormalities on the first breath image.

tially obstruct the pulmonary vasculature rather than the bronchi, resulting in an entire lung having decreased or absent perfusion with relatively preserved ventilation. Endobronchial lesions typically result in matched ventilation and perfusion defects since the airways are obstructed to that part of the lung.

17. **Can V/Q scans be performed in pregnant women?**
    In general, V/Q scans can be performed in pregnant women, especially since most of the radioactivity is confined to the lungs rather than the abdomen or pelvis. It is important to establish the need for a V/Q scan in this setting so that the patient can be informed that the risks of PE outweigh the relatively minor risks of low levels of radiation to the fetus from the scan. It is

Figure 53-7. V/Q scan shows relatively uniform ventilation (upper right corner) with a mild decrease in the left lung. Perfusion images in the lower two rows (uppermost row: anterior, posterior, right lateral and left lateral projections; lower row: left posterior oblique, right posterior oblique, right anterior oblique, and left anterior oblique projections) show markedly reduced perfusion in the entire left lung, which is much worse than the corresponding ventilation abnormality.

sometimes protocol to decrease the dose of MAA by half to further diminish the radiation exposure to the fetus.

18. **What does activity in the brain or kidneys imply on a V/Q scan?**
Most nuclear medicine departments will image the brain or kidneys to evaluate for a mechanical right-to-left shunt. Since MAA is too large to pass through the capillary beds of the lungs, all of the injected material should remain in the lungs unless there is a shunt that bypasses the lungs. Such a shunt is most commonly found in the heart (i.e., an atrial septal defect) or possibly as arteriovenous malformations in the lungs. Even though the shunt can be detected on a V/Q scan, it is difficult to adequately assess the severity of the shunt, which typically requires additional studies using other radiographic or ultrasound techniques.

19. **How quickly do perfusion defects associated with PE resolve?**
Studies have reported varying rates of resolution of perfusion defects associated with PE. Some perfusion defects can resolve within 24 hours, whereas others may persist indefinitely. For this

reason, some clinicians recommend obtaining a V/Q scan approximately 3 months after treatment of PE to determine the new "baseline" perfusion pattern of the patient. This scan can then be compared with future scans if a determination of new PE is needed because of acute pulmonary symptoms.

20. **How are V/Q scans used in patients who have had lung transplants?**
In the immediate postoperative period, the V/Q scan can be used to assess the transplanted lung for overall function and to confirm that it is working adequately. V/Q scans can also be used to assess patients for PE in the transplanted lung, much the same way they are used in nontransplant patients. V/Q scans can also be helpful to assess patients for worsening function that may be attributable to rejection or infection. Even though the exact V/Q findings are nonspecific, rejection can result in small perfusion defects that are associated with small vessel abnormalities. Worsening ventilation and perfusion can also be observed in transplant patients who are developing bronchiolitis obliterans, even though the chest x-ray may be unremarkable.

21. **What is a "stripe sign"? What does it signify on a V/Q scan?**
A "stripe sign" is a rim of activity that surrounds the edge of a perfusion defect, as shown in Figure 53-8. The implication of this sign is that a perfusion defect that is bordered by the stripe sign is not the result of a PE. The physiologic basis of this interpretation is that perfusion defects related to PE should extend all the way to the periphery of the lung. If there is a stripe of perfused tissue distal to the perfusion defect, then it most likely does not represent PE.

Figure 53-8. This perfusion image in the right posterior projection demonstrates a "stripe sign," in which there is decreased activity centrally with a rim around the activity posteriorly and inferiorly. The implication is that this does not represent a PE since PE should result in a perfusion defect that extends to the periphery of the lung.

22. **What are the causes of matched ventilation and perfusion defects?**
Most conditions associated with matched ventilation and perfusion defects arise from diseases affecting the airways with subsequent physiologic shunting away from the underventilated regions. The most common causes of matched defects include COPD, bronchitis and bronchiectasis, and asthma. Other causes include those due to pleural effusions, mucous plugging, tumors, blebs and bullae, and pneumonia.

23. **What are possible causes of unilateral decreases in lung perfusion with relatively preserved ventilation?**
The most common cause of unilaterally decreased lung perfusion is a proximal mass lesion, such as lung cancer, which affects perfusion more than ventilation due to the more compressible nature of blood vessels compared with that of the rigid bronchi. Patients with congenital heart disease, such as Blalock-Taussig shunt or an absent pulmonary artery, can also have a similar pattern. A PE in the central pulmonary artery is another cause of unilateral perfusion decrease. A similar pattern can also be observed in patients who have undergone unilateral lung

transplant. Interestingly, the perfusion pressure in the pulmonary arteries of patients with COPD may be relatively normal, and therefore, the perfusion in the transplanted lung in the immediate postoperative period may only be 50–60% but will increase with time. On the other hand, patients with pulmonary hypertension will have a significant improvement with the lung transplant, which will receive up to 90% of the perfusion in the early postoperative period.

BIBLIOGRAPHY

1. Jacobson AF, Patel N, Lewis DH: Clinical outcome of patients with intermediate probability lung scans during six-month follow up. J Nucl Med 38:1593–1596, 1997.

2. PIOPED Investigators: Value of the ventilation/perfusion in acute pulmonary embolism: Results of the prospective investigation of pulmonary embolism diagnosis (PIOPED). JAMA 263:2753–2759, 1990.

3. Remy-Jardin M, Remy J, Deschildre F, et al: Diagnosis of pulmonary embolism with spiral CT: Comparison with pulmonary angiography and scintigraphy. Radiology 200:699–706, 1996.

4. Trujillo NP, Pratt JP, Tahisani S, et al: DTPA aerosol in ventilation/perfusion scintigraphy for diagnosing pulmonary embolism. J Nucl Med 38:1781–1783, 1997.

5. Worsley DF, Alavi A: Radionuclide imaging of acute pulmonary embolism. Semin Nucl Med 33(4):259–278, 2003.

CHAPTER 54

THYROID SCINTIGRAPHY

Andrew Newberg, MD

1. **What patient preparation is required before thyroid scanning?**
   Patients should fast after midnight or, at a minimum, for 4 hours before receiving the radioactive iodine (I)-123 pill to maximize absorption through the gut. Patients should also avoid ingesting foods containing high amounts of iodine since they will saturate the iodine stores in the body and thyroid and diminish the uptake of the radioactive iodine. Foods such as shellfish and seaweed, as well as supplements containing large amounts of iodine, should be avoided. Patients should also discontinue taking any medication that will affect thyroid function, particularly thyroid replacement medication (for at least 2 weeks); thyroid-blocking medication (propylthiouracil or methimazole for at least 5 days); and other medications, such as amiodarone, that contain substantial amounts of iodine. Finally, patients should not be scanned if they have received iodinated contrast agents as recently as 1 month before the scan (although sometimes the effects of such contrast agents on the thyroid can be seen as long as 3 months later).

2. **Which isotopes can be used for imaging the thyroid? How do they compare physiologically?**
   The most common radioactive materials used in thyroid imaging are the various isotopes of iodine. I-123 is the most commonly used isotope because of its excellent image quality and relatively low radiation exposure. Isotopes I-125 and I-127 are not typically used because of their high radiation exposure and poorer image quality. I-131 is still used for thyroid imaging in patients with thyroid cancer. Its higher photon energy theoretically makes it easier to detect cancer foci in the deep soft tissues in the body. However, I-131 releases a higher radiation exposure to patients, and the image quality is not as good as I-123. All of the iodine tracers are trapped by the thyroid and undergo organification into the thyroid hormones. The other primary tracer for thyroid imaging is technetium (Tc)-99m pertechnetate. This material is only trapped (not organified) by the thyroid and can provide high-quality images. However, the amount of uptake of the Tc-99m tracer cannot be used to plan I-131 therapy, as is the case with the iodine tracers.

3. **What are normal thyroid scan and iodine uptake results?**
   Thyroid images are obtained 24 hours after the administration of I-123 or approximately 30 minutes after Tc-99m. The gland should appear uniform throughout with smooth contours. The isthmus and pyramidal lobes can be observed, although they are more commonly seen in patients with Graves' disease. Iodine uptake values are usually obtained at 2 and 24 hours after administration of the I-123 pill. The 2-hour uptake should be between 2–10%, and the 24-hour uptake is usually between 10–30%. These values may differ slightly, depending on the uptake probe that is used, so it is always important to know what a particular institution considers to be the normal range (Fig. 54-1).

4. **Can a patient with normal I-123 uptake still have Graves' disease?**
   The important point here is that the iodine uptake refers to the activity of the gland and not to whether the person is hyperthyroid. Thus, even though a person may have normal scan results and uptake values, if the thyroid function tests indicate that the patient is hyperthyroid, a normal

Figure 54-1. Normal thyroid scan (clockwise from top left: anterior view, anterior view with marker in sternal notch, right anterior oblique view, and left anterior oblique view).

iodine uptake is still too high. A hyperthyroid patient should have a gland that is almost completely shut down. An uptake of 20–30% is much too high if a patient is hyperthyroid with an undetectable thyroid-stimulating hormone (TSH) level. In such a setting, a patient with normal scan results can still have Graves' disease.

5. **What are possible outcomes after I-131 therapy for Graves' disease?**
   There are three possible outcomes. A patient may be hypothyroid if the dose is sufficient to destroy most of the thyroid tissue and function. A patient may be euthyroid if the dose diminishes the function of the thyroid, but there is sufficient activity to maintain normal circulating levels of thyroid hormone. Finally, a patient may be undertreated (i.e., remain hyperthyroid), with the gland continuing to produce high levels of thyroid hormone. In the hypothyroid case, patients typically begin undergoing thyroid replacement therapy. In the hyperthyroid case, patients usually require re-treatment with a higher dose of I-131. The likelihood of each outcome depends on the range of doses given. Lower doses will result in fewer hypothyroid patients, with

more patients requiring re-treatment for persistent hyperthyroidism. Higher doses will result in more patients being hypothyroid, and thus fewer needing to be re-treated.

6. **How is a patient with a hot nodule treated for hyperthyroidism? Why is such a patient more likely to end up euthyroid?**

   Hot nodules are typically treated with I-131 therapy but are more resistant. Therefore, it is usually recommended that the dose be higher than that used for treating a patient with Graves' disease. However, the overall approach to therapy is relatively the same, including the preparation and radiation precautions that will be followed after the dose is given. The reason that patients with hot nodules have a higher likelihood of ending up euthyroid is that the hot nodule typically causes a suppression of the remainder of the gland. This protects the gland from the I-131 therapy. When the nodule is eliminated by the I-131, the patient's thyroid function drops, and eventually the TSH level begins to rise. This will stimulate the remaining thyroid tissue to begin producing thyroid hormone again. Since most of the suppressed tissue was protected, the patient may be able to make normal amounts of thyroid hormone (Fig. 54-2).

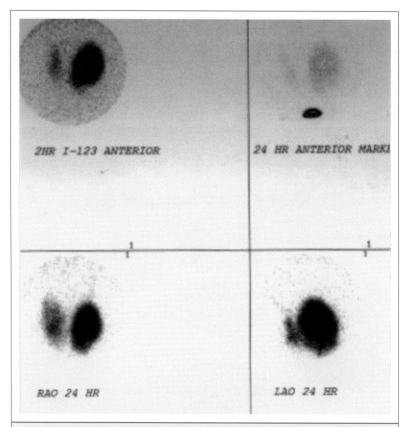

Figure 54-2. Thyroid scan shows a large "hot" nodule in the left lobe with suppression of the right lobe (clockwise from top left: anterior view, anterior view with marker in sternal notch, right anterior oblique view, and left anterior oblique view).

7. **What are the typical radiation safety precautions that patients must follow after I-131 therapy?**

   For approximately 5 days, patients treated with I-131 must do the following: sleep alone if possible; avoid kissing and sexual intercourse; minimize time with pregnant women and young children; minimize close contact with others; use good hygiene habits; wash hands thoroughly after each toilet use; use a separate bathroom, if possible; flush the toilet two times after each use; drink plenty of liquids; use disposable eating utensils; use separate bath linens; launder linens and underclothing separately initially; maintain a toothbrush in a separate holder; if possible, not prepare food for others; not apply cosmetics or lip balm; and wipe the telephone mouthpiece with a tissue after each use. In addition, nursing women should completely discontinue breastfeeding until their next child, and all women should not attempt to become pregnant for at least 90 days.

8. **When should a patient with multinodular goiter be treated with I-131?**

   Typical indications are either symptomatic hyperthyroidism or symptomatic mass effect related to the enlarged thyroid. Hyperthyroid patients can usually be treated with I-131, although with usually 2–3 times the dose as that for a patient with Graves' disease because the multinodular gland can be more refractory to the effects of I-131. Patients with compression of the airway or other vital structures in the neck or chest from an enlarged thyroid can be treated either surgically or with I-131. I-131 therapy is much less invasive and usually results in substantial shrinkage of the gland, which may obviate the need for surgery. However, some clinicians are concerned that potential inflammatory response from high levels of I-131 may result in clinical worsening (Fig. 54-3).

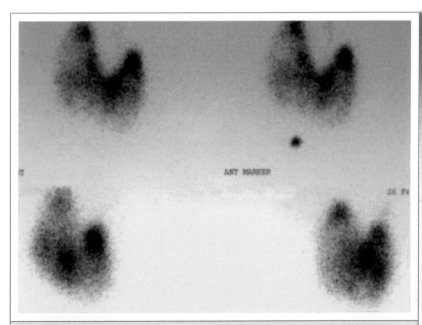

Figure 54-3. Thyroid scan shows multinodular goiter with numerous hot and cold regions (clockwise from top left: anterior view, anterior view with marker in sternal notch, right anterior oblique view, and left anterior oblique view).

9. **What factors affect the likelihood that a cold nodule represents thyroid cancer?**
Several factors relating to patient demographics, patient history, and features of the nodule affect the probability that a cold nodule may harbor cancer. Younger male patients with cold nodules are more likely to have cancer than older female patients with similar findings. Exposure to radiation in the neck is an important risk factor for cancer. Cold nodules in the setting of a multinodular goiter are substantially less likely to be cancer than other cold nodules. Finally, ultrasound findings of mixed cystic and solid components within a cold nodule are also more suggestive of thyroid cancer (Fig. 54-4).

Figure 54-4. Thyroid scan shows a large cold nodule in the right pole (clockwise from top left: anterior view, anterior view with marker in sternal notch, right anterior oblique view, and left anterior oblique view).

10. **Why can I-131 be used to treat thyroid cancer if the original nodule is cold?**
Although a cold nodule does not appear to take up any of the radioactive iodine on scintigraphy, its inactive appearance is in comparison to the background activity of the normal gland. In general, thyroid cancer cells will take up the iodine, but not as well as normal tissues. For this reason, thyroid cancer appears cold on the scan, but it can still take up enough iodine for therapy to be effective. To enhance the therapeutic effects of I-131 therapy, the normal thyroid is surgically removed. By eliminating much of the normal thyroid tissue, there is a better chance for any remaining thyroid cancer cells to take up the I-131. The hope is that by removing the thyroid and keeping the patient off thyroid replacement hormones, the TSH level will be greater than 30 miU/mL, which should maximally stimulate any thyroid cancer cells to take up the I-131. Patients

are also usually prescribed a low-iodine diet to "starve" any thyroid cells, further maximizing uptake of the I-131.

11. **What foods should be avoided as part of a low-iodine diet?**
A low-iodine diet is highly restrictive since many foods contain iodine. Foods to be avoided include most dairy products (milk, yogurt, ice cream, cheese), luncheon meats, bacon, hot dogs, fish, shellfish, noodles, pasta, cereals, pastry, breads, packaged rice, canned juices, canned fruits, canned or frozen vegetables, cocoa mixes, diet bars, jams/jellies, nuts, mustard, olives, candy, pretzels, and any snack foods. Patients can eat small portions fresh chicken, fresh potatoes, fresh fruit, all fresh vegetables except spinach, sweet butter, vegetable oils, onion or garlic powder, fresh herbs, and popcorn with no salt.

12. **What is the general management plan for patients diagnosed with thyroid cancer?**
Usually, patients who are diagnosed with thyroid cancer initially undergo surgery to remove the gland. Occasionally, one lobe is removed first and then, if cancer is detected, the other lobe is removed. However, most of the time, when cancer has already been definitively diagnosed with biopsy, as much of the gland is removed as possible. The patient then goes to the nuclear medicine department for a scan and therapy. The pretherapy scan usually demonstrates some uptake in the thyroid bed since it is difficult to surgically remove all of the gland, especially when it is adjacent to critical structures in the neck. Therapy is performed using I-131, given as an oral dose. The purpose of this therapeutic dose is to ablate any remaining normal thyroid tissue (some of which is usually left by the surgeon due to its proximity to critical structures in the neck) and to eliminate any remaining thyroid cancer cells. Patients are then followed up at regular intervals with neck and whole body iodine scans and serum measures of thyroglobulins. Patients can be re-treated with I-131 if there is a recurrence (Fig. 54-5).

Figure 54-5. Anterior view of an I-123 whole body scan of a patient with thyroid cancer after surgical resection. The scan of this patient who is now presenting for I-131 therapy shows two foci in the neck of residual thyroid tissue. The activity in the nasopharyngeal area, gut, and bladder represents areas of normal excretion of the I-123.

13. **What does "stunning" mean with regard to I-131 scanning?**
Several studies have suggested that a typical I-131 imaging dose of 4 mCi will actually have a small therapeutic effect on the thyroid and will therefore "stun" the thyroid cells, thereby making them slightly resistant to the larger therapeutic dose. For this reason, some clinicians have recommended using I-123 for whole body imaging before I-131 therapy to avoid this effect.

14. **What range of doses of I-131 is typically recommended for therapy for thyroid cancer in patients with the scans in Figures 54-6 and 54-7?**
The range of doses given to patients being treated for thyroid cancer depends on the extent of the cancer as well as the institution. Either way, there is usually a graded scale of doses that increases for worsening extent of disease. An example of the dose ranges is given in the Key Points.

KEY POINTS: TYPICAL DOSE RANGES FOR I-131 THERAPY

1. 60-100 mCi for low-risk disease

2. 125 mCi for lymph node involvement

3. 150 mCi for lung involvement

4. 175 mCi for bone involvement

Figure 54-6. Anterior view of an I-123 whole body scan of a patient with thyroid cancer after surgical resection. The scan of this patient who is now presenting for I-131 therapy shows multiple foci in the neck, which are consistent with lymph node involvement.

15. **How does a recombinant human thyrotropia (Thyrogen) scan work?**

    A Thyrogen scan is usually performed in the second year of follow-up for patients treated with I-131 for thyroid cancer. A Thyrogen scan is performed by subcutaneously administering a synthetic version of TSH on two consecutive days and then performing the iodine scan to detect thyroid tissue. Usually, patients stop taking thyroid medications to ensure that the TSH is maximally stimulating any residual thyroid tissue so that it can be detected on the scan. By giving the patient TSH, a similar physiologic state is obtained.

16. **What are possible causes of a thyroid scan in which there is no uptake or minimal uptake by the thyroid?**

    When there is no uptake observed on a scan, there are several potential causes. Patients may have thyroiditis, in which the inflammatory process has destroyed most functioning tissue. Such patients can be hyperthyroid or hypothyroid. Other causes of minimal uptake in the thyroid gland include exogenous sources of thyroid hormone (some patients take thyroid hormone as a form of diet pill) or iodine (e.g., recent iodinated contrast, drugs containing iodine such as amiodarone, high-salt or seafood diets, and alternative medicine supplements). Exogenous sources of thyroid tissue, such as struma ovarii (thyroid tissue in a monodermal ovarian teratoma), should also be considered in such patients.

Figure 54-7. Anterior and posterior views of an I-123 whole body scan of a patient with thyroid cancer after surgical resection who is now presenting for I-131 therapy. The scan shows multiple foci of intense activity in the neck, mediastinum, thorax, abdomen, and right humerus. These findings suggest widespread disease with bone involvement.

17. **How is fluorodeoxyglucose positron emission tomography (FDG PET) useful in the management of thyroid cancer?**

    In general, PET has no application in the initial diagnosis of thyroid carcinoma because there is overlap of FDG uptake between benign and malignant thyroid tumors. However, PET can be very useful in patients previously treated for thyroid cancer who now have rising tumor markers and an I-131 scan with negative results. FDG PET can be a useful adjunct imaging modality to help detect sites of tumor recurrence. The sensitivity for detection of recurrence with FDG PET is improved with hormonal withdrawal or administration of recombinant TSH. FDG PET also has a role in the management of patients with anaplastic, Hürthle cell, or medullary carcinoma since these tumors are not iodine avid.

BIBLIOGRAPHY

1. Alnafisi NS, Driedger AA, Coates G, et al: FDG PET of recurrent or metastatic 131I-negative papillary thyroid carcinoma. J Nucl Med 41(6):1010–1015, 2000.

2. Dworkin HJ, Meier DA, Kaplan M: Advances in the management of patients with thyroid disease. Semin Nucl Med 25(3):205–220, 1995.

3. Leslie WD, Peterdy AC, Dupont JO: Radioiodine treatment outcomes in thyroid glands previously irradiated for Graves' hyperthyroidism. J Nucl Med 39:712–716, 1998.

4. Shankar LK, Yamamoto AJ, Alavi A, Mandel SJ: Comparison of I 13I scintigraphy at 5 and 24 hours in patients with differentiated thyroid cancer. J Nucl Med 43(1):72–76, 2002.

5. Singer PA, Cooper DS, Daniels GH, et al: Treatment guidelines for patients with thyroid nodules and well differentiated thyroid cancer. Arch Intern Med 156:2165–2172, 1996.

CHAPTER 55

GI/GU SCINTIGRAPHY

Andrew Newberg, MD

1. **What should patients know about a renal scan? What preparation should they be given?**
   In general, there is little in the way of patient preparation for a renal scan, although patients should be well hydrated. Patients should refrain from taking furosemide, which is sometimes given during the scan to help evaluate for obstruction. Angiotensin-converting enzyme (ACE) inhibitors should also be avoided since they can alter the kidney's ability to regulate perfusion; however, captopril may be given during the study to help assess for renovascular disease. The scan itself usually takes approximately 30 minutes and begins with an injection of a radiopharmaceutical agent followed by imaging in the posterior view for native kidneys and the anterior view for transplants.

2. **What are the normal findings in a renal scan?**
   The perfusion component, measured during the first minute after injection of the tracer, should reveal renal perfusion occurring within several seconds of the aortic activity. Renal blood flow should be symmetric and greater than that in the spleen and liver (each kidney receives approximately 10% of cardiac output compared with less than 5% for the liver and spleen). Cortical images are obtained usually every minute for approximately 25 minutes. Cortical uptake should be symmetric with no focal defects. Activity should be observed entering the collecting system by 5 minutes (the cortical transit time [how long it takes for urine to appear in the collecting system]). Urine should flow freely into the bladder without significant retention or obstruction (Fig. 55-1).

3. **What are causes of focal areas of decreased flow within a kidney?**
   Most causes involve a mass effect, such as a cyst, abscess, or tumor (benign or malignant), that has altered renal morphologic features. Scarring in the kidney can result from chronic pyelonephritis or chronic ureteral reflux. Other causes of focal decreases in blood flow include infarction of part of the kidney or a hematoma associated with trauma or surgery. Such abnormalities can be either unifocal or multifocal, and all should be evaluated with anatomic imaging such as ultrasound or computed tomography (CT).

4. **An increase in size of one or both kidneys may be associated with what processes?**
   A common cause of a unilateral large kidney is compensatory hypertrophy for an absent or poorly functioning contralateral kidney. Hydronephrosis can also result in an enlarged kidney and may affect one or both kidneys. Patients with polycystic disease can also have kidneys that appear enlarged and often have multiple cold defects associated with cysts. Renal vein thrombosis can also result in enlargement of a kidney related to the engorgement of blood associated with the obstruction on the venous side.

5. **What are causes of a unilateral small kidney on the renal scan?**
   Several clinically important processes may be associated with a small kidney:
   - Dysplastic kidney
   - Postinflammatory atrophy

Figure 55-1. *(A)* Normal renal scan (posterior view) with symmetric and prompt flow into both kidneys on the blood flow phase. *(B)* Delayed images demonstrate activity entering into the collecting systems by 4 minutes with adequate and symmetric excretion into the bladder. There is only mild retention of activity in the collecting systems on the last image.

- Postobstructive atrophy
- Renal artery stenosis
- Radiation nephritis

Correlation with clinical history and anatomic imaging such as ultrasound or CT can help to differentiate the etiologic factor. Bilateral small kidneys are usually a manifestation of end-stage renal disease (ESRD), which can be caused by many processes.

6. **What are potential causes of nonvisualization of a kidney?**

Nonvisualization of a kidney on renal scan can be expected when a patient has had a nephrectomy, renal agenesis, posttraumatic or postsurgical damage to the kidney's vascular supply, or other vascular or obstructive processes. Vascular disorders that result in nonvisualization of a kidney include renal artery occlusion, which can be in the artery itself or from an abdominal aortic aneurysm, and renal vein occlusion. Neoplastic disease can also impair renal function or perfusion, resulting in nonvisualization. Finally, chronic obstruction, such as ureteropelvic junction obstruction, can eventually result in absent flow and function in a kidney (Fig. 55-2).

Figure 55-2. There is no visualization of the left kidney in this renal scan of a patient after nephrectomy for renal cell carcinoma. The right kidney appears slightly enlarged and has a normal cortical transit time.

7. **How do processes that decrease the activity in both kidneys differ from those that affect a single kidney?**

Processes affecting both kidneys are often more systemic. For example, glomerulonephritis can cause decreased flow in both kidneys. Acute or chronic renal failure also results in decreased flow and function in both kidneys. Acute tubular necrosis similarly results in decreased flow and function in the kidneys, although the function is typically more severely impaired. Of course there can always be bilateral vascular or obstructive processes, and these should also be considered. Finally, technical factors, such as injecting the wrong tracer or acquiring images on the wrong photopeak, can be considered if the kidneys are not visualized (Fig. 55-3).

DYNAMIC   1 MIN REFRAMED IMAGES

Figure 55-3. Delayed images from a renal scan in a patient with chronic renal failure show bilaterally decreased uptake in the kidneys and no clear evidence of function. Note that the kidneys have less activity than the liver and spleen, confirming the overall poor renal flow and function. Typically each kidney receives approximately 10% of cardiac output, whereas the liver and spleen each receive less than 5%. Thus, normal kidneys should have more activity than that in the liver and spleen.

8. **How is a captopril renal scan used to evaluate for renal artery stenosis?**
   A renal scan in a patient with renal artery stenosis often appears within normal limits since the renin-angiotensin system causes a vasoconstriction of the efferent arterioles, which helps maintain the pressure across the glomeruli, thus preserving renal function. A renal scan performed after the administration of captopril or another ACE inhibitor reveals abnormal flow and function since the regulatory mechanism of angiotensin is blocked by the ACE inhibitor. Therefore, a scan using diethylenetriaminepentaacetic acid (DTPA) after captopril should show evidence of diminished flow and function in a kidney with renal artery stenosis compared with the renal scan without captopril. The overall sensitivity and specificity of this test have generally been approximately 90% and 95%, respectively. With the advent of magnetic resonance (MR) angiography, there has been considerably less use of the captopril renal scan, but it is still sometimes helpful in evaluating the functional relevance of partially stenotic renal arteries.

9. **Why are renal scans obtained 1 day after transplant?**
   A renal scan within 1 day of surgical transplant can be very useful for detecting overall flow in the transplanted kidney to ensure that the artery is patent. The renal scan can also be used to help evaluate the extent of acute tubular necrosis (ATN), which occurs in virtually every

transplant, although it is much more common and severe in cadaveric transplants compared with living related transplants. ATN on a renal scan typically is diagnosed when there is relatively normal flow but diminished cortical transit of the tracer. The normal cortical transit time is usually less than 5 minutes; thus, ATN can be evaluated based on the delay in cortical transit, with severe ATN showing no significant cortical function. A renal scan can also help with the evaluation of hyperacute rejection, which would appear as near-absent perfusion of the kidney. Renal scans can also provide information regarding possible obstruction or leak of urine (leaks most often occur several days after transplant) (Fig. 55-4).

DYNAMIC   1 MIN REFRAMED IMAGES

Figure 55-4. Renal scan (anterior projection) in a patient 1 day after transplant from a living related donor. The uptake is good, and the cortical transit is within 5 minutes with good excretion into the bladder.

10. **How is ATN differentiated from rejection in transplant patients?**
Clinically, ATN occurs almost immediately, whereas chronic rejection occurs over several days to weeks or even longer. ATN can occur later, although it is usually associated with some specific event that might damage the kidney. ATN usually takes up to several weeks or months to resolve after transplantation.
Renal scan findings are often different for ATN and rejection, with ATN having normal or only slightly diminished perfusion of the kidney with a delayed cortical transit time. Rejection usually is associated with diminished flow with mildly impaired cortical function. Of course, in severe

rejection, both flow and function are markedly reduced. In both cases, when minimal or no urine is produced, it is impossible to exclude a leak or urinary tract obstruction since both of these entities require some radioactive urine to be produced. It is also possible to have both ATN and rejection superimposed, and this is particularly the case when a bone scan reveals diminished flow and function. A clinician may have to treat such patients for both conditions (Fig. 55-5).

11. **What type of renal scan is used to evaluate for cortical scarring related to pyelonephritis or vesicoureteral reflux? How does it work?**
   Pyelonephritis can result in scarring, hypertension, proteinuria, and renal failure. Renal scarring from vesicoureteral reflux accounts for 10–20% of patients with ESRD. A renal scan with dimercaptosuccinic acid (DMSA) is more sensitive than ultrasound or IV urography for the detection of parenchymal involvement. DMSA binds to the renal cortex and is essentially not excreted into the urine. This allows for imaging of the cortex to evaluate for areas of abnormally decreased activity. Imaging typically is performed approximately 20 minutes after injection, and single photon emission computed tomography imaging is performed to provide tomographic images for evaluation.

12. **What are the current uses of a liver/spleen scan?**
   In current nuclear medicine practice, liver/spleen scans are primarily used to evaluate liver function associated with cirrhosis, in which there is decreased uptake in the liver and a "colloid shift" to the spleen and bone marrow. Liver/spleen scans can help to assess patients for focal nodular hyperplasia, which results in focal areas of increased uptake in the liver. Liver/spleen scans can also be used to assess splenic function. This last indication may be in the setting of trauma or surgery that may have damaged the spleen, or it may be used to seek out additional splenic tissue in patients with heterotaxia (Fig. 55-6).

13. **What conditions result in a hot quadrate lobe and a hot caudate lobe on the liver/spleen scan?**
   Superior vena cava obstruction results in increased activity in the quadrate lobe. This occurs because collateral thoracic and abdominal vessels communicate with a recanalized umbilical vein, resulting in a hot quadrate lobe relative to the other areas of the liver. On the other hand, Budd-Chiari syndrome (hepatic vein thrombosis) appears as increased uptake in the caudate lobe, which has preserved function due to direct venous drainage into the inferior vena cava. The remainder of the liver is decreased in activity due to impaired function.

14. **What is the diagnostic pattern of activity on a red blood cell scan in a patient with a hemangioma in the liver?**
   The diagnosis of hemangiomas in the liver using tagged red blood cell imaging is based on identifying an early photopenic area with delayed filling because of the altered vasculature in the hemangioma. However, as blood slowly accumulates in the hemangioma, it has difficulty exiting the lesion due to the altered vasculature of the hemangioma. Thus, the same area eventually has increased activity on delayed images. The reported sensitivity for planar imaging is approximately 55% and for tomographic imaging is 88%.

15. **What is the best test for the detection of splenic tissue?**
   The heat denatured red cell scan is the most sensitive and specific for the evaluation of splenic tissue. Autologous red blood cells are incubated at 50°C for 30 minutes and then reinjected. The main indications for performing such a study are to evaluate patients with heterotaxia, patients who may have ectopic splenic tissue, and patients with sickle cell disease to assess for splenic function.

Figure 55-5. DTPA renal scan (anterior projection) in a patient 1 day after cadaveric renal transplant showing good flow *(A)* but no clear evidence of function *(B)*. This constellation of findings is consistent with ATN. An obstruction or a leak cannot be adequately assessed on this scan due to the overall poor renal function. Chronic rejection *(C)*, in a different patient, typically reduces flow and function to the point that severe rejection demonstrates no significant flow in the transplanted kidney.

post

liversplee

A

ant   post

B

Figure 55-6. Normal colloid distribution on anterior and posterior projections of a liver/spleen scan
(A) with the most activity in the liver, followed by the spleen. Only approximately 5% of the activity is
in the bone marrow. This can be compared with a patient with mild colloid shift with a larger spleen
(B) with similar uptake to the liver and overall more prominent bone marrow activity.

16. **What functions of the hepatobiliary system can be evaluated using
    iminodiacetic acid tracers?**
    Hepatocellular function can be evaluated since the tracer uptake by the liver depends on overall
    function. If the activity in the cardiac blood pool disappears within 5 minutes, hepatocellular
    function is considered to be normal. A longer time to clearance suggests hepatocellular dysfunc-
    tion. The patency of the common bile duct and cystic duct can also be evaluated. This helps to
    diagnose acute and chronic cholecystitis. Finally, a leak or extrabiliary collection can be
    assessed (Fig. 55-7).

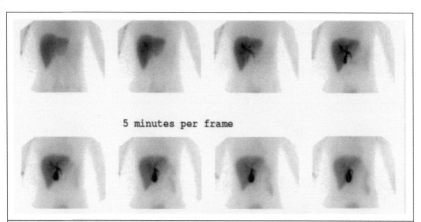

5 minutes per frame

Figure 55-7. Normal hepatobiliary scan (5 minutes per image) using technetium (Tc)-99m mebrofenin (Choletec) shows good hepatocellular function associated with elimination of the cardiac blood pool by 5 minutes. The gallbladder is observed by 20 minutes, and activity is observed in the bowel by 25 minutes.

17. **When should cholecystokinin (CCK) or morphine sulfate be used in relation to a hepatobiliary scan?**
    CCK should be used before the administration of a radiopharmaceutical agent when a patient has not eaten in more than 24 hours. The reason for the use of CCK is that the gallbladder can become filled with sludge with prolonged fasting, and this can result in false-positive scans. The IV infusion of CCK over about 15–30 minutes (faster infusions can result in nausea and vomiting) before beginning the hepatobiliary scan causes contraction of the gallbladder, which will then fill with the radioactive tracer as it expands. Morphine augmentation is used if, after the 1-hour scan, there is nonvisualization of the gallbladder. Morphine should be given only if the common bile duct is patent. Morphine causes contraction of the sphincter of Oddi, which results in a back pressure that can open a functionally closed cystic duct. If there is still nonvisualization of the gallbladder at the end of an additional 30 minutes of imaging after morphine is given, then the result is consistent with acute cholecystitis.

18. **What can a gallbladder ejection fraction study show?**
    A gallbladder ejection fraction study can be performed in patients with a normally filling gallbladder who continue to have right upper quadrant symptoms. At the end of the standard hepatobiliary scan, CCK (or sometimes a fatty meal) is administered, and images are obtained for another 30 minutes. The counts in the pre-CCK and post-CCK scans can be compared to provide a gallbladder ejection fraction. A normal value is considered to be greater than 30–35%; however, the distribution of values makes a normal range difficult to determine. If the ejection fraction is less than this value, gallbladder dysfunction is suspected. Cystic duct syndrome is considered if the gallbladder does not contract in a uniform manner or even expands after administration of CCK.

19. **What are the causes of nonvisualization of the gallbladder on a hepatobiliary scan?**
    The most common cause is acute cholecystitis (Fig. 55-8). However, a number of other potential causes, including various diseases and congenital problems, must be considered in the evaluation:
    - Chronic cholecystitis
    - Complete common duct obstruction

- Prolonged fasting
- Severe hepatocellular disease
- Acute pancreatitis
- Cholecystectomy
- Agenesis of gallbladder

60 SEC/FR ANTERIOR

Figure 55-8. Hepatobiliary scan shows good liver uptake but no evidence of gallbladder activity. If the gallbladder is still not visualized on morphine augmentation or delayed images, the scan findings are highly suggestive of acute cholecystitis.

20. **What are the causes of a false-negative scan (i.e., visualization of the gallbladder even in the presence of acute cholecystitis)?**
There are several reasons why the gallbladder, or a structure appearing to be the gallbladder, can be observed on a hepatobiliary scan. False-negative results occur most commonly when the patient has acalculous cholecystitis. However, several other structures, such as the bowel, a duplicate gallbladder, or another abnormality of the biliary tree, can demonstrate activity in the region of the gallbladder even though the patient actually has acute cholecystitis. Another interesting cause of false-negative results is perforation of the gallbladder, which subsequently lowers the pressure and relieves the obstruction, thereby allowing the radioactive tracer to enter into the gallbladder region.

KEY POINTS: CAUSES OF FALSE-NEGATIVE HEPATOBILIARY ✔ SCANS

1. Acalculous cholecystitis
2. Loop of bowel
3. Dual gallbladder
4. Biliary duplication cyst
5. Right hydronephrosis
6. Gangrenous cholecystitis after perforation
7. Partial cystic duct obstruction
8. Intermittent obstruction from stone

21. **What is the "rim sign"? What does it imply?**
The rim sign refers to an area of increased activity in the liver region surrounding the gallbladder. The implication is that there is hyperemia or inflammation associated with acute cholecystitis. This hyperemia appears as a rim of increased activity immediately adjacent to the gallbladder. However, the diagnosis of acute cholecystitis still depends on nonvisualization of the gallbladder.

22. **When a biliary leak occurs, where are the possible sites to observe the leak?**
A biliary leak can occur anywhere along the biliary tree. However, leaks usually occur in areas of surgical interventions or anastomoses. When performing a hepatobiliary scan to look for a leak, it is important to perform the test in the standard manner. However, additional images of surgical drains and anterior views with the patient in lateral decubitus positions will help to assess for subtle leaks. Surgical drains should be evaluated for activity, and it is important to know where these drains are actually located. Drains in the surgical bed that have activity suggest a leak in that area. Drains in the biliary tree should naturally have activity. Decubitus views are obtained to assess for activity in free abdominal fluid, which would help to confirm a leak (Fig. 55-9).

23. **How is biliary atresia differentiated from neonatal hepatitis on a hepatobiliary scan?**
In both disorders, the bilirubin level is extremely high, making adequate visualization of activity entering into the small bowel difficult to assess. During the initial hour of imaging, activity is usually seen in the liver with persistent cardiac blood pool activity. Delayed imaging at 4 hours and sometimes 24 hours is required to determine whether any activity is observed entering into the bowel. If any activity does enter the bowel, biliary atresia can be excluded and the diagnosis of neonatal hepatitis can be made. However, absence of activity in the small bowel can still be related to either disorder because if insufficient activity is sent into the biliary system by the liver, it is not possible to evaluate for potential complete obstruction.

24. **What are the typical findings of a positive gastrointestinal (GI) bleed?**
In general, a positive GI bleeding scan requires that there be a focus of growing intensity that moves through the bowel. Thus, a focus that only increases in activity can sometimes be a false positive and attributable to kidney activity or hyperemia in the bowel or some other vascular structure. It is also important to observe the initial site in which the focus occurs since the primary importance of this study is to determine localization of the bleed.

Figure 55-9. Hepatobiliary scan in a patient after liver transplant *(A)*. The liver has relatively preserved function. The gallbladder is not visualized secondary to the surgery. However, there is an accumulation of activity lateral to the left lobe of the liver that appears to be filling the left colic gutter. Anterior images taken with the patient in lateral decubitus positions *(B)* reveal that there is radioactivity in the free fluid in the abdomen, which is consistent with a large leak.

25. **Contrast the differences between the sulfur colloid scan and the tagged red cell scan for detecting GI bleeding.**

    Both radiopharmaceutical agents are labeled with technetium (Tc)-99m. Sulfur colloid scans can be started immediately when the patient arrives in the nuclear medicine department, since the agent can be prepared ahead of time. The sulfur colloid remains in the intravascular space for approximately 25 minutes. Therefore, an active bleed can be detected quickly. An intermittent bleed might be missed if the patient bleeds after more than 25 minutes post-injection of the sulfur colloid. Since sulfur colloid does not remain in the intravascular space, if there is a negative scan the first time, a repeat scan can be performed any time when the patient begins to bleed again.

A tagged red cell scan requires drawing some of the patient's blood, which must then be labeled, a process that takes 15–20 minutes. After injection of Tc-99m–labeled red blood cells, the activity persists in the intravascular space, and therefore, imaging can be performed continuously for up to several hours after injection. This can help to detect intermittent bleeds. However, if the initial scan results are negative, then a repeat scan cannot be performed for approximately 24 hours so that the Tc-99m decays sufficiently. Otherwise, the bowel will have too much activity.

26. **How does a gastric emptying study work? What are the normal rates for emptying?**
   A gastric emptying study involves the ingestion of a standardized meal consisting of some food source that is tagged with a radioactive label. The most common meal today consists of egg whites tagged with Tc-99m–labeled sulfur colloid. Meals must be standardized for content and calories so that an adequate comparison is made. Imaging usually is performed over 90–180 minutes. Images may be obtained throughout that time period or at regular intervals. Images are usually either obtained in both the anterior and posterior views or a single left anterior oblique view. The importance of these views is that food enters the stomach posteriorly and moves anteriorly. Therefore, images must take into account movement within the stomach and differentiate it from actual emptying. The rate of gastric emptying is dependent on the particular methods and meal used, but the normal half emptying time of the stomach is usually between 50 and 100 minutes.

27. **What physiologic factors normally affect gastric emptying?**
   A number of factors can affect gastric emptying. Factors that increase the rate include the patient positioned upright, younger male patients, higher liquid content of food, smaller size of food particles, larger volume of food, and lower fat content. Factors that can slow the rate include the patient positioned supine, older female patients, higher solid content of food, larger size of food particles, smaller volume of food, and higher fat content. Other factors that can cause variable responses include the hormonal and metabolic state of the patient, stress, and drugs. For these reasons, it is imperative that a standardized meal and acquisition protocol be used and compared with normal values established for that specific technique.

BIBLIOGRAPHY

1. Datz FL: Considerations for accurately measuring gastric emptying. J Nucl Med 32:881–884, 1991.

2. Dubovsky EV, Russell CD, Bischof-Delaloye A, et al: Report of the Radionuclides in Nephrourology Committee for evaluation of transplanted kidney (review of techniques). Semin Nucl Med 29(2):175–188, 1999.

3. Emslie JT, Zarnegar K, Siegel ME, et al: Technetium-99m–labeled red blood cell scans in the investigation of gastrointestinal bleeding. Dis Colon Rectum 39:750–754, 1996.

4. Krishnamurthy S, Krishnamurthy GT: Biliary dyskinesia: Role of the sphincter of Oddi, gallbladder and cholecystokinin. J Nucl Med 38(11):1824–1830, 1997.

5. O'Reilly P, Aurell M, Britton K, et al: Consensus report on diuresis renography for investigating the dilated upper urinary tract. J Nucl Med 37:1872–1876, 1996.

6. Ponzo F, Zhuang H, Liu FM, et al: Tc-99m sulfur colloid and Tc-99m tagged red blood cell methods are comparable for detecting lower gastrointestinal bleeding in clinical practice. Clin Nucl Med 27(6):405–409, 2002.

7. Taylor A, Nally J, Aurell M, et al: Consensus report on ACE inhibitor renography for detecting renovascular hypertension. J Nucl Med 37:1876–1882, 1996.

CHAPTER 56

NUCLEAR CARDIOLOGY

Andrew Newberg, MD

1. **How would you prepare a patient for a nuclear medicine stress test?**
Patients should be informed that the test takes approximately a half day and consists of two parts. There is typically a resting part and a stress part. The placement of an IV catheter (usually inserted at the beginning of the day) is required to administer the radiopharmaceutical agent. The order of the study can be either rest-stress or stress-rest, although the higher dose is given for the second scan, and therefore, the stress test is often performed second to have the best image quality. Scans are obtained approximately 30–60 minutes after injection of the radiopharmaceutical agent, and each scan takes approximately 15–30 minutes. The patient should not eat or drink the night before the examination. Patients are commonly asked to stop taking their medications unless there is some reason (e.g., very high blood pressure or serious arrhythmias) that requires the stress test to be performed while the patient continues to take medications.

2. **What are the different types of radiopharmaceutical agents available for stress testing?**
There are three basic categories: thallium, technetium (Tc)-99m–labeled compounds, and positron emission tomography (PET) compounds. Table 56-1 compares thallium and Tc-99m compounds. The most commonly used Tc-99m compounds are tetrofosmin and sestamibi, which both have similar imaging and chemical characteristics. Tc-99m compounds generally provide more flexibility in terms of imaging times. Due to the photon energy and the number of photons emitted, Tc-99m compounds are generally easier to use for image acquisition and analysis. PET radiopharmaceutical agents, such as nitrogen (N)-13 ammonia and fluorine (F)-18 fluorodeoxyglucose (FDG), can be used to evaluate myocardial perfusion and glucose metabolism, respectively. N-13 has a short (20-minute) half-life, so there are some logistical limitations in using PET for cardiac imaging.

TABLE 56-1. COMPARISON OF Tc-99m COMPOUNDS AND THALLIUM FOR CARDIAC IMAGING

	Tc-99m Compounds	Thallium
Energy	140 keV (ideal for gamma camera)	69–83 keV (suboptimal for gamma camera)
First-pass studies of ventricular function	Possible with these agents	Not feasible
Gated imaging	Readily accomplished	Count rate marginal for gated imaging
Stress-rest imaging	Two injections required	Can be accomplished with one injection

3. **What are the three types of stress tests?**

The three basic types of stress tests are exercise, dipyridamole (Persantine) or adenosine, and dobutamine. Exercise stress tests are typically performed using a treadmill with several possible protocols that sequentially increase the speed and grade of the treadmill. An alternative exercise test uses a stationary bicycle. The goal is to raise heart rate to 85% of the patient's age-predicted maximum, although others have used a combination of heart rate and blood pressure as a target. Persantine is an inhibitor of adenosine deaminase that results in increased adenosine within the epicardial coronary arteries. The result is a relative decrease in perfusion to areas in which there is a significant obstruction in the coronary arteries. Finally, dobutamine, an adrenergic agonist, causes increased heart rate and increased inotropic contraction of the heart, simulating exercise.

4. **What are contraindications for an exercise stress test?**

Any patient with significant musculoskeletal problems that would prevent him or her from achieving maximal heart rate should undergo pharmacologic stress testing. Patients with certain ongoing arrhythmias, such as ventricular tachycardia, supraventricular tachycardia, new onset atrial fibrillation, or heart block, should receive treatment for those arrhythmias before the stress test is rescheduled. Known atrial fibrillation that is adequately treated is not a contraindication. Patients with severe pulmonary disease, severe hypertension (i.e., systolic blood pressure >210 and diastolic blood pressure >110), abdominal aortic aneurysms, symptomatic aortic stenosis, unstable angina, or active ischemia on electrocardiogram (ECG) should also be excluded.

5. **What are the contraindications for pharmacologic stress tests?**

Persantine stress tests should not be performed in patients with severe reactive airway disease, particularly when a patient demonstrates active wheezing on physical examination. However, patients who use inhalers but who otherwise have stable airway disease can often safely undergo Persantine stress tests. Any patient taking Persantine or methylxanthines should not have a Persantine stress test unless the medication can be stopped for at least 24–48 hours. Furthermore, all patients who are to undergo Persantine studies should abstain from caffeine for 24 hours since caffeine blocks the effect of Persantine and adenosine. Dobutamine stress tests have similar contraindications to those of exercise testing, except that musculoskeletal problems are not an issue.

6. **Should patients taking medications that can affect the heart be given stress tests?**

In general, any patient can undergo a cardiac stress test. In patients taking medications for blood pressure, such as beta blockers or calcium channel blockers, the medication may prevent the patient from achieving the necessary heart rate. In such patients, it is recommended that the medications be stopped for approximately 24 hours before the study. However, if a patient has severe hypertension, the patient may need to be tested while taking the medication for this condition, since without the medication, the blood pressure would be too high to safely proceed with the study.

7. **Under what conditions would you stop an exercise stress test?**

An exercise stress test should generally have the following endpoints:

- The patient cannot continue because of dyspnea, chest pain, fatigue, or musculoskeletal problems.
- The patient has a hypertensive response.
- The patient develops ST-segment depressions greater than 3 mm.
- The patient develops ST-segment elevation, heralding a possible myocardial infarction.
- The patient develops the onset of a potentially dangerous arrhythmia, such as ventricular tachycardia, ventricular fibrillation, very rapid supraventricular tachycardia, or heart block.

8. **Which territories are supplied by which coronary arteries?**
   The three main branches of the coronary arteries are the left anterior descending (LAD) artery, the left circumflex artery, and the right coronary artery. The LAD supplies the anterior wall, including the anterolateral region; septum; and in most cases, the apex. The right coronary artery supplies the inferior wall and, in a "right dominant" system, can wrap around the apex to include part of the inferoapical wall. The left circumflex artery supplies the lateral wall. Smaller branches of these major arteries can supply smaller segments of individual walls (Fig. 56-1).

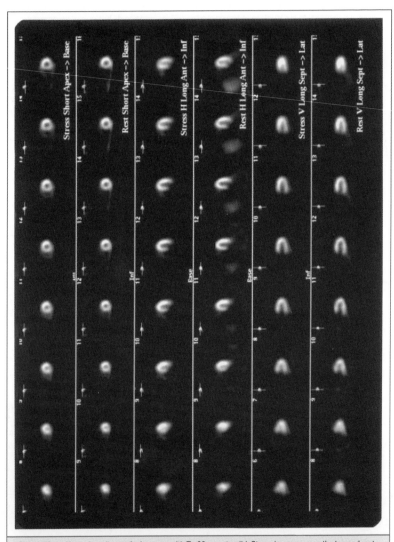

Figure 56-1. Normal cardiac perfusion scan with Tc-99m sestamibi. Stress images are on the top and rest images are on the bottom of each pair of projections. The short axis (from apex to base) demonstrates the classic "doughnut" appearance, with the anterior wall at the top of the cardiac image, the lateral wall to the right, the inferior wall at the bottom, and the septum to the left. The horizontal long axis shows the septum on the left of the cardiac image, the apex at the top of the image, and the lateral wall to the right. The vertical long axis shows the anterior wall on the top of the image, the apex at the right of the image, and the inferior wall at the bottom. On this normal scan, the level of activity is uniform throughout all walls.

9. **What is the implication of a "fixed" defect?**

A fixed defect implies that there is a lack of perfusion during both the rest and stress components of the scan (i.e., there is no difference between the two scans). Fixed defects can often be caused by artifact, such as when part of the heart is attenuated, or blocked, by a structure between the heart and the scanner. The most common structures that cause fixed defects via attenuation include the diaphragm (inferior wall) and breast tissue (anterior wall and apex). When fixed defects are associated with an actual cardiac pathologic condition, they are related to scarring or infarction. An infarct should have decreased perfusion during both stress and rest images since it is dead tissue (Figs. 56-2 and 56-3).

Figure 56-2. Cardiac perfusion scan with Tc-99m sestamibi reveals a lateral wall perfusion defect on both the stress and rest images in the short axis and the horizontal long axis *(arrows)*. Since this perfusion defect is observed on both stress and rest images, it is a fixed defect and implies a prior infarct with near absent perfusion in the scar.

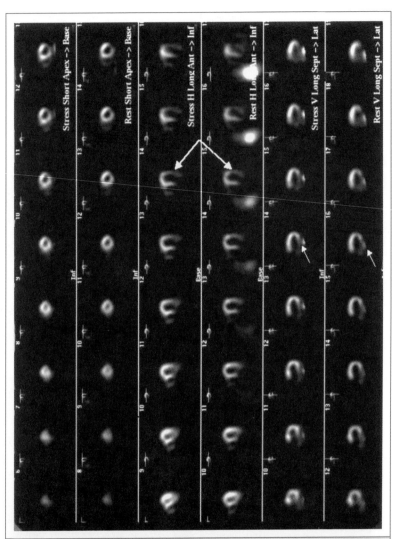

Figure 56-3. Cardiac perfusion scan with Tc-99m sestamibi reveals a fixed inferolateral wall perfusion defect. There is decreased perfusion in the lateral wall on the horizontal long axis *(large arrows)* and decreased perfusion in the inferior wall on the vertical long axis *(small arrows)*. The defect can also be observed on the short-axis views. It is typically important to confirm any finding on other projections to ensure that it is a real defect rather than from artifact. This fixed defect represents a prior infarction.

10. **What methods are available to correct for attenuation artifact?**

Two common methods are used to correct for attenuation artifact. One method directly corrects this problem by using an external radioactive source that is transmitted through the patient. This source is used to map the patient's body structures to assess their ability to attenuate radioactive photons. By creating an attenuation map, the computer can then combine the attenuation map with the emission images to correct for missing counts. The resulting image appears to "fill in" the areas that have attenuation artifact and eliminate the defects altogether.

A second method involves performing an ECG-gated study, obtaining images throughout the cardiac cycle. The ECG is monitored, and the R-R interval is divided into 8 or 16 equal segments during which the scan is acquired. The result is a sequence of images that can be played back to back to observe the wall motion throughout the R-R cycle. By obtaining the end diastolic and end systolic volumes, an ejection fraction and regional wall motion can be determined. If a fixed defect is observed to move and thicken normally, it is most likely normal myocardium that has an apparent defect related to attenuation. If a fixed defect does not appear to move, then it is most likely related to a scar. Thus, gating helps to assess whether a defect is related to attenuation artifact or whether it is a real perfusion defect.

11. **How do stress imaging studies compare with routine stress ECG studies in the evaluation of coronary artery disease (CAD)?**
In general, a routine stress ECG is relatively sensitive, with positive ECG stress test results indicating a high likelihood for CAD. However, the accuracy is significantly reduced in patients with abnormal baseline ECGs or a previous history of CAD or if a patient does not achieve 85% of the maximal heart rate for patient age. In these patients, a stress imaging study has a sensitivity of approximately 92% and a specificity of about 72% for detecting CAD. The relative prevalence of CAD in the specific patient population is also a factor. For example, women have a much higher rate of false-positive stress test results because their prestudy risk is much lower than that for male patients.

12. **What is the implication of a reversible defect?**
A reversible defect implies a lack of perfusion during the stress component but normal perfusion during rest. Reversible defects can be caused by attenuation artifact but must always be assumed to be related to CAD, in which the stenotic artery cannot accommodate the extra perfusion demand during stress. The importance of a reversible defect is that the myocardium is intact but is at risk for coronary events. It typically requires a stenosis of at least 50–70% for perfusion to be affected during the stress test. Reversible defects also usually mandate further study with coronary angiography to assess for the extent of blockage of the artery (Fig. 56-4).

13. **Why is transient left ventricular cavity dilation a poor prognostic sign?**
Transient left ventricular cavity dilation refers to the cavity appearing larger on stress images than on resting images. This is in contrast to an individual who has fixed cavity dilation that may be associated with a cardiomyopathy. The implication of transient left ventricular cavity dilation is that during stress, the perfusion abnormalities result in worsening myocardial function such that the heart cannot maintain its usual contractile state and then dilation occurs. This is a poor prognostic sign since there is significant cardiac function and structure that is at risk for an ischemic event.

KEY POINTS: REVERSIBLE DEFECT ON CARDIAC NUCLEAR SCANNING

1. Reversible defect equals lack of perfusion during stress and normal perfusion during rest.
2. Reversible defect implies vessel stenosis of at least 50–70%.
3. Coronary angiography is indicated for further evaluation.

14. **How might a left bundle-branch block (LBBB) on ECG affect imaging findings?**
An LBBB on ECG can cause perfusion defects in the septum during exercise. Therefore, a reversible defect can be observed in patients with LBBB. The cause of this defect has not been

Figure 56-4. Cardiac perfusion scan with Tc-99m sestamibi shows a perfusion defect in the anterior and apical regions on the stress images in both the short axis and vertical long axis *(solid arrows)*. The site of the stress perfusion defect appears to be normal on the resting images *(dotted arrow)*, suggesting that the defect is reversible. The implication is that there is significant atherosclerosis in the artery supplying this territory, which in this case is the left anterior descending artery. It should also be noted that the overall left ventricular cavity size appears dilated on the stress images compared with that on the resting images (see particularly the short axis and vertical long axis images), a finding that implies left ventricular dysfunction during stress.

completely elucidated, although it may be associated with altered depolarization of the septum due to the conduction abnormality or related to left ventricular dilation and dysfunction associated with the LBBB. To minimize the problem of perfusion defects associated with LBBB, a Persantine or adenosine stress test can be performed.

15. **How is a thallium resting-redistribution scan performed? How are the results of a resting-redistribution scan used clinically?**

In a resting-redistribution scan, the patient receives an injection of thallium at rest and then undergoes scanning approximately 15 minutes later. The subject is then scanned approximately 4 hours later and sometimes 24 hours after injection. Images are reconstructed in the typical tomographic projections. The images are evaluated for perfusion and for reversibility of defects observed on the initial scan. The general idea is that a patient with known CAD has several segments of the myocardium that have undergone ischemic injury. The question is whether these segments are viable, which can be determined either because they have some perfusion on initial images or they demonstrate some degree of reversibility. Areas of the myocardium that demonstrate this type of viability will typically respond well after revascularization by regaining some degree of function. Areas that are not viable will typically not respond to revascularization. Therefore, resting-redistribution studies can help to determine what parts of the heart and, hence, what vessels might be the best targets for revascularization.

16. **What is the difference between hibernating and stunned myocardium?**

Stunned myocardium refers to relatively preserved myocardial perfusion as measured by SPECT or PET imaging, normal or decreased glucose metabolism on FDG PET scans, and decreased wall motion on echocardiography. The implication is that there was an ischemic event that caused a reduction in myocardial wall function, even though perfusion and metabolism are now reestablished. The stunning should resolve as long as perfusion is maintained. On the other hand, *hibernating myocardium* refers to decreased perfusion with relatively preserved glucose metabolism and decreased wall motion. The implication is that there is a chronic ischemia that is resulting in decreased flow and function even though the myocardium is still viable. Hibernating myocardium should respond well to attempts to revascularize the region, which would return flow and eventually reverse the functional deficits.

17. **How is an MUGA scan performed?**

The multiple-gate acquisition (MUGA) scan involves the radioactive tagging of the patient's red blood cells (RBCs) so that the blood pool remains radioactive throughout the study (Fig. 56-5). Labeling can be performed either in vitro or in vivo. The in vitro labeling requires blood to be drawn from the patient first, and then the labeling is performed in the laboratory and reinjected into the patient. Alternatively, the RBCs can be labeled in the patient by first injecting stannous pyrophosphate, which allows the RBCs to take up the Tc-99m. Once the patient's RBCs are labeled, images are usually acquired in the left anterior oblique projection and the anterior projection for approximately 15 minutes while the ECG is monitored. The R-R interval is divided into 8 or 16 segments, during which image acquisition occurs. The result is that the activity in the ventricle can be measured throughout the cardiac cycle, and the end diastolic (ED) and end systolic (ES) activity levels can be assessed as well as regional wall motion. The ejection fraction is calculated based on the following equation:

$$(ED - ES) / (ED - BG)$$

The background (BG) counts are also important since placement of the background region over an area with significant activity (e.g., the aorta) will result in a falsely elevated calculated ejection fraction.

18. **How is an MUGA scan used clinically?**

The MUGA scan is primarily used in the evaluation of myocardial wall motion and determination of left ventricular ejection fraction. Both of these can now be assessed with echocardiography, which can also be used to evaluate the structure and function of the heart's valves. For this reason, MUGAs are used relatively infrequently. The principal use is for the determination of ejection fraction in cancer patients before and after they undergo chemotherapy. Patients taking chemotherapeutic agents that can affect cardiac function, such as doxorubicin (Adriamycin),

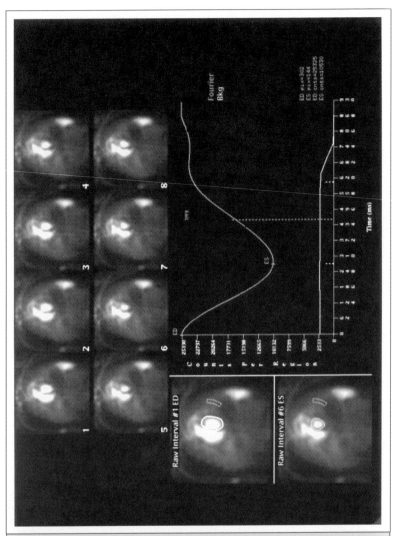

Figure 56-5. A normal MUGA scan showing eight images (top) ranging from end diastole (ED) to end systole (ES) with a subsequent decrease in the overall cavity size and counts. To the left are two images that include regions drawn around the left ventricle on both ED and ES, as well as a background region. These regions help to establish the curve that represents the normal number of counts throughout the cardiac cycle. The background counts are the curve at the bottom. The ejection fraction is calculated on the basis of the ED and ES counts in the left ventricle, which in this case was 61%.

need to have serial measures of cardiac function with the initial scan before therapy. MUGA scans provide true quantitative information regarding ejection fraction since the actual counts of activity within the left ventricular cavity can be assessed (echocardiography determines ejection fraction by estimation). General guidelines suggest that if the ejection fraction falls to less than 40% or has a decrease of more than 15%, the patient should not continue chemotherapy with the same agent.

BIBLIOGRAPHY

1. Bolli R: Myocardial 'stunning' in man. Circulation 86:1671–1691, 1992.

2. Brown KA, Altland E, Rowen M: Prognostic value of normal technetium–99m-sestamibi cardiac imaging. J Nucl Med 14:554–557, 1994.

3. Freeman LM, Blaufox MD: Cardiovascular nuclear medicine, Parts 1 and 2. Semin Nucl Med 19, 1999.

4. Rahimtoola SH: The hibernating myocardium. Am Heart J 117:211–221, 1989.

5. Santano-Boado C, Candell-Riera J, Castell-Conesa J, et al: Diagnostic accuracy of technetium-99m–MIBI myocardial SPECT in women and men. J Nucl Med 39:751–755, 1998.

6. Schwaiger M: Myocardial perfusion imaging with PET. J Nucl Med 35:693–698, 1994.

PEDIATRIC THORACIC RADIOLOGY

D. Andrew Mong, MD

1. **What is the embryologic relationship between the lungs and the gastrointestinal tract?**
   The lung bud is an outpouching of the primitive foregut, appearing during the fourth week of development. This intricate relationship is the basis for tracheoesophageal fistulas (see Chapter 58).

2. **Describe the histologic stages of lung development.**
   The lung bud progressively ramifies during embryologic development, undergoing a pseudo-glandular stage (weeks 5–17); a canalicular stage (weeks 16–25); a terminal sac stage (weeks 25–40); and an alveolar stage, which begins late in fetal life and continues until approximately 8 years.

3. **What is surfactant? Why is it important?**
   Surfactant is produced by type II pneumocytes, which begin to form at approximately 6 months of gestation. It is a complex substance containing phospholipids and apoproteins, which act to reduce surface tension and prevent alveolar collapse.

4. **Describe the pertinent findings on a normal neonatal chest radiograph.**
   The appearance of the thymus is variable but may be visible until 2 years of age. The "sail sign" refers to the thymus creating a triangular shadow of soft tissue along the mediastinal border on chest x-ray. Always check for the side of the aortic arch (normally left-sided). This may be difficult to do in newborns and may need to be inferred by observing that the descending aorta runs to the left of the spine and that the trachea is mildly deviated to the right. Look at heart size. Unlike adults, the cardiac-thoracic ratio may be up to 60%. The apex of the heart should be on the left (levocardia). Pulmonary vascularity should be assessed. This may be difficult, but some clues to increased vascularity include seeing vessels behind the liver shadow or noting that the right descending pulmonary artery is larger in diameter than the trachea. Look at the bones (especially the vertebrae for any segmental anomalies), and note whether the humeral heads have ossified (this happens at 40 weeks of gestation). Look under the diaphragm for organomegaly and the position of the stomach bubble (normally in the left upper quadrant.) Since you will not forget to look at the lung fields, try to make yourself do that last.

5. **What is neonatal respiratory distress syndrome (RDS)? How does it appear radiographically?**
   RDS is a syndrome of premature infants, usually born at less than 36 weeks of gestation, that occurs as a result of surfactant deficiency from underdeveloped type II pneumocytes. This leads to elevated alveolar surface tension and diffuse microatelectasis. The resulting radiographic appearance is a diffuse, symmetric ground-glass appearance to the lung parenchyma with low lung volumes (Fig. 57-1).

6. **How is RDS treated? What are the potential consequences?**
   Maternal steroids have been shown to promote surfactant production if preterm delivery is imminent. Exogenous surfactant administration is beneficial. Infants may require intubation.

Intubation may lead to air leaks in the form of pneumothoraces; pneumomediastinum; or pulmonary interstitial emphysema, which appears as linear interstitial lucencies. Long-term consequences of barotrauma and increased oxygen exposure include neonatal chronic lung disease, which may manifest as diffuse interstitial thickening and hyperaeration.

Figure 57-1. Frontal chest radiograph of a premature infant with diffuse ground-glass lung disease and low lung volumes, which is indicative of RDS. (Courtesy Richard Markowitz, Children's Hospital of Philadelphia.)

7. **In addition to RDS, what are other neonatal diffuse lung diseases? How might they be differentiated clinically?**
Other neonatal diffuse lung diseases include transient tachypnea of the newborn (TTN), congestive heart failure (CHF), neonatal pneumonia, and meconium aspiration. Neonatal pneumonia may occur in the preterm or term infant. Meconium aspiration and TTN are generally diseases of term infants, and CHF and pneumonia may occur in either.

KEY POINTS: CAUSES OF NEONATAL DIFFUSE LUNG DISEASE

1. Respiratory distress syndrome

2. Transient tachypnea of the newborn

3. Congestive heart failure

4. Pneumonia

5. Meconium aspiration

8. **What is the mechanism behind meconium aspiration? How does it appear radiographically?**
Perinatal hypoxia may lead to both a deep gasping reflex and premature passage of meconium, which combine to cause aspiration. Meconium aspiration may cause hyperaeration (sometimes the sole radiographic appearance), scattered areas of atelectasis, and ropelike perihilar radiations.

9. **What is TTN? How does it appear on a chest radiograph?**
TTN results from inadequate clearance of fetal serum from the lung parenchyma during the transition to aerated lung at birth. A primary stimulus for clearance is passage during the birth canal, so infants delivered by cesarean section are at increased risk. This is usually a benign process that resolves within 2–3 days, although in rare cases, infants may require intubation.

Radiographically, it appears as mild CHF, with an enlarged heart, increased interstitial markings, and pleural effusions.

10. **Name the major causes of CHF in a newborn.**

TTN, as described, may look like CHF. Causes of CHF in the newborn include constitutional problems, such as anemia, hypoglycemia, sepsis; primary pump problems, such as hypoplastic left heart; outflow obstructions, such as aortic stenosis or coarctation of the aorta; inflow problems, such as cor triatriatum or mitral valve stenosis; and extracardiac shunts, such as a vein of Galen malformation or a hepatic hemangioendothelioma.

11. **What is the role of the radiologist in assessing suspected congenital heart disease (CHD)?**

Even though magnetic resonance (MR) examination of the heart (beyond the scope of this chapter) may be used to assess cardiac chamber size and position, wall thickness, the presence of intracardiac shunts, and the position of the coronary arteries, the initial role of the radiologist is to evaluate the chest radiograph and to provide an ordered, logical differential diagnosis. It is usually not possible to give a precise diagnosis in these cases.

12. **What are the most common acyanotic CHDs?**

The first consideration in diagnosing CHD should be whether the infant is clinically cyanotic. Acyanosis implies a left-to-right shunt, and the most common causes include atrial septal defect (ASD), ventricular septal defect (VSD), patent ductus arteriosus (PDA), and endocardial cushion defects. These typically cause enlargement of specific chambers in the heart due to decompression of some chambers and overload in others. A VSD, for example, will result in an enlarged right ventricle, main pulmonary artery, and left atrium, but the left ventricle will be normal in size as blood is shunted away from it. An ASD will typically result in an enlarged right atrium and right ventricle but a normal-sized left atrium.

13. **How does assessment of pulmonary blood flow aid in the diagnoses of cyanotic CHD?**

Cyanosis implies either admixture of oxygenated and deoxygenated blood, which would appear as increased blood flow in the heart, or that blood is shunted away from the lungs, which would appear as decreased blood flow. Assessment of blood flow includes looking for shunt vessels at the periphery of the lung fields or behind the liver shadow.

14. **Which CHDs appear with cyanosis and increased pulmonary blood flow?**

These include total anomalous pulmonary venous return, truncus arteriosus, transposition of the great vessels, tricuspid atresia, and single ventricle. Hypoplastic left heart syndrome may also appear with CHF and cyanosis.

15. **What is the importance of a right-sided aortic arch?**

A right-sided arch may demonstrate mirror-image branching or an aberrant left subclavian artery (see question 18). A right-sided arch may be associated with tetralogy of Fallot or truncus arteriosus. If you see a right-sided aortic arch, look for other anomalies and consider recommending echocardiography.

16. **What are the major surgical diseases of the neonatal chest?**

Surgical neonatal chest disease is generally a focal process and includes entities such as congenital diaphragmatic hernia (CDH), congenital cystic adenomatoid malformation (CCAM), pulmonary sequestration, and congenital lobar emphysema. Even though these entities may appear solid at birth, CDH, CCAM, and congenital lobar emphysema will usually aerate over time. Pulmonary sequestrations and certain types of CCAM will remain solid unless there is superinfection (Fig. 57-2).

17. What is the most common cause of a neonatal pleural effusion?

A chylothorax. The etiologic factor of these effusions is uncertain, but it may be secondary to birth trauma of the thoracic duct. These are typically treated conservatively, with drainage of the effusion and administration of a medium-chain triglyceride diet.

18. Describe the two main types of vascular rings.

Vascular rings may cause constriction of the trachea and esophagus, creating stridor or dysphagia. A ring around the trachea and esophagus may be formed by a double aortic arch or by a right-sided arch with an aberrant left subclavian artery. In the latter case, the ring is completed by the ligamentum arteriosum. A vascular ring may be suspected if lateral compressions on the trachea on a chest radiograph are noted. Traditionally, rings were evaluated with a barium swallow, which would show a posterior external compression on the esophagus (with either type of ring). Today, these are often evaluated with MR imaging.

Figure 57-2. CCAM may be seen as several large cysts, multiple small cysts, or microscopic cysts that appear solid. The appearance of this frontal chest radiograph could also be due to congenital lobar emphysema. (Courtesy Richard Markowitz, MD, Children's Hospital of Philadelphia.)

KEY POINTS: CAUSES OF FOCAL NEONATAL LUNG DISEASE

1. Congenital diaphragmatic hernia

2. Congenital cystic adenomatoid malformation

3. Congenital lobar emphysema

4. Pulmonary sequestration

19. How does a pulmonary sling cause symptoms?

A pulmonary sling refers to anomalous origin of the left pulmonary artery from the right pulmonary artery, with the left artery coursing abnormally between the trachea and esophagus. Patients typically present with wheezing or even respiratory distress. There is a high association with complete cartilaginous rings of the trachea (as opposed to the incomplete horse-shoe cartilaginous components in a normal patient), which are often the cause of the patient's symptoms.

20. **How do heterotaxia syndromes manifest in the lungs?**
Heterotaxia syndromes refer to situs ambiguous, when the organs conform neither to the normal situs solitus confirmation nor to the situs inversus (complete mirror image.) In heterotaxia, the liver is midline and the stomach bubble may be to the right or left of midline. Heterotaxia syndromes are typically divided into polysplenia and asplenia. In polysplenia, both the abdomen and chest are "left-sided." Findings include multiple spleens, azygous continuation of the inferior vena cava, and absence of the gallbladder. In the chest, polysplenia syndrome includes two "left-sided lungs," so there are bilateral bilobed lungs with hyparterial bronchi (under the pulmonary arteries). In asplenia, the abdomen and chest are right-sided. The spleen is absent. In the chest, asplenia syndrome includes two right-sided lungs that have three lobes and eparterial bronchi (above the pulmonary arteries). Both asplenia and polysplenia are associated with gastrointestinal malrotation and CHD, although CHD in polysplenia tends to be milder than in asplenia.

21. **Describe how chlamydial pneumonia presents clinically and radiographically.**
Chlamydial pneumonia is a disease of neonates, usually presenting within the first 2 weeks of life, often with associated conjunctivitis. Chest radiographs usually demonstrate hyperinflation and ill-defined linear markings, sometimes creating a shaggy appearance of the cardiac border.

22. **What are the pulmonary and extrapulmonary manifestations of cystic fibrosis?**
Cystic fibrosis is an autosomal recessive disorder of abnormal chloride ion transport, which results in backup of thick mucous secretions in various organs. In the lungs, this manifests as repeated infections that result in bronchiectasis, predominantly in the upper lobes. On plain films, bronchiectasis may appear as multiple lucent holes or a tram-track appearance of the bronchi, which may be fluid filled. On computed tomography (CT) examination, bronchiectasis is defined as bronchi that are larger in diameter than the adjacent pulmonary arteries. Extrapulmonary manifestations include neonatal meconium ileus (small bowel obstruction at the terminal ileum from inspissated meconium), chronic pancreatitis, and cirrhosis. Check for an enlarged spleen, which may result from portal hypertension. This may be manifest on a chest radiograph as medial deviation of the stomach bubble in the left upper quadrant.

23. **What are the findings of primary tuberculosis of the lungs in a pediatric patient?**
These are nonspecific, as in an adult, but can include mediastinal and/or hilar adenopathy, pulmonary parenchymal disease, and pleural effusion.

24. **Who suffers from acute chest syndrome?**
Patients with sickle cell anemia. *Acute chest syndrome* refers to alveolar edema, which appears radiographically as scattered dense areas of consolidation. This is usually difficult to differentiate from bacteria pneumonia.

25. **What is lymphocytic interstitial pneumonia (LIP)?**
LIP is a lymphoproliferative response in the chest, often to HIV. Radiographically, LIP appears as multiple interstitial nodules. This pattern is much more common in children than in adults. The differential diagnosis of multiple pulmonary nodules includes Langerhans' cell histiocytosis, miliary infections such as tuberculosis or histoplasmosis, hypersensitivity pneumonitis, viral etiologies such as varicella, and metastatic disease.

26. **How should a suspected aspirated foreign body be evaluated?**
A nonradiopaque aspirated foreign body in a mainstem bronchus may produce a ball-valve effect, trapping air unilaterally and creating a large lucent lung compared with the contralateral normal size. These findings may be subtle, but if suspected, expiratory films may make them

more obvious because the unaffected lung will lose volume, whereas the affected lung will not. Decubitus films may also exaggerate this difference, with the unaffected lung losing volume when it is in the dependent position. Air trapping may also be demonstrated by fluoroscopy.

27. **What is Swyer-James syndrome?**
The hypothesized pathogenesis of Swyer-James syndrome involves a viral infection that arrests growth of an affected lung through an obliterative bronchiolitis. This results in hyperlucency from air trapping and diminished arterial flow. Traditionally, this was thought to be a unilateral process, but CT examinations often demonstrate scattered areas of bilateral air trapping.

28. **What are important structures to identify on a lateral view of the neck?**
Assess the prevertebral soft tissues. Soft tissue swelling in this area could be due to retropharyngeal abscess, edema, hematoma, or soft tissue mass. The epiglottis should be triangular or flat, not bulbous or thumblike (which would indicate epiglottitis!), and the aryepiglottic folds should not be thickened. Look for enlargement of the adenoid tissue and tonsils. Assess the caliber of the trachea, which should not change abruptly. You may identify sloughed membranes within the lumen from bacterial tracheitis. A frontal radiograph is often useful in identifying croup, characterized by symmetric subglottic narrowing that creates the steeple sign from loss of the normal subglottic shoulders (Figs. 57-3 and 57-4).

Figure 57-3. Abnormal bulbous thickening of the epiglottis *(arrows)*. This finding reflects epiglottitis, an emergency requiring intubation. (Courtesy Richard Markowitz, Children's Hospital of Philadelphia.)

Figure 57-4. Frontal plain film of the soft tissues of the neck shows the classic steeple sign *(arrows)* of croup, with loss of the normal subglottic shoulders.

BIBLIOGRAPHY

1. Alford BA, McIlhenny J: An approach to the asymmetric neonatal chest radiograph. Radiol Clin North Am 37(6):1079–1092, 1999.

2. Berdon WE: Rings, slings, and other things: Vascular compression of the infant trachea updated from the mid-century to the millennium—the legacy of Robert E. Gross, MD, and Edward B.D. Neuhauser, MD. Radiology 216(3):624–632, 2000.
3. Gibson AT, Steiner GM: Imaging the neonatal chest. Clin Radiol 52(3):172–186, 1997.
4. Strife JL, Sze RW: Radiographic evaluation of the neonate with congenital heart disease. Radiol Clin North Am 37(6):1093–1107, 1999.

CHAPTER 58

PEDIATRIC GASTROINTESTINAL RADIOLOGY

Kerry Bron, MD, and Avrum N. Pollock, MD

1. **What are the most common causes of small bowel obstruction in a child?**
   AAIIMM is a mnemonic that makes it easy to remember the causes.
   A = *A*dhesions, usually postsurgical
   A = *A*ppendicitis
   I = *I*ntussusception
   I = *I*ncarcerated inguinal hernia
   M = *M*alrotation with volvulus or bands
   M = *M*iscellaneous, such as Meckel's diverticulum or intestinal duplication

2. **What is intussusception? What causes it?**
   Intussusception is a condition in which a proximal portion of the bowel (intussusceptum) tele-scopes into the adjacent distal bowel (intussuscipiens). When the inner loop and its mesentery become obstructed, a small bowel obstruction occurs. In most cases this condition is idiopathic. In <5% of cases, the intussusception contains a lead point, such as a polyp, Meckel's diverticulum, or hypertrophic lymphatic tissue. Most intussusceptions are ileocolic.

3. **What are the clinical signs of intussusception?**
   The classic clinical triad of intussusception is intermittent colicky abdominal pain, current jelly stools, and a palpable abdominal mass. However, fewer than 50% of patients present with these symptoms. Children often cry and are very irritable during bouts of abdominal pain and then become drowsy and lethargic. Vomiting and fever may also occur. Intussusception is most common in children between the ages of 3 months and 4 years, with a peak incidence at 3–9 months. It is more common in boys.

4. **How is intussusception diagnosed radiographically?**
   The most accurate technique for the diagnosis of intussusception is ultrasound. The characteris-tic sonographic appearance is a mass that measures 3–5 cm, which is easily detectable. On the transverse scan the mass has a "target" appearance that contains echogenic fat. The "pseudokidney" sign appears in the longitudinal direction. A barium enema can also be used to diagnose intussusception.

   Although the plain film has been used in the past to diagnose intussusception by detection of a soft tissue mass in the right upper quadrant and lack of large bowel gas, particularly in the right upper quadrant, studies have shown poor interobserver agreement and predictive value of only approximately 50%.

5. **How is an intussusception treated? How can one tell that an intussusception has been successfully reduced?**
   An intussusception is treated by air enema with fluoroscopic guidance or hydrostatic enema using barium or water-soluble contrast (Fig. 58-1). The advantages of the air enema are that it is quicker, less messy, easier to perform, and delivers less radiation to the patient. The only con-traindications to enema reduction of intussusception are pneumoperitoneum or peritonitis. The air enema generates pressure up to 120 mmHg to reduce the intussusception.

If a successful air reduction has been performed, fluid with air bubbles should be seen passing through the ileocecal valve into the terminal ileum. If a successful reduction with contrast has been performed, contrast must reflux into multiple loops of small bowel. If reflux into the small bowel is not seen, the intussusception may not have been completely reduced and a distal lead point may have been overlooked.

Figure 58-1. Spot radiograph from a contrast enema examination demonstrates intussusception, with the lead point outlined by the barium.

6. **Describe the "double bubble" sign, and name the conditions in which it is found.**

   The "double bubble" sign is found on plain radiographs and represents an air- or fluid-filled distended stomach and duodenal bulb (Fig. 58-2). It is seen in malrotation, duodenal atresia, and jejunal atresia.

7. **What is malrotation of the intestines?**

   Malrotation of the intestines is a misnomer since it is really nonrotation or incomplete rotation of the bowel. To understand malrotation, one must first consider normal embryologic rotation of the intestines. During normal embryologic development in the first trimester, the mid-gut leaves the abdominal cavity, travels into the umbilical cord, and then returns to the abdominal cavity. As the intestines return, the proximal and distal parts of the mid-gut rotate around the superior mesenteric artery axis 270 degrees in a counterclockwise direction. The ligament of Treitz (duodenojejunal junction) lands in the left upper quadrant, and the cecum comes to rest in the right lower quadrant.

Figure 58-2. Plain film of the abdomen in a child with duodenal atresia, demonstrating a dilated stomach and duodenal bulb, the "double bubble" sign.

   In malrotation, this intestinal rotation and fixation occur abnormally. If normal rotation does not occur, the cecum is not anchored in the right lower quadrant and may be midline or in the upper abdomen. The small bowel is not anchored in the left upper quadrant and may lie entirely in the right abdomen.

KEY POINTS: INTUSSUSCEPTION

1. A relatively common cause of small bowel obstruction in children

2. Idiopathic in children, unlike in adults

3. Usually ileocolic

4. Diagnosed by ultrasound

5. Treated with air enema or contrast barium enema

---

8. **What are Ladd's bands?**
   Ladd's bands are dense peritoneal bands that develop as an attempt to fix the bowel to the abdominal wall in malrotation. They may extend from the malpositioned cecum across the duodenum to the posterolateral abdomen and porta hepatis in either incomplete rotation or nonrotation and can cause extrinsic duodenal obstruction.

9. **How does a mid-gut volvulus occur? Why is this an emergency?**
   Lack of attachment of the mid-gut to the posterior abdominal wall allows the mid-gut to twist on a shortened root mesentery, which results from lack of complete rotation (Fig. 58-3). This twisting is called a *volvulus,* and it causes small bowel obstruction with concomitant obstruction to the lymphatic and venous supply of the bowel and eventually to the arterial supply, which leads to ischemia and necrosis. If it is not repaired within several hours, all of the intestine supplied by the superior mesenteric artery will infarct.

Figure 58-3. Spot radiograph from an upper gastrointestinal (GI) examination demonstrating the "corkscrew" finding of a mid-gut volvulus.

10. **Does a patient with malrotation always present with clinical symptoms, and what is the clinical presentation?**
    Not all patients with malrotation are symptomatic because not all develop a mid-gut volvulus or extrinsic duodenal obstruction from Ladd's bands. Patients with incomplete rotation who have intestinal obstruction usually present within the first week or first month of life (75% of patients). They present with an acute onset of bilious vomiting, which is a surgical emergency. Some patients present later in childhood with intermittent mechanical obstruction, which manifests as cyclic vomiting. Malrotation in the remainder of patients is often found incidentally when the patients are studied for other complaints.

11. **Which study is the gold standard for diagnosing malrotation?**
    The upper gastrointestinal (GI) examination. To confirm normal rotation of the bowel, the ligament of Treitz, which attaches the third and fourth parts of the duodenum, must be visualized to the left of midline. If there is malrotation, the ligament of Treitz may be located to the right of

midline or in the midline. Often, there is inversion of the superior mesenteric artery and vein, which can be visualized on computed tomography.

12. **What other anomalies are associated with malrotation?**
Duodenal atresia or stenosis, Meckel's diverticulum, omphalocele, gastroschisis, polysplenia/asplenia syndromes, situs ambiguous, Bochdalek's hernia, and renal anomalies.

KEY POINTS: MALROTATION OF THE INTESTINES

1. Causes small bowel obstruction through a mid-gut volvulus and Ladd's bands

2. Causes altered GI anatomy, with the ligament of Treitz not situated in the left upper quadrant and the cecum not in the right lower quadrant

13. **What is the clinical presentation of pyloric stenosis?**
Hypertrophic pyloric stenosis, which is the most common GI surgical disease of infancy in the United States, presents most commonly during the second to sixth weeks of life, with a peak incidence at 3 weeks of age and rare presentation after 3 months of life. The major symptom is progressive nonbilious vomiting, which starts as simple regurgitation and progresses to projectile vomiting. This progressive vomiting leads to dehydration and hypochloremic metabolic alkalosis and weight loss. The condition is more common in boys. A palpable "olive" representing the thickened pylorus muscle is present in the right upper quadrant approximately 80% of the time if the infant can be examined in a calm manner with decreased stomach distention.

14. **If the "olive" cannot be palpated, how can pyloric stenosis be diagnosed with radiologic studies?**
The evaluation can begin with a supine or prone plain film of the abdomen, which can exclude other diagnoses that could be causing similar obstructive symptoms. It will also reveal a markedly dilated stomach, soft tissue mass projecting into the gastric antrum, and paucity of gas in the distal bowel. The suspicion of pyloric stenosis can be confirmed with either ultrasound or fluoroscopy. Ultrasound is the imaging test of choice because it directly visualizes the hypertrophied pylorus muscle without radiation (Fig. 58-4), whereas the upper GI series infers the presence of pyloric stenosis indirectly. With ultrasound, the pylorus muscle is seen as a hypoechoic structure greater than

Figure 58-4. Ultrasound examination of the pylorus demonstrates hypertrophic pyloric stenosis. The thickened walls of the pylorus *(asterisks)* surround the central lumen *(arrows)*.

4 mm thick surrounding an echogenic compressed pyloric channel. Although less sensitive, the pyloric channel length is another measurement used to make the diagnosis. A length greater than 17 mm is considered diagnostic for pyloric stenosis.

15. **What is Meckel's diverticulum?**
    Meckel's diverticulum is the most common anomaly of the GI tract. It is a persistence of the omphalomesenteric duct at its junction with the ileum. It can be remembered by the rules of two: It occurs in 2% of the population; 2% develop complications; complications usually occur before 2 years of age; and it is located within 2 feet of the ileocecal valve. The most common complication of Meckel's diverticulum is painless GI bleeding, which occurs secondary to irritation or ulceration from production of hydrochloric acid by the gastric mucosa that lines it.

16. **How is Meckel's diverticulum diagnosed?**
    Meckel's diverticulum is detected by a nuclear medicine scan with technetium 99m pertechnetate. The tracer accumulates within the diverticulum, usually appearing at or approximately at the same time as activity in the stomach, with gradually increasing intensity, which verifies the presence of ectopic gastric mucosa.

17. **What are the most common causes of GI bleeding in children?**
    The differential diagnosis depends on the age of the patient (Table 58-1).

TABLE 58-1. COMMON CAUSES OF GI BLEEDING IN CHILDREN			
Newborn and Neonate (<1 mo)	**Young Infant (1–3 mo)**	**Older Infant (3 mo–1 yr)**	**Child (1–10 yr)**
Swallowed maternal blood	Esophagitis	Esophagitis	Esophagitis
Anal fissure	Intussusception	Anal fissure	Esophageal varices
Necrotizing enterocolitis	Anal fissure	Colon polyp	Colon polyp
Hemorrhagic disease of the newborn	Gangrenous bowel	Intussusception	Anal fissure
Allergic or infectious colitis	Meckel's diverticulum	Gangrenous bowel	Foreign body
		Foreign body	Crohn's disease
			Ulcerative colitis

18. **What causes necrotizing enterocolitis (NEC)? Who develops this condition?**
    NEC is a multifactorial condition that has traditionally been thought to be caused by hypoxia, infection, and enteral feeding. The pathology of NEC resembles that of ischemic necrosis. It may be that the main pathologic trigger in NEC is injury to the intestinal mucosa, which can be caused by different factors in different patients. Approximately 80% of patients who develop NEC are premature infants. Older infants who develop NEC usually have severe underlying medical problems such as Hirschsprung's disease or congenital heart disease. Patients with this condition present with abdominal distention, vomiting, increased gastric residuals, blood in the stool, lethargy, apnea, and temperature instability.

19. **What findings of NEC can be seen on x-ray, and what is the role of the radiologist?**
    The radiographic findings of NEC are very nonspecific when the condition is first suspected. Films are obtained serially; the role of the radiologist is to try to diagnose the condition before bowel perforation occurs. In early NEC, the most commonly detected abnormality is diffuse gaseous distention of the intestine. A more useful sign of early NEC is loss of the normal symmetric bowel gas pattern, with a resulting disorganized or asymmetric pattern. In more advanced NEC, the finding of pneumatosis intestinalis (intramural gas) is pathognomonic for the

condition (Fig. 58-5). Gas in the portal venous system is another pathognomonic finding in NEC, which occurs in 10–30% of cases. Babies at risk for imminent perforation often have portal venous gas. They may have the persistent loop sign, which is a dilated loop of intestine that remains unchanged over 24–36 hours. Another grave sign is a shift from a pattern of generalized dilation to asymmetric bowel dilation. Ascites is another sign of impending perforation. Once pneumoperitoneum develops, this is a definite sign that the bowel has perforated and the baby must have surgery.

20. **What are other causes of pneumoperitoneum in infants and children?**
The most common causes are surgery and instrumentation. Pneumoperitoneum can be found after laparotomy, after paracentesis, or after resuscitation. Also, distal bowel obstruction from conditions such as Hirschsprung's disease or meconium ileus and dissection of air from pneumomediastinum, a ruptured ulcer, or Meckel's diverticulum can cause pneumoperitoneum.

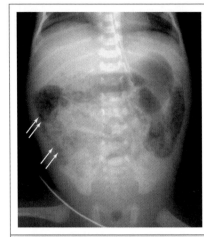

Figure 58-5. Plain film radiograph of the abdomen in a patient with NEC. The mottled pattern of air in the bowel wall *(arrows)* is typical of NEC.

21. **What is Hirschsprung's disease?**
Hirschsprung's disease is a condition of distal aganglionic bowel that results from the lack of Auerbach's (intermuscular) and Meissner's (submucosal) plexuses. This leads to a functional obstruction of the distal bowel. It usually presents in the first 48 hours of life with the failure to pass meconium, or it may present with abdominal distention, bilious vomiting, or diarrhea. More than 80% of patients present in the first 6 weeks of life.

22. **What are the x-ray findings of Hirschsprung's disease? Is this condition diagnosed definitively by imaging?**
The most typical plain film finding of Hirschsprung's disease is a dilated colon proximal to the distal and smaller aganglionic segment. X-rays may also demonstrate a high-grade distal bowel obstruction. Radiologic diagnosis of Hirschsprung's disease requires a contrast enema (Fig. 58-6). Spot radiographs are obtained in the lateral and oblique projections, and the examination is stopped

Figure 58-6. Lateral spot radiograph from a barium enema examination in a patient with Hirschsprung's disease demonstrates a transition zone (from dilated to nondilated bowel) in the distal colon.

after a transition zone has been identified. The barium enema can demonstrate the transition zone, which is situated between a narrowed aganglionic segment and the distended proximal bowel. The x-ray transition zone may be visualized more distally than the histologic transition zone secondary to stool dilating the proximal part of the aganglionic segment. To make a definitive diagnosis of Hirschsprung's disease, a rectal biopsy must be obtained that shows lack of ganglion cells.

23. **Name the types of tracheoesophageal fistulas (TEFs). How common is each type?**
    The most common type of TEF is esophageal atresia with distal esophageal communication with the tracheobronchial tree (Fig. 58-7). This accounts for more than 80% of cases. The next most common type is esophageal atresia without a TEF, which accounts for almost 10% of cases. The H-type fistulas occur between an otherwise intact trachea and esophagus and account for approximately 5% of cases. Esophageal atresias occurring with both proximal and distal communication with the trachea are found in fewer than 2% of cases, and esophageal atresia with proximal communication is rare. TEF is associated with the VACTERL syndromes (in which affected patients manifest at least three of the following: *v*ertebral anomalies, *a*nal atresia/imperforate anus, *c*ardiac anomalies, *t*racheo*e*sophageal fistula, *r*enal anomalies, and *l*imb anomalies).

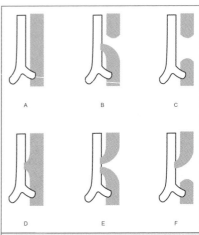

Figure 58-7. Different types of TEFs. (A) Normal relationship of the esophagus anterior to the trachea: no atresia or fistula. (B) Esophageal atresia with distal TEF—most common (>80%). (C) Esophageal atresia with no TEF (~10%). (D) H-type fistula with no esophageal atresia (~5%). (E) Esophageal atresia with proximal and distal fistulas (<2%). (F) Esophageal atresia with a proximal fistula (1%).

24. **What are the plain film findings in TEF?**
    In a patient with esophageal atresia (and no fistula or a proximal fistula), the plain x-ray may reveal a gasless abdomen. A nasogastric tube may be seen coiled in the proximal esophagus. Patients with esophageal atresia with a distal TEF or an H-type fistula may present with a distended abdomen. Aspiration is a risk for all patients with esophageal atresia.

25. **How can a plain x-ray help to differentiate a coin in the esophagus from a coin in the trachea?**
    On a plain chest x-ray, a coin in the esophagus will be visualized as a round object en face (a full circle can be seen) (Fig. 58-8), and a coin in the trachea will lie sagittally and appear end-on in a posteroanterior film.

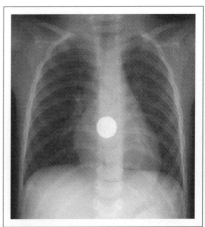

Figure 58-8. Posteroanterior plain film of the chest demonstrates a coin in the esophagus.

BIBLIOGRAPHY

1. Buonomo C: The radiology of necrotizing enterocolitis. Radiol Clin North Am 37:1187–1197, 1999.

2. Daneman A, Alton D: Intussusception: Issues and controversies related to diagnosis and reduction. Radiol Clin North Am 34:743–755, 1996.

3. Hayden K: Ultrasonography of the acute pediatric abdomen. Radiol Clin North Am 34:791–806, 1996.

4. Hernanz-Schulman M: Imaging of neonatal gastrointestinal obstruction. Radiol Clin North Am 37:1163–1185, 1999.

5. Kirks DR: Practical Pediatric Imaging: Diagnostic Imaging of Infants and Children, 3rd ed. Philadelphia, Lippincott-Raven, 1997.

6. McAlister W, Kronemer K: Emergency gastrointestinal radiology of the newborn. Radiol Clin North Am 34:819–844, 1996.

7. Merten D: Practical approaches to pediatric gastrointestinal radiology. Radiol Clin North Am 31:1395–1407, 1993.

CHAPTER 59

PEDIATRIC URORADIOLOGY

Richard D. Bellah, MD

1. **What is the role of the radiologist in pediatric urinary tract infection (UTI)?**
   UTIs that occur and recur in some children are the result of many interrelated factors, most of which the radiologist cannot assess. Generally speaking, UTI results when bacterial virulence outweighs host resistance. One important factor affecting host resistance that the radiologist can assess is whether there is impairment of unidirectional flow of urine out of the urinary tract, resulting in urinary stasis and predisposing infants and children to UTI.

2. **What conditions can be detected radiologically that impair normal urinary flow?**
   Urinary tract obstruction (congenital), vesicoureteral reflux (VUR), and dysfunctional voiding (e.g., neurogenic bladder) (Fig. 59-1).

3. **Which imaging tests should be used to diagnose these conditions?**
   Renal and bladder sonography and voiding cystourethrography (VCUG).

4. **Why is renal and bladder sonography used?**
   Renal and bladder sonography should be used to detect hydronephrosis due to obstruction or VUR and to assess for any renal parenchymal damage that may have been caused by prior infections.

5. **When should renal and bladder sonography be performed?**
   Sonography should be performed within several weeks after an initial UTI is diagnosed, but sooner if the child fails to respond to conventional antibiotic therapy. (Also, as a result of the routine use of prenatal sonography, hydronephrosis is often detected in utero, and UTI can be prevented by prophylactically administering antibiotics to the infant.)

Figure 59-1. Dysfunctional voiding. Fluoroscopic spot view of the bladder and urethra at VCUG shows mild bladder wall trabeculation. A small amount of VUR is seen on the right *(arrow)*. The urethra has a "spinning top" configuration.

6. **How is VCUG performed?**
   The bladder is catheterized using sterile technique, and under fluoroscopy, the bladder is filled to capacity with iodinated contrast. The catheter is then removed, and the child voids on the fluoroscopy table. During the procedure, the anatomy of the lower urinary tract and bladder function are examined, a series of radiographic images are obtained, and the presence or absence of reflux of contrast (i.e., VUR) into the ureters is determined.

7. How is VCUG modified in infants?

A cyclic study is typically performed. Infants usually void around the small catheter that is placed through the urethra into the bladder; thus multiple cycles of voiding and bladder filling are studied. This also increases the probability that reflux, if present, will be elicited.

8. When should VCUG be performed?

VCUG should be performed after a first UTI in both boys and girls and generally after the bladder infection is treated.

In *boys,* routine fluoroscopic VCUG is recommended as the initial examination, particularly to study the urethral anatomy (e.g., to look for valves in the posterior urethra, a common cause of lower urinary tract obstruction in young boys).

In *girls,* either routine VCUG can be done or a voiding urethrogram can be performed by instilling a radionuclide into the bladder. The latter procedure is performed in the nuclear medicine department; images are obtained with a gamma camera, and reflux is detected when the radionuclide (which is diluted in the sterile saline that is placed in the bladder via a catheter) reaches the ureter during the instillation of contrast and/or during voiding.

9. What are the pros and cons of a radionuclide cystogram compared with fluoroscopic VCUG?

Fluoroscopic VCUG provides anatomic detail but at a much higher radiation dose. The radionuclide cystogram is highly sensitive for detecting reflux because the child is continuously monitored by the gamma camera, but at the expense of good anatomic detail. The radionuclide cystogram is particularly useful for follow-up studies that assess for resolution of previously detected VUR and is also useful for screening siblings of patients with known reflux.

10. What is primary VUR?

VUR occurs either primarily or secondarily. Primary reflux is due to "immaturity" or abnormality of the ureterovesical junction (UVJ), which allows urine to ascend into the ureters during bladder filling or voiding. Generally, reflux is related to ureteral orifice size as well as the length of the ureter as it tunnels into the bladder.

11. What is secondary VUR?

Secondary reflux occurs as the result of an abnormality of the UVJ, such as a distal ureteral diverticulum or a ureterocele (an outpouching of the ureter that extends into the bladder). Secondary reflux may also occur as a result of bladder outlet obstruction or due to a neurogenic bladder.

12. How is primary reflux graded?

Primary reflux is graded on a scale from 1 to 5, based on the degree of ureteral and pelvicaliceal (renal collecting system) filling and dilation (Fig. 59-2). In addition to providing the referring physician with a visual description of the degree of reflux, assigning a grade also gives the clinician an idea of the likelihood of spontaneous resolution (e.g., 80% of grade 2 reflux resolve within 3 years).

GRADES OF REFLUX

Figure 59-2. Grading of primary VUR. Reflux is graded according to the degree of ureteral and pelvicaliceal filling. The higher the grade, the less likelihood of spontaneous resolution.

13. **What is dysfunctional voiding?**
Dysfunctional voiding may be due to either a neurogenic bladder or the so-called "pediatric unstable bladder." The bladder may show variable degrees of thickening, trabeculation, and alteration in contour and storage capacity (*see* Fig. 59-1). Bladder-sphincter dyssynergia may be indicated by the presence of a dilated posterior urethra caused by the external sphincter failing to relax as the bladder neck opens. This often leads to high-pressure voiding, incomplete emptying, and urine retention.

14. **What diagnostic tests are useful for the detection of acute and chronic pyelonephritis in children?**
Renal cortical scintigraphy (nuclear scan), contrast-enhanced computed tomography (CT), and renal sonography. Pyelonephritis may be difficult to diagnose accurately, especially in infants and young children who cannot give a history. It may be difficult to distinguish between uncomplicated UTI and pyelonephritis (with or without subsequent complications such as renal abscess) on the basis of physical examination, history, and laboratory studies. Therefore, imaging plays an important role in the work-up of children with known or suspected UTI.

15. **What are the findings on a renal nuclear scan in acute and chronic infection?**
A renal cortical nuclear scan reveals parenchymal defects in children with acute infection due to focal areas of edema and inflammation. These defects revert to normal if the process completely resolves. However, in chronic infection or chronic pyelonephritis secondary to reflux nephropathy, residual areas of scar appear as persistent cortical defects on follow-up examinations.

16. **What are the CT findings associated with pyelonephritis?**
A contrast-enhanced CT is somewhat less sensitive than a renal cortical nuclear scan for the detection of acute infection. Acute infection is seen as wedge-shaped areas of decreased density in the kidney. Areas of scar related to prior infection can also be identified. CT is particularly helpful when abscess formation is suspected.

17. **How useful is renal sonography in the work-up of suspected pyelonephritis?**
Gray-scale sonography is limited in its ability to depict acute pyelonephritis. The sensitivity of ultrasound, however, is increased when power Doppler ultrasound is used (Fig. 59-3). The latter technique is an advance in Doppler ultrasound, which depicts normal and abnormal blood flow in a manner that is independent of the direction of the flow; therefore, power Doppler is more sensitive than routine color Doppler. Renal sonography may also be used to assess for significant renal scarring due to chronic pyelonephritis. Small focal scars may be difficult to detect with sonography, however.

18. **What are the most common forms of congenital hydronephrosis?**
   - Ureteropelvic junction (UPJ) obstruction
   - UVJ obstruction, commonly referred to as "primary obstructive megaureter"
   - VUR

Figure 59-3. Acute pyelonephritis. Power Doppler sonography demonstrates a focal area of decreased perfusion within the upper pole of the kidney *(open arrows)*. This finding corresponds to an area of pyelonephritis.

- Renal and ureteral duplication anomalies
- Posterior urethral valves
- Prune-belly syndrome

19. **When should a postnatal renal and bladder sonogram be obtained in a patient with congenital hydronephrosis?**
A postnatal renal and bladder sonogram should be performed on any infant with dilation of the renal pelvis that is detected prenatally on sonography, if the renal pelvis measures ≥4 mm before 33 weeks of gestation and ≥7 mm after 33 weeks of gestation. A renal pelvic diameter less than 4 mm seen on sonography at birth has been shown to normalize spontaneously within 1 year. In boys with bilateral hydroureteronephrosis, this sonogram should be obtained soon after birth to assess for posterior urethral valves. Otherwise, the initial sonogram should be done at 5–7 days after birth (when the glomerular filtration rate is greater than it is immediately after birth).

20. **What are the roles of nuclear medicine, VCUG, IV urography, and MR in congenital hydronephrosis?**
VCUG should be performed to assess for reflux and to determine whether posterior urethral valves are present (in boys). Utilization of nuclear renal scintigraphy and IV urography varies from patient to patient and from institution to institution. Renal scintigraphy provides quantitative information regarding the effect of obstruction on renal function; for example, the function of the obstructed kidney can be compared with the opposite kidney before and after surgical treatment. The IV urogram provides less quantitative information but provides better anatomic detail. It serves best as a "road map" for the surgeon and gives information about anatomy and function after surgery. Recent studies have shown that functional MR with gadolinium is a promising technique, not only because it provides the advantage of exquisite anatomic detail, but, like renal scintigraphy, it can provide information of differential perfusion and function.

21. **What are posterior urethral valves?**
At the distal end of the verumontanum, several folds, or plicae, arise and pass caudally to encircle a portion of the membranous urethra. These plicae occur normally and vary in the extent to which they encircle the urethra. When they fuse anteriorly, they form the most common type of posterior urethral valves (type 1) (Fig. 59-4). Type 2 posterior urethral valves are mucosal folds that extend from the proximal end of the verumontanum toward the bladder neck; their very existence is controversial. Type 3 valves refer to a urethral diaphragm that occurs below the caudal end of the verumontanum.

22. **How are posterior urethral valves detected?**
Posterior urethral valves, which are the most common cause of bladder outlet obstruction in infant boys, cause changes in the bladder that are detected by sonography and cystography. These changes include enlargement, thickening, sacculation, and trabeculation of the bladder. Dilation of the posterior (prostatic) urethra above the valve can

Figure 59-4. Posterior urethral valves. Fluoroscopic spot view shows a dilated posterior urethra. Valves *(arrow)* are identified at the distal end of the verumontanum *(v)*.

be seen on both prenatal and postnatal sonograms as well as with VCUG. Hydroureteronephrosis is often present, either due to reflux or high pressures in the bladder. If rupture of a caliceal fornix occurs, urinary ascites and/or a urinoma can develop. Posterior urethral valves are confirmed cystoscopically and are treated with fulguration or incision.

23. **What is primary megaureter?**

    Primary megaureter results from an abnormal proportion of muscle fibers and fibrous tissue in the distalmost 3–4 cm of the ureter. When primary megaureter is obstructive, the degree of obstruction is variable and seems to improve in many cases over time. Most often, this condition is detected incidentally on prenatal sonography. Postnatal sonography and urography reveal a variable degree of dilation of the ureter and collecting system on the affected side (Fig. 59-5). Occasionally, a short, narrow segment of ureter may be seen through sonography at the UVJ. VCUG typically shows absence of reflux, although reflux may be present in 10% of cases.

Figure 59-5. Primary obstructive megaureter. IV urogram shows mild bilateral pevlicaliectasis. Moderate ureterectasis is most significant in the distal one half of the ureters.

24. **What are common forms of a duplex kidney?**

    A duplex kidney (duplication of the kidney, collecting system, and ureters) arises from abnormal development of the ureteric bud. Although various degrees of duplication may be present, in the full-blown condition, the kidney is large and there are separate collecting systems and ureters that drain the upper and lower poles of the kidney.

25. **What is the "Weigert-Meyer" rule?**

    According to this rule, when there is a complete duplication of the kidney, the lower pole ureter inserts normally into the bladder. The upper pole ureter inserts ectopically into the bladder, in a location that is medial and caudal to the insertion of the lower pole ureter.

26. **Are the collecting systems and ureters dilated in a duplicated system?**

    The appearance depends on whether there is reflux into the lower pole ureter and the exact site of the ectopically inserting upper pole ureter. In the typical situation, which is often bilateral, the distal ureters are contained within a common sheath and either come together or insert separately but are close together in the trigone of the bladder. If the upper pole ureter is associated with a ureterocele (a localized dilation of the distal ureter), the ureterocele can protrude through the bladder to the urethra and present as a perineal mass. If a ureterocele is present, the upper pole of the kidney may be obstructed (the "drooping lily" effect on the lower pole collecting system) or may be small and dysplastic, causing little or no effect on the lower pole. If a uretero-cele is not present, the upper pole moiety may insert in an ectopic location and have a stenotic insertion, causing obstruction (boys and girls), or may present with urinary dribbling (girls only) due to an ectopic insertion into the urethra, vagina, or perineum.

27. **What is the most common scrotal mass?**
The most common cause of a scrotal mass is probably a hydrocele, which is a collection of fluid outside the testicle, between layers of the tunica vaginalis. It may be congenital or may be asso-ciated with trauma, torsion, or hemorrhage.

28. **What are the main differential considerations of a painful scrotum?**
Testicular torsion and epididymitis/orchitis. Testicular torsion is a surgical emergency and can be confirmed or excluded either with color Doppler ultrasound or a nuclear scan (using tech-netium pertechnetate as the radiopharmaceutical agent). Epididymitis is much more common in the postpubescent male than in younger children and is identified on sonography by swelling of and increased flow in the epididymis. The cause of epididymitis is often bacterial, and there may be associated infection in the testicle.

KEY POINTS: PEDIATRIC URORADIOLOGY

1. Congenital urinary tract obstruction, VUR, and dysfunctional voiding can be diagnosed with renal and bladder sonography and VCUG.

2. Primary VUR is graded on a scale of 1 to 5, depending on the degree of ureteral and pelvicaliceal filling and dilation.

3. Renal cortical scintigraphy, contrast-enhanced CT, and renal sonography may be used to diagnose pyelonephritis in children.

4. Sonography and cystography can detect bladder outlet obstruction due posterior urethral valves, which is the most common cause of bladder outlet obstruction in boys.

5. The main differential considerations of a painful scrotum are testicular torsion and epididymitis/orchitis.

6. Testicular torsion is a surgical emergency and can be confirmed or excluded with either color Doppler ultrasound or a nuclear scan with technetium pertechnetate.

29. **If epididymitis is present in an infant, what should be suspected as the etiologic factor?**
Epididymitis is rare in infants and is usually associated with an anatomic abnormality of the gen-itourinary system, such as a dysplastic kidney with an ectopic ureter. Renal and bladder sono-graphy as well as VCUG are therefore indicated.

30. **What is the most common testicular tumor in children?**
Yolk sac tumors. They occur more commonly than teratomas and are seen primarily during the first 2 years of life. Most children with yolk sac tumors have elevated alpha-fetoprotein levels, whereas those with teratomas do not.

31. **What are the most common testicular tumors in adolescents?**

    Germ cell tumors (Fig. 59-6), but the most common histologic types are seminomas, choriocarcinomas, teratocarcinomas, and tumors with mixed histologies.

32. **What urinary problems occur in children with spina bifida?**

    There is an increased incidence of renal anomalies in children with myelomeningocele, including fusion anomalies (e.g., a horseshoe kidney), renal dysplasia, and agenesis. The most significant problems, however, relate to the abnormal innervation of the bladder.

Figure 59-6. Testicular germ cell tumor. Transverse sonogram of the scrotum in an infant shows a normal right (R) testis and massive enlargement of the left (L) testis *(arrows)*.

33. **What are the specific problems in spina bifida that are related to the neurogenic bladder?**

    The neurogenic bladder fails to store urine correctly, which may cause leaking, does not empty properly due to bladder-sphincter dyssynergia, and experiences uninhibited contractions, which may also cause leaking (Fig. 59-7). High storage pressures can result in reflux and hydronephrosis.

34. **What are the goals of therapy for urinary tract dysfunction in a patient with spina bifida?**

    The goals are to decrease storage pressure, either with frequent intermittent catheterization, vesicostomy, and/or bladder augmentation, and to keep the patient "dry" through continent diversion. Cystography is performed to assess bladder size, storage capacity, and the volume at which leakage occurs and to detect any reflux. Renal and bladder sonography is routinely performed every 6 months to assess for hydronephrosis, stones, and the ability of the patient to empty the bladder with self-catheterization.

Figure 59-7. Neurogenic bladder. VCUG in a patient with meningomyelocele shows a "pinecone" bladder with marked trabeculation and sacculation. When the patient attempts to void, there is dilation of the posterior urethra (u) with contraction of the external sphincter. A small amount of reflux is seen in the distal left ureter *(arrow)*.

35. **What is the triad of prune-belly syndrome?**
Absent or deficient abdominal musculature, cryptorchidism, and urinary tract abnormalities (Fig. 59-8).

36. **What urinary tract abnormalities are associated with prune-belly syndrome?**
They are diverse and include marked hydroureteronephrosis as well as marked bladder and urethral dilation, reflux, renal dysplasia, prostatic hypoplasia, urachal abnormalities, and microphallus. The clinical features often parallel the degree of urinary tract involvement. Newborns with severe renal dysplasia may have Potter's syndrome (oligohydramnios, pulmonary hypoplasia). Children with urinary tract dilation and/or reflux need to be closely monitored for infection.

Figure 59-8. Prune-belly syndrome. VCUG demonstrates megacystis as well as bilateral pelvicaliectasis and ureterectasis with significant ureteral tortuosity.

37. **What is a basic classification for cystic kidney diseases affecting infants, children, and adolescents?**
Cystic renal diseases can be classified as genetic or nongenetic. The most common cause of nongenetic cystic disease is multicystic dysplastic kidney (MCDK).

38. **What is the most common sonographic appearance of MCDK?**
Most commonly, MCDK is the result of atresia of the renal pelvis, and the kidney appears on sonography as multiple cysts of varying sizes that do not communicate with each other; there is no definable renal pelvis. The less common form is the hydronephrotic form, which has a central renal cyst. MCDK is associated with other abnormalities of the urinary tract, especially a contralateral UPJ obstruction and contralateral VUR.

39. **What are the other forms of nongenetic cystic renal disease?**
Simple renal cyst (rare in children), medullary cystic disease, caliceal diverticulum, and cystic renal dysplasia (associated with urinary tract obstruction).

40. **What are the genetic forms of cystic renal disease?**
Autosomal dominant polycystic kidney disease (ADPCKD), autosomal recessive polycystic kidney disease (ARPCKD), glomerulocystic kidney disease, congenital nephrosis, and cystic kidney disease associated with syndromes (e.g., tuberous sclerosis).

41. **Does "adult-type" ADPCKD occur in infants and young children?**
ADPCKD has been recognized at sonography both prenatally and postnatally. The appearance can closely mimic that of ARPCKD, in which both kidneys can appear large and echogenic. Small, sonographically resolvable cysts can be seen in either syndrome in the newborn period. More commonly, ADPCKD is suspected if sonography reveals progressive development of multiple cortical and medullary renal cysts. This may be found incidentally or in a child referred for hypertension and hematuria. Careful examination of the family history and sonographic screening of the family are recommended to detect for any evidence of cystic kidney disease in parents who may be unaware of their own subclinical disease.

42. **What imaging findings may help distinguish ADPCKD from ARPCKD in the infant or young child (Fig. 59-9)?**

The renal sonographic appearances of the two syndromes can be quite similar. The kidneys are often large and echogenic with each type. Careful inspection with sonography can occasionally detect tubular ectasia in echogenic renal pyramids, which is typical of ARPCKD. Sonographically resolvable cysts are more suggestive of autosomal dominant disease. Additionally, the liver should be examined for abnormal echotexture caused by hepatic fibrosis and biliary ectasia, which is often associated with autosomal recessive disease. In adolescents with ARPCKD, the renal involvement is less marked than the liver disease, which causes portal hypertension and splenomegaly. Excretory urography (or CT) can occasionally be helpful to distinguish the recessive from the dominant disease. In the former, there is delay and prolongation of the nephrogram; the contrast is taken up by dilated tubules

Figure 59-9. Autosomal recessive polycystic kidney disease. *(A)* Sagittal sonogram of right kidney *(arrows)* shows marked enlargement with heterogeneous echogenicity. Small (1 mm) cystic elements are seen within the renal parenchyma. *(B)* Transverse sonogram of liver. Parenchyma shows increased liver echotexture due to hepatic fibrosis. Minimal ectasia of the intrahepatic biliary tree *(small arrows)* can be seen adjacent to the left portal vein.

and has a spoked-wheel appearance. These findings are typically absent in the dominant disease, in which excretion is prompt.

43. **What are five hereditary syndromes associated with renal cysts?**
Tuberous sclerosis, von Hippel-Lindau disease, Zellweger's (cerebrohepatorenal) syndrome, Jeune's syndrome (thoracic asphyxiating dystrophy), and Meckel-Gruber syndrome.

44. **What conditions cause echogenic renal pyramids in the infant?**
Nephrocalcinosis (due to renal tubular acidosis, hypercalcemia, or furosemide therapy), renal tubular ectasia (ARPCKD), and Tamm-Horsfall protein deposition (transient phenomenon).

45. **What is the most common solid renal mass in infants?**
The fetal renal hamartoma, also known as the "mesoblastic nephroma." Infants usually present with a palpable renal mass. Hematuria, hypertension, and hypercalcemia may also be present. The tumor is composed of monotonous sheets of spindle-shaped cells and usually occupies most of the kidney. The tumor appears large and solid at sonography. The mass is usually resected, and the prognosis is excellent. Less common causes of solitary renal masses in infants include nephroblastomatosis and the malignant rhabdoid tumor.

46. **What is the role of imaging in infants with ambiguous genitalia?**
    Evaluation is indicated when the testes cannot be palpated and when there is severe hypospadias, incomplete scrotal fusion, fused labia, a micropenis, or clitoral enlargement. These conditions can be classified as true hermaphroditism, female pseudohermaphroditism, male pseudohermaphroditism, and gonadal dysgenesis, depending on further clinical, laboratory, and surgical investigations.

    Figure 59-10. Urogenital sinus in ambiguous genitalia. Retrograde genitogram shows low confluence *(arrow)* of the urethra as well as the vagina (v) and cervical impression (c).

    Sonography is the simplest method of identifying the internal anatomy by detecting the presence or absence of a uterus and gonads. This is usually combined with a retrograde genitogram performed under fluoroscopy that further defines the relationship of the urogenital sinus to the urethra and vagina (Fig. 59-10).

47. **What is nephroblastomatosis?**
    Multiple or diffuse rests of nephrogenic tissue. They are persistent embryonal remnants in the kidney that are apparent precursors to Wilms' tumor. The involved kidneys are typically enlarged and have a lobulated configuration. Ultrasound, CT, and magnetic resonance can be used to identify and monitor the condition of children with nephroblastomatosis (Fig. 59-11). The following are several conditions in which children may have nephroblastomatosis and can develop Wilms' tumor: hemihypertrophy, Drash syndrome (pseudohermaphroditism), aniridia, and a positive family history of Wilms' tumor/nephroblastomatosis.

Figure 59-11. Nephroblastomatosis. *A,* Sonogram of the right kidney shows significant renal enlargement with loss of normal cortical medullary differentiation (the left kidney has a smaller appearance). *B,* CT (enhanced) demonstrates loss of normal intrarenal architecture with diffuse infiltration of both kidneys by intralobar nephroblastomatosis.

48. **What are the two major types of nephroblastomatosis?**

Perilobar and intralobar. The perilobar form is limited to the periphery of the kidney, whereas the intralobar form can be found anywhere within a renal lobe as well as within the renal pelvis and collecting system. Nephroblastomatosis may remain dormant, mature, involute, develop hyperplastic overgrowth, or become neoplastic (Wilms' tumor).

49. **How can nephroblastomatosis be distinguished from a Wilms' tumor?**

With difficulty. Generally, a Wilms' tumor is suspected when a lesion noted by either ultrasound or CT is greater than 3 cm and has a spherical configuration. Many lesions previously thought to be small or medium-sized Wilms' tumors, especially in cases of bilateral or multicentric tumor, may actually represent hyperplastic nephroblastomatosis. Biopsy is of limited value in distinguishing the hyperplastic form from Wilms' tumor, and serial imaging is critical in determining whether surgery should be performed.

50. **What is the Mayer-Rokitansky-Küster-Hauser syndrome?**

Vaginal atresia with other variable müllerian duct abnormalities such as a bicornuate or septated uterus. The fallopian tubes, ovaries, and broad ligaments are normal. Unilateral renal or skeletal anomalies are associated in 50% and 12% of cases, respectively.

51. **How is pelvic sonography used in the evaluation of a child with precocious puberty?**

Uterine and ovarian volumes are larger than normal in true isosexual precocious puberty, whereas enlargement of only the ovary has been reported with pseudosexual precocity. True isosexual precocity is due to the premature activation of the hypothalamic pituitary gonadal axis, whereas pseudosexual precocity refers to pubertal changes occurring independent of these actions, as in the case of a functional ovarian cyst or tumor. Multiple, small (less than 1 cm) cysts can be seen in the ovaries of normal children, as well as in children who have precocious puberty. However, the best predictor of true precocious puberty is bilateral ovarian enlargement, but unilateral ovarian enlargement associated with larger cysts is more related to pseudosexual precocity.

BIBLIOGRAPHY

1. Beckwith JB: Precursor lesions of Wilms' tumor: Clinical and biological implications. Med Pediatr Oncol 21:158–168, 1993.
2. Bjorgvinsson E, Majd M, Eggli KD: Diagnosis of acute pyelonephritis in children: Comparison of sonography and Tc99m-DMSA scintigraphy. Am J Roentgenol 157:539–543, 1991.
3. Blickman JG, Lebowitz RL: The coexistence of primary megaureter and reflux. Am J Roentgenol 143:1053–1057, 1984.
4. Corteville JE, Gray DL, Crane JP: Congenital hydronephrosis: Correlations of fetal ultrasonographic findings with infant outcome. Am J Obstet Gynecol 165:384, 1991.
5. Cremin BJ: A review of ultrasonic appearances of posterior urethral valves and ureteroceles. Pediatr Radiol 16:357–364, 1986.
6. Fotter R, Kopp W, Skein E, et al: Unstable bladder in children: Functional evaluation by modified voiding cystography. Radiology 161:811–813, 1986.
7. Greskovich FJ III, Nyberg LM Jr: The prune belly syndrome: A review of its etiology, defects, treatment and prognosis. J Urol 140:707–712, 1988.
8. Jain M, LeQuesne GW, Bourne AJ, Henning P: High-resolution ultrasonography in the differential diagnosis of cystic diseases of the kidney in infancy and childhood: Preliminary experience. J Ultrasound Med 16:235–240, 1997.
9. Kaplan BS, Kaplan P, Rosenberg HK, et al: Polycystic kidney diseases in childhood. J Pediatr 115:867–879, 1989.

10. King LR, Siegel MJ, Solomon AL: Usefulness of ovarian volume and cysts in female isosexual precocious puberty. J Ultrasound Med 12:577–581, 1993.

11. Lebowitz RL, Mandell J: Urinary tract infection in children: Putting radiology in its place. Radiology 165:1–9, 1987.

12. Nunn IN, Stephens FD: The triad syndrome: A composite anomaly of the abdominal wall, urinary system, and testes. J Urol 86:782–794, 1961.

13. Rosenberg HK, Sherman NH, Tarry WF, et al: Mayer-Rokitansky-Kuster-Hauser syndrome: US aid and diagnosis. Radiology 161:815–819, 1986.

14. Saxton HM, Borzyskowski M, Mundy AR, Vivian GC: Spinning top urethra: Not a normal variant. Radiology 168:147–150, 1988.

15. Sutherland RS, Mevorach RA, Baskin LS, Kogan BA: Spinal dysraphism in children: An overview and an approach to prevent complications. Urology 46:294–304, 1995.

CHAPTER 60

PEDIATRIC NEURORADIOLOGY

D. Andrew Mong, MD, and Avrum N. Pollock, MD

1. **How does myelinated brain differ from nonmyelinated brain on an infant magnetic resonance image (MRI)? Where do you expect to see myelinization occur first?**

   Myelinated brain white matter, as in adults, appears hyperintense relative to gray matter on T1-weighted images and hypointense on T2-weighted images. In nonmyelinated brain, this pattern is reversed. Myelinization of the infant brain occurs in a predictable pattern, beginning in the brain stem and cerebellum and then progressing to the posterior limb of the internal capsule, optic pathways, and parietal lobes. This pattern of change occurs from caudal to cephalad, dorsal to ventral, and central to peripheral. Myelinization should appear complete on MR by 24 months but may be incomplete in the terminal zones up to approximately 4–5 years of age and in rare cases not until the first decade.

2. **What are migrational anomalies of the central nervous system (CNS)?**

   Normal neuronal migration occurs during fetal brain development as neurons migrate from the germinal matrix to the cortex along radial glial fibers. Partial or total arrest of this process leads to a migrational anomaly. These anomalies may include subependymal heterotopias (abnormal gray matter lining the ventricles), band heterotopias (an extra band of gray matter exists partially or completely underneath a normal-appearing cortex and a strip of white matter), schizencephaly (a cleft lined by gray matter extending from the outer cortex to the ventricles), polymicrogyria (too many gyri), pachygyria (abnormally thickened gyri), or lissencephaly (complete absence of gyri). Children typically present with developmental delay or seizures (Fig. 60-1).

Figure 60-1. Axial T2-weighted image through the level of the basal ganglia demonstrates abnormally thickened and enlarged large gyri *(arrows)* of the frontal cortex, which is consistent with pachygyria.

3. **Name the three kinds of holoprosencephaly.**

   Holoprosencephaly refers to incomplete differentiation of the fetal prosencephalon (forebrain) into separate ventricles. This may manifest as *alobar*, resulting in one ventricle and fusion of the thalami, *semilobar* (two hemispheres posteriorly but not anteriorly), or *lobar* (the mildest form, which may present with only mild midline abnormalities, such as absence of the septum pellucidum and subtle incomplete visualization of the interhemispheric fissure associated with an azygous anterior cerebral artery). The mildest form along the continuum is thought to include septo-optic dysplasia.

4. **What is the differential diagnosis for what appears to be massively dilated ventricles on a prenatal ultrasound?**
   This may be secondary to holoprosencephaly, hydranencephaly, or hydrocephalus. Hydranencephaly results from massive necrosis of the cerebral hemispheres and may be secondary to vascular disease with bilateral internal carotid occlusion, infection, or trauma with severe hydrocephalus. There is usually has a thin residual remnant of cerebral cortex applied to the inner table of the calvarium. The most common causes of prenatal hydrocephalus include Arnold-Chiari malformation II, intracranial hemorrhage, aqueductal stenosis, and Dandy-Walker malformation.

5. **Describe the classification of germinal matrix hemorrhage.**
   The germinal matrix lies in the caudothalamic groove. This is a highly vascular region of the prenatal and premature brain and is therefore prone to hemorrhage, with rupture of the thin venules subsequent to decreased perfusion or oxygenation. Morbidity and mortality can be predicted based on the grade of the hemorrhage. Grade I hemorrhage is confined to the germinal matrix. Grade II hemorrhage extends into the lateral ventricle. Grade III hemorrhage expands into and dilates the lateral ventricle. Grade IV hemorrhage extends into the adjacent parenchyma. Ultrasound of the premature infant's head through the anterior fontanelle is the modality of choice for diagnosis and follow-up of germinal matrix hemorrhage.

KEY POINTS: GRADING OF GERMINAL MATRIX HEMORRHAGE IN NEONATES

1. Grade I: confined to the caudothalamic groove

2. Grade II: extension into the lateral ventricle

3. Grade III: extension into and dilation of the lateral ventricle

4. Grade IV: extension into the adjacent parenchyma

6. **How does the premature brain respond to ischemic injury?**
   Periventricular leukomalacia is characterized by ischemia in an endarterial distribution, namely in the watershed regions of white matter that surround the ventricles. Ultrasound examination may show increase in periventricular echogenicity soon after the initial insult. Cystic change in these regions can be seen later in the subacute stage, as the white matter begins to be resorbed. MRI will show abnormal periventricular signal intensity as well as volume loss. Before 28 weeks of gestation, however, the developing brain does not display a leukomalacic response, and only volume loss results. This may take the form of dilated ventricles and expanded extra-axial spaces, or even porencephalic cysts (expanded cystlike dilations from the ventricles, which may reach the cortex). A porencephalic cyst can be differentiated from schizencephaly by noting that, in the former entity, there is no gray matter lining the cyst.

7. **Describe the three main types of Chiari malformation.**
   - *Chiari I* malformation involves herniation of the cerebellar tonsils into the foramen magnum (greater than 5 mm in patients younger than 15 years old) (Fig. 60-2).
   - *Chiari II* is more severe, involving herniation of the medulla and vermis as well as elongation and downward displacement of the brain stem. Chiari II is virtually always associated with a meningomyelocele. Prenatal ultrasound may show crowding of the posterior fossa ("banana sign" appearance of the cerebellar hemispheres as they wrap around the brain stem). Lacunar skull (Lückenschädel) may also be demonstrated in Chiari II but is thought to be due to a bony dysplasia rather than the copper-beaten appearance associated with increase in intracranial

pressure. Lacunar skull appears on plain film as multiple focal areas of thinning in the skull, which resolves with age.
- *Chiari III* involves herniation of contents of the posterior fossa through the occiput or upper cervical canal via a bony defect (i.e., akin to an encephalocele).

Figure 60-2. Sagittal T1-weighted image through the craniocervical junction shows inferior displacement of the cerebellar tonsils *(arrow)* below the level of the foramen magnum.

8. **How does the corpus callosum develop? Why is this important?**
    The corpus callosum develops front to back, except for the rostrum (anterior genu, body, splenium, and rostrum last). This is important because an in utero insult may result in destruction of part of the corpus callosum. If posterior portions of the corpus callosum are present and anterior portions are not, this means that they were present at one point and were destroyed. If posterior portions are absent instead, this may mean that they did not develop.

9. **What entity does not follow the normal rule of corpus callosum development?**
    Holoprosencephaly, previously described, may follow an atypical pattern of corpus callosum development, in which the posterior portions develop and the anterior portions do not. This is termed *atypical callosal dysgenesis*.

10. **What are the TORCH infections? How do they appear radiographically?**
    The *TORCH* acronym stands for infections caused by *t*oxoplasmosis, *o*ther (varicella), *r*ubella, *c*ytomegalovirus (CMV), and *h*erpes/*H*IV. It is often not possible to distinguish these radiographically. Intracranial calcification patterns may aid in differentiating them. CMV calcifications are classically present only in the periventricular (circumventricular) regions, whereas toxoplasmosis and rubella will also have basal ganglia and cortical calcifications. CMV may also be associated with migrational abnormalities previously discussed. HIV infection may present as atrophy with bilateral basal ganglia calcifications. Cerebral atrophy may be present in any infection.

11. **List the CNS manifestations of neurofibromatosis type I (NF-1).**
    Patients with NF-1 may have plexiform neurofibromas, which will be present along a nerve distribution and insinuate within the fascial planes of the head and neck. Sphenoid wing dysplasia, with its resultant harlequin eye appearance, is also a common finding. Nonspecific areas of high T2 signal may be present (NF spots) in the basal ganglia, brain stem, and cerebellum and are referred to as "spongiform dysplasia." Gliomas may develop anywhere along the optic pathway.
    In the spine, patients with NF-1 may develop lateral meningoceles, which herniate from the thecal sac into the thorax. Plain films of the spine may also demonstrate posterior vertebral body scalloping (from dural ectasia) or enlargement of the neural foramina (from neurofibromas) and inferior rib notching/remodeling due to the growth of the neurofibromas along the course of the intercostal nerves.

KEY POINTS: CNS MANIFESTATIONS OF NF-I ✓

1. Plexiform neurofibromas

2. Optic pathway gliomas

3. NF spots in the basal ganglia

4. Sphenoid wing dysplasia

5. Lateral meningoceles

6. Dural ectasia and posterior vertebral scalloping

7. Enlargement of the neural foramina from neurofibromas

12. **How is neurofibromatosis type II (NF-2) different from NF-1?**

The gene for NF-2 is on chromosome 22, as opposed to chromosome 17 for NF-1. NF-2 tumors can be remembered with the mnemonic *MISME,* which stands for *m*ultiple *i*nherited *s*chwanno-mas, *m*eningiomas, and *e*pendymomas. Classically, these appear as bilateral cerebellopontine angle tumors, representing bilateral acoustic schwannomas (but may involve any of the cranial nerves), which is diagnostic of NF-2.

13. **What is tuberous sclerosis (TS)?**

TS is an autosomal dominant disorder with variable expressivity, which manifests as hamartomatous lesions in multiple organ systems. TS consists of the clinical triad of seizures, adenoma sebaceum, and mental retardation. In the CNS, this includes subependymal nodules and subcortical tubers. The tubers have a typical appearance of wispy high signal on T2-weighted images in the subcortical white matter. Giant cell astrocytomas may occur at the foramen of Monroe and cause an obstructive hydrocephalus. Extra-CNS involvement includes angiomyolipomas (fat-containing masses) in the kidneys, rhabdomyomas of the heart, and cystic lung disease as well as bony involvement (Fig. 60-3).

14. **Describe the manifestations of Sturge-Weber syndrome.**

Sturge-Weber syndrome, also known as "encephalotrigeminal angiomatosis," includes venous angiomatous malformations within the leptomeninges and choroid plexus with an associated port-wine stain in the distribution of a branch of the trigeminal nerve on the side of the hemispheric involvement. On cross-sectional imaging, there will be a focal

Figure 60-3. Axial T2-weighted image through the brain demonstrates dark subependymal nodules *(arrows)* lining the lateral ventricles and wispy high signal in scattered subcortical areas, representing hamartomas.

region of leptomeningeal enhancement, often overlying a region of cortical atrophy. There is usually also abnormal enhancement in the enlarged ipsilateral choroid plexus. Computed tomography (CT) examination will also detect "tram-track" subcortical calcifications and ipsilateral hemispheric volume loss, which is not seen in early infancy because they take some time to occur.

15. **What are the most common brain tumors in infants?**
Although pediatric tumors in general are more likely to occur in the posterior fossa, in infants up to 2 years old, the most common individual tumors are supratentorial. These include teratoma, astrocytomas (e.g., glioblastoma multiforme), choroid plexus papilloma/carcinomas (in the lateral ventricles), and primitive neuroectodermal tumors.

16. **Name the major posterior fossa tumors in children.**
The majority of pediatric brain tumors are infratentorial. These include pilocytic astrocytoma, fibrillary astrocytoma, medulloblastoma, and ependymomas.

17. **What are the typical tumors that occur in the suprasellar region of a child?**
Craniopharyngiomas are cystic lesions that often contain calcium (Fig. 60-4). These may be confused with Rathke's cleft cysts, which are remnants of Rathke's pouch, the structure that forms the anterior portion of the pituitary gland. Other tumors include those of hypothalamic origin (gliomas or hamartomas), optic nerve tumors (such as those seen in NF-1), germinomas arising from the pituitary stalk, and pituitary adenomas. Langerhans cell histiocytosis (eosinophilic granuloma) can present as thickening of the infundibulum and loss of visualization of the normal posterior pituitary bright spot and is associated with a clinical history of growth delay.

Figure 60-4. Coronal T1-weighted image after the administration of intravenous contrast shows a ring-enhancing craniopharyngioma in the suprasellar region.

18. **Why is thickening of the pituitary stalk an important finding?**
The pituitary stalk is considered thickened if it is greater than 2 mm at the insertion of the gland. Close interval follow-up is warranted because this thickening may be a manifestation of a germinoma or Langerhans cell histiocytosis. Alternatively, the thickening may be idiopathic.

19. **What is the differential diagnosis for a pediatric cystic neck mass?**
This is a broad differential that may be narrowed by location. Type II branchial cleft cysts (the most common) are suprahyoid lesions that classically push the sternocleidomastoid muscle posteriorly and have a tongue of tissue arising between the external and internal carotid arteries. Thyroglossal duct cysts are remnants of the thyroglossal duct and are found in the midline, usually at or below the hyoid bone beneath the strap muscles. Teratomas or dermoids may occur anywhere, but can be identified by the presence of fat and/or calcium. Lymphangiomas have a typical appearance of a cystic mass, often with septations, that insinuates through fascial planes (sometimes inferiorly into the mediastinum).

20. **What is the differential diagnosis for leukocoria?**
Leukocoria is defined as an abnormal white papillary reflex. Retinoblastoma is the most concerning cause. Other causes include congenital cataract, infection (e.g., toxocariasis), persistent hyperplastic primary vitreous, retinopathy of prematurity, and Coat's disease (fusiform dilation of retinal vessels, often with associated retinal detachment and subretinal exudate). Historical clues are helpful in differentiating these entities. The average age of patients with retinoblastoma is 13 months, whereas Coat's disease generally occurs in boys older than 4 years old, and toxocariasis occurs generally after 6 years of age. The presence of calcification may aid in the diagnosis on CT since 95% of retinoblastomas contain calcium.

21. **What is meant by *trilateral retinoblastoma*?**
Bilateral retinoblastomas will often occur in the familial form of the disease, which is characterized genetically as a mutation in the Rb1 tumor suppressor gene. These patients are also at risk for developing a third primitive intracranial neoplasm, usually in the pineal gland, the so-called third-eye. *Trilateral retinoblastoma* therefore involves tumor in both eyes as well as in the pineal gland. As in the retina, even a fleck of calcium in the pineal gland of a child younger than 6 years old should be considered suggestive of neoplasm.

22. **What is fibromatosis colli? Describe its imaging characteristics.**
Fibromatosis colli is benign focal or fusiform enlargement of the sternocleidomastoid muscle in infants that usually regresses by 6–8 months of age and is thought to be due to trauma to the sternocleidomastoid muscle or to an in utero positioning abnormality. Ultrasound of the muscle demonstrates either diffuse enlargement or a focal hyperechoic mass. If there is question about the diagnosis, MR may be of use. MR should demonstrate low signal on T2-weighted images, which represents fibrosis in the sternocleidomastoid muscle.

23. **Where do cholesteatomas typically arise? What is the role of the radiologist in their evaluation?**
A cholesteatoma is squamous epithelium that is trapped in the skull base, often creating expansion and erosion of adjacent bony structures. Cholesteatomas may be congenital, in which case they are well defined and rounded and typically occur in the anterior mesotympanum or in the region of the eustachian tube, near the cochlear promontory. Cholesteatomas may also occur as a result of tympanic membrane perforation (i.e., acquired), in which case they typically occur in the epitympanum, adjacent to the scutum and involving Prussak's space, or into the posterior middle ear. CT examination of the temporal bones often cannot be used to distinguish between cholesteatoma and fluid or inflammatory tissue, but it is often helpful in defining whether there are effects on adjacent bony structures. Radiologists may therefore comment on the integrity of the ossicles, erosion of the scutum, the presence or absence of labyrinthine fistulas, or defects in the roof of the middle ear (tegmen tympani). MR is not as helpful for evaluating bony structures but may be an important problem-solving tool if there are questions concerning intracranial extension.

24. **What is the role of the radiologist in the evaluation of sacrococcygeal teratoma?**
The presence of a sacrococcygeal teratoma may be detected in utero with ultrasonography or fetal MRI. Since the mass may be cystic, the differential diagnosis may include a meningocele (outpouching of meninges through a defect in the posterior elements in the lumbosacral spine). High-output cardiac failure caused by a teratoma may result from flow to the mass, leading to hydrops fetalis; placentomegaly; and polyhydramnios, which may necessitate cesarean section or fetal surgery. MRI may be useful in the evaluation of these masses since the prognosis and surgical approach may depend on which components of the mass are within the abdomen and pelvis. Lesions confined to the true pelvis tend to be benign histologically, whereas those that extend beyond the confines of the sacrum tend to be malignant.

BIBLIOGRAPHY

1. Parazzini C, Baldoli C, Scotti G, Triulzi F: Terminal zones of myelination: MR evaluation of children aged 20-40 months. Am J Neuroradiol 23(10):1669–1673, 2002.

2. Roach ES: Neurocutaneous syndromes. Pediatr Clin North Am 39(4):591–620, 1992.

3. Roland EH, Hill A: Germinal matrix-intraventricular hemorrhage in the premature newborn: Management and outcome. Neurol Clin 21(4):833–851, vi–vii, 2003.

4. Truhan AP, Filipek PA: Magnetic resonance imaging: Its role in the neuroradiologic evaluation of neurofibromatosis, tuberous sclerosis, and Sturge-Weber syndrome. Arch Dermatol 129(2):219–226, 1993.

5. Vezina LG: Diagnostic imaging in neuro-oncology. Pediatr Clin North Am 44(3):701–719, 1997.

PEDIATRIC MUSCULOSKELETAL RADIOLOGY

D. Andrew Mong, MD

1. **How does growing bone respond to trauma? How is this different from mature bone?**

   The cartilaginous physis separates the epiphysis from the metaphysis. Pediatric ligaments and tendons are relatively stronger than growing bone (unlike adults). Given an equivalent force applied to growing and mature bone, the growing bone has a higher likelihood of fracture. In addition, immature bone has a propensity to bow instead of break, which may cause buckles in one side of the cortex (torus fractures) or greenstick fractures (fracture of one cortex and bowing of the other). These patterns are not seen in mature bone.

2. **What is the significance of fractures of the physis? How are they classified?**

   The cartilaginous physis is vulnerable to injury, especially at its attachment to the metaphysis. Disruption of the physis may result in slower growth and even premature fusion, leading to limb length discrepancy. Physeal injuries are classified in the Salter-Harris scheme, increasing in severity from I to V. Type I is a fracture through the physis. The fracture line in type II includes the metaphysis and physis. The type III fracture includes the epiphysis and the physis. Type IV involves the metaphysis, physis, and epiphysis. Type V is a crush injury of the physis. Follow-up for Salter-Harris fractures may include magnetic resonance (MR) examination, which can delineate an abnormally fused physis in the healing phase that may need to be disrupted to allow future osseous growth (Fig. 61-1).

Figure 61-1. Salter-Harris fractures of the distal femur.

3. **What are secondary ossification centers, and why are they particularly important to understand in the setting of elbow trauma?**

   Secondary ossification centers appear and then later fuse with the primary ossification center on plain radiographs at predictable times during skeletal maturation. There are multiple secondary ossification centers about the elbow that appear at different ages. Their usual sequence can be remembered by the mnemonic *C-R-I-T-O-E: c*apitellum (1 year), *r*adial head (3 years), *i*nternal (medial) epicondyle (5 years), *t*rochlea (7 years), *o*lecranon (9 years), and *e*xternal (lateral) epicondyle (11 years) (Fig. 61-2). One important reason to understand this sequence is that a type I Salter-Harris fracture through the physis of the medial epicondyle may cause displacement of this ossification center into the region of the trochlea. This might create the false impression that the trochlear ossification center is present while the medial epicondylar ossification center has not yet appeared. Knowledge of this sequence will allow one to appropriately identify this appearance as a displaced fracture.

Figure 61-2. Frog-leg view of the left hip shows an open physis with inferior displacement of the femoral capital epiphysis compared with the metaphysis. (Courtesy Richard Markowitz, MD, Children's Hospital of Philadelphia.)

4. **How may subtle supracondylar fractures of the elbow be diagnosed?**
   Pediatric elbow fractures often occur in the supracondylar region, where the humerus is relatively flat. The anterior humeral line, drawn on the lateral view of the elbow along the anterior humerus, will normally intersect the middle third of the capitellum. This will likely be disrupted in supracondylar fractures. The presence of a joint effusion (hemarthrosis) is also extremely helpful and can be assessed by the presence of an elevated posterior fat pad, which will be displaced and visible on the lateral view if there is blood in the joint. Displacement of the anterior fat pad (sail sign) may also be seen with hemarthrosis, but this finding is less specific.

5. **Describe nursemaid's elbow.**
   Nursemaid's elbow is caused by radial head subluxation through the annular ligament of the elbow, resulting in abnormal positioning of the ligament between the radial head and capitellum. It is often caused by sudden traction on the forearm in a child between the ages of 1 and 3 years Radiographs may have normal results but are obtained to exclude fractures.

6. **What are the risk factors for developmental dysplasia of the hip (DDH)? When is DDH suspected clinically?**
   Risk factors for DDH include Caucasian race, female gender, torticollis, club foot, and breech birth. It is difficult to diagnose DDH in newborns up to 4 weeks old secondary to normal joint laxity, but this condition is suspected in infants with leg length discrepancy and asymmetric thigh creases. The Barlow maneuver on physical examination dislocates the femoral head rearward, and the Ortolani maneuver reduces the recently dislocated hip, often with a resultant "clunk."

7. **What are the potential complications of untreated DDH?**
   Leg length discrepancy, osteoarthritis, pain, gait disturbance, and decrease in agility.

8. **How is DDH diagnosed radiographically?**
   Traditionally, plain films have been used. While the femoral head begins to ossify during the first year (usually between 3 and 6 months), its location must be inferred in infants. The acetabulum is divided into quadrants by the horizontal Hilgenreiner's line, drawn through both triradiate cartilages, and the vertical Perkin's line, drawn through the lateral rim of the acetabulum. A normal femoral head should fall within the inner lower quadrant of these intersecting lines, whereas a femoral head in DDH will be displaced superolaterally. The acetabular angle should also be eval-

uated, drawn between Hilgenreiner's line and a line connecting the superolateral ridge of the acetabulum with the triradiate cartilage. This angle should be less than 30 degrees in neonates.

9. **How is DDH diagnosed sonographically?**
Ultrasound is now the preferred method of diagnosing DDH in children younger than 1 year old. The hip is studied in the coronal plane. The alpha angle is measured between the straight lateral margin of the ilium and a line from the inferior point of the ilium tangential to the acetabulum. This is a measure of acetabular depth and should be greater than 60 degrees. At least half of the femoral head should be seated within the acetabulum.

10. **What is Legg-Calvé-Perthes disease?**
This is idiopathic osteonecrosis of the femoral head, usually affecting children 3–12 years old with a mean age of 7 years. Plain radiographic findings include a small femoral head epiphysis, which may become fragmented, and widening of the articular space, which may be due to an associated joint effusion.

11. **Describe slipped capital femoral epiphysis (SCFE).**
SCFE is a hip disease of early adolescence (10–15 years), characterized by idiopathic posterior and inferior slippage of the capital femoral epiphysis on the femoral neck metaphysis. Complications include avascular necrosis of the femoral head or chondrolysis. Anteroposterior (AP) and frog-leg views of both hips should be obtained because the condition can be bilateral in up to 40% of cases. On the frog-leg view, a normal epiphysis will project superior to Klein's line, which is drawn along the superior surface of the femoral neck. In early SCFE, the epiphysis will be flush with this line (*see* Fig. 61-2).

KEY POINTS: CHARACTERISTIC AGES OF PEDIATRIC HIP DISORDERS

1. Developmental dysplasia is a disorder of infants.
2. Legg-Calvé-Perthes disease occurs in children 3–12 years of age.
3. Slipped capital femoral epiphysis occurs in children 10–15 years old. This disorder cannot occur once the physes have fused!

12. **How is SCFE treated?**
Treatment goals include the prevention of both further slippage and physeal plate closure. SCFE may be treated with internal fixation, bone graft, osteotomy, and cast immobilization. It is important to note that there is no attempt to reduce the slip because this may cause avascular necrosis.

13. **What are coxa vara and coxa valga?**
These are abnormalities of the femoral shaft to neck ratio. The normal ratio is 150 degrees at birth, decreasing to 120–135 degrees in adults. Coxa vara is an angle less than 120 degrees and may be secondary to trauma, tumor, SCFE, or a congenital abnormality. Coxa valga (greater than 150 degrees) is usually neuromuscular in origin but may also be seen in blood dyscrasias such as thalassemia.

14. **Describe Blount disease.**
    Blount disease is a varus deformity of the knee (i.e., the tibia is abnormally directed medially compared with the femur), resulting from growth disturbance of the medial aspect of the proximal tibial metaphysis. This may occur in infants, in which case it is often bilateral, or adolescents. Tibial osteotomy may be required for treatment because growth disturbance may result from abnormal tibial bowing.

15. **What is Osgood-Schlatter disease?**
    A common cause of knee pain in adolescence (11–14 years), Osgood-Schlatter disease is thought to result from repetitive traction through the patellar tendon onto the developing tibial tubercle. This can lead to partial avulsion through the ossification center and heterotopic bone formation. Even though the diagnosis may be made clinically, radiographs may aid in the exclusion of other etiologies of knee pain. Lateral radiographs may reveal irregular ossification of the proximal tibial tubercle, calcification and thickening of the patellar tendon, and soft tissue swelling.

16. **What is the difference between a triplane fracture and a juvenile Tillaux fracture of the ankle?**
    Both fractures occur after partial closure of the distal tibial physis. On frontal radiographs, the triplane fracture appears as a Salter III fracture through the epiphysis, and on the lateral radiograph, it appears as a Salter II fracture through the metaphysis. The juvenile Tillaux fracture is simply a Salter III fracture that occurs at the anterolateral aspect of the distal tibia. This occurs because the physis fuses from medial to lateral, leaving the lateral aspect more vulnerable to injury.

17. **What is Freiberg's infraction?**
    Freiberg's infraction is an idiopathic osteochondrosis of the head of a metatarsal bone (usually the second), which results in flattening and osteosclerosis of the metatarsal head. It is usually seen in adolescents (13–18 years).

18. **What are craniosynostoses?**
    A craniosynostosis represents premature closure of a suture of the skull. This results in cessation of growth of the skull perpendicular to the suture line and abnormal compensatory growth along the axis of the closed suture. For this reason, sagittal craniosynostosis results in an elongated skull in the AP dimension (scaphocephaly) (Fig. 61-3). Plagiocephaly results from premature closure of one coronal suture, resulting in abnormal bulging on the opposite forehead. Premature closure of the metopic suture results in trigonocephaly, which appears as a triangular keel-shaped forehead. Cloverleaf skull (Kleeblattschädel) results from premature closure of the coronal, lambdoid, and posterior sagittal sutures, with bulging of the vertex of the brain through the squamosal, anterior sagittal, and metopic sutures.

Figure 61-3. Markedly increased AP diameter from premature closure of the sagittal suture, creating a boat-shaped skull, or scaphocephaly.

19. Give the differential diagnosis for vertebra plana.

Flattening of a vertebral body (vertebra plana) in a child should first and foremost bring to mind the diagnosis of Langerhans cell histiocytosis. Other diagnostic possibilities in the pediatric population include leukemia, lymphoma, metastatic disease, infection, and storage diseases.

20. When and where do pediatric primary tumors of bone occur?

Ewing's sarcoma and osteosarcoma are the most common primary pediatric bone tumors and typically occur between the ages of 10 and 25 years. The most common sites are the pelvis, thigh, lower leg, upper arm, and ribs, but soft tissue may also be the primary site of involvement. Ewing's sarcoma typically does not have a matrix and appears as a permeative aggressive lesion, often with associated periosteal reaction. Most osteosarcomas occur in the metaphysis, typically about the knee. Although the appearance of osteosarcomas is quite variable, they often produce a characteristic fluffy osteoid matrix.

21. How should a suspected osteoid osteoma be evaluated?

Osteoid osteoma is a benign neoplasm with a nidus of osteoid-rich tissue that typically causes an intense sclerotic reaction in surrounding bone. An osteoid osteoma may occur in the cortical, cancellous, or periosteal regions of any bone (or rarely in adjacent soft tissues). Most patients are between the ages of 10 and 30 years and will often give a typical history of night pain relieved by aspirin. Radionuclide bone scan may point to the abnormality before any changes are apparent on plain film and should be performed on any patient with a painful scoliosis in whom osteoid osteoma in the spine is the working diagnosis. If plain films do not reveal the lucent nidus surrounded by sclerotic bone, a computed tomography scan is the preferred next step since intracortical tumors may be missed on MRI.

22. What is rickets? How does it appear radiographically?

Rickets is a relative or absolute deficiency in vitamin D, which causes a decrease in ossification. It is almost exclusively seen in children younger than 2 years. Bone density will overall be decreased, but the more specific signs include loss of the zone of provisional calcification within the metaphysis of long bones. This leads to metaphyseal irregularity, cupping, and fraying with an associated widened physis. These changes are seen best in the distal radius, which is why films of the wrists are ordered to evaluate rickets (Fig. 61-4). Another classic appearance is the "rachitic rosary," which is enlargement of the costochondral joints in the chest.

Figure 61-4. Frontal plain film of the hand shows cupping and fraying of the metaphyses *(arrows)* from rickets. (Courtesy Richard Markowitz, MD, Children's Hospital of Philadelphia.)

23. Describe the bony changes of sickle cell anemia.

Sickle cell anemia is secondary to a disorder of "sickling" of red blood cells due to abnormal hemoglobin molecules. Clumped, sickled cells form venous (and sometimes arterial) thromboses, affecting multiple organs. Osseous manifestations include patchy sclerotic changes in bone from infarctions. A more specific sign includes a "Lincoln log" appearance of the vertebral bodies, with squarelike depressions seen in both the superior and inferior end plates on a lateral spine film. Avascular necrosis of the hips may also be seen. Affected patients are prone to osteomyelitis from *Staphylococcus aureus* and *Salmonella*. On MR, it can be difficult to distinguish infarction from osteomyelitis because both may produce signal abnormalities in marrow (bright T2 signal) along with adjacent soft tissue changes. *Dactylitis* is a nonspecific term referring to inflammation of a digit, which may also be seen in sickle cell anemia and be secondary to infarction or infection. Finally, because of the chronic anemia, sickle cell patients have an increased red-to-yellow marrow ratio, which may be inferred on a lateral skull radiograph by the widening of the diploic space (Fig. 61-5).

Figure 61-5. Sagittal T1-weighted image of the brain shows widening of the diploic space *(arrows)* of the skull from marrow expansion in a sickle cell patient. This finding is not specific for sickle cell anemia and may be found in other severe anemias, such as thalassemia or iron deficiency anemia.

24. **What is the most common dwarfism, and what are its manifestations?**
    Achondroplasia. This is a rhizomelic (shortening of the proximal bones) auto-somal dominant disorder. Typical charac-teristics include a large head with frontal bossing, a trident configuration of the hands, genu varum (bowed legs), and an exaggerated lumbar lordosis (with posterior scalloping of the vertebral bodies). On a frontal radiograph of the lumbosacral spine in a normal patient, the distance between the pedicles will gradually widen from L1 to L5, whereas an achondroplastic dwarf will demonstrate a decrease in the interpedicular distance of the caudal spine. Other radi-ographic findings include a notchlike sacroiliac groove and metaphyseal flaring of the long bones.

25. **What is the differential diagnosis for dense metaphyseal bands? How does one know when they are abnormally dense?**
    Dense metaphyseal bands may be a normal variant, so it is important to look at areas that do not have a lot of bone turn-over to see whether they are affected as well. Specifically, the metaphy-ses of the fibula are good areas to check. A major concern is heavy metal poisoning (specifically lead intoxication). Lead poisoning can be diagnosed by noting not only the metaphyseal bands but also the radiopaque lead chips seen on a frontal plain view of the abdomen floating in the child's intestines. Other etiologic factors include stress lines, treated rickets, scurvy, hypervita-minosis D, or treated leukemia.

BIBLIOGRAPHY

1. England SP, Sundberg S: Management of common pediatric fractures. Pediatr Clin North Am 43(5):991–1012, 1996.
2. Kao SC, Smith WL: Skeletal injuries in the pediatric patient. Radiol Clin North Am 35(3):727–746, 1997.
3. Lemyre E, Azouz EM, Teebi AS, et al: Bone dysplasia series. Achondroplasia, hypochondroplasia and thanatophoric dysplasia: Review and update. Can Assoc Radiol J 50:185–197, 1999.
4. Lins RE, Simovitch RW, Waters PM: Pediatric elbow trauma. Orthop Clin North Am 30(1):119–132, 1999.

CHAPTER 62

IMAGING OF CHILD ABUSE

D. Andrew Mong, MD, and Avrum N. Pollock, MD

1. **What are key history and physical examination findings that may raise suspicion of the possibility of nonaccidental trauma (NAT)?**
   Historic red flags that should lead the clinician and radiologist to consider child abuse include injuries that are not commensurate with the development of the child, a delay in seeking care, or vague or changing stories given by caretakers. Superficial physical examination findings that the clinician may convey to the radiologist include bruises in various stages of healing; "pattern injuries," such as those from cigarette burns; and signs of neglect.

2. **What diagnostic algorithm might the clinician and radiologist apply if skeletal injury from child abuse is suspected?**
   In addition to radiographs of any specific injuries, a skeletal survey should be performed on all children younger than 2 years. This includes plain frontal radiographs of the chest, arms, hands, pelvis, legs, ankles, and feet and frontal and lateral radiographs of the skull and entire spine. A "babygram" (frontal radiograph of the chest and abdomen) is not adequate. A nuclear medicine bone scan may be performed if these findings are equivocal for abuse or if there is a high index of clinical suspicion and the skeletal survey does not reveal an abnormality (Fig. 62-1).

3. **Describe shaken infant syndrome.**
   Shaken infant syndrome occurs when an infant or young child is shaken forcefully. This creates shearing forces that may cause classic patterns of injury seen in the chest and brain. Long bone injuries with resultant metaphyseal corner fractures are due to twisting/torsion type injuries that can occur with or without shaken baby/shaken impact syndrome but are a separate injury, mechanism, and type of NAT.

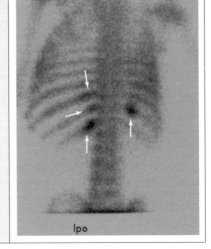

Figure 62-1. Posterior view of a technetium-labeled methylene diphosphonate bone scan demonstrates multiple posterior rib fractures *(arrows)*.

lpo

4. **What are metaphyseal corner fractures?**

   Metaphyseal fractures result from shearing forces of NAT and appear as metaphyseal corner fractures or bucket-handle fractures, the same fractures seen in different projections/obliquities. These fractures may heal quickly. They typically appear as lucent areas extending across the metaphysis, nearly perpendicular to the long axis of the bone. They are highly specific for child abuse (Fig. 62-2).

5. **Name other pediatric fractures with high specificity for child abuse.**

   Posterior rib fractures are another aspect of shaken infant syndrome that occur when adult hands forcefully grab the infant's chest while shaking the infant, resulting in a levering/fulcruming effect of the posterior ribs against the costal processes of the adjacent vertebral bodies. These fractures are specific for abuse and may be detected incidentally on a routine chest radiograph obtained for an unrelated reason or when the patient presents with dyspnea/respiratory distress secondary to the underlying central nervous system injury sustained due to violent shaking. Other suspicious fractures include those of the scapula, spinous processes, or sternum or compression fractures of the vertebral bodies (Fig. 62-3).

Figure 62-2. Typical metaphyseal corner fracture *(arrows)* of the distal tibia.

Figure 62-3. Posterior rib fractures *(arrow).*

6. **What fractures have low specificity for child abuse?**

   Fractures of the long bones, clavicular fractures, and linear skull fractures.

7. **What features of skull fractures increase the likelihood of NAT?**

   Branching, multiple, depressed, or distracted fractures and fractures that cross suture lines are more likely to be caused by abuse than are linear skull fractures.

8. **What features of a fracture are useful in estimating its age?**

   Features that may be useful to the radiologist include sclerosis at the fracture margin, the presence or absence of periosteal reaction, callus formation, bony bridging, and bony remodeling. Multiple fractures of different ages are *highly* suggestive of NAT.

9. **Summarize common findings of head trauma in shaken infant syndrome.**

   Shearing forces may create subdural hematomas (SDHs). An interhemispheric SDH and posterior fossa/tentorial SDH are very suspicious areas of involvement. Severe cerebral edema, which may result from asphyxiation, has a typical appearance on unenhanced head computed tomography (CT), with loss of gray-white matter differentiation and edema of the cerebral cortex and central gray structures (basal ganglia and thalami). The cerebrum, therefore, will appear diffusely low in attenuation (Fig. 62-4).

10. **What is the most common cause of death in a patient who has suffered NAT?**
Injury to the central nervous system.

11. **How should imaging of the brain be applied in the setting of suspected abuse?**
Any child younger than 2 years in whom there is a clinical suspicion of abuse, even if asymptomatic, should receive a head CT because of the high incidence of occult brain trauma. Brain imaging should be considered in older children as well. Irritability, vomiting, altered state of consciousness, and irregular respira-tions are strong indications for imaging the brain. Magnetic resonance imaging (MRI) of the brain can be performed to detect more subtle shear type of injuries of the white matter not visible or evident on head CT and can also be used to date areas of hem-orrhage with greater accuracy.

Figure 62-4. Midline subdural hematoma *(arrow),* which is in a typical location seen in case of nonaccidental trauma. Also note that there is diffuse cerebral edema with loss of the gray-white differentiation.

12. **How is the age of intracranial blood determined on MRI examinations?**
Evolving blood products in cerebral or subdural hematomas go through various stages of signal intensity on T1- and T2-weighted MR images. Hyperacute hemorrhage (oxyhemoglobin) is dark on T1 and bright on T2. Acute hemorrhage (deoxyhemoglobin) is dark on T1 and T2. Early subacute hematoma (intracellular methemoglobin) is bright on T1 and dark on T2. Late subacute hematoma (extracellular methemoglobin) is bright on T1 and T2. Chronic hematoma (hemosiderin) is dark on both sequences.

13. **Describe possible bowel findings in cases of abuse.**
Bowel injuries typically occur in children older than 2 years who may have been punched or kicked, with resultant compression of the bowel loops against the spinal column. The duodenum and proximal small bowel are the most commonly affected areas of the small bowel and may demonstrate lacerations or intramural hematomas, which can cause obstruction if bleeding is severe. These injuries can be studied with an upper gastrointestinal or CT scan.

14. **What is the most common cause of pediatric pancreatitis? What are its radiologic manifestations?**
Trauma, either accidental or nonaccidental, is the most common cause. Pancreatic injury may be suspected with abdominal pain, fever, and vomiting. Pancreatitis may be detected with an elevation of amylase and lipase levels without any radiographic findings. On CT examination, pancreatitis may present as fullness of the pancreatic tissues, stranding in the adjacent mesenteric fat, or frank peripancreatic fluid collections. On CT examination, pancreatic lacera-tions appear as areas of linear discontinuation of pancreatic tissue, usually with surrounding fluid.

KEY POINTS: LESIONS THAT SHOULD PROMPT A WORK-UP FOR CHILD ABUSE ✔

1. Metaphyseal corner fractures (highly specific and sensitive for abuse)

2. Posterior rib fractures

3. Fractures of spinous processes, scapula, or sternum or compression fractures of vertebral bodies

4. Subdural hematomas, especially midline

5. Duodenal hematoma and pancreatitis

15. **Are multiple bruises and skeletal injuries always diagnostic of child abuse?**
No. Systemic disorders can also be responsible. Abnormalities of coagulation may mimic abuse and include entities such as leukemia, hemophilia, idiopathic thrombocytopenic purpura, or Henoch-Schönlein purpura. Metabolic/congenital abnormalities are also important mimickers to consider, including osteogenesis imperfecta, Menkes' kinky hair syndrome, Ehlers-Danlos syndrome, congenital syphilis, and rickets.

16. **How does congenital syphilis mimic child abuse?**
Both may produce metaphyseal fractures. In congenital syphilis, these are pathologic fractures secondary to fragmentation of the metaphysis from osteomyelitis. These findings are usually symmetric in a child with syphilis and asymmetric in an abused child. Syphilis may also be differentiated from child abuse through noting concomitant diaphyseal diffuse periosteal reaction along long bones, splenomegaly, and positive serologic test results.

17. **What is the differential diagnosis of periosteal reaction in a newborn?**
In addition to fractures from NAT, the differential diagnosis includes congenital infection (such as syphilis), neuroblastoma metastases, physiologic periosteal new bone formation, prostaglandin treatment, and Caffey's disease. Caffey's disease is a benign, self-limited periosteal reaction of uncertain etiology, usually involving the mandible, clavicles, and long bones.

18. **When does physiologic periosteal new bone formation occur?**
Periosteal new bone formation can occur symmetrically along shafts of long bones in newborns and resolves by 3 months of age. It is thought to be due to handling of the infant. There are no associated fractures.

19. **Can a metaphyseal corner fracture ever look like a metaphyseal lucent band?**
Yes. If a lucent metaphyseal band is identified, additional projections may identify it as a corner fracture. The differential diagnosis of a lucent metaphyseal band includes leukemia, lymphoma, metastatic disease (neuroblastoma), congenital infection, and scurvy.

20. **What is the legal responsibility of any U.S. physician who suspects child abuse?**
Child protection ordinances exist in all 50 states and require medical professionals to report suspected abuse to the local child protective service agency. Radiologists have the added onus of ensuring that high-quality films are obtained for the skeletal survey, which may be used in court.

BIBLIOGRAPHY

1. Lonergan GJ, Baker AM, Morey MK, Boos SC: From the archives of the AFIP. Child abuse: Radiologic-pathologic correlation. Radiographics 23(4):811–845, 2003.

2. Mogbo KI, Slovis TL, Canady AI, et al: Appropriate imaging in children with skull fractures and suspicion of abuse. Radiology 208:521–524, 1998.

3. Nimkin K, Kleinman PK: Imaging of child abuse. Radiol Clin North Am 39(4):843–864, 2001.

SOLITARY AND MULTIPLE PULMONARY NODULES

Drew A. Torigian, MD

CHAPTER 63

1. **What is a solitary pulmonary nodule (SPN)?**

   An SPN is a solitary focal lesion in the lung that is ≤3 cm. A solitary focal lesion that is >3 cm is considered to be a mass, and the majority of masses are malignant. Approximately 150,000 SPNs are detected annually in the United States, often incidentally on imaging. About 60% are benign, but up to 40% are malignant. Therefore, the goal of radiologic evaluation of an SPN is to noninvasively differentiate whether it is benign or malignant as accurately as possible. An SPN is the initial radiographic finding in up to 30% of patients with lung cancer, and the prognosis is partly dependent on the stage at presentation.

2. **List some causes of pulmonary nodules.**

   Primary lung carcinoma is the most common cause of an SPN, pulmonary granuloma is the second most common overall cause, and pulmonary hamartoma the third most common cause. See Table 63-1 for a more complete list. Many other entities can cause solitary or multiple pulmonary nodules including tumors (e.g., metastatic disease), infections, vasculitis, and inflammatory diseases (e.g., sarcoidosis, rheumatoid arthritis, or inhalational lung disease). Be careful about a "confluence of shadows" or overlap of normal vascular and osseous structures appearing to represent a nodule. Nipple shadows can also appear as nodules, but are usually seen at a similar level bilaterally.

3. **What is the general approach to the evaluation of an SPN?**

   The initial step is to determine whether a visualized "nodule" on chest radiography is truly a pulmonary nodule or a pseudolesion that mimics a nodule (some of the causes of a pseudolesion are listed in Table 63-1). If a "nodule" is due to a pseudolesion associated with bone, such as a rib fracture, it will have the same anatomic relationship to its bone of origin on radiographs with multiple views, whereas a true pulmonary nodule that overlaps with osseous structures one view will appear to move apart from these osseous structures on other views. Furthermore, radiopaque nipple markers can be used to distinguish pseudolesions due to nipples from true pulmonary nodules. Once a true pulmonary nodule has been confirmed, a more detailed investigation begins.

4. **What further diagnostic steps may be implemented in the work-up of indeterminate pulmonary nodules?**

   Thin-section unenhanced computed tomography (CT), CT nodule densitometry, 2-[^{18}F]-2-deoxy-D-glucose (FDG) positron emission tomography (PET), short-term follow-up chest radiography or CT, or tissue sampling are among some of the options available for the work-up of indeterminate pulmonary nodules. The choice is based on several factors, including the pretest probability of malignancy, the morphologic features of the nodules, and the patient's clinical history and current status. Thin-section unenhanced CT is useful for the identification of fat or certain patterns of calcification within a nodule that indicate benignity.

TABLE 63-1.   DIFFERENTIAL DIAGNOSIS OF PULMONARY NODULES

Neoplasia
Primary lung carcinoma (No. 1 cause of an SPN)
Metastasis
Lymphoma/post-transplant lymphoproliferative disorder
Carcinoid tumor
Primary lung sarcoma
Hamartoma (No. 3 cause of an SPN, No. 2 cause of a benign SPN)

Infection
Granuloma (No. 2 cause of an SPN, No. 1 cause of a benign SPN)
Bacterial
Viral
Fungal
Mycobacterial
Parasitic
Septic emboli (often multiple, peripheral, and cavitary)

Vascular
Pulmonary infarction (often peripheral and wedge-shaped, associated with pulmonary
    embolism)
Vasculitis
Arteriovenous malformation
Pulmonary venous varix (tubular and avidly enhancing on CT)
Pulmonary artery aneurysm

Inflammatory
Sarcoidosis
Inhalational lung disease
Hypersensitivity pneumonitis
Organizing pneumonia
Bronchiolitis
Langerhans' cell histiocytosis (associated with upper lobe predominant cystic interstitial
    lung disease in smokers)
Rheumatoid (necrobiotic) nodule
Inflammatory pseudotumor

Congenital
Intrapulmonary lymph node
Pulmonary sequestration (solid or cystic opacity most often in the lower lobes)
Bronchial atresia

TABLE 63-1.	DIFFERENTIAL DIAGNOSIS OF PULMONARY NODULES—CONT'D

Traumatic

Radiation therapy (typically has linear margins and a known history of prior radiation therapy)

Pulmonary contusion (associated with traumatic injury to the chest)

Pseudonodules

Rounded atelectasis ("folded lung," typically a subpleural opacity associated with pleural
thickening or effusion and a "comet-tail sign" of swirling bronchovascular structures
central to the opacity)

Pulmonary scarring

Mucoid impaction

Fluid in an interlobar fissure (often lenticular in shape on lateral chest radiography in the
location of a fissure)

Healing rib fracture

Bone island

Spinal osteophyte

Skin lesion

Nipple shadow

Pleural lesion

Mediastinal lesion

Overlap of vascular and osseous structures

5. **What are some potential "blind spots" on chest radiography and CT when trying to detect pulmonary nodules?**
On chest radiography, potential blind spots include the lung apices where the clavicles and ribs overlap, the hila and retrocardiac region where superimposed cardiovascular structures are located, and within the lung bases below the level of the anterior portions of the hemidiaphragms where abdominal soft tissue overlaps. On CT, potential "blind spots" include the central portions of the lungs (e.g., the hilar regions and the azygoesophageal recess) and the endoluminal portions of the trachea and bronchi.

6. **List some morphologic imaging features of nodules assessed on chest radiography and CT.**
   - Shape
   - Size/volume and change over time
   - Margins
   - Internal architecture
   - Presence of fat
   - Presence and pattern of calcification

7. **What morphologic imaging findings are more suggestive of a benign SPN?**
Small size and smooth, well-defined margins are suggestive of benignity, although 15% and 40% of malignant nodules are less than 1 and 2 cm in diameter, respectively, and 20% of malignant nodules have well-defined margins. Intranodular fat is a reliable indicator of a hamartoma, a benign lesion (Fig. 63-1). Central, diffuse solid, laminated, and "popcornlike" patterns of nodule calcification are indicative of benignity, with the first three typically seen in calcified granulomata and the

last in a pulmonary hamartoma (Fig. 63-2). Other patterns of calcification are nonspecific, and up to 15% of lung carcinomas may contain amorphous, stippled, or punctate and eccentric calcification. Avidly enhancing serpentine or tubular feeding arteries and an early draining vein associated with an enhancing nidus are pathognomonic of an arteriovenous malformation (Fig. 63-3). Small satellite nodules around the periphery of a smooth dominant nodule are strongly suggestive of a granulomatous infection. "Ground-glass" opacity surrounding a nodule (the "CT halo sign") is highly suggestive of angioinvasive opportunistic infection such as by aspergillosis, particularly in the setting of neutropenia (Fig. 63-4). A three-dimensional ratio of the nodule's largest axial diameter to the largest craniocaudal diameter >1.78:1 (i.e., a flattened configuration) is highly suggestive of benignity.

Figure 63-1. Hamartoma on CT. Smoothly marginated round SPN contains very low-density fat *(arrows)*, which is pathognomonic for a hamartoma.

A peripheral rim of enhancement or the "enhancing rim sign" of a nodule is also suggestive of benignity.

| Central | Diffuse solid | Laminated | Popcornlike |

Figure 63-2. Four benign patterns of nodule calcification.

8. **What morphologic imaging findings are more suggestive of a malignant SPN?**
Size greater than 2 cm is more suggestive of malignancy. Lobulated or spiculated margins with distortion of adjacent vessels are typically associated with malignancy, although a lobulated or spiculated margin is seen in up to 25% and 10% of benign nodules, respectively. The "corona radiata" sign consists of very fine linear strands extending outward from a nodule and is strongly suggestive of malignancy. Partly solid nodules (i.e., nodules composed of "ground-glass" and solid components) tend to be malignant and are most often due to bronchioloalveo-

Figure 63-3. Pulmonary arteriovenous malformation on CT. Note the tubular enhancing nidus in the right lung *(arrow)* that has enhancement similar to cardiac chambers. Multiple other images demonstrate an enhanced feeding artery and draining vein to and from the nidus (not shown).

lar cell carcinoma (BAC) or adenocarcinoma with BAC features. Internal inhomogeneity, particularly from cystic/bubbly lucencies or pseudocavitation, is strongly suggestive of malignancy, most often from BAC. Cavitary nodules with maximal wall thickness >15 mm and wall irregularity tend to be malignant, whereas those with wall thickness ≤4 mm tend to be benign.

9. **How does measurement of the doubling time of nodules aid in the determination of benignity?**
Doubling time, the time required for a nodule to double in volume (equivalent to an increase of about 26% in diameter), for most malignant nodules

Figure 63-4. Invasive aspergillosis with "halo sign" on CT. Note the pulmonary nodules surrounded by faint "ground-glass" opacities *(arrows)* due to pulmonary hemorrhage.

is between 1 and 15 months. However, nodules that double in volume more rapidly or more slowly than this are typically benign. Generally, lack of growth of a nodule over a 2-year period is strongly suggestive of benignity, although some malignant nodules, such as those due to BAC, bronchial carcinoid, or some pulmonary metastases, may take longer to grow. In general, follow-up CT scans for indeterminate pulmonary nodules are performed at 3, 6, 12, and 24 months after the initial CT scan to assess for interval growth.

10. **How does the degree of enhancement of pulmonary nodules on CT aid in the determination of benignity?**
The degree of enhancement of pulmonary nodules is directly related to the likelihood of malignancy and the vascularity of the nodules and may be determined through CT nodule densitometry. Nodule enhancement of less than 15 Hounsfield units (a measure of density) on CT after IV contrast material administration is strongly predictive of benignity, whereas enhancement of more than 15 Hounsfield units may indicate either malignancy or active inflammation. False-negative enhancement studies may occur occasionally when central necrosis, cavitation, or abundant mucin is present within a pulmonary nodule or if a pulmonary nodule is very small.

11. **How does 2-FDG PET aid in the differentiation of benign and malignant lung nodules?**
Malignant pulmonary nodules generally have increased glucose metabolism with increased uptake, trapping, and accumulation of 2-FDG, a radioisotopic glucose analog that can be seen on PET. Occasionally, active inflammatory granulomatous pulmonary nodules may demonstrate increased uptake of 2-FDG, although not as great in amount as in malignancy. However, lack of 2-FDG uptake in a ≥10 mm pulmonary nodule is strongly predictive of benignity, although malignant nodules that are due to BAC or bronchial carcinoid or that are <10 mm may have low or absent 2-FDG uptake. Dual-point 2-FDG PET with early and delayed imaging can further characterize pulmonary nodules since malignant nodules tend to accumulate radiotracer over time and benign nodules tend to gradually wash out radiotracer.

12. **Describe some clinical features that suggest whether a pulmonary nodule is more likely to be malignant and whether it is more likely to be due to lung carcinoma or a pulmonary metastasis if there is a history of extrapulmonary primary malignancy.**
Older patient age (>35 years old), history of prior malignancy, presence of symptoms and signs of malignancy such as hemoptysis, and history of tobacco use all increase the likelihood that an

SPN is malignant rather than benign. Most patients with a history of extrapulmonary primary malignancy and an SPN have a primary lung carcinoma rather than a pulmonary metastasis or benign lesion, although this varies depending on the type of primary malignancy. For example, a metastasis as the cause of an SPN in this setting is more common than primary lung carcinoma when the primary malignancy is due to melanoma, sarcoma, or testicular carcinoma. Multiplicity of pulmonary nodules also tends to make metastases more likely than lung carcinoma. Finally, primary lung carcinoma occurs more commonly in the upper lung fields, whereas pulmonary metastases occur more commonly in the lower lung fields. However, there are no definitive imaging criteria that can fully separate a pulmonary metastasis from a primary lung carcinoma as the etiologic factor for a pulmonary nodule.

13. **What minimally invasive procedures may be used to obtain tissue samples from a pulmonary nodule?**
Image-guided transthoracic needle biopsy is the procedure of choice for definitive characterization of peripheral pulmonary nodules, whereas bronchoscopic needle biopsy is typically used for the characterization of nodules that involve the central airways and lungs.

14. **What are some potential complications of transthoracic needle biopsy?**
Pneumothorax is the most common complication, occurring in up to 25% of cases, particularly when severe emphysema is present. Nondiagnostic or false-negative biopsy results, hemoptysis, hemorrhage, pain, infection, air embolus, and tumor seeding are less common complications. Avoiding crossing pulmonary fissures with the biopsy needle or avoiding multiple lung punctures decreases the incidence of pneumothorax.

15. **How important is lung carcinoma as a public health issue?**
Lung carcinoma is the most common cause of cancer-related death in both men and women and is the second most common cause of cancer in men and women after prostate cancer and breast cancer, respectively. More Americans will die of lung carcinoma than those with colon, breast, prostate, and pancreas cancers combined. Tobacco use is the No. 1 risk factor for lung carcinoma, and 85% of lung carcinoma deaths are due to smoking. The risk of developing lung carcinoma is proportional to the number of pack-years of smoking. Synchronous primary lung carcinomas occur in fewer than 5% of patients with lung carcinoma, but metachronous primary lung carcinomas may occur in up to 15%, with a latency of about 4–5 years. Overall, survival rates for patients with lung carcinoma are dismal (<15% at 5 years), although those with treated early-stage disease or with a BAC tumor subtype tend to have much better survival rates.

16. **What are the major histologic types and subtypes of lung carcinoma?**
Histologically, 75% are non–small cell lung carcinoma (NSCLC), for which the prognosis primarily depends on surgical stage at diagnosis, and 25% are small cell lung carcinoma (SCLC), which behave aggressively with early and wide dissemination. NSCLC may be subdivided into adenocarcinoma, squamous cell carcinoma, and large cell carcinoma subtypes, in order of decreasing frequency. BAC is a less aggressive subtype of adenocarcinoma that spreads along preexisting alveolar septa without lung parenchymal invasion.

17. **What are some differing features of the various histologic types and subtypes of lung carcinoma?**
Adenocarcinoma is the subtype least closely associated with tobacco use and tends to develop in the lung periphery, whereas squamous cell carcinoma is strongly associated with tobacco use, tends to develop centrally within a lobar or segmental bronchus, and is often cavitary. Large cell carcinoma is a histologic diagnosis of exclusion among the subtypes of lung carcinoma, is strongly associated with tobacco use, and often presents as a large peripheral lung mass. SCLC usually arises centrally within the chest with extensive metastatic lymphadenopathy involving the hila and mediastinum and only rarely cavitates, but it may present in a more limited form in one hemithorax or as an SPN (Fig. 63-5).

18. **What is a superior sulcus tumor?**

    Superior sulcus tumor (or *Pancoast tumor*) usually refers to a primary lung carcinoma that is located in the lung apex and involves the adjacent pleura, chest wall, brachial plexus, and/or subclavian vessels (Fig. 63-6). Typically, this manifests clinically as chest, shoulder, and arm pain with paresthesias, along with Horner's syndrome (ipsilateral ptosis, miosis, and anhidrosis) caused by invasion of the stellate ganglion. Squamous cell carcinoma is the most common subtype involved, and adenocarcinoma is the second most common.

Figure 63-5. SCLC on CT. Note the extensive left hilar and mediastinal lymphadenopathy, a common manifestation of SCLC on initial imaging.

19. **Name the major imaging findings related to lung carcinoma.**

    A pulmonary or endobronchial nodule or mass is seen that may be associated with obstructive atelectasis or pneumonitis; thoracic lymphadenopathy; pleural, mediastinal, or chest wall involvement; or distant metastatic disease (Figs. 63-7 and 63-8). Sometimes, obstructive segmental or lobar atelectasis may be the only sign of lung carcinoma on chest radiography, particularly if associated air bronchograms are not present. When obstructive

Figure 63-6. Pancoast tumor on chest radiography. Note the masslike opacity at the left lung apex *(arrows)* associated with destruction of the posterior left second rib.

Figure 63-7. *A,* NSCLC on chest radiograph. Note the right apical pulmonary mass (M) with lobulated margins. A small right apical pneumothorax is present due to recent percutaneous biopsy. *B,* NSCLC on CT. Note the right apical pulmonary mass (M) with a lobulated and spiculated border and the "corona radiata" sign of very fine linear strands extending outward from the mass *(arrows).*

atelectasis is associated with focal convexity centrally due to the nodule or mass with concavity more distally on chest radiography, an S-shaped smooth fissural margin may be seen that is known as the "S sign of Golden" (Fig. 63-9). Unilateral hilar lymphadenopathy; a unilateral pleural effusion (particularly when present on the left); abrupt cutoff of a bronchus (the "bronchial cutoff sign"); and obscuration of a hilar, mediastinal, or diaphragmatic structure (the "silhouette sign") are other chest radiographic findings of pulmonary malignancy. BAC may appear as a solitary nodule; multiple "ground-glass," solid, or mixed-density pulmonary nodules (Fig. 63-10); or solitary, multiple, or diffuse foci of chronic pulmonary consolidation.

Figure 63-8. Unresectable NSCLC associated with pulmonary artery invasion and lobar obstructive atelectasis on CT. Note the soft tissue mass *(M)* invading the left pulmonary artery *(arrow)* with associated left upper lobe atelectasis *(a)*. Also note the lack of air bronchograms, which is typical of obstructive atelectasis.

Figure 63-9. NSCLC causing lobar atelectasis with "S sign of Golden" on chest radiograph. Note the right upper lobe obstructive atelectasis with an S-shaped fissural margin *(white outline)* with focal convexity centrally due to the central mass and concavity more distally. Again, note the lack of air bronchograms, which is typical of obstructive atelectasis.

Figure 63-10. BAC subtype of NSCLC on CT. Note the SPN in the left lung with mixed "ground-glass" and solid density components.

20. **Describe the tumor node metastasis (TNM) staging system for NSCLC.**
    See Table 63-2.

TABLE 63-2. TNM STAGING SYSTEM OF NSCLC

T = Primary Tumor

T0: no evidence of primary tumor

T1: ≤3 cm, surrounded by lung/visceral pleural, no invasion of mainstem bronchus

T2: >3 cm, involvement of mainstem bronchus ≥2 cm from carina, invasion of visceral pleura; obstructive atelectasis of part of the lung

T3: invasion of chest wall, mediastinal pleura, diaphragm, parietal pericardium, mainstem bronchus <2 cm from carina; obstructive atelectasis of entire lung

T4: invasion of mediastinal structures, malignant pleural effusion, or satellite tumor in primary tumor lobe

N = Regional Lymphadenopathy

N0: no regional lymph node metastases

N1: ipsilateral hilar, peribronchial, or intrapulmonary lymphadenopathy

N2: ipsilateral mediastinal or subcarinal lymphadenopathy

N3: supraclavicular, scalene, contralateral mediastinal, or hilar lymphadenopathy

M = Distant Metastasis

M0: no distant metastasis

M1: distant metastasis

Stage 0: carcinoma in situ

Stage Ia: T1N0M0

Stage Ib: T2N0M0

Stage IIa: T1N1M0

Stage IIb: T2N1M0, T3N0M0

Stage IIIa: T3N1M0, T1–3N2M0

Stage IIIb: T4N0–3M0, T1–3N3M0

Stage IV: T0–4N0–3M1

Note that any N2 lesion is at least stage IIIa, any T4 or N3 lesion is at least stage IIIb, and any M1 lesion is stage IV. Also note that patients with stage 0–IIIa lesions are generally treated with surgery, whereas patients with stage IIIb and IV lesions are generally treated with medical therapy.

---

21. **When is NSCLC generally considered unresectable?**
    When NSCLC is stage IIIb (i.e., with the presence of invasion of vital mediastinal structures, associated malignant pleural effusion, satellite tumor in the primary tumor lobe, or unresectable lymphadenopathy) or stage IV (i.e., with the presence of distant metastases). Unfortunately, symptoms and signs are rarely present until the disease is advanced in stage and therefore more likely to be unresectable.

22. **Are there any reliable screening tests for lung carcinoma? What is the National Lung Screening Trial (NLST)?**

No. At this time, no laboratory or imaging screening test has been shown to decrease lung cancer mortality rates. The NLST is an ongoing multicenter prospective trial that is comparing screening with frontal chest radiography to screening with thin-section low-dose chest CT for a decrease in lung cancer–specific mortality. The trial will be concluded in the year 2010. Research is also currently ongoing in the search for biomarkers that could potentially be used as screening tools for the presence of lung carcinoma or as indicators of high risk for future development of lung carcinoma.

KEY POINTS: PULMONARY NODULES

1. Be aware of the major "blind spots" on frontal chest radiography: the lung apices where the clavicles and ribs overlap, the hilar regions where vascular structures abound, the retrocardiac region, and the lung bases where there is superimposition with the upper abdominal soft tissue.

2. If you see lobar or segmental atelectasis on chest radiography, particularly without air bronchograms, be suspicious of an obstructive endobronchial lesion such as a lung carcinoma, and at the minimum, get a short-term follow-up chest radiograph.

3. If a pulmonary infiltrate does not resolve over time despite treatment with antimicrobial agents, be suspicious of a potential bronchioloalveolar cell subtype of lung carcinoma.

4. The best way to prevent lung cancer is through prevention (i.e., by not smoking).

5. Although mucoid impaction of a bronchus may mimic a pulmonary nodule on chest radiography, one should exclude an endobronchial lesion as the cause for mucus retention in a bronchus if resolution is not seen on follow-up imaging.

23. **Name some treatment options for lung carcinoma.**

Surgical resection (typically lobectomy with lymph node resection), chemotherapy, and radiation therapy may be used depending on the stage of disease and the histology of the tumor. Cessation of tobacco use is also part of treatment. Newer techniques such as percutaneous ablation of focal lung or bronchial tumors are currently under investigation.

24. **Describe the imaging findings of pulmonary metastases.**

Solitary or multiple pulmonary and/or endobronchial nodules or masses are often seen, which may be ill defined or well circumscribed, "ground-glass" or solid in density, and often associated with metastases to other thoracic or extrathoracic anatomic locations. Depending on the underlying primary malignancy, the lesions may be homogeneous or heterogeneous with cystic, necrotic, calcific, or hemorrhagic change and may vary in size from very small (miliary) nodules to very large "cannonball" masses (Fig. 63-11). Interestingly,

Figure 63-11. Pulmonary metastases on CT. Note the multiple variably sized smoothly marginated nodules throughout lungs. Note also that the largest nodule *(arrow)* resembles a "cannonball."

pneumothorax is often associated with pulmonary metastatic disease from osteogenic sarcoma. Overall, the lungs are an extremely common site of metastatic disease.

25. **What is lymphangitic carcinomatosis?**

This is the hematogenous spread of metastatic disease to lung interstitium with subsequent lymphatic obstruction, interstitial edema, and fibrosis. Primary tumors of the breast, lung, stomach, pancreas, ovary, and cervix are often associated with lymphangitic carcinomatosis. On chest radiography, the lungs may appear clear, or they may demonstrate a central linear pattern of interstitial thickening that is commonly bilateral but asymmetric in distribution between the lungs. On CT, typical smooth or nodular thickening of the interlobular septa is seen often with peribronchovascular thickening and asymmetric involvement of the lungs bilaterally (Fig. 63-12).

Figure 63-12. Lymphangitic carcinomatosis on CT. Note the central linear pattern of interstitial lung disease with nodular thickening of the interlobular septa *(arrows)* asymmetrically involving the right lung more than the left lung. A left breast implant (b) is present, as this patient had breast carcinoma.

26. **What are pulmonary carcinoid tumors?**

These are rare neuroendocrine neoplasms that range from low-grade typical carcinoids to more aggressive atypical carcinoids. They are not related to tobacco use and occur slightly more commonly in women. The majority arise centrally in an endobronchial location and are commonly associated with segmental or lobar obstructive atelectasis or pneumonitis, whereas the remainder appear as well-circumscribed peripheral pulmonary nodules or masses. These lesions typically demonstrate avid enhancement, and up to 40% may be associated with internal calcification. Carcinoid syndrome is very uncommonly associated with pulmonary carcinoid tumors.

27. **What is a pulmonary hamartoma?**

This is the most common benign neoplasm of the lung and typically presents as an asymptomatic well-circumscribed SPN, typically during the fourth through seventh decades of life. Pathologically, they are mesenchymal tumors that have foci of mature cartilage separated by islands of fat and bronchial epithelium, often with fibrosis, calcification, and/or ossification. Typical CT findings include a smoothly marginated SPN that often contains visible fat or dense foci of calcification and/or ossification.

28. **What is congenital bronchial atresia?**

Congenital bronchial atresia is due to atresia or stenosis of a bronchus at or near its origin, most often seen in the apicoposterior segment of the left upper lobe. Imaging findings include hyperlucency with air trapping and decreased vascularity to the portion of lung supplied by the involved bronchus, along with a nonenhancing hilar mass (bronchocele) or nonenhancing branching soft tissue opacities usually with bronchial dilation due to mucoid impaction. Congenital bronchial atresia can appear as an SPN on chest radiography.

BIBLIOGRAPHY

1. Henschke CI, Yankelevitz DF, Mirtcheva R, et al: CT screening for lung cancer: Frequency and significance of part-solid and nonsolid nodules. Am J Roentgenol 178:1053–1057, 2002.

2. Jemal A, Tiwari RC, Murray T, et al: Cancer statistics, 2004. CA Cancer J Clin 54:8–29, 2004.

3. Leef JL 3rd, Klein JS: The solitary pulmonary nodule. Radiol Clin North Am 40:123–143, ix, 2002.

4. Matthies A, Hickeson M, Cuchiara A, Alavi A: Dual time point 18F-FDG PET for the evaluation of pulmonary nodules. J Nucl Med 43:871–875, 2002.

5. Takashima S, Sone S, Li F, et al: Small solitary pulmonary nodules (≤1 cm) detected at population-based CT screening for lung cancer: Reliable high-resolution CT features of benign lesions. Am J Roentgenol 180:955–964, 2003.

6. Tan BB, Flaherty KR, Kazerooni EA, Iannettoni MD: The solitary pulmonary nodule. Chest 123:89S–96S, 2003.

7. Tang AW, Moss HA, Robertson RJ: The solitary pulmonary nodule. Eur J Radiol 45:69–77, 2003.

CHAPTER 64

INTERSTITIAL LUNG DISEASE

Wallace T. Miller, Jr., MD, and Drew A. Torigian, MD

1. **What radiographic features distinguish interstitial diseases from airspace diseases?**

There are two primary characteristics that radiographically distinguish interstitial from airspace diseases. First, interstitial diseases displace little of the air within the lung, whereas airspace diseases displace large amounts of air. Thus, interstitial diseases change the overall opacity of the lung very little, whereas airspace diseases in most cases dramatically increase the opacity (whiteness) of the lung on chest radiography. Secondly, interstitial diseases appear as increases in small nodules (generally <5 mm in diameter) and/or thin lines (<5 mm in width) within the lung, whereas airspace disorders appear as indistinctly marginated patches of opacity. See Figure 64-1 for the normal appearance of the lungs on frontal chest radiography.

Figure 64-1. Normal frontal chest radiograph of the lungs. Note the normal sharp delineation of branching vessels from the bilateral hila outward.

2. **What factors influence the likelihood of one interstitial disease over another interstitial disease?**

There are three primary factors that affect the likelihood of a given interstitial disease. The first and most important is the relative incidence of a given disease in the general population. In general, typical presentations of common diseases are most likely, followed by atypical presentations of common diseases, followed by typical presentations of uncommon diseases, followed by atypical presentations of uncommon diseases. Secondly, the clinical history of the patient will strongly influence the likelihood of any given diagnosis. Lastly, the radiographic pattern of the interstitial disease will influence the likelihood of any given diagnosis.

3. **What is the most common interstitial abnormality identified on chest radiography?**

Interstitial pulmonary edema, usually caused by congestive heart failure, is the most common interstitial abnormality encountered in daily practice. Therefore, a diagnosis of interstitial pulmonary edema should be considered in all cases of interstitial abnormality detected on a chest radiograph. In many cases, it might be advisable to diurese the patient and repeat the chest radiograph as the first diagnostic test.

4. **What are the most common interstitial abnormalities other than interstitial pulmonary edema?**

Idiopathic pulmonary fibrosis and sarcoidosis are the most common chronic interstitial disorders in the United States and should be among the first diagnoses entertained when encountering a chest radiograph with an interstitial abnormality.

5. **What radiographic characteristics help determine the diagnosis of interstitial disorders?**
The interstitial abnormalities may be roughly subdivided into those that produce small round opacities ("nodular" interstitial diseases) and those that produce small networks of holes ("reticular" interstitial diseases). In this chapter, we will describe one nodular pattern of interstitial disease and the three following reticular patterns of interstitial disease: the peripheral reticular pattern, the linear pattern, and the cystic pattern.

6. **What is the appearance of the nodular interstitial pattern on chest radiography?**
A normal chest radiograph will typically demonstrate many small nodular opacities that represent normal blood vessels end on. In most cases, these small nodules can be recognized as blood vessels because they overlap with a small line of similar diameter, which represents an adjacent branch of the pulmonary vascular tree. The nodular pattern of interstitial lung disease appears as increased numbers of small nodular opacities (<10 mm in diameter) that are randomly distributed throughout the lung parenchyma.

Figure 64-2. Nodular pattern of interstitial lung disease.

These small nodules will not overlap with the normal vascular lines of the lung (Figs. 64-2 and 64-3).

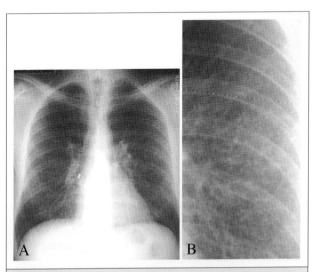

Figure 64-3. *A,* Nodular pattern of interstitial lung disease due to cryptococcal infection on a frontal chest radiograph. Note the subtle, tiny nodular densities throughout lung fields bilaterally. *B,* Nodular pattern of interstitial lung disease caused by cryptococcal infection on a magnified view of a chest radiograph. Note the subtle, tiny nodular densities throughout lung.

7. **What disorders cause nodular interstitial diseases?**

There are three broad groups of disorders that cause nodular interstitial diseases: granulomatous lung diseases, nodular pneumoconioses, and small metastases.

8. **Discuss some granulomatous lung diseases that cause nodular interstitial disease.**

Sarcoidosis is the most common granulomatous interstitial lung disease to cause a micronodular pattern. This idiopathic disorder typically presents in middle-aged individuals, especially those of African-American descent. Miliary infections also cause a small nodular pattern and are typified by miliary tuberculosis but also include miliary spread of histoplasmosis, cryptococcosis, coccidioidomycosis, and blastomycosis. These infections typically affect immunocompromised individuals, such as those with HIV infection, those who have undergone organ transplantation, or those with a history of chronic steroid use. Many physicians are unaware that extrinsic allergic alveolitis or hypersensitivity pneumonitis causes a granulomatous interstitial fibrosis but may also produce an interstitial nodular pattern of lung disease. Langerhans cell histiocytosis (LCH), also known as "eosinophilic granuloma of the lung," may also produce a nodular pattern of interstitial lung disease. In the great majority of cases, pulmonary LCH is associated with a history of smoking and typically presents as persistent cough and/or dyspnea in young and middle-aged adults. In the early stages of disease, the patient will develop small nodular areas of interstitial fibrosis. As the disorder progresses, cystic lesions may develop in association with an obstructive lung disease.

9. **Discuss some pneumoconioses and tumors that lead to nodular interstitial lung disease.**

The pneumoconioses that may produce a micronodular interstitial pattern are silicosis, coal workers' pneumoconiosis, talcosis, and berylliosis. Pneumoconioses are diffuse interstitial lung diseases due to inorganic dusts, most often related to occupational exposures. Mining, sandblasting, gravestone engraving, and pottery are some of the occupations in which workers may be exposed to silica dust with resultant silicosis; as identified in the name, coal workers' pneumoconiosis is seen in coal miners. Berylliosis is an uncommon chronic pneumoconiosis that may be encountered in individuals who mine beryllium, manufacture beryllium ceramics, or who previously manufactured beryllium lighting (these types of lights are no longer manufactured because of the high risk of acute and chronic berylliosis). Talcosis may occur as a result of the mining of talc or excessive inhalation of talcum powder and in IV drug abusers. Thyroid carcinoma is the prototypical tumor that produces thousands of tiny micronodular metastases and may appear as a nodular interstitial lung disease. Breast cancer may also produce this pattern of metastasis; other primary tumors will rarely produce a micronodular pattern of lung metastasis.

10. **What is the chest radiographic staging system for sarcoidosis, and what is the clinical significance?**

Table 64-1 lists the staging system for sarcoidosis. The higher the stage of sarcoidosis, the greater the likelihood that the patient will experience chronic respiratory deficits.

11. **Name some examples of hypersensitivity pneumonitis (extrinsic allergic alveolitis).**

Farmer's lung is the prototypical example of a hypersensitivity pneumonitis. There are a wide variety of other hypersensitivity pneumonitides. Some of the many other causes are listed in Table 64-2. These disorders represent an allergic lung reaction to a wide variety of organic dusts that can initially manifest as capillary leak pulmonary edema but chronically result in granulomatous interstitial fibrosis. In most cases, the offending antigens are microorganisms that grow within decaying vegetable matter. Antigens from these organisms are delivered to the lung via inhalation of dust or aerosolized contaminated water. Notable exceptions to this general concept

TABLE 64-1. CHEST RADIOGRAPHIC STAGING SYSTEM FOR SARCOIDOSIS

Stage	Radiographic Appearance
0	Chest radiograph appears normal
I	Chest radiographic evidence of hilar or mediastinal lymphadenopathy without evidence of interstitial disease
II	Chest radiographic evidence of hilar or mediastinal lymphadenopathy and evidence of interstitial lung disease
III	Chest radiographic evidence of interstitial disease without evidence of hilar or mediastinal lymphadenopathy
IV	Chest radiographic evidence of interstitial fibrosis with distortion of pulmonary structures, such as blood vessels, without evidence of hilar or mediastinal lymphadenopathy

TABLE 64-2. CAUSES OF HYPERSENSITIVITY PNEUMONITIS

Exposures	Causes
Occupational	**Organic dust**
Farmer's lung	Hay
Baker's lung	Flour
Sugar cane worker's lung	Sugar cane dust
Cotton worker's lung	Cotton dust
Mushroom worker's lung	Mushrooms
Hobbies	
Bird fancier's lung	Bird feathers
Other exposures	
Down pillows and comforters	Bird feathers
Hot tubs	Aerosolized water
Humidifiers	Aerosolized water

are the bird-related hypersensitivity pneumonitides. In bird fancier's lung, hypersensitivity occurs against bird-related antigens, such as those found in bird feathers.

12. **Why do IV drug abusers get talcosis?**
Not all IV drug abuse will result in talcosis. The process that can result in talcosis is the IV injection of oral medications. These medications are ground into a fine powder, suspended in fluid, and injected intravenously. Pills contain inorganic fillers, including talc and methylcellulose, which are inorganic substances that embolize to the lung microvasculature and result in a foreign body giant cell granulomatous reaction, which may appear as small nodules on chest radiography.

13. **What radiographic feature of the nodular pneumoconioses is most strongly associated with respiratory deficits?**

Progressive massive fibrosis (PMF), also know as "conglomerate masses," is the radiographic feature most strongly associated with respiratory deficits. In PMF, the small nodular areas of fibrosis associated with the nodular pneumoconioses progressively coalesce into large (>3 cm) fibrotic masses. These masses are typically found in the upper lung zones and result in fibrotic distortion of the surrounding lung parenchyma. All of the nodular pneumoconioses can cause PMF, but it is most strongly associated with silicosis. Many patients with simple silicosis (nodular interstitial disease without PMF) will be clinically asymptomatic. However, nearly all patients with complicated silicosis (nodular interstitial disease with PMF) will complain of dyspnea. The causes of the nodular interstitial pattern are reviewed in Table 64-3.

TABLE 64-3. CAUSES OF NODULAR INTERSTITIAL LUNG DISEASE PATTERN

Category	Diseases
Granulomatous diseases	Sarcoidosis
	Miliary infections
	Tuberculosis
	Histoplasmosis
	Coccidioidomycosis
	Cryptococcosis
	Blastomycosis
	Hypersensitivity pneumonitis
	LCH (eosinophilic granuloma)
Nodular pneumoconiosis	Silicosis
	Coal workers' pneumoconiosis
	Berylliosis
	Talcosis
Metastasis	Thyroid carcinoma
	Other malignancies

14. **What are the radiographic characteristics of the peripheral reticular pattern?**

The peripheral reticular pattern has two distinguishing features: (1) the small size of the holes (typically <5 mm) seen within a network of fine crisscrossing linear opacities and (2) the peripheral and basilar distribution of the network. Thus, the network typically is seen filling the costophrenic angles on both frontal and lateral chest radiographs (Figs. 64-4 and 64-5).

Figure 64-4. Peripheral reticular pattern of interstitial lung disease.

Figure 64-5. *A,* Peripheral reticular pattern of interstitial lung disease due to IPF on a frontal chest radiograph. Note the peripheral and basilar distribution. *B,* Magnified view of a chest radiograph. Note the network of fine crisscrossing linear opacities in peripheral and basilar distribution of the lungs forming small holes between opacities.

15. **Which diseases cause the peripheral reticular pattern?**
    Even though a variety of disorders may occasionally result in the peripheral reticular pattern, the vast majority of cases are caused by idiopathic pulmonary fibrosis (IPF), a connective tissue disorder, or asbestosis.

16. **What demographic features can help distinguish the cause of the peripheral reticular pattern?**
    Asbestosis and IPF are disorders of the elderly, usually in individuals older than 50, whereas connective tissue disorders tend to affect younger individuals, often in their 30s and 40s. Patients must have had an extensive exposure to asbestos dust to acquire asbestosis. Therefore, nearly all patients with asbestosis will have an occupational exposure to asbestos, such as from mining, roofing, car brake shoe repair, shipyard work, or boiler making. Asbestosis is almost exclusively seen in men because few women have sufficient asbestos dust exposure to acquire the disease. Connective tissue disorders are more commonly encountered in women, and therefore more patients with connective tissue–related interstitial disease are women.

17. **Which connective tissue disorders can result in interstitial disease?**
    Scleroderma, or progressive systemic sclerosis (PSS), has the highest incidence of interstitial fibrosis among all connective tissue disorders. Rheumatoid arthritis (RA) has the highest prevalence of interstitial disease because it is among the most common connective tissue disorders and may occasionally cause interstitial fibrosis. Dermatomyositis/polymyositis may also result in interstitial fibrosis. By virtue of its potential to overlap with PSS, RA, or dermatomyositis/polymyositis, mixed connective tissue disorder (MCTD) may also cause interstitial fibrosis. Systemic lupus erythematosus (SLE) is among the most prevalent connective tissue disorders but only rarely produces clinically significant interstitial fibrosis. Although pathologic and radiologic studies may demonstrate mild abnormalities, it is quite rare for patients with SLE to have respiratory symptoms related to interstitial fibrosis. When these disorders cause

interstitial fibrosis, they produce a peripheral reticular interstitial pattern on chest radiography.

18. **Are there any imaging features that can help distinguish the cause of the peripheral reticular pattern?**
In most cases, there will be no imaging features that will help distinguish the different causes of the peripheral reticular pattern. However, occasionally, there will be extrapulmonary findings that will help in the differential diagnosis of the peripheral reticular pattern. Approximately two thirds of patients with asbestosis also have asbestos-related pleural plaques. Patients with PSS may have a radiographically identifiable dilated esophagus as a result of the CREST syndrome. CREST is a mnemonic that stands for *c*alcinosis cutis, *R*aynaud's phenomenon, *e*sophageal dysfunction, *s*clerodactyly, and *t*elangiectasia. Patients with RA may have erosions of the distal clavicles as a result of acromioclavicular arthritis. The causes of the peripheral reticular pattern of interstitial lung disease are reviewed in Table 64-4.

TABLE 64-4.	CAUSES OF THE PERIPHERAL RETICULAR INTERSTITIAL LUNG DISEASE PATTERN

Idiopathic pulmonary fibrosis
Connective tissue disorders
    Scleroderma, or PSS
    RA
    Polymyositis/dermatomyositis
    MCTD
    SLE
Asbestosis

19. **What are the imaging characteristics of the linear pattern on chest radiography?**
The lines demonstrable on a normal chest radiograph represent the branching pulmonary arteries and veins. These begin centrally and radiate from the hilum toward the periphery of the lung. The linear pattern appears as increased numbers of lines radiating from the hilum of the lung, like an explosion of lines from the central hila bilaterally. In addition, the linear pattern may produce Kerley's B lines. These are thin horizontal lines 1–2 cm long, extending from the lateral chest wall toward the central lung (Figs. 64-6 and 64-7). The most common cause of the linear pattern is congestive heart failure, and to the degree that an interstitial abnormality resembles congestive heart failure, it is more likely to represent the linear pattern of interstitial disease. Novice readers should take care not to overdiagnose the linear interstitial pattern. There is a wide variation in the normal appearance of chest radiographs. If you are unsure of whether there is an interstitial abnormality present on a chest radiograph, it is usually best to assume that the examination is normal.

Figure 64-6. Linear pattern of interstitial lung disease.

Figure 64-7. *A,* Linear pattern of interstitial lung disease due to congestive heart failure on a frontal chest radiograph. Note the symmetrically increased number of lines radiating from the bilateral hila. *B,* Central linear pattern of interstitial lung disease caused by congestive heart failure on a magnified view of a chest radiograph. Note the symmetrically increased number of lines radiating from the bilateral hila.

20. **What disorders cause the linear pattern of interstitial disease?**
Congestive heart failure and other causes of interstitial pulmonary edema are the most common causes of the linear pattern. In nearly all cases, the presence of a linear interstitial pattern should be assumed to represent interstitial pulmonary edema. Lymphangitic carcinomatosis is the most common chronic cause for the linear pattern. This is a form of hematogenous metastasis that grows along the interstitial framework of the lung rather than growing concentrically as nodules. Breast and lung cancers are the malignancies most likely to cause a pattern of lymphangitic metastasis. Gastric, pancreatic, and ovarian carcinomas are some other causes of lymphangitic carcinomatosis. Sarcoidosis will typically cause peribronchial granulomata, which may also result in interstitial lung disease with a pattern of lines radiating from the hilum of the lung, producing a linear pattern. Very rarely, some diffuse pneumonias such as *Mycoplasma, Pneumocystis*, and viral pneumonia will appear as a linear interstitial pattern.

21. **Are there any imaging clues that may help to distinguish the cause of the linear interstitial pattern?**
In most cases, there will be no imaging clues that help to distinguish the cause of the linear pattern of interstitial disease. One notable exception is the recognition of a markedly asymmetric linear pattern, in which one lung is considerably more affected than the other. This imaging finding is virtually always associated with lymphangitic carcinomatosis. Causes of the linear interstitial pattern include:
- Interstitial pulmonary edema
- Lymphangitic carcinomatosis
- Sarcoidosis
- Diffuse pneumonia

22. **What are the imaging characteristics of the cystic pattern of interstitial lung disease?**
This pattern is characterized by a group of curved lines that produce a network of fine ring shadows in the more central lung. Although a reticular pattern, the cystic pattern is quite distinct

from the peripheral reticular pattern. In the cystic pattern, the holes are, on average, approximately 10 mm in diameter, which are much larger than those seen in the peripheral reticular pattern. Furthermore, the rings of the cystic pattern are distributed in the more central lung, whereas the peripheral reticular pattern characteristically affects the subpleural and basilar lung (Figs. 64-8 and 64-9).

23. **What disorders produce the cystic interstitial pattern?**
The cystic interstitial pattern is the least common of the interstitial pat-

Figure 64-8. Cystic pattern of interstitial lung disease.

Figure 64-9. *A,* Cystic pattern of interstitial lung disease due to eosinophilic granuloma on a frontal chest radiograph. Note the network of fine ring shadows in the more central lung and the larger holes between opacities (compared with the smaller holes in peripheral reticular pattern). *B,* Cystic pattern of interstitial lung disease due to eosinophilic granuloma on a magnified view of a chest radiograph. Note the network of fine ring shadows in the more central lung and the larger holes between opacities (compared with the smaller holes in peripheral reticular pattern). *C,* Cystic pattern of interstitial lung disease due to eosinophilic granuloma on CT. Note the multiple cysts of variable size throughout the lungs.

terns on chest radiography, and the most common cause of the cystic pattern is not interstitial lung disease but emphysema. Emphysema will usually appear as a decrease in the number and conspicuity of the normal lines seen on chest radiography. However, it has been recognized for many years that, occasionally, emphysema will appear as an increase in the number and conspicuity of interstitial lines. When emphysema does this, it appears in the cystic interstitial pattern. Diffuse bronchiectasis may also appear as many ring shadows distributed throughout the lung parenchyma. Two rare disorders that may also cause this pattern are LCH (which was previously discussed along with the nodular pattern) and lymphangioleiomyomatosis (LAM). LAM is a rare hormonally mediated disorder of young and middle-aged women. Proliferation of interstitial smooth muscle results in air trapping and production of small uniform cystic spaces in the lung. Table 64-5 lists the causes of the cystic interstitial lung disease pattern.

KEY POINTS: INTERSTITIAL LUNG DISEASE

1. Interstitial pulmonary edema, usually due to congestive heart failure, is the most common interstitial abnormality encountered in daily practice.

2. The nodular pattern of interstitial lung disease appears as increased numbers of nodular opacities (<10 mm) that are randomly distributed throughout the lung parenchyma. The three broad groups of disorders that cause nodular interstitial disease are granulomatous lung diseases, nodular pneumoconioses, and small metastases.

3. The two distinguishing features of the peripheral reticular pattern of interstitial lung disease are the small size of the holes (typically <5 mm) seen within a network of fine crisscrossing linear opacities and a peripheral and basilar distribution of this network. The vast majority of cases will be caused by IPF, a connective tissue disorder, or asbestosis.

4. The linear pattern of interstitial lung disease appears as increased numbers of lines radiating from the hila centrally. This pattern also may produce peripheral Kerley's B lines. The most common cause of this pattern is congestive heart failure, although lymphangitic carcinomatosis is the most common chronic cause of this pattern.

5. The cystic pattern is characterized by a group of curved lines that produce a network of fine ring shadows in the more central lung with larger holes than those seen in the peripheral reticular pattern. The most common cause of this pattern is emphysema.

TABLE 64-5.   CAUSES OF THE CYSTIC INTERSTITIAL LUNG DISEASE PATTERN

Emphysema
LCH (eosinophilic granuloma)
LAM
Diffuse bronchiectasis
    Cystic fibrosis
    Dysmotile cilia syndrome
    Allergic bronchopulmonary aspergillosis
    Immunodeficiency states
        Common variable immunodeficiency
        Hyperimmunoglobulin E syndrome
        Other

24. **What disorders cause diffuse bronchiectasis?**

Although a variety of disorders may result in bronchiectasis, only a few diseases cause wide-spread bronchiectasis that involves the majority of the lung parenchyma. The most common of these is cystic fibrosis. Other diseases include dysmotile cilia syndrome; allergic bronchopulmonary aspergillosis; and a variety of immunodeficiency states, such as common variable immunodeficiency syndrome, natural killer cell deficiency, and hyperimmunoglobulin E syndrome.

25. **Are there any imaging features that help to distinguish the cause of the cystic pattern?**

In many cases, the disorders that cause the cystic pattern will produce radiographically indistinguishable disease. One notable exception is diffuse bronchiectasis. The cystic spaces caused by bronchiectasis typically produce thick-walled, distinct ring shadows, whereas the other disorders often cause very faint rings (*see* Table 64-5 for causes of the cystic interstitial pattern).

26. **When is computed tomography (CT) scanning indicated for the evaluation of interstitial lung disease?**

CT is both more sensitive and more specific than chest radiography for interstitial abnormalities. Thus, in many advanced cases with obvious chest radiographic findings, no further imaging will be necessary. However, patients with apparently normal or minimally abnormal chest radiographs in whom there is a clinical suspicion of interstitial lung disease should receive a thin-section chest CT to better evaluate for the presence of interstitial lung disease. Furthermore, patients with chest radiographs that are nonspecific may benefit from a CT study, which in many cases will allow for a narrower differential diagnosis. Lastly, CT provides improved characterization of the extent of disease. Therefore, in cases in which therapeutic decisions will be based on imaging evidence of progression, stability, or regression of disease, CT scanning is indicated.

27. **What type of CT scan is indicated for the evaluation of interstitial lung disease?**

CT scanning has inherently less spatial resolution than standard chest radiography. Since interstitial diseases are typified by very fine spatial abnormalities, it is necessary to maximize the spatial resolution of CT images. This is done by minimizing the collimation of the CT scanner. Collimation, at most, should be 1.5 mm. Many multislice spiral scanners obtain images at this resolution in nearly all studies, although older single-slice spiral and nonspiral scanners require special imaging protocols to minimize the slice collimation. These imaging protocols are often called "high-resolution" scans because of the improved spatial resolution that is characteristic of the studies.

BIBLIOGRAPHY

1. Kazerooni EA: High-resolution CT of the lungs. Am J Roentgenol 177:501–519, 2001.
2. Miller WT Jr: Radiographic evaluation of diffuse interstitial lung disease: Review of a dying art. Semin Ultrasound CT MR 23:324–338, 2002.
3. Muller N, Fraser R, Colman N, Pare PD: Radiologic Diagnosis of Diseases of the Chest. Philadelphia, W.B. Saunders, 2001.
4. Webb WR, Muller NL, Naidich D: High-Resolution CT of the Lung, 3rd ed. New York, Lippincott-Raven, 2001.

CHAPTER 65

MEDIASTINAL DISEASES

Drew A. Torigian, MD, and Wallace T. Miller, Jr., MD

1. **Describe the anatomy of the mediastinum.**

   The mediastinum is located centrally within the thorax between the pleural cavities laterally, the sternum anteriorly, the spine posteriorly, the thoracic inlet superiorly, and the diaphragm inferiorly. It is usually divided into anterior, middle, and posterior "compartments" to help categorize tumors and diseases by their site of origin and location. Lesions that arise in these different compartments are generally related to the anatomic structures located within the compartments. Figure 65-1, *A*, shows the normal appearance of the mediastinum on frontal chest radiography.

2. **What are the three compartments of the mediastinum?**

   The anterior mediastinal compartment is the space posterior to the sternum and anterior to the heart and trachea extending from the thoracic inlet to the diaphragm and contains the thymus gland, thyroid gland, fat, and lymph nodes. The middle mediastinal compartment is the space that contains the heart and pericardium along with the ascending aorta and aortic arch, brachiocephalic vessels, venae cavae, main pulmonary arteries and veins, trachea and bronchi, fat, and lymph nodes. The posterior mediastinal compartment is the space posterior to the middle mediastinal compartment that contains the descending thoracic aorta, esophagus, azygos and hemiazygos veins, autonomic ganglia and nerves, thoracic duct, fat, and lymph nodes. Figure 65-1, *B*, delineates the three compartments of the mediastinum on lateral chest radiography.

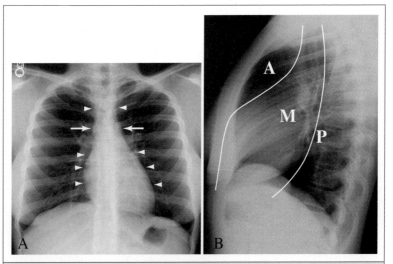

Figure 65-1. *A,* Normal frontal chest radiograph. Note the normal width of the mediastinum *(between arrows)* and the sharp demarcation of mediastinal contours *(arrowheads)* against the adjacent lungs. *B,* Normal lateral chest radiograph. Note the lines separating the anterior (A), middle (M), and posterior (P) compartments of the mediastinum.

3. **What is the differential diagnosis of major anterior mediastinal lesions?**
   In the list below, an asterisk (*) indicates the most common causes:
   1. *Thymic masses*
      - Lymphoma*
      - Thymoma* (Fig. 65-2)
      - Thymic carcinoma (Fig. 65-2)
      - Thymic carcinoid
      - Thymolipoma
      - Thymic cyst
      - Thymic hyperplasia
   2. *Thyroid masses*
      - Thyroid goiter*
      - Thyroid cyst
      - Thyroid adenoma
      - Thyroid carcinoma

Figure 65-2. *A,* Right anterior mediastinal mass due to mixed thymoma and thymic carcinoma on a frontal chest radiograph. Note the ovoid mass (M) overlying the right cardiac border that is partially obscured *(arrow). B,* Right anterior mediastinal mass due to mixed thymoma and thymic carcinoma on a lateral chest radiograph. Note the ovoid mass (M) overlying the anterior aspect of the heart. *C,* Right anterior mediastinal mass due to mixed thymoma and thymic carcinoma on computed tomography (CT). Note the ovoid enhancing soft tissue mass (M) in the right anterior mediastinum.

3. *Germ cell tumors*
   - Teratoma and teratocarcinoma*
   - Seminoma
   - Mixed germ cell tumors

4. **What is the differential diagnosis of major middle mediastinal lesions?**
   In the list below, an asterisk (*) indicates the most common causes:
   - Goiter
   - Lymphadenopathy
   - Metastatic disease* (lung cancer is the most common etiologic factor)
   - Lymphoma (non-Hodgkin's lymphoma and Hodgkin's lymphoma) or leukemia*
   - Granulomatous infection (fungus, tuberculosis [TB], nontuberculous mycobacterium)
   - Sarcoidosis
   - Inhalational lung disease (silicosis, coal workers' pneumoconiosis, or berylliosis)
   - Castleman's disease
   - Aortic abnormalities: aneurysm,* dissection,* traumatic aortic rupture (Fig. 65-3)
   - Bronchopulmonary foregut cysts
   - Tracheal tumor
   - Esophageal abnormalities: neoplasms (carcinoma, leiomyoma, leiomyosarcoma), achalasia
   - Hiatal hernia* (often contains an air-fluid level)
   - Cardiac tumor
   - Left ventricular or thoracic aortic aneurysm or pseudoaneurysm
   - Pulmonary artery aneurysm
   - Neurogenic tumor of the vagus nerve

A

B

Figure 65-3. *A,* Mediastinal hematoma and left hemothorax due to traumatic aortic transection on a supine frontal chest radiograph. Note the widening of the mediastinum *(between arrows)* and increased density of the left hemithorax due to the layering hemothorax behind the left lung. *B,* Mediastinal hematoma and left hemothorax on CT due to traumatic aortic transection. Note the high-density mediastinal hemorrhage (h) and the left hemothorax (H) along with the abnormal contour of the transected descending thoracic aorta *(arrow).*

5. **What is the differential diagnosis of major posterior mediastinal lesions?**
   In the list below, an asterisk (*) indicates the most common causes:
   - Neurogenic tumors* (peripheral nerve, sympathetic ganglion, or parasympathetic involvement)
   - Primary or metastatic bone tumor of the thoracic spine
   - Osteomyelitis or paraspinal abscess of the thoracic spine
   - Extramedullary hematopoiesis

6. **What is the differential diagnosis of fat-containing mediastinal lesions?**
   - Lipoma
   - Mature teratoma

- Thymolipoma
- Well-differentiated liposarcoma
- Mediastinal lipomatosis
- Fat-containing hernia (hiatal, Bochdalek's, or Morgagni's hernia)
- Posterior mediastinal angiomyolipoma

7. **What is the differential diagnosis of cystic mediastinal lesions?**
   1. Cysts with a thin, smooth wall
      - Pericardial cyst
      - Bronchogenic cyst
      - Esophageal duplication cyst
      - Thymic cyst
      - Neurenteric cyst
      - Mediastinal pancreatic pseudocyst
      - Intrathoracic meningocele
   2. Cysts with a thick wall, mural nodularity, or internal septations
      - Thymic teratoma
      - Any mediastinal tumor with necrosis or cystic change
      - Mediastinal abscess

8. **Name different collections that may occur within the mediastinum.**
   - Fluid: mediastinal edema or pericardial effusion
   - Blood: mediastinal hematoma or hemopericardium
   - Pus: mediastinal abscess, pericardial abscess, or acute mediastinitis
   - Air: pneumomediastinum and pneumopericardium
   - Fat: mediastinal lipomatosis
   - Fibrosis: fibrosing mediastinitis
   - Cells: mediastinal tumor

9. **What clinical symptoms and signs can be associated with mediastinal lesions?**
   Compression or invasion of the trachea or bronchi, recurrent laryngeal nerve, or esophagus may produce cough, dyspnea, chest pain, respiratory infection, hoarseness, or dysphagia. Compression or invasion of the adjacent cardiovascular structures may produce superior vena cava syndrome; cardiac dysrhythmias; constrictive pathophysiology; cardiac tamponade; or rarely, sudden death. Interestingly, about 75% of asymptomatic patients with mediastinal tumors have benign lesions, whereas about 66% of symptomatic patients with mediastinal masses have malignant lesions.

10. **What is a thymoma?**
    A thymoma is a rare tumor that is the most common primary tumor of the thymus and the most common primary tumor of the anterior mediastinum. It occurs in men and women equally and most often occurs after age 40. It is an epithelial neoplasm composed of a mixture of epithelial cells and mature lymphocytes. About 33% are invasive, and the remainder are encapsulated. Complete surgical resection is the major treatment for a thymoma. Radiation therapy or chemotherapy may be used for an invasive thymoma, an incompletely resected thymoma, or a disseminated thymoma. Most patients with an encapsulated thymoma will be cured with surgical resection, and many with a microscopically invasive thymoma will be cured with surgery and adjunctive radiation therapy. However, those with macroscopic invasion will often have a prolonged course with slowly growing metastatic disease.

11. **Describe the clinical presentation of a thymoma.**
    Most patients are asymptomatic, although 33% may be symptomatic because of compression or invasion of adjacent structures. Up to 50% may have a paraneoplastic syndrome such as

myasthenia gravis, hypogammaglobulinemia, or pure red blood cell aplasia. About 30–50% of patients with a thymoma may develop myasthenia gravis, whereas 15% of patients with myasthenia gravis have a thymoma. Ten percent with a thymoma may develop hypogammaglobulinemia, whereas 5% with hypogammaglobulinemia have a thymoma. Five percent with a thymoma may develop red cell aplasia, whereas 50% with red blood cell aplasia have a thymoma.

12. **List the imaging findings of a thymoma.**

One typically sees a well-defined, rounded, or lobulated anterosuperior mediastinal soft tissue mass arising from one of the thymic lobes with asymmetric growth toward one side of the midline, often with necrotic, cystic, hemorrhagic, or calcific changes. About 33% of thymomas invade through the capsule with involvement of the mediastinal fat, pleura, pericardium, great vessels, right atrium, or lung, less commonly with extension through the diaphragm into the peritoneal cavity or retroperitoneum. Metastatic disease is most commonly to the pleura, often mimicking malignant pleural mesothelioma with unilateral pleural thickening, masses, or diffuse nodular circumferential pleural thickening encasing the ipsilateral lung. Uncommonly, pleural effusions, lymphadenopathy, or distant hematogenous metastases are present (see Fig. 65-2).

13. **What is thymic carcinoma?**

Thymic carcinoma is an aggressive epithelial malignancy that often includes early local invasion, lymphadenopathy, and distant metastatic disease. Squamous cell carcinoma and lymphoepithelioma-like carcinoma are the most common cell types and most often occur in middle-aged men. On imaging, thymic carcinomas are commonly large, poorly defined, infiltrative anterior mediastinal masses that may have cystic or necrotic changes, often with pleural and pericardial effusions. Treatment and prognosis depend on the stage and histologic grade of the tumor.

14. **What is thymic carcinoid?**

Thymic carcinoid is a rare neuroendocrine tumor that typically affects men in the fourth to fifth decades of life. About 50% of patients will have endocrine abnormalities, most commonly Cushing's syndrome resulting from ectopic adrenocorticotropic hormone production or multiple endocrine neoplasia syndrome. Classic carcinoid syndrome due to serotonin secretion is rarely associated with thymic carcinoid. Symptoms and signs due to local mass effect and invasion may also occur. A large lobulated and usually invasive anterior mediastinal mass is seen that may be associated with cystic, necrotic, hemorrhagic, or calcific change. Lymphadenopathy and distant metastases may be seen in up to 75% of cases. Complete surgical excision is the treatment of choice, and radiotherapy and chemotherapy may be used for more advanced disease.

15. **What is thymolipoma?**

Thymolipoma is a rare, benign, slow-growing thymic neoplasm that may occur in any age group, although young adults are most commonly affected. It is a large, soft, encapsulated mass composed of mature adipose cells and thymic tissue. About 50% of patients are asymptomatic. On imaging, thymolipoma is a large anterior mediastinal mass that commonly droops into the anteroinferior mediastinum, may occupy one or both hemithoraces, and is characterized by its ability to conform to adjacent structures and to change in shape after changes in patient positioning. Predominant fat density and intermixed soft tissue density foci are seen on CT. Complete surgical resection is curative.

16. **What is a mediastinal germ cell tumor?**

Mediastinal germ cell tumors are a heterogeneous group of benign and malignant neoplasms that originate from primitive germ cells left over in the mediastinum during early embryogenesis. The anterior mediastinum is the most common extragonadal primary site of germ cell tumors. They usually occur in young adults, and even though mature teratomas occur equally in men and women, the majority of malignant germ cell tumors occur in men. Alpha-fetoprotein and beta-human chorionic gonadotropin serum levels may be positive with malignant mediastinal germ cell tumors. Primary testicular or ovarian germ cell tumor should be excluded when a mediastinal germ cell tumor is discovered because the mediastinum may be a site of metastasis from gonadal germ cell tumors.

17. What is a mediastinal teratoma?
Teratoma is the most common mediastinal germ cell tumor, composed of tissues from more than one of the three primitive germ cell layers (teeth, skin, and hair from ectoderm; cartilage and bone from mesoderm; and bronchial, intestinal, or pancreatic tissue from endoderm). Most teratomas are well differentiated and benign (mature) but rarely contain fetal tissue (when immature, in which case they may recur or metastasize). Mediastinal teratomas occur most commonly in children and young adults. Although usually asymptomatic, large tumors may cause symptoms due to local mass effect. On imaging, mature teratoma appears as a lobulated, well-defined heterogeneous anterior mediastinal mass usually located to one side of the midline with fat density foci along with multilocular cysts, dense teeth, calcification, or bone. The presence of fat, fluid, and soft tissue elements with or without calcification within an anterior mediastinal mass is virtually diagnostic of a mediastinal teratoma. Surgical excision is curative.

18. List a rare but highly specific clinical presentation of mediastinal teratoma.
Expectoration of hair (trichoptysis) or sebum is a rare but pathognomonic sign of ruptured mediastinal teratoma. This is due to secretion of digestive enzymes by intestinal mucosa or pancreatic tissue in the tumor, precipitating rupture into the bronchi.

19. What is mediastinal thyroid goiter?
This is an encapsulated, lobulated heterogeneous enlargement of part or all of the thyroid gland, most commonly in asymptomatic women with a palpable cervical goiter. Occasionally, local compressive symptoms are present. Twenty percent extend inferiorly into the thorax, usually into the left anterosuperior mediastinum, and less commonly into the middle or posterior mediastinal compartment. On imaging, a well-defined, lobulated heterogeneous lesion, often in the anterosuperior mediastinum, with areas of cystic, hemorrhagic, or calcific change is seen, often with tracheal displacement in the neck. Tracheal displacement on a chest radiograph is indicative of a mass of thyroid origin in the vast majority of cases and, in most cases, will represent a goiter. On CT, identification of contiguity of the mass with the thyroid gland establishes origin from the thyroid gland. Surgical resection is the treatment of choice for symptomatic lesions, although most patients with a goiter will be asymptomatic and require no therapy other than iodine or hormonal replacement.

20. Define mediastinal lipoma and mediastinal lipomatosis.
- A *lipoma* is a benign, well-circumscribed mesenchymal tumor that originates from adipose tissue, predominantly occurring in the anterior mediastinum often without clinical symptoms or signs. On imaging, it is generally a well-circumscribed, oval or round homogeneous fat density lesion.
- *Mediastinal lipomatosis* is due to excessive unencapsulated infiltrative fat deposition within the mediastinum. It is commonly associated with obesity and chronic exogenous corticosteroid administration and appears as widening of the mediastinum on radiography and as an increase in mediastinal fat on CT.

21. What is Hodgkin's lymphoma?
Hodgkin's lymphoma represents about 25–30% of lymphomas. Up to 85% of patients with mediastinal involvement by lymphoma have Hodgkin's lymphoma. Hodgkin's lymphoma occurs with a bimodal age distribution, with peaks during adolescence/early adulthood and after the fifth decade of life, most often occurring above the diaphragm. On pathology, the diagnosis is established by identification of Reed-Sternberg cells, generally in a background of inflammation and fibrosis. On imaging, one generally sees enlarged lymph nodes or conglomerate masses,

sometimes with hemorrhagic, necrotic, cystic, or calcific change and almost always involving the anterior mediastinum, often involving contiguous nodal groups. Avid uptake of 18-fluorodeoxyglucose (FDG) on positron emission tomography (PET) imaging is often seen.

22. **What is non-Hodgkin's lymphoma?**
Non-Hodgkin's lymphoma may occur in all age groups, although older patients tend to be affected most commonly. The majority of patients present with advanced disease. On pathology, one sees a predominance of malignant lymphocytes that are generally homogeneous and uniformly cellular. On imaging, one may see enlarged lymph nodes anywhere within the thorax, but extranodal disease is common, generally appearing as homogeneous soft tissue masses that may involve nearly any organ in the body. Cystic, necrotic, or calcific changes are uncommon but may occasionally be seen. Avid uptake of 18-FDG on PET imaging is often present.

23. **What are the most common causes of mediastinal lymphadenopathy?**
The four most common causes of radiographically detectable mediastinal lymphadenopathy are sarcoidosis, lymphoma, metastatic tumor, and granulomatous infections. In younger patients with bilateral hilar and mediastinal lymphadenopathy, sarcoidosis should be the diagnosis of exclusion because, by a large margin, it is the most common cause. In older individuals, lymphoma and metastatic tumor will be the most common causes of mediastinal lymphadenopathy. It would seem logical that any pulmonary infection could lead to mediastinal lymphadenopathy; however, only the granulomatous infections commonly cause mediastinal and/or hilar lymphadenopathy. These include primary tuberculosis, histoplasmosis, cryptococcosis, and coccidioidomycosis.

24. **Which vascular disorders can appear as mediastinal masses?**
Aortic aneurysm, aortic dissection, and traumatic aortic rupture can appear as a mediastinal mass, most often projecting from the left side of the mediastinum on chest radiography. Cross-sectional imaging will demonstrate enlargement of the aorta in the setting of aortic aneurysm and sometimes in the setting of the latter two conditions. Also, mediastinal hematoma may be seen if aortic rupture has occurred.

25. **Describe the congenital foregut cysts.**
Bronchogenic cysts represent 50–60% of all mediastinal cysts, esophageal duplication cysts represent 5–10%, and neurenteric cysts represent 2–5%. About 85% of bronchogenic cysts are located close to the trachea, mainstem bronchi, or carina, and 15% may occur in the lungs. Esophageal duplication cysts are almost always found within the esophageal wall or adherent to the esophagus. Neurenteric cysts may occur in isolation within the mediastinum or may be connected by a fibrous tract to the spine. On imaging, cysts are generally round, smooth, thin-walled lesions that contain simple fluid or sometimes complex fluid. Symptoms may occur from compression of mediastinal structures or superinfection.

26. **What is a mediastinal pancreatic pseudocyst?**
It is an encapsulated collection of pancreatic secretions that does not have an epithelial lining and is almost always located in the inferior-posterior mediastinum. A mediastinal pancreatic pseudocyst is due to extension of fluid through the esophageal or aortic hiatus of the diaphragm in the setting of pancreatitis.

27. **What is pneumomediastinum?**
Pneumomediastinum is air within the mediastinum. On imaging, one sees streaky linear or curvilinear lucent gas in the mediastinum that outlines mediastinal structures (Fig. 65-4). Whereas pneumopericardium (air within the pericardial space) is confined to the distribution of the pericardial reflection, pneumomediastinum may occur anywhere within the mediastinum. The causes of pneumomediastinum include:

- Air trapping: emphysema, asthma
- Straining against a closed glottis: vomiting, parturition, weight-lifting, marijuana use
- Blunt/penetrating trauma or iatrogenic injury to the trachea, bronchi, or esophagus
- Barotrauma: mechanical ventilation, sudden drop in atmospheric pressure, coughing
- Erosion of the trachea or esophagus by tumor
- Esophageal rupture: Boerhaave's syndrome, alcoholism, diabetic ketoacidosis
- Extension of air from pneumothorax, pneumoperitoneum, or pneumoretroperitoneum

28. **What is a mediastinal abscess?**
A mediastinal abscess is a loculated collection of pus. Major causes of mediastinal abscess include surgery, esophageal perforation, tracheobronchial perforation, spread of infection from a contiguous location, or penetrating trauma. On imaging, one may see a loculated fluid collection that tends to have a thick, enhancing wall and which may contain gas. In general, acute infection of the mediastinum is often fulminant and life-threatening and therefore is treated urgently.

Figure 65-4. Pneumomediastinum on a frontal chest radiograph after a recent coronary artery bypass graft. Note the streaky linear and curvilinear lucent gas in the mediastinum that outlines the mediastinal structures, such as the thoracic aorta *(arrow)*.

29. **What is fibrosing mediastinitis?**
Fibrosing mediastinitis is an uncommon benign disorder characterized by proliferation of dense mediastinal fibrous tissue. It typically occurs in young patients who present with symptoms and signs due to obstruction of vital mediastinal structures. Fibrosing mediastinitis is sometimes related to histoplasmosis infection but is often idiopathic in etiology. On imaging, one often sees nonspecific mediastinal widening, sometimes with hilar involvement, by focal or diffuse confluent soft tissue that is commonly calcified. Encasement, narrowing, or occlusion of the mediastinal airway or vascular structures is also often seen.

30. **What are neurogenic tumors?**
Neurogenic tumors are the most common cause of posterior mediastinal masses. Schwannoma and neurofibroma arise from peripheral nerves, most commonly in adults, whereas ganglioneuroma, ganglioneuroblastoma, and neuroblastoma arise from sympathetic ganglia, more commonly in children. Paragangliomas arise from paraganglia and are less common. Schwannomas and neurofibromas are the most common mediastinal neurogenic tumors and are benign. Schwannomas are encapsulated tumors composed of Schwann cells and loose reticular tissue; arise from the nerve sheath; and are often heterogeneous with hemorrhagic, cystic, necrotic, calcific, or fatty change. Neurofibromas are usually homogeneous nonencapsulated tumors composed of Schwann cells, nerve fibers, and fibroblasts.

31. **Describe the imaging appearance of neurogenic tumors.**
On imaging, peripheral nerve neurogenic tumors may appear as lobulated spherical or fusiform masses in the paraspinal region of the thorax, sometimes with a dumbbell configuration if there is extension into a neural foramen. A plexiform neurofibroma, pathognomonic for neurofibromatosis type 1 (NF-1), usually involves an entire nerve trunk or plexus. Associated smooth pressure erosions of the adjacent inferior rib surfaces and vertebrae or enlargement of the neural foramina may also be seen. Neurogenic tumors that arise from the sympathetic ganglia tend to appear as vertically oriented, elongated paraspinal masses with tapered borders.

KEY POINTS: MEDIASTINAL DISEASES

1. Lesions that arise in the different compartments of the mediastinum are generally related to the anatomic structures located within the compartments.

2. The majority of patients with asymptomatic mediastinal tumors have benign tumors, whereas the majority of patients with symptomatic mediastinal tumors have malignant tumors.

3. Thymoma is the most common primary tumor of the anterior mediastinum and of the thymus.

4. Primary testicular or ovarian germ cell tumor should be excluded when a mediastinal germ cell tumor is discovered.

5. Neurogenic tumor is the most common mass of the posterior mediastinum.

32. **What is an intrathoracic meningocele?**
An intrathoracic meningocele is an anomalous herniation of leptomeninges through an intervertebral foramen or a defect in the vertebral body, commonly associated with NF-1. On imaging, one sees a well-circumscribed, smooth lobulated or round paraspinal cystic lesion with enlargement of the intervertebral foramen or associated vertebral and rib anomalies or scoliosis. Diagnosis is confirmed by filling of the lesion with intraspinal contrast material on CT or fluoroscopy.

33. **How do osseous tumors and infection within the posterior mediastinum differ on imaging?**
In general, tumors of the thoracic spine are centered on the vertebrae without narrowing of the intervening disc spaces, whereas infections tend to be centered on the intervertebral disc spaces with disc space narrowing and involvement of the adjacent vertebral end plates.

34. **What is extramedullary hematopoiesis?**
Extramedullary hematopoiesis is due to proliferation of blood-forming elements in patients with thalassemia or other anemias and occurs most commonly in the liver and spleen, and sometimes in the chest. On imaging, multiple lobulated masses along the thoracic spine or along the ribs may be seen with pressure erosions, sometimes with associated splenomegaly.

BIBLIOGRAPHY

1. Gaerte SC, Meyer CA, Winer-Muram HT, et al: Fat-containing lesions of the chest. Radiographics 22(Suppl):S61–S78, 2002.

2. Jeung MY, Gasser B, Gangi A, et al: Imaging of cystic masses of the mediastinum. Radiographics 22(Suppl):S79–S93, 2002.

3. Muller N, Fraser R, Colman N, Pare PD: Radiologic Diagnosis of Diseases of the Chest. Philadelphia, W.B. Saunders, 2001.

4. Rossi SE, McAdams HP, Rosado-de-Christenson ML, et al: Fibrosing mediastinitis. Radiographics 21:737–757, 2001.

5. Strollo DC, Rosado-de-Christenson ML, Jett JR: Primary mediastinal tumors. Part I: Tumors of the anterior mediastinum. Chest 112:511–522, 1997.

6. Strollo DC, Rosado-de-Christenson ML, Jett JR: Primary mediastinal tumors. Part II: Tumors of the middle and posterior mediastinum. Chest 112:1344–1357, 1997.

7. Zylak CM, Standen JR, Barnes GR, Zylak CJ: Pneumomediastinum revisited. Radiographics 20:1043–1057, 2000.

CHAPTER 66

PLEURAL DISEASES

Drew A. Torigian, MD, and Wallace T. Miller, Jr., MD

1. **Describe the normal pleural anatomy and physiologic features.**
   The pleural space is a potential space that contains 2–10 mL of pleural fluid between visceral and parietal pleural layers that essentially represents interstitial fluid from the parietal pleura (an ultrafiltrate of plasma). The pleural space is contiguous with the interlobar fissures of the lungs. The pleura is a thin, serous layer that covers the lungs (visceral pleura) and is reflected onto the chest wall and pericardium (parietal pleura). The visceral pleura is supplied by the pulmonary arterial system and drains into the pulmonary venous system, whereas the parietal pleura is supplied by systemic arterial system and drains into the systemic venous system. Figure 66-1 shows the normal appearance of the pleura on chest radiography.

2. **What are the major tumors that may affect the pleura?**
   - Malignant pleural mesothelioma
   - Localized solitary fibrous tumor of the pleura
   - Pleural metastases
   - Pleural lymphoma

3. **What are the major substances that may collect within the pleural space?**
   - Fluid: pleural effusion (plasma ultrafiltrate, chyle, bile, urine, gastrointestinal contents, or ascites)
   - Blood: hemothorax
   - Air: pneumothorax
   - Pus: empyema
   - Cells: pleural tumor
   - Fibrosis: fibrothorax

Figure 66-1. *A,* Normal frontal chest radiograph of the pleura. Note the sharp lateral costophrenic angles *(arrows)* bilaterally and the clear demarcation of the hemidiaphragms. *B,* Normal lateral chest radiograph of the pleura. Note the sharp posterior costophrenic angles *(arrows)* bilaterally and the clear demarcation of the hemidiaphragms.

4. **What is the differential diagnosis of major causes of pleural effusion?**
   See Table 66-1.

TABLE 66-1.   DIFFERENTIAL DIAGNOSIS OF PLEURAL EFFUSION
Congestive heart failure*
Malignancy
Metastases*
Malignant mesothelioma
Lymphoma
Trauma
Thoracic or abdominal surgery*
Inflammatory disease
Infection (bacterial, mycobacterial, viral, fungal, parasitic)
Parapneumonic effusion*
Empyema
Collagen vascular disease: systemic lupus erythematosus, rheumatoid arthritis, systemic sclerosis
Hypoalbuminemia
Cirrhosis*
Nephrotic syndrome
Acute pulmonary embolism
Abdominal pathologic conditions*
Ascites
Pancreatitis
Peritonitis
Other inflammatory conditions of the abdomen
Other unusual causes
Lymphangioleiomyomatosis (associated with chylous effusions)
*Most common causes.

5. **List the major mechanisms of pleural effusion formation.**
   - Increased hydrostatic pressure in the microvascular circulation (e.g., congestive heart failure)
   - Decreased oncotic pressure in the microvascular circulation (e.g., hypoalbuminemia)
   - Decreased pressure in the pleural space (e.g., with pulmonary atelectasis or restrictive lung disease)
   - Increased permeability of the microvascular circulation (e.g., from pleural inflammation or neoplasm)
   - Impaired lymphatic drainage from the pleural space caused by blockage in the lymphatic system
   - Transit of fluid from the peritoneal cavity through the diaphragm to the pleural space

6. **What are the two major types of pleural effusion?**
   - *Transudates* are usually caused by increased systemic or pulmonary capillary pressure and decreased osmotic pressure, resulting in increased filtration and decreased absorption of

pleural fluid. Major causes are cirrhosis, congestive heart failure, nephrotic syndrome, and protein-losing enteropathy. Protein levels are less than 3 g/dL.

- *Exudates* occur when the pleural surface is damaged with associated capillary leak and increased permeability to protein or when there is decreased lymphatic drainage or decreased pleural pressure. Major causes are infection, malignancy, collagen vascular disease, or acute pulmonary embolism. Protein levels are more than 3 g/dL, the pleural protein–to–serum protein ratio is greater than 0.5, and the pleural lactate dehydrogenase to serum lactate dehydrogenase ratio is greater than 0.6.

7. **What are the major imaging findings of simple nonloculated pleural effusions on erect chest radiography?**

The most common imaging finding of a pleural effusion is blunting of the lateral costophrenic sulcus on erect frontal chest radiography or blunting of the posterior costophrenic sulcus on erect lateral chest radiography. A pleural effusion usually has a sharply marginated, concave-upward curved border between the lung and pleural space, which is known as the "meniscus sign." Since the posterior costophrenic angle is more dependent than the lateral costophrenic angle, smaller pleural effusions will be more apparent on the lateral view (with >75 mL of fluid) than on the frontal view (with >200 mL of fluid). Moderate to large pleural effusions usually obscure the ipsilateral hemidiaphragm (Fig. 66-2). Less common manifestations of pleural effusions include apparent elevation and medial flattening of the hemidiaphragm with lateral displacement of the diaphragmatic apex and an increase in distance (>2 cm) between the inferior surface of the lung and the gastric bubble on the left. The lateral decubitus view is the most sensitive radiographic view for detection of a pleural effusion and can detect as little as 5 mL of pleural fluid.

8. **What are the major imaging findings related to simple nonloculated pleural effusions on portable supine and semierect chest radiography?**

A little understood fact is that blunting of the costophrenic angles is a rare manifestation of pleural effusions on portable supine and semierect chest radiographs. On these views, pleural effusions most often appear as increased opacity of the hemithorax without obscuration of vascular markings or of the ipsilateral hemithorax because fluid layers in the posterior

Figure 66-2. *A*, Pleural effusion due to end-stage liver disease on a frontal chest radiograph. Note the blunting of the lateral costophrenic angle with a meniscus sign and obscuration of the right hemidiaphragm. *B*, Pleural effusion due to end-stage liver disease on a lateral chest radiograph. Note the blunting of the right posterior costophrenic angle with a meniscus sign and obscuration of the right hemidiaphragm. Compare with the unobscured left hemidiaphragm and left posterior costophrenic angle *(arrows)*, where no left pleural effusion is present.

pleural space dependently behind the more anterior nondependent lung. If the patient is supine, this will appear as a uniform haze of the ipsilateral hemithorax. On semierect radiographs, the density produced by the pleural effusion will increase from superior to inferior because free-flowing pleural fluid falls dependently into the more inferior portions of the pleural space. Rarely, if the patient is imaged in the Trendelenburg position, the pleural fluid will collect as a crescentic opacity over the lung apex, which is known as an *apical cap*.

9. **What are the major imaging findings associated with complex loculated pleural effusions?**
Complex pleural effusions (often seen with exudative effusions) are often located in nondependent portions of the pleural space and do not shift freely in the pleural space on lateral decubitus chest radiography due to adhesions between the visceral and parietal pleurae. Computed tomography (CT) scans may also sometimes demonstrate associated pleural thickening. Occasionally, loculated pleural fluid in the interlobar fissure may mimic a pseudomass on chest radiography, often appearing as a poorly marginated opacity on frontal chest radiography and as an elliptical opacity in the location of a major or minor interlobar fissure on lateral chest radiography.

10. **List the differential diagnosis of major causes of hemothorax.**
   - Trauma (blunt or penetrating or iatrogenic) (most common cause)
   - Bleeding diathesis (e.g., anticoagulation, protein S or C deficiency)
   - Malignancy
   - Infection
   - Acute pulmonary embolism
   - Thoracic aortic rupture (from [pseudo]aneurysm, dissection, penetrating aortic ulcer, or transection)

11. **What is pneumothorax?**
Pneumothorax is air within the pleural cavity. This occurs either through a communication between the outside world and the pleural space via a defect in the chest wall or through a communication between the air-containing bronchi or alveoli and the pleural space via a defect in the visceral pleura. Free intrapleural air preferentially moves to the nondependent aspects of the pleural spaces (apicolateral location on erect chest radiography and basilar or anteromedial location on supine chest radiography).

12. **What are the radiographic imaging findings of pneumothorax?**
The pathognomonic finding is a thin, sharply defined, visceral pleural "white" line between radiolucent lung (with vascular markings) and radiolucent "black" free air in the peripheral pleural space (without vascular markings). On supine chest radiography, one may see sharp visualization of the right cardiac border, superior and inferior vena cavae, left subclavian artery, and the anterior junction line; a deep lucent cardiophrenic sulcus ("deep sulcus sign"); hyperlucency at the lung bases; and associated atelectasis of the adjacent lung.

13. **How much air in a pneumothorax is required for radiographic visualization? What radiographic maneuvers can be performed to demonstrate a subtle pneumothorax?**
On erect chest radiographs, small amounts of air (about 50 mL) are generally visible at the lung apex, whereas on supine radiographs, about 500 mL of air is needed to be visible. Expiratory chest radiography or contralateral decubitus chest radiography (i.e., left side down if looking for a right pneumothorax and vice versa) can often demonstrate a small pneumothorax that may not be seen on standard inspiratory frontal chest radiography. Alternatively, cross-table lateral chest radiography with the patient in the supine position can also demonstrate a subtle pneumothorax.

14. **What is a tension pneumothorax?**

Uncommonly, air in the pleural space can develop positive pressure, most often as a result of mechanical ventilation, and can compress the mediastinum with resultant decreased venous return to the heart. This can be a medical emergency because rapid cardiopulmonary compromise and death may ensue if the patient is not immediately treated. The radiographic clues to a tension pneumothorax are the presence of a pneumothorax in association with contralateral mediastinal shift and inferior displacement of the ipsilateral hemidiaphragm (Fig. 66-3). However, these findings are not diagnostic of a tension pneumothorax, which can occur without these findings. The diagnosis is based on radiographic recognition of a pneumothorax and clinical findings of hypotension and tachycardia. Immediate decompression by needle thoracentesis through the second rib interspace in the mid-clavicular line or with chest thoracostomy is typically performed for emergent treatment of a tension pneumothorax.

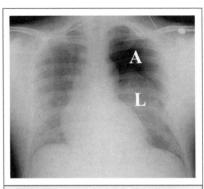

Figure 66-3. Tension pneumothorax on a frontal chest radiograph. Note the thin, sharply defined, visceral pleural "white" line between radiolucent lung (L) and radiolucent "black" free air (A) in the peripheral pleural space, in addition to rightward mediastinal shift and inferior left hemidiaphragmatic shift due to air under tension.

15. **What is the differential diagnosis of major causes of pneumothorax?**

In the following list, an asterisk (*) indicates the most common causes:

- Idiopathic*: most often due to rupture of an apical bleb
- Trauma*: blunt or penetrating injury, iatrogenic injury (e.g., central venous line placement), barotrauma (mechanical ventilation)
- Obstructive lung disease (e.g., chronic obstructive pulmonary disease, asthma)
- Cystic lung disease (e.g., eosinophilic granuloma, lymphangiomyomatosis, tuberous sclerosis)
- Bronchiectasis or cavitary lung disease (e.g., cystic fibrosis, tuberculosis, *Pneumocystis carinii* pneumonia)
- Advanced interstitial lung disease with honeycombing (e.g., usual interstitial pneumonitis, sarcoidosis, chronic hypersensitivity pneumonitis)
- Adult respiratory distress syndrome
- Endometriosis (e.g., catamenial pneumothorax)
- Bronchopulmonary fistula (e.g., after lung surgery or transplantation)

16. **When should treatment of a patient with a pneumothorax be considered?**

Many pneumothoraces will resolve spontaneously, and therefore only patients at risk for complications of the pneumothorax require intervention. Generally, treatment with chest thoracostomy is necessary if the patient has respiratory compromise as a result of the pneumothorax. Findings such as shortness of breath, dyspnea, hypoxemia, or hypotension indicate the need for drainage of the pneumothorax. If the pneumothorax increases in size on serial chest radiographs, then treatment will also be necessary. If clinical and radiographic findings indicate a tension pneumothorax, decompression and drainage of the pneumothorax are necessary. Finally, most patients receiving positive pressure ventilation require chest tube drainage because of the increased risk of developing a tension pneumothorax.

17. **How is the diagnosis of an empyema obtained? When is empyema usually treated?**

    Diagnosis is made when pleural fluid is grossly purulent, has a positive Gram stain or culture, or when the white blood cell count is greater than 5×10^9 cells. Anaerobic bacteria, usually streptococci or gram-negative rods, are responsible in about 75% of cases. Chest radiographic findings of empyema are similar to those of other loculated pleural fluid collections. CT findings may include increased density of the fluid caused by protein, cells, or hemorrhage; septations and loculation; foci of gas; thickened enhancing pleural surfaces (the "split-pleura sign"); or increased density of the extrapleural fat. Empyemas with pH less than 7.0 or a glucose level less than 40 mg/dL must be treated with chest thoracostomy. If simple drainage fails or if a fibrinous peel forms on the lung, decortication is usually curative.

18. **What is empyema necessitatis?**

    This is an uncommon complication of an empyema in which the inflammatory process within the pleural space decompresses and extends into the soft tissues of the chest wall, forming a subcutaneous abscess, which may or may not communicate directly with the skin surface. The most common etiologic factor is tuberculosis, and the most common clinical presentation is a palpable mass in the chest wall, sometimes with a cutaneous fistula. This extension into the chest wall will usually not be evident on chest radiographs but may be detected with CT or magnetic resonance imaging (MRI) of the thorax.

19. **List some causes of pleural calcification.**
    - Chronic infection/inflammation (tuberculosis, bacterial empyema)
    - Chronic hemothorax
    - Asbestos exposure

20. **What are pleural plaques?**

    Pleural plaques are collections of hyalinized collagen in the parietal pleural that are the most common benign finding of prior asbestos exposure. These are virtually pathognomonic for confirming prior asbestos exposure, and typically appear more than 20 years after such exposure. When noncalcified, they appear as small plateau-shaped areas of pleural thickening when seen in profile and may mimic pulmonary nodules when seen face on. However, they often calcify. With a tangential view on chest radiography, a linear or curvilinear calcification along the pleural surface will be seen, whereas when seen en face, irregular linear, stippled, or geographic calcification overlying the hemithorax will be seen (Fig. 66-4).

Figure 66-4. Calcified asbestos-related pleural plaques on a frontal chest radiograph. Note the linear or curvilinear dense calcifications along the lateral aspects of the hemithoraces (seen tangentially) and irregular geographic calcifications overlying the hemithoraces (seen en face).

21. **What is malignant mesothelioma?**

    Malignant mesothelioma is an uncommon neoplasm that arises from the parietal pleura or, rarely, from the pericardium or peritoneum. Histologic subtypes include epithelioid, sarcomatoid (fibrous), and mixed (biphasic), with epithelioid being the most common. About 2000–3000 new cases are diagnosed in the United States each year. This is the most common primary pleural malignancy, and its incidence has been increasing over the past 30 years.

22. **What are some risk factors for the development of malignant pleural mesothelioma?**
    Exposure to asbestos is the most important risk factor (amphibole fibers, including crocidolite and amosite, are the most potent causes). Other minerals and the simian virus 40 (SV 40) are also risk factors. About 80% of cases occur in patients with a history of asbestos exposure, with a lifetime risk of 10%. The latency period after exposure is an average of 40 years, with a range of approximately 15–65 years.

23. **What are some symptoms and signs of malignant pleural mesothelioma?**
    Nonspecific dull chest or shoulder pain, shortness of breath, dyspnea, dry cough, fatigue, weight loss, digital clubbing, hypertrophic osteoarthropathy, superior vena cava syndrome, lymphadenopathy, chest wall masses, dysrhythmias, pleural effusion, pericardial effusion, ascites, or bowel obstruction due to spread to the peritoneal cavity may be seen. Chest wall pain is an important sign of chest wall involvement by tumor. Malignant mesothelioma should be considered in any patient with either pleural effusion or pleural thickening, especially if chest pain is present.

24. **What are the imaging findings of malignant pleural mesothelioma?**
    The most common chest radiographic finding of mesothelioma is a loculated pleural effusion. Unilateral pleural masses or plaquelike or nodular, irregular pleural thickening with encasement of the entire lung are also common findings that are highly suggestive of mesothelioma. Extension into the interlobar fissures, lung, mediastinum, chest wall, diaphragm, and biopsy tracts may occur. As a result of constriction of the lung by adherent pleural tumor, ipsilateral volume loss of the hemithorax with ipsilateral mediastinal shift, narrowing of the intercostal spaces, and elevation of the ipsilateral hemidiaphragm are commonly present (Fig. 66-5). Pleural calcification due to prior asbestos exposure is seen in up to two thirds of cases, and intrathoracic lymphadenopathy, extension to the peritoneum or retroperitoneum, and hematogenous metastases anywhere in body may also be seen on CT or MRI in later stages.

Figure 66-5. *A,* Right malignant pleural mesothelioma on a frontal chest radiograph. Note the diffuse nodular right pleural thickening and decreased volume of the right hemithorax relative to the left hemithorax. *B,* Right malignant pleural mesothelioma on CT. Note the diffuse nodular right pleural thickening and decreased volume of the right hemithorax relative to the left hemithorax.

25. **What diagnostic tests may be used in the diagnosis or staging of malignant pleural mesothelioma?**
    Chest radiography, CT, MRI, fluorodeoxyglucose positron emission tomography (18-FDG PET), ultrasound (US), thoracentesis, and biopsy are diagnostic tools that are used. Chest radiography

may sometimes have normal results, and negative pleural biopsy and cytology results do not exclude mesothelioma. However, US, CT, and 18-FDG PET scanning may be used to guide biopsy and increase diagnostic yield. CT and MRI are nearly equivalent in staging accuracy, but MRI is superior to CT for diaphragmatic, endothoracic fascial, or focal chest wall invasion and is often used as a problem-solving tool after CT. 18-FDG PET scanning is also useful in staging and preoperative evaluation and has increased accuracy for detecting malignant lymphadenopathy or occult extrathoracic metastases. Metabolic activity on 18-FDG PET scanning and patient survival are inversely proportional.

26. What is the prognosis for malignant pleural mesothelioma?
Prognosis is generally poor, with a median survival of 8–18 months, since the tumor is generally progressive. Favorable prognostic factors include limited extent of disease and an epithelioid histologic subtype. Unfavorable prognostic factors include sarcomatoid or mixed histologic subtypes; more advanced stages of disease, such as with intrathoracic lymphadenopathy; extensive pleural involvement; distant metastatic disease; and older age.

27. Describe the general treatment approach to malignant pleural mesothelioma.
Radical surgery (either radical pleurectomy-decortication or extrapleural pneumonectomy with removal of the pleura, mediastinal lymph nodes, ipsilateral pericardium, and diaphragm) is considered when there is epithelioid mesothelioma without lymphadenopathy. Radiotherapy, chemotherapy, and photodynamic therapy may also be used with surgery as adjuvant treatments, but no treatment so far has conclusively improved survival significantly beyond palliative care. Talc pleurodesis or video-assisted thorascopic pleurectomy may also be used to control pleural effusions and are safer than open pleurectomy and decortication. Radiotherapy may be used palliatively to relieve pain in about 50% of cases or can be used prophylactically at biopsy sites to prevent seeding by tumor. Pain medications are used as needed.

28. What is localized fibrous tumor of the pleura?
This is a rare mesenchymal neoplasm that most commonly affects the pleura, uncommonly affects the lungs and mediastinum, and rarely involves extrathoracic sites. It is unrelated to asbestos exposure and may either be benign (about 90%) or malignant (about 10%). The majority of patients present in the fifth through eighth decades of life and have a much better

KEY POINTS: PLEURAL DISEASES

1. If you see a pneumothorax on chest radiography that is associated with contralateral mediastinal shift and inferior displacement of the ipsilateral hemidiaphragm, immediately notify the physician caring for the patient because a tension pneumothorax may be present, requiring emergent treatment to prevent rapid death.

2. Malignant mesothelioma is the most common primary malignancy of the pleura and is most often related to prior asbestos exposure.

3. Malignant mesothelioma should be considered in any patient with either pleural effusion or pleural thickening, especially if chest pain is present.

4. Normal chest radiography and negative pleural biopsy and cytology results do not exclude malignant mesothelioma.

5. Paraneoplastic syndromes such as hypoglycemia, digital clubbing, and hypertrophic osteoarthropathy may suggest the diagnosis of localized fibrous tumor of the pleura when associated with an intrathoracic mass.

prognosis than those with malignant pleural mesothelioma. Eighty percent of these neoplasms arise from the visceral pleura, and 20% arise from the parietal pleura, although a small number are intrapulmonary in location. Between 20% and 50% are pedunculated, and they are composed of spindle-shaped fibroblast-like cells with a variable amount of collagenous stroma, vascularity, and myxoid or cystic degeneration.

29. Name some clinical presentations of localized fibrous tumor of the pleura.
Up to 50% may be asymptomatic, and symptoms and signs, when present, may include cough, dyspnea, hemoptysis, chest pain, and sensation of a mass. Paraneoplastic syndromes such as hypoglycemia, digital clubbing, and hypertrophic osteoarthropathy are uncommon but may be associated with an intrathoracic mass.

30. What are the imaging features of localized fibrous tumor of the pleura?
Typically, a well-defined, usually sharply marginated, lobulated, and solitary lesion is identified within the thorax adjacent to the chest wall or diaphragm. It may be very small or massive. When large, it can fill the inferior aspect of the hemithorax and resemble an elevated hemidiaphragm. The tumor typically is connected to the chest wall by a thin pedicle or stalk. Therefore, changes in patient positioning, such as with decubitus radiographs, may result in changes in position of the mass within the thorax. On CT or MRI, intense enhancement, myxoid or cystic degeneration, hemorrhage, or calcification may be seen, and no imaging findings other than metastatic disease can help differentiate between benignity and malignancy of the lesion.

31. What is the treatment for localized fibrous tumor of the pleura?
Treatment involves surgical resection, which is often curative, although some patients will have local recurrence, malignant transformation, or distant metastatic disease. Complete surgical excision is overall the best prognostic indicator.

BIBLIOGRAPHY

1. Au VW, Thomas M: Radiological manifestations of malignant pleural mesothelioma. Australas Radiol 47:111–116, 2003.

2. Gallardo X, Castaner E, Mata JM: Benign pleural diseases. Eur J Radiol 34:87–97, 2000.

3. Lee KH, Song KS, Kwon Y, et al: Mesenchymal tumours of the thorax: CT findings and pathological features. Clin Radiol 58:934–944, 2003.

4. Muller N, Fraser R, Colman N, Pare PD: Radiologic Diagnosis of Diseases of the Chest. Philadelphia, W.B. Saunders, 2001.

5. Parker C, Neville E: Lung cancer. Part 8: Management of malignant mesothelioma. Thorax 58:809–813, 2003.

6. Peek GJ, Morcos S, Cooper G: The pleural cavity. BMJ 320:1318–1321, 2000.

7. Rosado-de-Christenson ML, Abbott GF, McAdams HP, et al: From the archives of the AFIP: Localized fibrous tumor of the pleura. Radiographics 23:759–783, 2003.

8. Sahn SA, Heffner JE: Spontaneous pneumothorax. N Engl J Med 342:868–874, 2000.

9. Statement on malignant mesothelioma in the United Kingdom. Thorax 56:250–265, 2001.

10. van Ruth S, Baas P, Zoetmulder FA: Surgical treatment of malignant pleural mesothelioma: A review. Chest 123:551–561, 2003.

11. Wang ZJ, Reddy GP, Gotway MB, et al: Malignant pleural mesothelioma: Evaluation with CT, MR imaging, and PET. Radiographics 24:105–119, 2004.

CHAPTER 67

TUBES, LINES, AND CATHETERS

Drew A. Torigian, MD

1. **What is the radiographic appearance of an endotracheal tube (ETT)? Where is it optimally placed?**
    An ETT is usually seen by a thin, radiopaque line along its length, and its position should be determined relative to the carina, which if not seen on chest radiography can be approximated by following the course of the mainstem bronchi medially at the T5–T7 level. The tip of the tube should be about 5–7 cm above the carina when the patient's head is in neutral position and below the thoracic inlet, since flexion and extension of the neck cause the tube to move about 2 cm higher or lower, respectively. The optimal width of the tube should be between one half and two thirds of the tracheal width (generally <3 cm), and the inflated cuff should not distend the trachea because tracheal injury could occur.

2. **Describe how an ETT may be malpositioned. List other potential complications of ETT placement.**
    If the tube is inserted beyond the carina (i.e., with unilateral bronchial intubation), preferential hyperaeration and potential barotrauma of the intubated lung (more commonly the right) and hypoaeration and atelectasis of the contralateral lung may occur (Fig. 67-1). If the tube is not advanced far enough, inadvertent extubation or possible vocal cord damage due to pressure from the inflated cuff may occur. Esophageal intubation may also be encountered, which is detected clinically by gurgling sounds and distention of the stomach as air is insufflated and radiographically by lateral extension of the tube margins beyond the tracheal margins, visualization of the tracheal air column to the side of the tube, gastric distention, and lung hypoinflation (Fig. 67-2). Other complications include pharyngeal, laryngeal, or tracheobronchial injury (particularly if placed too high or if the cuff is overinflated [Fig. 67-3]); aspiration; sinusitis; and dislodgement of teeth.

Figure 67-1. Malpositioned ETT and peripherally inserted central catheter (PICC). Note the tip of the ETT within the proximal right mainstem bronchus *(thick white arrow)* with complete atelectasis (A) of left lung. Also note the right PICC *(arrowheads)* malpositioned within the right internal jugular vein. An appropriately placed nasogastric tube enters the abdomen *(thin dark arrows)*.

3. **What is the optimal positioning of a tracheostomy tube?**
    A tracheostomy tube tip is optimally located between one half and two thirds of the distance from the stoma to the carina. The tube itself should overlie the trachea, and the width of the tube should be about two thirds of the tracheal width. See Figure 67-8 for the normal radiographic appearance of a tracheostomy tube.

4. **Name potential complications after tracheostomy tube placement.**
   Potential complications include injury of the recurrent laryngeal nerve with resultant vocal cord paralysis; injury of the lung apex with pneumothorax or pneumomediastinum formation; injury of the trachea with tracheal malacia or stricture formation; and soft tissue infection, leading to tracheal ulceration and perforation with tracheoinnominate artery fistula, tracheoesophageal fistula, or cervical abscess formation.

Figure 67-2. Malpositioned ETT. Note the left lateral extension of the ETT tip *(thick white arrow)* and balloon cuff *(arrowheads)* beyond the tracheal margins *(thin arrows)*, with visualization of the tracheal air column to the right side of the ETT.

5. **What is the radiographic appearance and ideal positioning of a nasogastric tube (NGT) or orogastric tube (OGT)?**
   Radiographically, a thin, radiopaque curvilinear strip is visualized along the entire length of the tube (see Fig. 67-1). The tube should extend inferiorly along the midline of the chest, with its tip located at least 10 cm within the stomach, since multiple side holes are usually present from about 10 cm proximal to its distal end.

6. **Describe the radiographic appearance and optimal location of an enteral feeding tube (FT).**
   On plain film radiography, a radiopaque marker at the tip of the tube is generally seen and should be located beyond the gastric pylorus within the duodenum, optimally at the duodenojejunal junction (ligament of Treitz). On frontal radiography, the tube gener-

Figure 67-3. Malpositioned ETT with cuff overinflation. Note the ETT tip *(thick white arrow)* above the thoracic inlet (level of clavicles) with overinflation of the balloon cuff *(arrowheads)* distending the trachea. Extensive lucencies in the chest wall and neck reflect subcutaneous emphysema and pneumomediastinum, respectively. Bilateral thoracostomy tubes and a Swan-Ganz catheter (SGC) *(thin dark arrows)* are in the appropriate position.

ally curves to follow the C-shaped loop of the duodenum, and on lateral radiography the tube curves posteriorly from the gastric antrum into the duodenum before it enters the retroperitoneal second portion of the duodenum.

7. **List ways in which an NGT, OGT, or FT may be malpositioned, including other potential complications.**
   Coiling within the pharynx or esophagus may be seen even if the tip is in the appropriate position and may lead to vomiting and subsequent aspiration (Fig. 67-4). If a tube is located above the gastroesophageal junction, vomiting and subsequent aspiration may again occur. With tracheobronchial placement, the tube follows the course of the trachea and bronchi, sometimes

with lung perforation and location within the pleural space, leading to intrabronchial infusion of feedings, pneumonia, lung abscess, empyema, hydropneumothorax, or pneumothorax (Fig. 67-5). Esophageal perforation is a rare, serious complication, but extra-esophageal tube location is not generally appreciated on frontal radiography unless other views or water-soluble contrast injection are performed, which typically show a tube that does not follow the expected course of the esophagus, a widened mediastinum, pneumomediastinum, a unilateral pleural effusion, or contrast leak from the esophagus into other thoracic compartments.

Figure 67-4. Malpositioned NGT. Note that the NGT is curled within the pharynx and upper thoracic esophagus.

8. **If an NGT, OGT, or FT is misplaced within the tracheobronchial tree, what should one do before removing the tube?**
One should have a thoracostomy tube set ready at the patient's bedside before removing the tube, just in case a pneumothorax suddenly develops due to lung perforation with a tear in the visceral pleura.

9. **When is a thoracostomy tube generally used?**
A thoracostomy tube is generally placed for drainage of air (pneumothorax), particularly when persistent (i.e., with a bronchopleural fistula), large, increasing, or symptomatic (i.e., under tension); fluid (pleural effusion); blood (hemothorax); chylous fluid (chylothorax); or pus (empyema)

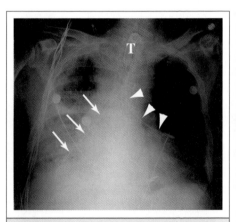

Figure 67-5. Malpositioned NGT and FT. Note the NGT *(arrows)* in the distal right bronchus and the FT *(arrowheads)* in the middle left bronchus. Patchy opacity in the right lung represents pneumonia. An appropriately positioned tracheostomy tube (T) is present overlying the trachea.

from the pleural space. It may also be placed for drainage of a lung abscess.

10. **What is the radiographic appearance of a thoracostomy tube, and where should its tip be located?**
A curvilinear radiopaque stripe that has a short-segment interruption in it at the level of its proximal drainage hole is typically seen on radiography; the tube should curve gently within the thorax (*see* Fig. 67-3). For drainage of a pneumothorax, the tube should be positioned near the lung apex at the anterior axillary line and directed anterosuperiorly, whereas for drainage of a pleural effusion, the tube should be positioned at the midaxillary line and directed posteroinferiorly through the sixth through eighth intercostal spaces. In either case, the proximal side hole should always be located medial to the ribs within the pleural space. Computed tomography

(CT) is indicated when a thoracostomy tube does not drain air or fluid properly and the chest radiograph is noncontributory.

11. **List potential complications of thoracostomy tube placement.**

Persistent pneumothorax and extensive subcutaneous emphysema may occur if side holes are located external to the rib cage and pleural space (Fig. 67-6). Lung laceration with bronchopleural fistula may also occur with a persistent pneumothorax, pneumomediastinum, and extensive subcutaneous emphysema and is more commonly seen with preexisting lung disease or pleural adhesions. Laceration or injury of an intercostal artery, phrenic nerve, thoracic duct, diaphragm, liver, spleen, stomach, mediastinum, heart, breast, or pectoralis muscle may also occur (Fig. 67-7). Placement within an interlobar fissure is common, may cause poor tube function, and is best seen on CT. Soft tissue or pleural infection may occur adjacent to the tube insertion site. Unilateral reexpansion pulmonary edema may be seen with rapid pleural decompression, and rapid development of an infiltrate at the tip or side holes may be due to pulmonary infarction from suction of lung tissue. High insertion in the posterior chest wall may lead to Horner's syndrome, and recurrence of a pleural collection, a pleurocutaneous fistula, or retention of a tube fragment are potential complications after tube removal.

Figure 67-6. Malpositioned thoracostomy tube. Note the side hole (S) of the thoracostomy tube externally located to the rib cage, leading to extensive streaky lucencies in the chest wall due to subcutaneous emphysema.

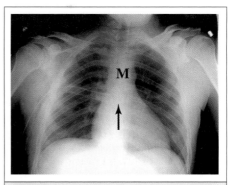

Figure 67-7. Malpositioned thoracostomy tube. Note the medially malpositioned thoracostomy tube tip (arrow) located over the mediastinum (M).

12. **How can one decrease the chance of injury to an intercostal artery or vein during thoracostomy tube placement?**

Place the tube just superior to a rib to avoid the neurovascular bundle that is located at the inferior aspect of each rib.

13. **Discuss the basic normal venous anatomy of the chest.**

The deeply situated brachial veins and the superficially situated basilic and cephalic veins of the upper extremities converge centrally to form the axillary veins. The axillary veins become the subclavian veins beyond the lateral aspects of the first ribs, and the superficially located external jugular veins drain from the neck into the subclavian veins. More centrally, the subclavian veins and internal jugular veins from the neck converge to form the brachiocephalic veins (longer on the left than on the right), which then join to form the superior vena cava (SVC), finally leading to the right atrium. The vertical portion of the azygos vein is located to the right of the thoracic spine and drains superiorly to its horizontal portion, which drains into the posterior SVC above the right mainstem bronchus. The hemiazygos venous system is located toward the left of the thoracic spine and has variable communication with the azygos system.

14. **What is the radiographic appearance and optimal location of a central venous line (CVL) and a peripherally inserted central catheter (PICC)?**
    A CVL appears as a thin, moderately radiopaque linear or curvilinear tube that extends centrally from a subclavian or internal jugular vein when in the chest, whereas a PICC appears as an even thinner, faintly radiopaque linear or curvilinear tube that extends from the upper extremity (since it is placed peripherally within the lower arm or upper forearm usually via the basilic vein) centrally into the chest. The optimal location of the tip of a CVL and PICC is within the SVC (see Fig. 67-9 for the normal radiographic appearance of a CVL).

15. **What are potential complications of CVL or PICC placement?**
    Early complications include pneumothorax, which is very common and more commonly encountered in the subclavian approach; malpositioning within a vein or artery or in the heart; arterial injury with pseudoaneurysm formation or thromboembolism; venous injury; perforation through a vein with extravascular malpositioning in the pleural space, mediastinum, or soft tissue; cardiac injury with risk of myocardial perforation and cardiac tamponade; hemorrhage or hematoma; air embolism; and catheter knotting, fracture, and embolism. Late complications include catheter occlusion, migration, knotting, fracture, and embolism; venous thrombosis; soft tissue infection; bacteremia/septicemia; and cardiac dysrhythmias, which usually occur with low right atrial placement.

16. **List locations where a CVL or PICC may be malpositioned when inserted through a vein.**
    For a PICC or subclavian vein CVL, malpositioning may occur in the ipsilateral internal jugular vein (*see* Fig. 67-1); contralateral subclavian vein; internal jugular vein; right atrium (Fig. 67-8); right ventricle; pulmonary artery; inferior vena cava; hepatic vein; axillary vein; subclavian vein; brachiocephalic vein; azygos vein; or branch vessels, including the external jugular vein, inferior thyroidal vein, superior intercostal vein, internal thoracic vein, or pericardiacophrenic vein. For an internal jugular vein CVL, malpositioning within the ipsilateral subclavian vein may also occur. Intracardiac malpositioning of a CVL inserted via the subclavian vein approach is more common when inserted on the right (30%) than on the left (12%).

Figure 67-8. Malpositioned PICC. Note the distal portion of the PICC *(arrows)* curled within the right atrium. Also note the appropriately placed tracheostomy tube (T) with overlying tracheostomy collar *(arrowheads).*

17. **Name some clues of inadvertent arterial puncture with a CVL, PICC, or Swan-Ganz catheter (SGC).**
    At the time of catheter placement, bright red and pulsatile backflow of blood may be seen, although in patients with hypoxia or hypotension, the blood may be nonpulsatile and dark,

mimicking venous blood. On chest radiography, arterial location of a catheter should be suspected when the course of the catheter follows the expected course of an artery rather than a vein or when the tip is located in a midsternal or left paravertebral location. Confirmation of an arterial puncture may be performed by analysis of blood gas levels of blood samples drawn through the catheter.

18. **What should one consider in the differential diagnosis for rapid development of an ipsilateral pleural effusion or mediastinal widening after CVL, PICC, or SGC placement?**
Rapid development of an ipsilateral pleural effusion or mediastinal widening after venous catheter placement should make one consider (1) perforation of a vein by the catheter, with the tip located in the pleural space or mediastinum after catheter infusion, or (2) vessel injury by the catheter with associated hemithorax or mediastinal hematoma. Pneumothorax is also often associated with vessel injury in this setting.

19. **If air embolism is suspected during catheter placement, what should one do to treat the patient? How does one prevent air embolism during catheter placement in the first place?**
When air embolism is suspected (usually when a sucking sound during patient inspiration is heard through a catheter at the time of placement or if inadvertent injection of air through a catheter occurs), the patient should immediately be placed in the left lateral decubitus position (i.e., left side down) to keep the air trapped in the right heart chambers, supplemental oxygen should be administered, and vital signs should be monitored. Air embolism during line placement is easily prevented by keeping one's finger over the open end(s) of the catheter until the catheter is flushed with saline and capped.

20. **Describe the radiographic appearance of an SGC and its optimal location.**
An SGC (or pulmonary arterial catheter) appears as a thin, moderately radiopaque curvilinear tube that originates centrally from a subclavian or internal jugular vein and passes successively through the brachiocephalic vein, SVC, right atrium, right ventricle, and pulmonary outflow tract, with its tip optimally located in the main, right, or left pulmonary artery or within a proximal lobar pulmonary arterial branch (see Fig. 67-3). When a balloon at the tip is inflated for pulmonary capillary wedge pressure measurement, a 1-cm round radiolucency at the catheter tip may be seen radiographically. A thin, short linear tubular radiopacity is also generally seen at the skin entry site, which is the vascular sheath that surrounds the SGC. The SGC can be removed while the sheath still remains in place.

21. **What are potential complications of SGC placement?**
Potential complications of SGC placement include those listed previously for CVL or PICC placement as well as malpositioning within the right atrium (Fig. 67-9), right ventricle, pulmonary outflow tract, or peripheral pulmonary arterial branch (Fig. 67-10); curling within cardiac chambers with associated cardiac injury, thrombus formation, or atrial or ventricular cardiac dysrhythmias; tricuspid or pulmonic valve injury; pulmonary arterial injury/rupture, occasionally with formation of either a pseudoaneurysm or a pulmonary artery to bronchial fistula; pulmonary thromboembolism; and pulmonary infarction.

22. **Why can pulmonary infarction occur as a complication of SGC placement?**
Pulmonary infarction in the setting of SGC placement results from obstruction of pulmonary blood flow, either due to tip placement too peripherally within a pulmonary arterial branch or persistent inflation of the balloon at the catheter tip. In general, the extent of pulmonary infarction is directly related to the caliber of the occluded vessel and to the portions of lung supplied by it. Typically, if the tip of an SGC is seen to be more than 2 cm lateral to the pulmonary hilum on frontal chest radiography, it is too peripheral in location and should be pulled back. Furthermore, the balloon should be inflated only during the measurement of wedge pressures.

23. **How does an intra-aortic counterpulsation balloon (IACB) work? What are the major indications and contraindications for placement?**

    An IACB is inserted percutaneously via the common femoral artery and subsequently passes through the external iliac artery, common iliac artery, and abdominal aorta to finally reach the descending thoracic aorta. A long, inflatable balloon approximately 3 cm long is present around the distal catheter that is repeatedly inflated during early diastole and deflated during early systole at each cardiac cycle.

Figure 67-9. Malpositioned SGC. Note the SGC curled within the right atrium *(thick arrows)* with its tip in the SVC. An appropriately positioned ETT (E), NGT *(thin arrows)*, and CVL *(arrowheads)* are also present.

    This helps to increase myocardial oxygenation and decrease myocardial oxygenation demand, mainly through improved coronary and peripheral arterial blood flow and decreased cardiac afterload. The IACB is often used in critically ill patients with left ventricular failure, unstable angina, acute myocardial ischemia/infarction associated with percutaneous transluminal angioplasty, or severe mitral regurgitation. Major contraindications to IACB placement include severe aortic insufficiency, aortic dissection, severe peripheral vascular disease, or contraindication to systemic anticoagulation.

Figure 67-10. Malpositioned SGC. Note the tip of the SGC *(arrow)* overlying the peripheral left superior pulmonary arterial branch.

24. **Describe the radiographic appearance of an IACB and its optimal position.**

    The distal tip of an IACB is seen as a small, radiopaque rectangle and should be located on frontal chest radiography just distal to the left subclavian artery within the proximal descending thoracic aorta below the level of the aortic knob.

25. **What are the potential complications of an IACB?**

    Potential complications include arterial injury and hemorrhage; aortic dissection; arterial thromboembolism with secondary limb, visceral, or cerebral ischemia; malpositioning within the aorta proximal to the left subclavian artery or far distal to the aortic arch; venous malpositioning; balloon rupture with potential air embolism if helium gas is used for balloon inflation; thrombocytopenia; soft tissue infection or hematoma formation at the percutaneous site of insertion; or bacteremia/septicemia. When the balloon is located proximal to the left subclavian artery, potential occlusion of the arterial branch vessels of the aortic arch (i.e., the innominate, left common carotid, and left subclavian arteries) is possible, and when the balloon is located far distal to the aortic arch, counterpulsation will be less effective and potential occlusion of the visceral branch vessels is possible.

KEY POINTS: TUBES, LINES, AND CATHETERS

1. If you see focal ovoid lucency surrounding an ETT or tracheostomy tube with an associated bulge in the adjacent tracheal walls, suspect overinflation of the cuff and notify the clinical staff immediately.

2. If an NGT, OGT, or FT is seen to extend into a distal bronchus, lung, or pleural space, notify the clinical staff immediately and suggest that tube removal be performed only after a thoracostomy tube set is at the bedside in case a significant pneumothorax develops.

3. Rapid development of an ipsilateral pleural effusion or mediastinal widening after venous catheter placement should lead one to consider venous perforation, with the tip located in the pleural space or mediastinum after catheter infusion, or vessel injury with associated hemithorax or mediastinal hematoma.

4. When air embolism is suspected during line placement or use, the patient should immediately be placed in the left lateral position to keep the air trapped in the right heart chambers, supplemental oxygen should be administered, and vital signs should be monitored.

26. **What is the radiographic appearance of a transvenous pacemaker or automatic implantable cardioverter defibrillator (AICD)?**
The power/generator pack for a transvenous pacemaker or AICD is located subcutaneously in the pectoral area of the anterior chest wall and appears as a radiopaque, round or ovoid structure that is about 5 cm in diameter on frontal chest radiography. The metallic lead(s) appears as a dense, thin curvilinear radiopacity (associated with thicker short segments of spring defibrillation coils in the case of an AICD) that generally extends through the subclavian or internal jugular vein from the generator pack to pass through the brachiocephalic vein and SVC, subsequently terminating in the right atrium, right ventricle, and/or coronary sinus (*see* Fig. 67-11, *A,* for the normal radiographic appearance of a dual-chambered transvenous pacemaker).

27. **Where should the leads of a transvenous pacemaker or AICD be located?**
A right atrial lead (usually in the right atrial appendage) curves around the right side of the heart on frontal chest radiography just below the SVC. On frontal chest radiography, a right ventricular lead should project slightly to the left of midline over the ventricular apex, and on lateral chest radiography it should project anteriorly and inferiorly near the ventricular apex. However, a lead within the coronary sinus projects superiorly and to the left over the heart on frontal chest radiography, and on lateral chest radiography it is directed posteriorly along the course of the atrioventricular groove.

28. **What are potential complications of transvenous pacemaker/AICD placement?**
Potential complications of transvenous pacemaker/AICD placement include all those of SGC, CVL, and PICC placement previously listed as well as hematoma or abscess formation about the generator pack; lead malpositioning, redundancy, tautness, dislodgement, migration, or fracture with or without embolism (Figs. 67-11 and 67-12); twiddler's syndrome; cardiac perforation; loss of pacing or cardioversion/defibrillation function; or induction of cardiac dysrhythmias. Cardiac perforation by a lead should be suspected on chest radiography

Figure 67-11. *A,* Normal radiographic appearance of a transvenous pacemaker. Note that the power/generator pack *(P)* over the left pectoral area appears as a radiopaque ovoid structure connected to leads, with one tip in the right atrium *(thick arrow)* overlying the right side of the heart and another tip in the right ventricle *(thin arrow)* overlying the ventricular apex. *B,* Dislodgement of the right atrial lead of the pacemaker with migration to the right ventricle. Note that the new position of the right atrial lead *(thick arrow)* (compared with [A]) is similar to that of the right ventricular lead *(thin arrow).*

(particularly on the lateral view) if the lead extends beyond the margin of the cardiac silhouette.

29. **What is twiddler's syndrome?**
    Twiddler's syndrome is a rare disorder in which a patient causes malfunction of a transvenous pacemaker or AICD by manipulating or "twiddling" with the pacing generator pack, which may be facilitated by a large pocket for the generator pack or loose subcutaneous tissue, leading to dislodgement of the pacing leads. Chest radiography is the key to diagnosis and typically shows twisting or coiling of the lead(s) about the axis of the pacemaker as well as possible lead fracture, displacement, or migration.

Figure 67-12. Fracture of pacemaker lead. Note the discontinuity *(arrow)* of one of the pacemaker leads.

BIBLIOGRAPHY

1. Cardall TY, Chan TC, Brady WJ, et al: Permanent cardiac pacemakers: Issues relevant to the emergency physician. Part I. J Emerg Med 17:479–489, 1999.

2. Dunbar RD: Radiologic appearance of compromised thoracic catheters, tubes, and wires. Radiol Clin North Am 22:699–722, 1984.

3. Gayer G, Rozenman J, Hoffmann C, et al: CT diagnosis of malpositioned chest tubes. Br J Radiol 73:786–790, 2000.

4. Gilbert TB, McGrath BJ, Soberman M: Chest tubes: Indications, placement, management, and complications. J Intensive Care Med 8:73–86, 1993.
5. Henschke CI, Yankelevitz DF, Wand A, et al: Chest radiography in the ICU. Clin Imaging 21:90–103, 1997.
6. Levy H: Nasogastric and nasoenteric feeding tubes. Gastrointest Endosc Clin North Am 8:529–549, 1998.
7. Peterson JC, Cook DJ: Intra-aortic balloon counterpulsation pump therapy: A critical appraisal of the evidence for patients with acute myocardial infarction. Crit Care 2:3–8, 1998.
8. Stone GW, Ohman EM, Miller MF, et al: Contemporary utilization and outcomes of intra-aortic balloon counterpulsation in acute myocardial infarction: The benchmark registry. J Am Coll Cardiol 41:1940–1945, 2003.
9. Zarshenas Z, Sparschu RA: Catheter placement and misplacement. Crit Care Clin 10:417–436, 1994.

OBSTETRIC ULTRASOUND: FIRST-TRIMESTER IMAGING

CHAPTER 68

Courtney Woodfield, MD, and Beverly G. Coleman, MD

1. **Should a first-trimester pelvic ultrasound be performed transabdominally or transvaginally?**

   A transabdominal pelvic ultrasound provides an overall view of the pelvis and is typically performed first, even without a full urinary bladder. If a normal intrauterine pregnancy is identified transabdominally, a transvaginal ultrasound may not be necessary. However, if an intrauterine pregnancy and/or the adnexa are not well visualized transabdominally, a transvaginal ultrasound should be performed. The transvaginal approach uses a higher-frequency transducer that is placed in closer proximity to the uterus and adnexa, allowing for improved resolution and the earlier detection of an intrauterine pregnancy.

2. **What are the indications for a first-trimester ultrasound?**

   First-trimester ultrasound is performed when the pregnancy is high risk (e.g., pregnant by in vitro fertilization or ovulation induction, advanced maternal age, personal or family history of genetic disorders, exposure to teratogens) or when a patient with a positive serum beta-human chorionic gonadotropin (HCG) level presents with vaginal bleeding, pelvic pain, or an adnexal mass.

3. **List seven causes of vaginal bleeding in the first trimester.**
   - Implantation bleed
   - Subchorionic hemorrhage
   - An embryonic pregnancy/blighted ovum
   - Embryonic demise
   - Spontaneous abortion
   - Ectopic pregnancy
   - Molar pregnancy

4. **Name three possible causes of a positive serum ß-HCG level and an empty uterus on ultrasound.**
   - Early normal intrauterine pregnancy (<5 weeks)
   - Complete spontaneous abortion
   - Ectopic pregnancy

5. **During a routine first-trimester ultrasound, what sonographic features should be documented?**
   - Presence and location of a gestational sac
   - Presence or absence of an embryo and yolk sac
   - Sonographic gestational (menstrual) age based on the mean gestational sac diameter and, when possible, the embryonic crown rump length
   - Embryonic cardiac activity and heart rate
   - Number of gestations
   - Uterine, adnexal, and cul-de-sac findings

6. **When should a gestational sac be seen with transabdominal and transvaginal ultrasound?**
   By 5 weeks (serum ß-HCG level of 1000–2000 mIU/mL), a gestational sac of approximately 5 mm should be seen transabdominally or transvaginally.

KEY POINTS: SONOGRAPHIC FEATURES OF A NORMAL EARLY INTRAUTERINE PREGNANCY

1. Double decidual sac sign present by 5–6 weeks

2. Yolk sac visible by a mean gestational sac diameter of 8 mm transvaginally and 20 mm transabdominally

3. Embryo visible by a mean gestational sac diameter of 16 mm transvaginally and 25 mm transabdominally

4. Embryonic cardiac activity detected by a crown rump length of ≥5 mm

7. **Describe the sonographic features of a normal gestational sac.**
   Before 5 weeks, a small, hypoechoic saclike structure may be seen within the thickened, echogenic decidual reaction of the endometrium (the intradecidual sac sign) (Fig. 68-1). By 5–6 weeks, the gestational sac appears as a smooth, round or ovoid, anechoic structure along the upper uterine body surrounded by a 2-mm-thick hyperechoic rim of decidual reaction (the double decidual sac sign). The gestational sac grows at a rate of 1.1 mm/day.

Figure 68-1. Sagittal transvaginal image of the uterus demonstrates the intradecidual sac sign of an early intrauterine pregnancy, with a hypoechoic saclike structure *(arrow)* of less than 5 mm located within the thickened, echogenic decidual reaction of the endometrium *(arrowhead)*.

8. **What comprises the double decidual sac sign?**
   Visualization of the echogenic decidual reaction of early pregnancy as two or three separate layers is indicative of the double decidual sac sign.
   Decidua vera lines the endometrial cavity, and decidua capsularis surrounds the gestational sac. The decidua basalis arises at the site of implantation and contributes to placental formation. When a small amount of hypoechoic fluid in the endometrial cavity separates the echogenic decidual layers of the endometrium and gestational sac, the double decidual sac sign is produced (Fig. 68-2). The double decidual sign is highly suggestive of an intrauterine pregnancy.

9. **When should a yolk sac and an embryo be seen with transabdominal and transvaginal ultrasound?**
   The mean gestational sac sizes at which a yolk sac and an embryo should be seen (also known as the "discriminatory sac sizes") are outlined in Table 68-1. Figure 68-3 depicts the normal early gestational ultrasound appearance of an embryo and a yolk sac.

10. **At what point should embryonic cardiac activity be detected sonographically?**
Embryonic cardiac activity should be detectable transvaginally when the embryonic crown rump length is ≥5 mm. Absence of sonographically detectable embryonic cardiac activity when the crown rump length is >5 mm is compatible with embryonic demise. Between 5 and 8 weeks, the heart rate is usually ≥100 beats per minute (bpm). From 8 weeks to term, the average heart rate is 140 bpm (range, 120–180 bpm). The thresholds for bradycardia based on embryonic size are listed in Table 68-2.

Figure 68-2. Coronal pelvic ultrasound image of a normal early intrauterine gestational sac with separation of the hyperechoic decidual endometrial and gestational sac layers, creating the double decidual sac sign *(arrows)*.

11. **Describe the sonographic features and significance of an abnormal gestational sac.**
On ultrasound examination, an irregularly shaped gestational sac that is low-lying and surrounded by a weakly echogenic and thin rim of decidual reaction is 90–100% predictive of an abnormal intrauterine pregnancy. A mean gestational sac diameter that is greater than the embryonic crown rump length by less than 5 mm, which is known as *first-trimester oligohydramnios,* is also associated with a poor pregnancy outcome.

Figure 68-3. Transvaginal ultrasound of a normal 9-week intrauterine pregnancy shows a well-defined embryo *(arrows)* and yolk sac *(arrowhead)* with normal separation of the amnion (A) and chorionic (C) sacs.

TABLE 68-1.	MEAN GESTATIONAL SAC SIZES AT WHICH A YOLK SAC AND AN EMBRYO SHOULD BE SEEN			
	Mean Transvaginal Gestational Sac Diameter (mm)	Mean Transabdominal Gestational Sac Diameter (mm)	Serum ß-HCG level (mIU/mL)*	Gestational Age (wk)
Yolk sac visible	8 mm	20 mm	7200	5–6
Embryo visible	16 mm	25 mm	10,000	>6

*Second International Reference Preparation.

TABLE 68-2.　THRESHOLDS FOR BRADYCARDIA BASED ON EMBRYONIC SIZE

Crown Rump Length (mm)	Bradycardia (beats/min)
<5	<80 bpm
5–9	<100 bpm
10–15	<110 bpm

Nonvisualization of an embryo when the mean gestational sac diameter is ≥25 mm transabdominally and ≥16 mm transvaginally is reported to be 100% predictive of an abnormal intrauterine pregnancy.

12. **What are the sonographic findings of an abnormal yolk sac?**
   A yolk sac that is large (>6 mm), fragmented, or calcified is suggestive of an abnormal intrauterine pregnancy (Fig. 68-4).

13. **Name six types of early pregnancy complications, and describe their sonographic appearances.**
   See Table 68-3 and Figure 68-5.

14. **What is an ectopic pregnancy?**
   A pregnancy located anywhere outside of the endometrial cavity. Ectopic

Figure 68-4. Transabdominal pelvic ultrasound of an early failed intrauterine pregnancy with a calcified yolk sac *(arrow)* and embryonic remnant *(arrowhead)*.

pregnancies occur with a frequency of approximately 14 in 1000 pregnancies. An ectopic pregnancy most commonly occurs in the fallopian tube (95–97% of cases), typically in the isthmic or ampullary portion of the tube. Other sites include the interstitial portion of the fallopian tube (2–5%), the ovary (1%), the cervix (<0.1%), and the abdominal cavity (<0.1%).

15. **Who is at increased risk for an ectopic pregnancy?**
   Patients with a history of prior ectopic pregnancy, pelvic inflammatory disease, fallopian tube surgery, in vitro fertilization, or use of an intrauterine contraceptive device.

16. **What is the classic clinical presentation of an ectopic pregnancy?**
   Approximately 45% of patients with ectopic pregnancies present with the clinical triad of vaginal bleeding, pelvic pain, and a palpable adnexal mass.

17. **List four possible sonographic findings associated with an ectopic pregnancy**
   - Embryo located outside of the uterus (5–10% of cases) is 100% diagnostic of an ectopic pregnancy
   - Complex or solid adnexal mass (Fig. 68-6)
   - Moderate to large amount of pelvic free fluid, especially if it is particulate
   - Empty uterus in conjunction with a serum ß-HCG level that is above the level at which a gestational sac should be seen.

TABLE 68-3. SONOGRAPHIC APPEARANCE OF SIX TYPES OF EARLY PREGNANCY COMPLICATIONS

Type of Abortion	Definition	Ultrasound Findings
Threatened abortion	Vaginal bleeding with a closed cervical os	Ranges from a live embryo to a small, empty gestational sac to a normal empty uterus
Abortion in progress	Intrauterine gestation in the process of being expelled	Irregular gestational sac in the lower uterus/cervix with or without a live embryo
Incomplete abortion	Incomplete passage of gestational tissues	Thickened endometrium with or without fluid and debris; areas of increased endometrial vascularity
Complete abortion	Expulsion of all gestational tissues	Normal empty uterus, which may be mildly vascular
Blighted ovum	Failed or abnormal embryonic development	Empty gestational sac or sac with abnormal yolk sac and no embryo; any abnormal gestational sac development
Embryonic demise	Lack of embryonic growth and absent expected cardiac activity	Embryo without cardiac activity

18. **What is a pseudogestational sac?**
In the setting of an ectopic pregnancy, a variable amount of fluid or hypoechoic debris may accumulate within the endometrial cavity, giving rise to a pseudogestational sac of an ectopic pregnancy (Fig. 68-7). This collection of fluid and debris may be surrounded by a single, thin, echogenic rim of decidual reaction because of stimulation of the endometrium by the circulating hormones of an ectopic pregnancy. Up to 5% of ectopic pregnancies have a pseudogestational sac.

19. **What and how common are heterotopic pregnancies?**
A heterotopic pregnancy occurs when there are concurrent intrauterine and extrauterine gestations. Patients who are pregnant by in vitro fertilization or the use of ovulation induction have a higher incidence of multiple gestations and are also at increased risk for ectopic and heterotopic pregnancies. The frequency of heterotopic pregnancies in the general population is approximately 1 in 7000 pregnancies. A higher heterotopic pregnancy rate of 1% has been reported in patients pregnant by in vitro fertilization.

Figure 68-5. Sagittal transvaginal color Doppler ultrasound of an incomplete abortion with increased vascularity, fluid, and echogenic debris *(arrows)* along the endometrium.

Figure 68-6. Coronal grayscale *(A)* and Doppler *(B)* transvaginal ultrasound images of an ectopic (ECT) right adnexal pregnancy seen as a tubal ring separate from the right ovary (OV). There is also a small amount of adjacent particulate free fluid (FF).

20. **What is a molar pregnancy?**

    A molar pregnancy is the most common and most benign form of the gestational trophoblastic diseases and is characterized by the proliferation of placental tissue after the abnormal fertilization of an empty ovum by one (complete mole, no fetus) or two (partial mole, fetus present) sperm. Patients characteristically present with markedly elevated serum ß-HCG levels, an enlarged uterus, hyperemesis gravidarum, preeclampsia, and/or vaginal bleeding.

21. **What is the sonographic appearance of a molar pregnancy?**

    The edematous placental tissue and prominent chorionic villi of a molar pregnancy classically have a "snowstorm" appearance on ultrasound. The endometrial canal

Figure 68-7. Sagittal transvaginal ultrasound of a pseudogestational sac *(arrows)* of an ectopic pregnancy with echogenic material consistent with hemorrhage filling the endometrial cavity.

is filled with hyperechoic placental tissue with good through-transmission and numerous small cystic villi, which may be too small to visualize (Fig. 68-8). A complete mole involves the entire placenta without a fetus. A partial mole involves a portion of the placenta and has an associated fetus, usually with multiple anomalies. Early first-trimester molar pregnancies can mimic blighted ova.

Figure 68-8. Sagittal midline transvaginal pelvic ultrasound of an endometrial cavity filled with heterogeneous cystic and solid placental tissue *(arrows),* which is characteristic of a complete molar pregnancy.

BIBLIOGRAPHY

1. Lazarus E: What's new in first trimester ultrasound. Radiol Clin North Am 41(4):663–679, 2003.
2. Lyons EA, Levi CS, Dashefsky SM: The first trimester. In Rumack CM, Wilson SR, Charboneau JW (eds): Diagnostic Ultrasound, 2nd ed. St. Louis, Mosby, 1998, pp 975–1011.
3. Middleton WD, Kurtz AB, Hertzberg BS: The first trimester and ectopic pregnancy. In: Ultrasound: The Requisites, 2nd ed. St. Louis, Mosby, 2003, pp 342–373.

CHAPTER 69

OBSTETRIC ULTRASOUND: SECOND-TRIMESTER IMAGING

Ross I. Silver, MD, and Beverly G. Coleman, MD

1. **What are the components of the basic (level 1) second-trimester ultrasound?**
   The components of a basic second-trimester ultrasound include documentation of the fetal heart rate; number and lie of fetus(es); estimation of the amniotic fluid volume; location and appearance of the placenta and its relationship to the internal os; gestational age; evaluation of the uterus and adnexa; and assessment of fetal anatomic characteristics, including the cerebral ventricles, four-chamber heart, spine, stomach, urinary bladder, umbilical cord, and kidneys.

2. **How is the normal amniotic fluid volume estimated?**
   To calculate the amniotic fluid index (AFI), the anteroposterior diameters of the largest empty fluid pocket (no umbilical cord or fetal parts) in each quadrant are added together. The AFI is normally between 7 and 25 cm. In addition, each individual pocket of fluid should be between 2 and 8 cm. Fluctuations outside of this range define oligohydramnios (too little amniotic fluid) or polyhydramnios (too much amniotic fluid).

KEY POINTS: COMPONENTS OF A BASIC SECOND-TRIMESTER ULTRASOUND

1. Documentation of fetal heart rate, number and lie of fetus(es)

2. Estimation of amniotic fluid volume

3. Location and appearance of the placenta and its relationship to the internal os

4. Gestational age

5. Evaluation of the uterus and adnexa

6. Fetal anatomic characteristics

3. **What are the major causes of polyhydramnios?**
   One third of cases of polyhydramnios are idiopathic and not associated with other anomalies. Two thirds of cases are associated with maternal problems, fetal problems, or both. These include gestational diabetes, multiple gestations, structural abnormalities of the fetus that impair swallowing of amniotic fluid (obstruction of the upper gastrointestinal tract, chest narrowing or masses, and severe central nervous system abnormalities), and fetal hydrops.

4. **What is the dreaded complication of oligohydramnios?**
   The lungs need an adequate supply of amniotic fluid for proper development; however, oligohydramnios leads to pulmonary hypoplasia, which, depending on the severity, can be a major cause of fetal morbidity and mortality.

5. **If the placenta appears to be covering the internal os, what entity may be present?**

This is called *placenta previa,* which occurs in 1 in 200 to 400 deliveries, more commonly after a previous cesarean section. If the placenta extends to the edge of the internal os, a marginal previa is present. If the placenta partially covers the os, this is called a *partial previa,* and if it completely covers the internal os, a complete previa is present. A fourth type, a central previa, occurs when a complete previa is centrally located over the internal os. Placenta previa can lead to maternal hemorrhage secondary to premature detach-

Figure 69-1. Sagittal transvaginal ultrasound demonstrates a complete placenta previa. The placenta completely covers the internal os *(arrow).*

ment of the placenta. It can also be a cause of premature delivery and perinatal mortality (Fig. 69-1).

6. **A pregnant woman presents with vaginal bleeding, pelvic pain, and tenderness over the uterus. What entity must be considered?**

This is a common presentation of placental abruption, a serious condition that can cause morbidity in the fetus and, less commonly, in the mother. Risk factors include maternal hypertension, collagen vascular disease, and abdominal trauma. Ultrasound can detect placental abruption by demonstrating blood behind a placenta that has separated from the uterine wall. Blood has a variable ultrasound appearance, depending on the age of the bleed, that ranges from hypoechoic or completely anechoic in the acute and chronic phases to hyperechoic and heterogeneous in the subacute phase.

7. **What is an "hourglass" deformity of the cervix?**

An hourglass deformity is a severe form of incompetent cervix that occurs when the internal cervical os is open and the endocervical canal is dilated to the external os. Clinically, the amniotic membranes bulge into the vagina. Spontaneous pregnancy loss usually cannot be avoided (Fig. 69-2).

Figure 69-2. Sagittal transvaginal ultrasound demonstrates the "hourglass" deformity of an incompetent cervix *(arrow).*

8. **Can the presence of a single umbilical artery be normal?**

Yes. Normal umbilical cords most commonly have three vessels (two arteries and one vein). A two-vessel cord does not necessarily imply fetal abnormality. In single gestations, approximately 50% of two-vessel cords (one artery and one vein) have no associated abnormalities. In multiple gestations, a two-vessel cord is a more common normal variant. Of the abnormalities that may exist with a two-vessel cord, fetal structural abnormalities and growth retardation are the most common. The posterior fossa, face, extremities, and heart should be thoroughly evaluated in pregnancies with a single umbilical artery (Fig. 69-3).

9. **What is the most accurate measurement to assess gestational age in the second trimester?**
The biparietal diameter (BPD) is accurate from approximately 5–7 days up to 24 weeks. It is measured in the transverse plane from the outer edge of the closer temporoparietal bone to the inner edge of the farther temporoparietal bone. The thalamus should be visualized when measuring the BPD. The head circumference is as accurate as the BPD and is measured at the same level. The femur length is as accurate as the BPD after 26 weeks (Fig. 69-4, *A*).

Figure 69-3. Transabdominal ultrasound demonstrates a normal three-vessel cord with a single umbilical vein *(arrow)* and two umbilical arteries *(arrowheads)*.

10. **How is the abdominal circumference obtained, and why is it used?**
The abdominal circumference is measured in the transverse plane at the fetal liver, with the umbilical portion of the left portal vein in the center of the abdomen. The abdominal circumference is not as accurate as the BPD and femur length are for estimating gestational age. Instead, it is commonly used to determine proportionality with the head. A head:abdominal circumference ratio is used for this purpose. Normally, the head is larger than the body in the second and early third trimester, with a reversal of this ratio at term (Fig. 69-4, *B*).

Figure 69-4. Measurements of normal gestational age. *A,* BPD (+) and thalami *(arrows). B,* Abdominal circumference (+), portal vein *(long arrow),* stomach *(short arrow),* and aorta *(arrowhead).*

11. **What is the difference between symmetric and asymmetric intrauterine growth retardation (IUGR)?**

Asymmetric IUGR makes up 90% of cases and is due to diminished blood supply and nourishment to the fetus. The abdominal circumference is disproportionately affected compared with the head and femur. It is usually diagnosed in the third trimester. Symmetric IUGR is usually diagnosed in the first or early second trimester and is due to decreased cellular growth, usually secondary to an insult to the mother or fetus early in the pregnancy. The head and body are equally affected in symmetric IUGR.

12. **What percentage of cardiac anomalies can be detected by the four-chamber view alone?**

Approximately 70% of cardiac anomalies can be detected with this view, including abnormalities of cardiac position (situs inversus), septal abnormalities (ventricular septal defect), and masses (rhabdomyomas). The percentage of detected anomalies can be increased to 80% with the addition of a short-axis view of the great vessels at the base of the heart, a view of the right ventricular outflow tract, and a long-axis view of the left ventricular outflow tract (Fig. 69-5).

Figure 69-5. Transabdominal ultrasound demonstrates a normal four-chamber view of the heart. Apex of the heart *(arrow)*.

13. **Describe the classic sonographic features of fetal hydrops.**

Whether the cause is immune or nonimmune, the appearance of fetal hydrops is the same: fluid in the serous cavities, including ascites; pleural and pericardial effusions; skin thickening; placental enlargement; and polyhydramnios. However, not all of these features may be present in any one case. In addition, hepatomegaly may be seen, particularly with immune hydrops.

14. **What is the most common intrathoracic/extracardiac fetal anomaly?**

Congenital diaphragmatic hernia (CDH) occurs in 1 of every 2000–3000 live births. Ninety percent of these are Bochdalek hernias, which are posterolateral in location. The remaining 10% are called Morgagni hernias, which occur in an anteromedial location. With a Bochdalek hernia, ultrasound shows the normal stomach bubble located in the chest and the heart is displaced upward and to the right. The presence of peristalsing, fluid-filled bowel loops in the chest is diagnostic. The spleen and left lobe of the liver may also be present in the thorax. Morgagni hernias are more subtle and difficult to diagnose (Fig. 69-6).

Figure 69-6. Transabdominal ultrasound demonstrates congenital diaphragmatic hernia. The heart *(long arrow)*, stomach *(short arrow)*, and liver *(arrowhead)* are in the thorax.

15. **Name the four types of anterior abdominal wall defects. Which are most common?**
    The four defects are omphalocele, gastroschisis, pentalogy of Cantrell, and limb-body wall complex. Omphalocele and gastroschisis are the most common, occurring in 1 in 4000 live births and 1 in 10,000 live births, respectively. The latter two are extraordinarily uncommon and are associated with a very poor prognosis.

16. **Which abdominal wall defect is covered by a membrane?**
    Omphalocele is defined as the hernia-tion of abdominal contents into the base of the umbilical cord and is cov-ered by a thin amnioperitoneal mem-brane. Either the liver and small bowel or small bowel alone can be contained within the defect. Gastroschisis is not covered by a membrane, and the typi-cal appearance is that of free-floating loops of bowel (Fig. 69-7).

17. **How can the abdominal cord insertion (ACI) help in the diagnosis of anterior abdominal wall defects?**
    An omphalocele is centrally located, and the umbilical cord typi-

Figure 69-7. *A,* Transabdominal ultrasound demonstrates an abdominal wall defect consistent with omphalocele *(arrowhead). B,* Omphalocele with a covering membrane *(arrow).*

cally inserts into the anterior portion of the defect. A pathognomonic feature of omphalocele is the presence of a "cyst" of Wharton's jelly at the site of cord insertion. A distinguishing feature of gas-troschisis is that the defect is paraumbilical, usually to the right of the ACI. Documentation of the ACI is an important part of all second-trimester ultrasounds. Color flow may be needed to visualize the ACI in some cases (Fig. 69-8).

18. **Which has a worse prognosis: omphalocele or gastroschisis?**
    Omphalocele has a worse prognosis because it is associated with a signifi-cantly increased incidence of chromo-somal abnormalities (approximately 12%). This is much greater with omphaloceles that contain only bowel. Other structural abnormalities, includ-ing cardiac, thoracic, gastrointestinal, genitourinary, and central nervous system, occur in 75% of cases. Gastroschisis is not associated

Figure 69-8. Transabdominal ultrasound shows a normal ACI *(arrow).*

with other abnormalities, although vascular compromise of the extruded bowel (both large and small bowel) may occur. Perforation of bowel may lead to an entity called *meconium peritonitis* (Fig. 69-9).

19. **Why might the urinary bladder *not* be visualized?**

    The bladder should be identified by 16 weeks. However, nonvisualization of the urinary bladder is not necessarily abnormal. Because of the normal cycling of the bladder, rescanning after initial nonvisualization every 15–20 minutes for 1 hour is recommended. If the bladder is still not present, then an abnormality likely exists, such as impairment of renal function from an intrinsic renal abnormality or upper urinary tract obstruction. Generalized growth retardation can also

Figure 69-9. Transabdominal ultrasound demonstrates gastroschisis. Free floating bowel loops are seen *(arrow)*. Doppler flow demonstrates the umbilical cord inserting to the side of the defect *(arrowhead)*.

lead to functional renal impairment. In bladder exstrophy, typically there is an infraumbilical wall defect with nonvisualization of the urinary bladder.

20. **A markedly distended bladder and ureters with bilateral hydronephrosis are visualized during a routine second-trimester ultrasound of a male fetus. What abnormality may be present?**

    This is the classic sonographic appearance of a severe, prolonged lower urinary tract obstruction. In a male fetus, this is most commonly caused by posterior urethral valves. In female fetuses, this is likely a result of urethral atresia. Cases of severe lower urinary tract obstruction are usually fatal due to marked oligohydramnios and the pulmonary hypoplasia that results (Fig. 69-10).

21. **Name the four patterns of limb shortening seen with skeletal dysplasias.**

    Skeletal dysplasias can be differentiated by determining which portion of the limb is affected. A micromelic pattern of shortening affects both the proximal and distal limbs. If only the proximal segment is shortened, a rhizomelic type of dysplasia is present. Less common patterns of dysplasia include the mesomelic pattern, in which only the forearm and foreleg are shortened, and the acromelic

Figure 69-10. *A,* Transabdominal ultrasound demonstrates a normal bladder *(arrow). B,* Lower urinary tract obstruction with distended bladder *(arrow)* and ureters *(arrowheads).*

pattern, in which only the distal segment is shortened. The most common type of skeletal dysplasia, heterozygous achondroplastic dysplasia, is characterized by a rhizomelic pattern of shortening.

22. **What would produce an enlarged cisterna magna on ultrasound?**
    A Dandy-Walker malformation causes an enlarged cisterna magna. From the inside of the occiput to the back of the cerebellar vermis, the cisterna magna normally measures 2–10 mm. Dandy-Walker malformations are caused by dysgenesis (Dandy-Walker variant) or agenesis of the cerebellar vermis and are associated with midline central nervous system abnormalities, including lateral and third ventricle hydrocephalus, encephalocele, and agenesis of the corpus callosum. Additional abnormalities of the body, including cardiac and renal abnormalities, may be found (Fig. 69-11).

Figure 69-11. *A,* Transabdominal ultrasound demonstrates a normal posterior fossa. Crosshairs measure the cerebellum *(+)* and cisterna magna *(x). B,* Dandy-Walker malformation with an absent vermis *(arrow)* and an enlarged cisterna magna *(arrowhead).*

23. **What is the significance of the nuchal skin?**
    Directly posterior to the occiput is a thin rim of soft tissue that normally measures ≤6 mm in the second trimester. An increased nuchal skin thickness greater than 6 mm is concerning for Down syndrome. The sensitivity of this finding is 50%, and the false-positive rate is less than 1%.

24. **Which open neural tube defect contains elements of spinal cord?**
    As *myelo* is the Latin prefix referring to the spine, a *myelo*meningocele contains spinal cord elements. The herniation of meninges alone through an open neural tube defect is known simply as a *meningocele*. On ultrasound, these defects usually appear as a cystic structure projecting through splayed posterior elements, most commonly in the lumbosacral region. If the cyst is completely anechoic, a meningocele is likely present. Hyperechoic strands representing neural elements within the cystic projection indicate that the likely diagnosis is myelomeningocele (Fig. 69-12).

25. **When an open neural tube defect is discovered, what else should be thoroughly evaluated?**
    The fetal head should be well evaluated whenever an open neural tube defect is discovered. These defects are almost always associated with Arnold-Chiari type II malformations, in which the cerebellar hemispheres herniate downward through the foramen magnum. Two ultrasound signs are associated with this malformation: the "banana sign" and the "lemon sign." With the banana sign, the cerebellum is shaped like a downward-curved C, and with the lemon sign, the bilateral frontoparietal bones are flattened. Both signs are sensitive and specific for open neural

Figure 69-12. *A,* Transverse transabdominal ultrasound view of a myelomeningocele. The posterior elements are splayed *(arrows). B,* Sagittal view of the spine demonstrates a low-lying, tethered spinal cord *(arrow)* and cystic mass arising from the spine *(arrowhead).*

tube defects; the banana sign is seen in more than 90% of cases, and the lemon sign is present in approximately 98% of cases.

BIBLIOGRAPHY

1. Brant WE: Ultrasound: The Core Curriculum. Philadelphia, Lippincott Williams & Wilkins, 2001, pp 25.
2. Callen PW: Ultrasonography in Obstetrics and Gynecology, 3rd ed. Philadelphia, W.B. Saunders, 1994.
3. Kurtz AB, Middleton WD: Ultrasound: The Requisites. St. Louis, Mosby, 1996, pp 153–179, 180–189, 207–340.

CHAPTER 70

VASCULAR ULTRASOUND

Denise S. White, DO, and Beverly G. Coleman, MD

1. **What is the incidence of deep venous thrombosis (DVT)?**

   The exact incidence of DVT is unknown due to the inherent difficulty in establishing the clinical diagnosis related to the nonspecific nature or lack of patient symptoms. However, recent data estimate the incidence of DVT to be about 80 cases per 100,000 persons annually, resulting in 600,000 hospitalizations for this diagnosis every year in the United States alone. Additionally, each year, approximately 200,000 deaths in the United States are attributed to pulmonary embolism resulting from DVT.

2. **How do patients with a lower extremity DVT present clinically?**

   No single physical finding or combination of signs and symptoms is sufficiently accurate to establish the diagnosis. The most common physical signs are edema, which is primarily unilateral; leg pain (present in about 50%), which is extremely nonspecific; leg tenderness (seen in about 75%); Homans' sign (calf pain with dorsiflexion of the foot), present in less than one third of patients with DVT; and increase in skin temperature with fever. Many patients are, however, asymptomatic, making the diagnosis even more difficult.

3. **Name the risk factors associated with the development of DVT.**

   Risk factors include malignancy, recent surgery, pregnancy, hypercoagulable states, stroke, trauma, cardiac failure, respiratory failure, immobilization, patient age <40, obesity, and oral contraceptive use.

4. **Describe how to perform an ultrasound examination of the lower extremity when looking for DVT.**

   Evaluation of the lower extremity for DVT may be performed in the ultrasound suite or portably at the patient's bedside. The patient is scanned with a linear array 7- to 10-MHz transducer in the supine position from the inguinal ligament to the proximal calf, with the leg mildly abducted and externally rotated and with slight knee flexion. The deep venous structures are evaluated with B-mode grayscale images in the transverse plane, compressing every 2 cm. Pulsed Doppler images are also obtained with and without augmentation maneuvers by manually squeezing the more distal portion of the extremity to assess flow. Color images are obtained to further evaluate patency of the lumen.

5. **How do the sonographic findings of acute and chronic DVT differ?**

   See Table 70-1 and Figures 70-1 and 70-2.

6. **How accurate is ultrasound in establishing the diagnosis of DVT?**

   In symptomatic patients, studies that have directly compared sonography with venography have shown average sensitivities and specificities of 95% and 98%, respectively. The results are, however, poorer in asymptomatic, high-risk, or postoperative patients. Collectively, results from six studies have shown a decrease in average sensitivity to 58%, whereas specificity was maintained at 98%. Reasons for the decrease in sensitivity in this group include small thrombus size, the nonocclusive nature of certain thrombi, and the higher prevalence of thrombus isolated to the calf.

TABLE 70-1	SONOGRAPHIC FINDINGS OF ACUTE AND CHRONIC DVT
Acute DVT	**Chronic DVT**
Loss of complete compressibility of the vein	Decreased venous diameter, atretic segment (most sensitive and specific sign)
Isoechoic/hypoechoic intraluminal thrombus	Thickened irregular venous wall
Venous enlargement	Echogenic weblike filling defect
Absent Doppler signal	Venous collaterals
Loss of phasicity	Calcification
Loss of flow augmentation	

Figure 70-1. Normal vein versus acute DVT. Left upper frame shows a normal anechoic vein (V) without compression, which is equal in size to the adjacent artery (A). Right upper frame with applied pressure demonstrates that the normal vein is completely compressible. Left and right lower frames, again performed with and without pressure, respectively, demonstrate echogenic thrombus distending the lumen of the vein (V) and loss of venous compressability, which is consistent with acute DVT.

7. **Name treatment options for patients with DVT.**
   Proper treatment of patients with DVT is important to help prevent a potentially fatal pulmonary embolism, to decrease associated morbidity, and to reduce the patient's chance of developing post-phlebitic syndrome. There are several available treatment options for acute DVT. Anticoagulation, the mainstay of initial therapy, begins with heparin (regular unfractionated or low molecular weight), with subsequent conversion to warfarin for 3–6 months. Catheter-directed thrombolysis can also be done, resulting in prompt resolution and restoration of normal venous flow. Surgical thrombectomy is also an option and is usually reserved for patients in whom limb salvage is at risk.

Figure 70-2. Chronic DVT. Note that an echogenic thrombus is identified within the lumen of the vein (V), as with acute DVT. There is, however, calcification *(arrows)* within this long-standing clot, a feature of chronic thrombus.

8. **What are the sonographic findings of a pseudoaneurysm (PSA)?**
   - Hypoechoic fluid collection immediately adjacent to the injured artery
   - Variable amount of peripheral thrombus
   - Swirling color flow (yin-yang) as blood flows in and out of the PSA
   - "To and fro" pattern of flow at the PSA neck on pulsed Doppler with a normal systolic upstroke as blood enters the PSA
   - Pandiastolic flow reversal due to the compliant nature of the PSA walls, as blood in the PSA cavity is ejected back into the artery during diastole (Fig. 70-3)

9. **How may a PSA be treated nonsurgically?**
   There are two nonsurgical methods for treatment of a PSA. Transcutaneous ultrasound-guided compression can be performed by applying pressure over the PSA neck. This is a time-consuming process and can be painful for the patient and fatiguing for the physician performing the compression. Success rates are variable and are better when the PSA is acute or subacute and when the neck is narrow. A second option is direct thrombin injection into the PSA under ultrasound guidance. When compared with transcutaneous ultrasound-guided compression, this technique is faster, less painful for the patient, and more successful (success rate is approximately 90%), and it does not require termination of anticoagulation therapy.

10. **List the differential diagnoses for a perivascular mass seen on grayscale imaging.**
    - *PSA:* a complication of arterial puncture/penetrating trauma, recognized by internal flow with features previously described
    - *Hematoma:* grayscale appearance may be identical to PSA, but a hematoma is avascular; transmitted pulsation from adjacent artery should not be mistaken for true flow
    - *Hyperplastic lymph node:* can be mistaken for a PSA because of the vascularity at its hilum, but it lacks a communicating neck, yin-yang flow, and "to and fro" pattern
    - *Arterial aneurysm:* when fusiform, it is easily recognized by its appearance/position within the arterial wall; when saccular, it can be difficult to differentiate from a PSA because they may share color Doppler flow patterns

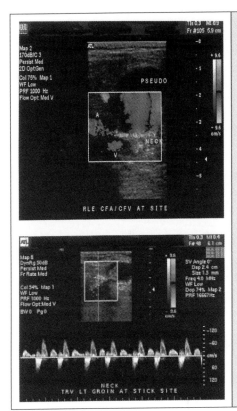

Figure 70-3. Pseudoaneurysm (PSA). Upper color Doppler image reveals characteristic yin-yang appearance as blood swirls within this posttraumatic groin PSA, which is labeled *"pseudo."* Note the thin linear attachment of the PSA to the adjacent artery (A), labeled *"neck."* Lower pulsed Doppler image at the neck of the PSA demonstrates normal antegrade systolic flow and diastolic flow reversal, the "to and fro" pattern.

11. **What are the characteristic findings of an arteriovenous fistula (AVF) on ultrasound?**
Color and pulsed Doppler imaging are extremely important to make this diagnosis since no grayscale abnormality is seen. With color imaging, a perivascular tissue vibration at the fistula site can be seen, resulting in a color bruit (Doppler artifact with random assignment of red and blue pixels in the perivascular soft tissue). Pulsed Doppler findings include localized low-resistance arterial flow, demonstrated by increased diastolic flow velocity and continuous forward flow throughout the cardiac cycle. This is in contrast to the normally absent or reversed diastolic flow seen in most peripheral arteries. On the venous end, localized turbulent/arterialized flow is seen due to direct arterial inflow (Fig. 70-4).

12. **Where in the femoral vasculature do AVFs most commonly occur?**
AVFs have increased in frequency due to the more common use of larger catheters and anticoagulation in a variety of vascular interventional procedures. Most AVFs are asymptomatic. When large, however, they can result in high-output cardiac failure or lower extremity ischemia. AVFs are almost always located distal to the femoral bifurcation. Above the bifurcation, the femoral artery and vein are positioned side by side. Below the femoral bifurcation, however, the femoral vein is posterior to the artery, making it more likely that AVF will develop, especially as complication of a procedure.

Figure 70-4. Arteriovenous fistula (AVF). The upper left image shows an example of a color bruit artifact (random assignment of extraluminal color pattern) in the region of an AVF, located above and to the right of the common femoral artery *(CFA)* in this image. The upper right panel shows abnormally low-resistance flow when Doppler sampled the affected artery. The lower right panel shows that there is abnormal pulsatility and arterialization of the venous waveform. The lower left panel shows that a sample taken at the site of the AVF resulted in a mixed low-resistance waveform.

13. **What are common indications for performing a carotid ultrasound examination?**
    - Evaluation of patients with a transient ischemic attack or cerebrovascular accident
    - Evaluation of a neck bruit or pulsatile neck mass
    - Postoperative follow-up after carotid endarterectomy
    - Preoperative screening before major cardiovascular surgical procedures

14. **Name the three components of a carotid ultrasound examination.**
    - *B-mode* is two-dimensional grayscale imaging in the transverse and longitudinal planes. It is used to identify wall thickening and the presence of plaque, to characterize plaque, and to estimate the degree of luminal narrowing.
    - *Spectral analysis* is a quantitative graphic display of the velocity and direction of flowing blood within a selected Doppler sample volume.
    - *Color Doppler* provides simultaneous hemodynamic and anatomic information by demonstrating flow direction, providing velocity information, and clarifying pulsed wave Doppler image mismatch.

15. **What spectral analysis findings are indicative of stenosis?**
    Depending on where the Doppler sample is obtained, the waveform findings are variable. There is an increase in resistance of flow proximal to the level of stenosis, which is manifested as decreased diastolic flow. At and distal to the level of stenosis, turbulence causes broadening of the spectral waveform. After the luminal diameter narrows approximately 40–50%, the velocity

increases with increasing severity of stenosis, except in some cases of critical stenosis (>95%), in which case the velocity may decrease or become normal again due to reduced flow volume.

16. **What parameters are used to grade the degree of carotid artery stenosis?**
    There are several parameters that can be used in isolation or in combination. They include the peak systolic velocity, end-diastolic velocity, ratio of internal carotid artery (ICA) to common carotid artery (CCA) peak systolic velocity, and the ratio of ICA to CCA end-diastolic velocity.

17. **What degree of carotid stenosis is considered clinically significant in the symptomatic and asymptomatic patient?**
    The North American Symptomatic Carotid Endarterectomy Trial (NASCET) and the European Carotid Surgery Trial (ECST), two large multicenter trials, have shown that carotid endarterectomy is more beneficial than medical management in symptomatic patients when the degree of ICA stenosis is between 70% and 99%. The Asymptomatic Carotid Atherosclerosis Study (ACAS) has shown that even asymptomatic patients with a stenosis greater than 60% can benefit from carotid surgery. It should be remembered that even patients with lesser degrees of stenosis with demonstrated carotid artery ulceration may also benefit from surgical management.

18. **In an area of critical stenosis, what is the significance of demonstrating a "string sign"?**
    When dealing with a critical stenosis (>95%), care must be taken to optimize flow sensitivity and gain settings to help facilitate the identification of a remaining trickle, or "string," of residual flow. This is important from a management standpoint because patients with a critical stenosis may be treated surgically, whereas those with complete occlusion are not operative candidates. With ultrasound, color and power Doppler are the best at differentiating critical stenosis with a remaining trickle of flow from complete carotid occlusion, which at times may be difficult to determine. When needed, angiography may be performed for confirmation.

19. **Name several potential pitfalls of carotid ultrasound.**
    - Elevated or low baseline velocities can cause an overestimation or underestimation of the degree of stenosis (seen with hypertension/contralateral stenosis or occlusion and decreased cardiac output/more proximal stenosis, respectively).
    - Tandem lesions (additional areas of stenosis) may not be identified and may reduce anticipated velocity shifts.
    - Paradoxic dampening of velocities may occur in a critical area of stenosis (>95%).
    - Underlying cardiac abnormalities, such as cardiac dysrhythmias, aortic valvular lesions, and severe cardiomyopathies, can cause significant alterations in the shape of the underlying carotid waveforms, and can also affect the systolic and diastolic velocities.

20. **Can ultrasound be used to make the diagnosis of subclavian steal syndrome?**
    Ultrasound is the preferred imaging modality for demonstrating subclavian steal syndrome, caused by stenosis or occlusion of the subclavian artery proximal to the origin of the vertebral artery. To maintain adequate perfusion, the distal subclavian artery and upper extremity receive blood via retrograde flow through the ipsilateral vertebral artery, bypassing the stenosis. This can lead to significant neurologic symptoms as blood is "stolen" through the circle of Willis from the contralateral vertebral artery. A spectrum of pulsed Doppler abnormalities can be seen, ranging from a transient decrease in midsystolic velocity (early) to complete flow reversal (late) in the ipsilateral vertebral artery.

21. **What does a parvus tardus waveform indicate?**

    Normal arterial waveforms have a rapid early systolic upstroke related to fast acceleration of blood at the initiation of systole and a significantly higher peak in systole when compared with diastole. Parvus tardus waveforms have a slow systolic upstroke and a systolic peak that is reduced in amplitude when compared with the amount of diastolic flow. This parvus (reduced) tardus (delayed) morphology is indicative of a significant, more proximal arterial stenosis (Fig. 70-5).

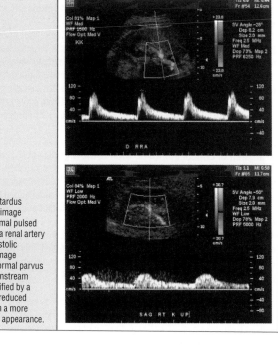

Figure 70-5. Parvus tardus waveform. The upper image demonstrates the normal pulsed Doppler waveform of a renal artery with a rapid, sharp systolic upstroke. The lower image demonstrates an abnormal parvus tardus waveform downstream from a stenosis, identified by a slower upstroke with reduced amplitude, resulting in a more rounded and flattened appearance.

22. **What is the role of ultrasound in establishing the diagnosis of renovascular hypertension?**

    Hypertension affects approximately 50 million people in the United States alone. A renal vascular cause is potentially curable, and even though only causative of only 1–5% of cases of hypertension, development of a screening test to identify patients with this etiologic factor is important. Duplex ultrasonography is a suitable screening test for this diagnosis because it is a relatively inexpensive, noninvasive modality that avoids the use of nephrotoxic contrast material, which is of obvious importance in patients with underlying renal disease. However, unlike other modalities, this examination is highly operator-dependent.

23. **What are the most common causes of renovascular hypertension?**

    In adults, the majority of cases are due to atherosclerosis (65%). Fibromuscular dysplasia is the next most common cause (30–35%), followed by a number of much less common etiologic factors, including aortic or renal artery dissection, aortic coarctation, vasculitides such as Takayasu's arteritis and polyarteritis nodosa, prior radiation therapy, renal artery aneurysm, and post-transplant stenosis.

KEY POINTS: CLINICAL CHARACTERISTICS OF RENOVASCULAR HYPERTENSION

1. Abdominal bruit

2. Onset of hypertension before age 25 or after age 50

3. Refractory hypertension (diastolic pressure >100 mmHg with patient taking three or more antihypertensive agents)

4. Worsening of hypertension after treatment with an angiotensin-converting enzyme inhibitor

5. Unexplained azotemia in an elderly hypertensive patient

24. **What parameters are used to make the diagnosis of renovascular hypertension on ultrasound?**

    The renal arteries are first localized using color Doppler, and then spectral analysis is performed. Using this information, several criteria have been suggested to establish this diagnosis and include elevated velocity (peak systolic velocity in the main renal artery >100 cm/sec), ratio of the main renal artery to aortic peak systolic velocity (>3.5), systolic acceleration time (<370–470 cm/sec), time of acceleration (>0.05–0.08. sec), and spectral analysis pattern recognition (parvus tardus waveform).

25. **How does sonography compare with other modalities in establishing the diagnosis of renovascular hypertension?**

    In establishing this diagnosis, sonography has the advantage of being relatively less expensive, does not require the use of a nephrotoxic contrast agent, and is often more accessible than other modalities. However, it is extremely operator dependent, has a higher technical failure rate (10–20%) than other modalities, and is limited in the evaluation of accessory renal arteries. Studies have shown that when done properly, its ability to accurately establish the diagnosis of renovascular hypertension is comparable with that of nuclear medicine, computed tomography angiography, and magnetic resonance angiography (Table 70-2).

TABLE 70-2. DIAGNOSTIC ACCURACY OF NONINVASIVE DETECTION OF RENOVASCULAR HYPERTENSION

	Sensitivity	Specificity
Duplex sonography	85–90%	95%
Captopril nuclear scan	90%	95%
Magnetic resonance angiography	95%	90%
Computed tomography angiography	92%	83%

WEBSITES

1. http://www.aium.org

2. http://www.jultrasoundmed.org

BIBLIOGRAPHY

1. Cronan JJ: Venous thromboembolic disease: The role of US. Radiology 186:619–630, 1993.

2. Freed KS, Brown LK, Carroll BA: The extracranial cerebral vessels. In Rumack CM, Wilson SR, Charboneau JW (eds): Diagnostic Ultrasound, 2nd ed. St. Louis, Mosby, 1998, pp 885–919.

3. Kawashima A, Sandler CM, Ernst RD, et al: CT evaluation of renovascular disease. Radiographics 20:1321–1340, 2000.

4. Lewis BD: The peripheral veins. In Rumack CM, Wilson SR, Charboneau JW (eds): Diagnostic Ultrasound, 2nd ed. St. Louis, Mosby, 1998, pp 943–958.

5. Middleton WD: Duplex and color Doppler sonography of postcatheterization arteriovenous fistulas. Semin Interv Radiol 7:192–197, 1990.

6. Polak JF: The peripheral arteries. In Rumack CM, Wilson SR, Charboneau JW (eds): Diagnostic Ultrasound, 2nd ed. St. Louis, Mosby, 1998, pp 921–941.

7. Soulez G, Oliva VL, Turpin S, et al: Imaging of renovascular hypertension: Respective values of renal scintigraphy, renal Doppler US, and MR angiography. Radiographics 20(5):1355–1368, 2000.

8. Weinmann EE, Salzman EW: Deep vein thrombosis. N Engl J Med 331:1630–1641, 1994.

CHAPTER 71

ABDOMINAL ULTRASOUND

Keith A. Ferguson, MD, and Susan Hilton, MD

1. **What anatomic landmarks can be used to determine in which hepatic segment an abnormality is located?**

   The hepatic veins can be useful in placing an abnormality within a segment (Fig. 71-1). The right hepatic vein separates the anterior and posterior segments of the right hepatic lobe. The middle hepatic vein separates the anterior segment of the right hepatic lobe from the medial segment of the left hepatic lobe, and the left hepatic vein separates the medial and lateral segments of the left hepatic lobe.

   Like the middle hepatic vein, the gallbladder separates the anterior segment of the right lobe and the medial segment of the left lobe. The ligamentum teres separates the medial and lateral segments of the left hepatic lobe.

Figure 71-1. Transverse image of the liver demonstrates the hepatic venous and segmental anatomy. The right hepatic vein (R) separates the right hepatic lobe into anterior (RA) and posterior (RP) segments. The middle hepatic vein (M) separates the anterior segment of the right hepatic lobe from the medial segment of the left hepatic lobe (LM), and the left hepatic vein (L) separates the left lobe into medial (LM) and lateral (LL) segments.

2. **What is the normal echogenicity of the liver?**

   The liver should normally be equal to or slightly more echogenic than the right kidney and less echogenic than the pancreas.

3. **Can one differentiate between hepatic and portal veins on ultrasound?**

   Yes. Because the portal veins travel with hepatic arteries and biliary radicles and are surrounded by periportal fibrofatty tissue, there is a rim of increased echogenicity surrounding the portal veins. The hepatic veins have no such echogenic rim.

4. **Name the common benign and malignant focal hepatic lesions.**

   See Table 71-1.

5. **What is the significance of a target lesion?**

   Features that characterize a target lesion are an echogenic center with a hypoechoic peripheral rim. This appearance is important because it is relatively specific for malignancy, most commonly metastatic disease and less commonly hepatocellular carcinoma. Hepatic adenomas can also have this appearance but are relatively rare.

TABLE 71-1.   CHARACTERISTICS OF COMMON FOCAL HEPATIC LESIONS

Lesion	Sonographic Appearance	Additional Information
Cysts	Anechoic lumen, imperceptible wall, increased through-transmission, well-defined posterior wall May contain septations	These characteristics apply to cysts in other organs as well (*see* Fig. 71-11 for an example of a renal cyst)
Fatty infiltration of the liver (Fig. 71-2)	Liver is more echogenic than the right kidney Common locations for focal fatty infiltration: adjacent to falciform ligament and anterior to the portal vein bifurcation	May be focal or diffuse
Hemangiomas (Fig. 71-3)	Homogeneously echogenic (typical hemangiomas) or echogenic periphery with hypoechoic center (atypical hemangiomas) Increased through-transmission in a minority of lesions	More common in women; 10% are multiple
Focal nodular hyperplasia	Variable appearance; central scar characteristic but rarely seen on ultrasound	Benign lesion composed of normal hepatocytes, Kuppfer cells, and bile ducts; more common in women
Adenomas	Variable appearance; when hemorrhagic, may have a complex or cystic appearance	Benign neoplasm composed of hepatocytes, but not Kuppfer cells or bile ducts; association with oral contraceptive pills Usually resected due to propensity to hemorrhage
Metastases	Wide range of appearances, including echogenic, calcified, or complex cystic lesions; usually multiple	Most common cause of focal solid liver lesions
Hepatocellular carcinoma	May be solitary, multifocal, or infiltrating; portal or hepatic vein invasion	Usually occurs in cirrhotic livers
Abscess	Complex cystic or solid appearance, increased through-transmission, gas in lesion may cause shadowing	Often occur secondary to seeding from intestinal sources

Figure 71-2. Diffuse fatty infiltration of the liver. *A*, Sagittal scan. The liver (L) is markedly more echogenic than the kidney (K). *B*, Transverse scan. There is decreased conspicuity of the portal vein *(arrow)*, and the sound beam fails to penetrate through the liver.

Figure 71-3. Hepatic hemangioma. On this sagittal scan, a well-circumscribed echogenic lesion *(arrow)* is seen in the left lobe of the liver, typical for hemangioma.

6. **What are the possible growth patterns of hepatocellular carcinoma? When should one highly consider the diagnosis?**

   Hepatocellular carcinoma may be solitary, multifocal, or infiltrative. Although sonographic features are generally nonspecific, invasion of the hepatic or portal veins is a feature commonly associated with hepatocellular carcinoma. True invasion can be differentiated from bland (nonneoplastic) thrombus by detecting arterial flow within the thrombus using Doppler imaging or by showing enhancement of the thrombus on computed tomography (CT) or magnetic resonance imaging (MRI).

   Additionally, hepatocellular carcinoma occurs almost exclusively in patients with cirrhosis, so the presence of a mass in a cirrhotic liver should be considered hepatocellular carcinoma until proven otherwise.

7. **What are the sonographic findings of cirrhosis?**
   A nodular liver surface is highly suggestive of cirrhosis. Findings of portal hypertension—including ascites, splenomegaly, portal vein enlargement, and recanalization of the paraumbilical veins—are also indicative of cirrhosis.

8. **In addition to location, what imaging features help to differentiate focal fatty infiltration from a mass lesion?**
   Focal fatty infiltration does not exert mass effect on the hepatic vessels and tends to have a more geographic distribution.

9. **Describe the sonographic appearance of gallstones.**
   A gallstone demonstrates a curvilinear, hyperechoic (bright) leading edge with posterior acoustic shadowing (Fig. 71-4). The posterior shadowing is caused by absorption of the sound beam by the gallstones and should be seen with stones bigger than 3 mm. Gallstones are also typically mobile, although they may occasionally adhere to the gallbladder wall.

Figure 71-4. Gallstones, sagittal scan. Characteristics of gallstones include a curvilinear, echogenic leading edge and posterior acoustic shadowing.

10. **What is meant by the WES sign?**
    The wall-echo-shadow (WES) sign may be seen when the gallbladder is completely filled with stones (Fig. 71-5). This sign consists of two curvilinear structures followed by a shadow. The first line is hypoechoic and represents the gallbladder wall. The second is echogenic, representing multiple gallstones, with their associated shadowing making up the third portion of the sign. The WES sign may be difficult to differentiate from a gas-filled bowel loop.

Figure 71-5. The WES complex consists of a hypoechoic line *(arrow)*, which represents the gallbladder wall, followed by an echogenic line *(*)*, which represents the leading edge of the gallstones, and posterior shadowing *(arrowheads)*.

11. **How does the sonographic appearance of gallstones differ from that of other intraluminal abnormalities?**
Like gallstones, tumefactive sludge (sludge balls) is typically mobile but does not shadow. Gallbladder polyps are nonmobile and do not shadow.

12. **What is the normal gallbladder wall thickness, and what diseases can produce gallbladder wall thickening?**
The normal thickness of the gallbladder wall is 3 mm or less. Gallbladder wall thickening may be seen in a number of disease processes, both of biliary and nonbiliary origin. Biliary causes of gallbladder wall thickening include acute or chronic cholecystitis, adenomyomatosis, AIDS cholangiopathy, sclerosing cholangitis, and gallbladder carcinoma. The nonbiliary causes include hepatitis, cirrhosis, portal hypertension, hypoproteinemia, and heart failure.

13. **Describe the sonographic signs of early or uncomplicated acute cholecystitis.**
Sonographic findings in early or uncomplicated acute cholecystitis may include gallstones (which may be impacted in the gallbladder neck or cystic duct), gallbladder wall thickening, and gallbladder distention. A sonographic Murphy's sign (focal tenderness over the gallbladder when compressed by the ultrasound transducer) may also be elicited. The combination of gallstones and a sonographic Murphy's sign has a positive predictive value of 92% and a negative predictive value of 95% for acute cholecystitis.

14. **What additional findings may be seen in advanced or complicated cholecystitis?**
Signs of advanced acute cholecystitis include pericholecystic fluid, a striated appearance of the thickened gallbladder wall, and intraluminal membranes caused by sloughed gallbladder mucosa (Fig. 71-6).

Emphysematous cholecystitis is most commonly seen in elderly patients with diabetes, in whom the gallbladder becomes infected by gas-producing organisms. The presence of gas in the gallbladder wall or lumen results in the presence of bright reflections along the nondependent portion of the gallbladder wall, with "dirty" posterior shadowing.

Figure 71-6. Cholecystitis. Sagittal *(A)* and transverse *(B)* scans. The gallbladder wall is thickened and striated *(arrows)*. Two gallstones (g) are present, one of which (denoted by the *asterisk*) is impacted in the gallbladder neck. The liver (L) and right kidney (K) are also seen.

15. **Describe the three sonographic appearances of gallbladder carcinoma. Which is the most common?**
Most commonly, gallbladder carcinoma appears as a soft tissue mass centered in the gallbladder fossa, completely or partially replacing the gallbladder lumen. In a minority of cases, gallbladder carcinoma may also appear as asymmetric gallbladder wall thickening or as a polypoid intraluminal mass. In the latter case, the mass is usually larger than 1 cm, which helps to distinguish it from benign cholesterol polyps.

16. **What malignancy has the highest propensity to metastasize to the gallbladder?**
Melanoma.

17. **What is the normal measurement of the common duct?**
The normal common duct (a term used to generally refer to both the common hepatic duct and common bile duct since these are difficult to distinguish sonographically) may vary in size based on the patient's age and cholecystectomy status and and where the measurement is taken. However, in general, the normal common duct should measure less than 7 mm in patients younger than 60. In older patients and patients who have had previous cholecystectomy, the common duct should measure less than 10 mm.

18. **Name three causes of extrahepatic biliary dilation.**
Choledocholithiasis, biliary stricture, and tumor within or adjacent to the biliary tree.

19. **Does a normal-appearing pancreas exclude the diagnosis of pancreatitis?**
No. Although the pancreas may be diffusely or focally enlarged and hypoechoic in patients with pancreatitis, it may also have a normal appearance.

20. **Since the pancreas may appear normal in pancreatitis, what is the role of sonography in patients suspected of having pancreatitis?**
One major role of sonography is to evaluate for the presence of stones in the biliary tree as the cause of pancreatitis, which may alter clinical management of a patient with pancreatitis. Additionally, sonography can evaluate for complications of pancreatitis, such as peripancreatic fluid collections and pseudocysts, thrombosis of the splenic or superior mesenteric vein, and pseudoaneurysm formation.

21. **What is the differential diagnosis of a hypoechoic pancreatic mass lesion?**
The top two considerations of a hypoechoic pancreatic mass lesion are pancreatic adenocarcinoma and focal pancreatitis (Fig. 71-7). A helpful finding in differentiating these is the presence of vascular encasement or metastases, which would support the diagnosis of adenocarcinoma. Pancreatic ductal dilation may be seen in either process, although the obstructed pancreatic duct in adenocarcinoma is typically smoothly dilated, whereas the duct in chronic pancreatitis most often has an irregular appearance. Other differential diagnostic considerations include islet cell tumors, pancreatic lymphoma, metastases, and peripancreatic lymph nodes.

22. **What are the two major types of cystic pancreatic neoplasm?**
Serous pancreatic cystadenoma, also known as "microcystic adenoma," usually presents as a large pancreatic mass made up of multiple small cysts. A calcified central scar may be present. This lesion is benign, most commonly located within the pancreatic tail and most commonly seen in elderly women.

Mucinous pancreatic tumors (macrocystic adenomas) either have malignant potential or are frankly malignant. They are typically made up of fewer larger cysts, which may contain internal septations or mural nodules. These are most common in middle-aged women and most often occur in the pancreatic body or tail.

Figure 71-7. Hypoechoic mass (M) in the pancreatic tail, transverse scan. The remainder of the pancreas (P) is normal in appearance. Note the liver (L) anterior to the pancreas and the splenic vein *(arrow)* posterior to the pancreas. A small portion of the pancreatic duct is seen *(arrowhead)*.

23. **What genetic diseases are associated with pancreatic cysts?**
    Von Hippel-Lindau disease is an autosomal dominant disease associated with pancreatic cysts and neoplasms, as well as cerebellar, retinal, and spinal cord hemangioblastomas; renal cysts; renal cell carcinoma; and pheochromocytoma. Autosomal dominant polycystic kidney disease may be associated with pancreatic cysts in less than 5% of cases.

24. **Describe the normal sonographic appearance of a kidney.**
    Kidneys have a more complex sonographic appearance than the other abdominal organs (Fig. 71-8). The central renal sinus is predominantly composed of fat and therefore appears hyperechoic on ultrasound. Occasionally, renal blood vessels or the collecting system may be seen as anechoic tubular structures within the sinus. The renal pyramids are hypoechoic triangular or slightly rounded structures that abut the renal sinus. The renal cortex is slightly more echogenic than the renal pyramids. The renal cortex should be equally or less echogenic than the liver and much less echogenic than the spleen. In normal adults, the kidneys should measure between 9 and 13 cm in length.

Figure 71-8. Normal sagittal image of the kidney. Note the normal renal architecture, which includes the echogenic renal sinus (S), the intermediately echogenic renal cortex (C), and the hypoechoic medullary pyramids *(arrows)*. The renal cortex is slightly less echogenic than the liver (L), which is normal.

25. **What is the main function of ultrasound in the setting of acute renal failure?**
    Ultrasound is very beneficial in determining whether urinary obstruction is present. Although urinary obstruction is a relatively uncommon cause of acute renal failure (accounting for approximately 5% of cases), early detection and treatment are critical to prevent permanent damage to the kidneys.

26. **What are the sonographic findings of obstruction?**

The sonographic hallmark for the diagnosis of obstruction is the detection of hydronephrosis (Fig. 71-9). A dilated renal collecting system appears as multiple anechoic structures conforming to the expected location of the renal calyces, all connecting with a dilated renal pelvis centrally. Patients with other processes, such as prior obstruction, pregnancy, bladder distention, vesicoureteral reflux, and diuresis, can also present with a dilated collecting system. The lack of ureteral jets in the bladder and elevated resistive indices can be helpful in differentiating acute obstruction from these other processes.

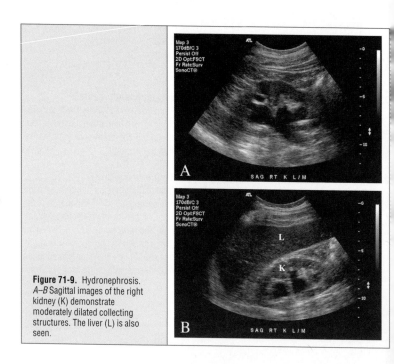

Figure 71-9. Hydronephrosis. *A–B* Sagittal images of the right kidney (K) demonstrate moderately dilated collecting structures. The liver (L) is also seen.

27. **Describe the sonographic appearance of renal calculi.**

Renal stones appear as hyperechoic foci within the renal sinus. Stones of sufficient size will demonstrate posterior acoustic shadowing, whereas smaller stones may not. Technical factors such as transducer frequency, focal zone depth, and beam width should be optimized to maximize the chance of detecting a shadow. Because the renal sinus is normally echogenic, renal stones are more difficult to detect sonographically than gallstones, which are surrounded by fluid. The composition of a renal calculus does not affect its sonographic appearance.

28. **What is the most common renal mass lesion?**

The ultrasound characteristics of simple cysts, liver, kidney, or elsewhere, are described in Table 71–1. They are present in up to 50% of people older than 50. The characteristics of simple cysts are described in the liver section. Cysts that contain thin internal septations, small peripheral thin calcification, or hemorrhagic or proteinaceous debris are termed *minimally complex cysts*, and, like simple cysts, are benign. The presence of thick septations or more extensive calcification is more suggestive of a cystic renal neoplasm and should be further evaluated with dedicated renal CT or MRI or followed up closely with ultrasound to evaluate for growth.

29. **Are any diseases associated with renal cysts?**
Yes. See Table 71-2 and Figure 71-10.

TABLE 71-2.	DISEASES ASSOCIATED WITH RENAL CYSTS		
Disease	**Cyst Characteristics**	**Associated Renal Abnormalities**	**Other Organ System Involvement**
Autosomal dominant polycystic disease	Multiple cysts of various sizes; hemorrhage into cysts common	Enlarged kidneys, renal failure, hypertension	Liver and pancreatic cysts, cerebral berry aneurysms
Acquired cystic disease	Multiple small cysts; hemorrhage common	Occurs in dialysis patients; kidneys are small and echogenic; increased risk of renal cell carcinoma	
Von Hippel-Lindau disease	Multiple bilateral renal cysts; risk of neoplasm arising in cyst walls	Multiple bilateral renal cell carcinomas	Cerebellar and spinal cord hemangioblastomas, retinal angiomas, pancreatic cysts and neoplasms, pheochromo-cytomas
Tuberous sclerosis	Cysts develop most commonly in infancy and childhood	Multiple bilateral angiomyolipomas	Mental retardation, seizures, central nervous system tumors, cardiac rhabdomyomas, pulmonary lymphangiomy-omatosis

Figure 71-10. Autosomal dominant polycystic kidney disease. Sagittal scan of the right kidney. The normal renal parenchyma is replaced by cysts of varying sizes.

30. **What is the most common solid renal mass? Describe its imaging features.**
Renal cell carcinoma is the most common solid renal mass. Most renal cell carcinomas are slightly hyperechoic or isoechoic to the renal parenchyma. Approximately 10% are hypoechoic, and another 10% are much more echogenic than the normal kidney. They may contain areas of calcification, necrosis, or hemorrhage. Predominantly cystic renal cell carcinomas also occur but are uncommon. Renal cell carcinoma has a propensity to invade the renal veins and inferior vena cava, and these should be evaluated in patients with a solid renal mass. Other neoplasms, both benign and malignant, may involve the kidney and produce a solid mass.

31. **What is the differential diagnosis for a markedly echogenic renal mass?**
Angiomyolipomas are usually well-defined, markedly hyperechoic renal masses. These benign lesions consist of varying degrees of fat, vessels, and muscle; it is the presence of fat that accounts for the hyperechoic appearance. However, as previously noted, a minority of renal cell carcinomas may also be much more echogenic than the renal parenchyma. Therefore, malignancy must also be considered in the differential diagnosis of a hyperechoic renal mass.
   The presence of posterior acoustic shadowing without calcification is more suggestive of angiomyolipoma, whereas areas of calcification or cystic regions would suggest renal cell carcinoma. Nevertheless, CT or MRI is usually indicated to further characterize these lesions.

KEY POINTS: DIAGNOSES TO CONSIDER FOR A SOLID RENAL MASS

1. Renal carcinoma is the most common cause.

2. Angiomyolipoma (AML) is usually hyperechoic, but some carcinomas mimic AML on ultrasound.

3. Other neoplasms include oncocytoma, renal lymphoma, transitional cell carcinoma of the renal collecting system, and metastasis to the kidney.

32. **Does pyelonephritis have a characteristic appearance on sonography?**
Most patients with pyelonephritis have normal-appearing kidneys on ultrasound. In more severe cases, there may be focal areas of masslike enlargement or heterogeneous echotexture of the kidneys. The most important role of sonography in pyelonephritis, however, is in excluding complications, such as renal or perinephric abscess or urinary obstruction.

33. **What is meant by renal parenchymal disease?**
Renal parenchymal disease, or medical renal disease, is a term used to describe kidneys of increased cortical echogenicity (Fig. 71-11). Kidneys that are more echogenic than the liver or equal to or greater than the spleen are too echogenic. Numerous disease processes result in this same sonographic appearance, and biopsy may be necessary to differentiate among them when clinically appropriate. Renal size is helpful to differentiate acute from chronic renal disease.

Figure 71-11. Renal parenchymal disease. Sagittal *(A)* and transverse *(B)* images demonstrate the right kidney to be much more echogenic than the liver. Also note the upper pole renal cyst, with its typical features of an anechoic lumen, well-defined posterior wall, and increased through-transmission *(arrows)*.

BIBLIOGRAPHY

1. Bennett GL, Balthazar EJ: Ultrasound and CT evaluation of emergent gallbladder pathology. Radiol Clin North Am 41(6):1203–1216, 2003.
2. Kurtz A, Middleton W: Ultrasound: The Requisites. St. Louis, Mosby, 1996.
3. Rumack CM, Wilson CR, Charboneau JW (eds): Diagnostic Ultrasound, 2nd ed. St. Louis, Mosby, 1998.

TRAINING PATHWAYS IN DIAGNOSTIC IMAGING

E. Scott Pretorius, MD

CHAPTER 72

1. **What is the usual training pathway to become a radiologist in the United States?**
   After medical school, candidates complete an internship (PGY-1). After internship, radiology residency is 4 years (PGY 2-5). Most residents choose to pursue fellowship subspecialist training after residency. In most cases, this takes 1 year (PGY-6), but most neuroradiology fellowships and pediatric radiology fellowships take 2 years.

2. **Do I have to match for a separate preliminary year?**
   In most cases, yes. There are a few radiology programs that are affiliated with specific preliminary years, but most allow candidates to train in any accredited PGY-1 year (most commonly transitional, medicine, or surgery; less commonly obstetrics/gynecology, pediatrics, family medicine, emergency medicine, or neurology). The American Board of Radiology (ABR) requires at least 9 months of clinical training. Candidates seeking board certification in radiology must complete both this clinical requirement and training requirements in diagnostic radiology. The requirement in clinical training may be met by internship in any of the fields mentioned above.

3. **Is it difficult to get a residency position in diagnostic radiology?**
   Yes. Diagnostic radiology has become one of the most competitive fields in which to match. It is not unusual for top programs to receive 100 applications for every open spot.

4. **What can I do to help my chances of matching in radiology?**
   For starters, do extremely well in medical school and score high on the United States Medical Licensing Examination (USMLE). Demonstrate commitment to the field by undertaking a research project in radiology. If you are interested in a particular program, try to make personal connections to people in that department. Some of the ways to do this include an audition elective rotation or a research project.

5. **What information should my personal statement contain?**
   Ideally, the personal statement includes information about how you came to this point in life—applying for radiology residency—and also tells something about where you expect your medical training to lead you. Do you see yourself in academic practice or private practice? What are your reasons for choosing radiology? Explain to your reader—without succumbing to arrogance—what personal qualities or achievements might separate you from other applicants.

6. **Does it matter who writes my letters of recommendation?**
   Many candidates aspire to have a letter from a particular well-known physician in their institution. That's fine, as long as he or she knows you well and is comfortable writing a very strong letter for you. In medicine, though, fame is often local or regional, and the surgeon who is "famous" in Los Angeles likely will be unknown to radiologists in Philadelphia. In general, you are better off soliciting letters from physicians who know you very well and who are comfortable writing very positive things about you.

7. **Do I need letters of recommendation from radiologists?**
   At least one of your letters should be from a radiologist. Without at least one such letter, it may appear that pursuing radiology is something that has only recently occurred to you and that you

have not investigated the field. You should not, however, feel that all of your letters need to come from radiologists. Again, you should choose people who know you very well.

If you are an MD PhD, at least one of your letters should come from someone who has worked with you on a clinical service. As spectacular as your research may be, you will be spending the majority of your residency working with patients and interacting with clinicians. Applicants who have only references from their laboratory experiences place themselves at a disadvantage.

8. **Are radiology positions offered outside of the National Resident Matching Program (NRMP) match?**
The vast majority of positions in radiology are offered through the NRMP match (www.nrmp.org). Positions available outside of the match very occasionally become available when residents choose to switch specialties or leave medicine altogether.

Residency programs that are part of the NRMP match are not allowed to offer positions to U.S. senior medical students outside of the match. International medical graduates or U.S. medical graduates who are not seniors (e.g., candidates who previously went unmatched or who matched in some other field but now wish to switch to radiology) may accept such offers. Such positions, however, are extremely rare.

9. **To how many residency programs should I apply?**
It depends on how competitive an applicant you are. If you are in the top 10% of your class in a good medical school with USMLE scores of 250 or more, you should feel comfortable applying to 12–15 top programs only. If you are a less competitive applicant, you should consider widening your application pool; 30 applications are not unreasonable for someone who is a good-but-not-spectacular applicant.

If you are in the bottom half of your class, even at a top-ranked school with average USMLE scores, you need to seriously consider less competitive residencies at regional or community hospitals. If you have geographic restrictions due to spouse, family, or some other reason, you should apply to absolutely every program in that geographic area and be willing to go anywhere you match. Almost all programs use the Electronic Residency Application Service of the Association of American Medical Colleges (www.aamc.org/students/eras/start.htm).

10. **To what kind of residency programs should I apply?**
Radiology residency programs are designed to train physicians for either academic medicine or private practice. If you want to work in academic medicine, you should go someplace where you will get dedicated research time, training in research methods, and opportunities to develop teaching skills. Such programs often offer opportunities to develop subspecialty interests during your residency training.

Programs such as these are not optimal for training people for private practice. For that, you are better off going to programs that focus on clinical work only. You want places that have few or no fellows so that all procedures are available for residents, since you will need those experiences to develop broad and versatile clinical skills.

11. **How do I become board-certified in diagnostic radiology?**
You must pass the written and oral examinations of the ABR (www.theabr.org). The written examination consists of a physics portion and a clinical portion. You may take the physics portion in your second, third, or fourth year of radiology training. The clinical written portion is taken in the fall of your fourth year, and the oral examination is taken in Louisville, Kentucky, in June of your fourth year of residency.

12. **I am an international medical graduate. What must I do to apply for a diagnostic radiology residency position in the United States?**
You must be a medical school graduate and be certified by the Educational Commission for Foreign Medical Graduates (www.ecfmg.org). You should take at least USMLE Step 1. If you

KEY POINTS: TRAINING PATHWAYS IN DIAGNOSTIC IMAGING

1. Not every residency is right for every person.

2. Consider your ultimate career goals and the residency's curriculum before ranking or applying to a program.

have completed a clinical year in your home country, that training, in most cases, can be counted as your clinical year toward ABR certification. Most radiology programs, though, are inundated with applicants and, in general, prefer candidates who have done some part of their training in the United States or Canada. You may, therefore, wish to complete a U.S./Canadian internship, even if you have completed similar training in your home country.

Some international medical graduate candidates may have completed all training requirements in diagnostic radiology in their home country. Even so, if such an individual wishes to become certified by the ABR, he or she must complete a U.S./Canadian residency or must serve as a resident and/or faculty member for 4 consecutive years in the same Accreditation Council for Graduate Medical Education/Royal College of Physicians and Surgeons of Canada (ACGME/RCPSC)–accredited institution to become eligible to take the ABR's examination (www.theabr.org/DRAppAndFeesinFrame.htm).

13. **What is a research track residency position?**
Research track residency positions allow candidates to use 1 of their 4 years of radiology training to do research. Such positions are relatively new but are increasing in number and are offered primarily by large, academic, research-driven departments. This is different from the Holman track, in which candidates complete 2 full years of research (www.theabr.org/Holman.htm).

14. **Do I have to complete a fellowship after residency?**
Fellowship is not required, but approximately 70% of residency graduates pursue fellowship training. Failure to complete a fellowship may place one at a competitive disadvantage in the job market. Fellowship training is virtually required at most academic institutions to secure an academic appointment.

15. **In what subspecialties is fellowship training offered?**
Interventional radiology, neuroradiology, thoracic imaging, musculoskeletal radiology, nuclear medicine, magnetic resonance imaging (MRI), breast imaging, abdominal imaging (ultrasound, computed tomography, and MRI), women's imaging (mammography, ultrasound, and usually MRI).

16. **What is the training pathway for nuclear medicine?**
Nuclear imaging is studied as part of diagnostic radiology residency and graduates of diagnostic radiology residencies may practice nuclear medicine. However, one may also pursue nuclear medicine alone. An internship (PGY-1) is required, and candidates then spend 2 more years (PGY-2 and 3) pursuing residency training in nuclear medicine.

17. **How I do I become board-certified in nuclear medicine?**
Candidates must pass the written examination of the American Board of Nuclear Medicine (ABNM). To be eligible, a candidate must have completed an intern year, followed by 2 years of training in a nuclear medicine residency. Candidates who have completed an internship and a diagnostic radiology residency may take the ABNM examination after completion of a 1-year

fellowship in nuclear imaging. Such candidates are eligible to seek board certification from both the ABR and ABNM.

18. **What is a certificate of added qualification (CAQ)?**
The ABR offers CAQs to appropriately trained persons in certain subspecialties, including nuclear radiology, vascular and interventional radiology, neuroradiology, and pediatric radiology. Attainment of this distinction requires completion of fellowship training, clinical experience, and passage of an oral examination.

WEBSITES

1. http://www.theabr.org
2. http://www.theabr.org/DRAppAndFeesinFrame.htm
3. http://www.ecfmg.org
4. http://www.aamc.org/students/eras/start.htm
5. http://www.theabr.org/Holman.htm
6. http://www.nrmp.org
7. http://www.abnm.org

CHAPTER 73

MEDICOLEGAL ISSUES IN DIAGNOSTIC IMAGING

Saurabh Jha, MBBS

"There but for the grace of God, go I."—John Bradford, Heretic, 1550 AD

1. **Define *medical negligence.***
   Negligence is the failure to possess and apply the knowledge that is possessed or applied by reasonable physicians practicing in similar circumstances.

2. **What must be proven for a physician to be found liable for malpractice?**
   - Establishment of a duty of care (i.e., physician-patient relationship)
   - Breach of the duty of care, or negligence
   - Adverse outcome with injury or harm
   - Direct causality between the negligence and outcome

KEY POINTS: LEGAL REQUIREMENTS FOR A FINDING OF MALPRACTICE

1. Establishment of a duty of care (i.e., physician-patient relationship)

2. Breach of the duty of care, or negligence

3. Adverse outcome with injury or harm

4. Direct causality between the negligence and outcome

3. **Outline the history behind current malpractice law. What is unique about the legal determination of medical negligence in the United States?**
   The relevant legal framework in the United States originates from the work of Sir William Blackstone, a renowned English legal scholar whose *Commentaries on the Laws of England,* published in 1768, described the term *mala praxis* for injuries resulting from professional neglect or want of skill, specifically by physicians. Malpractice is derived from this term.

   Malpractice law is part of the *tort,* or personal-injury, law. The *plaintiff* (injured party) files a suit against the *defendant* (physician) in a civil court in front of a *jury* composed of ordinary (not belonging to the medical profession) citizens. This adversarial system is different from the practice in countries such as the United Kingdom or Germany, where medical negligence is adjudicated by a panel of judges or medical experts.

4. **What factors have been responsible for the expansion of medical litigation in the United States?**
   The ethos of marketplace professionalism (no special status to medical societies) and antiegalitarian sentiments of the early 19th century forced physicians to raise the level of their professionalism and medical organizations to stipulate standards of practice that, ironically, would be

used against them. Medical innovations made physicians victims of their own advancement. Liability insurance ensured an available financial pool for compensation. Plaintiffs had nothing to lose by filing a lawsuit due to the contingent "no win–no fees" basis of legal representation and due to the fact that both adversarial parties had to bear their own legal costs regardless of the outcome.

5. **There can be no malpractice without established practice. Who sets the established practice? Who determines whether the established practice has been breached?**
   The expected standard may be defined in textbooks, other medical literature, or stated by professional organizations such as the American Medical Association and the American College of Radiology. It is the jury who decides whether a physician's conduct is below that expected of a reasonable physician. However, it is the *expert witness* (an individual of the same or similar clinical discipline as the defendant) who outlines the standard to which the physician should be held. The attorneys for both the plaintiff and defendant can retain an expert witness.

6. **Will a general radiologist who misses a lesion on a brain magnetic resonance (MR) image be held to the standard of a neuroradiologist?**
   No. The legal requirement is that the radiologist must possess the knowledge and skill that is ordinarily possessed by a reasonable peer. He or she is not required to possess the highest skill level to which some aspire. A general radiologist will be held to the standard of a reasonable generalist but not a specialist.

7. **The average plaintiff award in the United States is $3.5 million. What are the types of damage awarded by the jury? What is the aim of the award?**
   The ethos behind the jury award is restitution, not punishment. The award aims to compensate the patient and to deter further such episodes of negligence from occurring.
   Three types of damages are considered: (1) *economic losses,* such as the injured plaintiff's health care costs and loss of wages; (2) *noneconomic losses,* such as pain and suffering; and, very rarely, (3) *punitive* damages for cases in which the defendant demonstrated wanton disregard for the plaintiff's well-being.

8. **Can an exculpatory waiver signed by a patient shield the physician of a certain degree of liability?**
   It is common for instructional facilities for scuba diving, skydiving, and similar risky activities to ask participants to sign *exculpatory waivers* shielding them from lawsuits if injury or death results. Such a waiver implies a *"contract"* because the parties have theoretically agreed in advance on acceptable and unacceptable outcomes. However, the *patient-physician relationship* is not a contract but rather is a professional bond in which the physician assumes a position of responsibility as the possessor of knowledge and skill beyond the ordinary toward patients who may not know their own best interests. Thus, the signing of a waiver by a patient does not alter the legal course when medical negligence is alleged.

9. **A radiologist in an outpatient facility reads radiographs without ever meeting the patients. Does he or she still form a physician-patient relationship?**
   Although a physician-patient relationship typically is a consensual one, a radiologist forms that relationship when he or she renders an interpretation on an imaging study for the patient. This is true even if the radiologist never meets or speaks with the patient or referring physician. This is important to appreciate because the basis of any malpractice claim is the establishment of a duty of care by formation of a physician-patient relationship.

10. **It is estimated that in any given year a lawsuit may be brought against 1 in 10 radiologists. What are the most common reasons radiologists get sued?**
    There are three major categories:
    - Failure of diagnosis (includes perceptual errors, insufficient knowledge, incorrect judgment, and failure to correct poor patient positioning and exposure)
    - Failure to communicate findings in an appropriate and timely manner
    - Failure to suggest the next appropriate procedure

    Of these, failure to diagnose is the largest cause (70%), and two thirds of these cases are due to perceptual errors.

KEY POINTS: THE MOST COMMON REASONS RADIOLOGISTS ARE SUED

1. Failure to diagnose

2. Failure to communicate findings in an appropriate and timely manner

3. Failure to suggest the next appropriate procedure

---

11. **What are the groundbreaking findings of the Institute of Medicine's report *To Err is Human: Building a Safer Health System?***
    The report, published in 2000, received much media interest and put medical errors in the spotlight. On reviewing the 1984 patient files of New York hospitals and the 1992 files of Colorado and Utah hospitals retrospectively for adverse events, the report concluded that medical error alone could account for 44,000 to 98,000 deaths annually in American hospitals. This figure exceeds the number of deaths attributable annually to AIDS, motor vehicle accidents, or breast cancer.

12. **Radiology has its unique set of errors. What is the most common radiologic error? How often is this error estimated to occur?**
    Failure-to-diagnose errors, which are the most common, are of two major types: *cognitive,* in which an abnormality is seen but its nature is misinterpreted (e.g., an infiltrate on a chest x-ray that represents cancer is interpreted as pneumonia), and *perceptual,* or the "miss," in which a radiologic abnormality is simply not seen by the radiologist on initial interpretation.

    Since Garland's seminal study in 1944, in which he found significant interobserver and intraobserver variation in the interpretation of chest x-rays by radiologists, several studies have confirmed that perceptual errors occur at an alarmingly high frequency. A University of Missouri study in 1976 reported an average error rate of 30% among experienced radiologists interpreting chest, bone, and gastrointestinal radiographs.

13. **What is hindsight bias? Why is it important medicolegally?**
    Medicolegally, radiology is unique in that the evidence for examination (the image) remains for subsequent scrutiny, unlike physical examination findings or findings at endoscopy. It also lends itself to a phenomenon known as the *hindsight bias*—the tendency for people with knowledge of the actual event to believe falsely that they would have predicted the correct outcome.

    On 90% of chest films of patients with lung cancer that were reported as normal, the cancer was seen in hindsight. When a radiologist makes a perceptual error and the finding is subsequently seen, it is difficult to determine whether the finding was only seen in retrospect and in lieu of all the clinical information. In other words, it is difficult to determine when a "miss" is negligent and when it is simply an error of perception.

14. **What are some ways to minimize the occurrence of perceptual errors?**
    - Adequate radiographic technique
    - Appropriate clinical history: the knowledge of the site of pain reduces the "miss" of subtle fractures by 50%
    - Comparison with old studies whenever possible
    - Avoidance of *"satisfaction of search,"* where the presence of an overt finding diminishes the chances of making a second, more subtle finding
    - Double reading and spending more time examining the radiograph (controversial)
    - Computer-aided detection (still experimental)

15. **In 1997, the Wisconsin Court of Appeals issued a decision that has had a positive effect for radiologists sued for perceptual errors. Outline the decision.**
    Wisconsin's Medical Examining Board sought to revoke the medical license of a radiologist who had been sued for perceptual errors twice in a 10-year career. The case eventually reached the appeals court, which affirmed a decision in favor of the radiologist. The principles of the decision are as follows:
    - Medicine is not an exact science.
    - Error in and of itself is not negligence.
    - A "miss" may not constitute negligence, even if the finding could be determined by a majority of radiologists as long as the radiologist "conformed to the accepted standards of practice."

16. **What is the "Aunt Minnie" approach to film interpretation? How may this approach lead to errors in judgment?**
    The attachment of an interpretation to a radiographic finding with a strong preconceived notion is akin to spotting a familiar face: "I know that's my Aunt Minnie because it looks like my Aunt Minnie!" Researchers believe that such an approach results in errors in interpretation because the self-imposed–limited mindset leads to a failure to include a differential diagnosis. If a diagnosis is not considered, it is not investigated, and if it is not investigated, it is not found.

17. **How may errors in judgment be minimized?**
    - Analyze—not simply recognize—radiographic findings.
    - Keep an open mind; always try to incorporate a differential diagnosis.
    - Expand and maintain a comprehensive knowledge base.
    - Avoid *alliterative errors* (i.e., the influence of another radiologist's opinion). Look at a prior radiograph with a fresh set of eyes.

18. **Explain the following terms in the medicolegal context: proximate cause, law of intervening cause, and joint and several liabilities.**
    - *Proximate cause* is the connection between an alleged act of negligence and the injury sustained by a patient.
    - *Law of intervening cause* is when an intervening act of negligence breaks the causal link between the initial act of negligence and injury.
    - *Joint and several liabilities* is the fact that more than one person can be blamed for an injury (i.e., there can be multiple proximate causes).

    The effect imaging has in clinical decision-making makes radiologists quite vulnerable to erroneous medical decisions of their referring physicians if it can be shown that a radiographic report resulted in an error in subsequent clinical judgment. Radiologists may feel aggrieved at being named a co-defendant and thus ascribed a proximate cause for a plaintiff's injury, given that their report was followed by another's act of negligence, particularly since the referring physician has the bulk of clinical information. However, courts are generally reluctant to allow the law of intervening cause to apply. Their stance is well summarized in an appeals court decision:

Where an original act is negligent and in a natural and continuous sequence produces an injury that would not have taken place without the act, proximate cause is established, and the fact that some other intervening act contributes to the original act to cause injury does not relieve the initial offender from liability. . . .

19. **Explain the following terms in the medicolegal context: vicarious liability and respondeat superior. Who is responsible for the negligent action of a technologist?**

   - *Vicarious liability* is the placing of the negligence of one person on another.
   - *Respondeat superior* is a Latin term meaning "let the superior respond" and is a form of vicarious liability incurred by the employer (hospital or radiologist) due to the negligent acts of employees (nurses, physician assistants, or technologists), with the rationale that since an employer gains financial benefit through the actions of an employee, so should the employer be responsible for any harm as a result of an employee's actions.

   Negligence of the technologist will be vicariously incurred by the employer (i.e., the medical facility [hospital or private medical imaging group]) through the *respondeat superior* principle. However, if the negligence occurs during a procedure when a radiologist is normally present (e.g., fluoroscopy or interventional radiology), the supervising radiologist will be liable through a legal doctrine known as *"borrowed servant"* (the radiologist temporarily assumes authority over the actions of the technologist).

20. **What is meant by the term *res ipsa loquitur*? Give some examples.**

   Res ipsa loquitur means that the "situation speaks for itself" and is a legal concept that asserts that certain acts cannot, by definition, occur without negligence. In such situations, the burden of proof does not rest with the plaintiff. Medicolegal examples include retention of surgical instruments in the body; transfusion complications resulting from administration of the wrong person's blood; and, in radiologic practice, rectal perforation during a barium enema.

21. **A radiologist renders a report on an intensive care unit portable chest x-ray that reads, "Endotracheal tube in the right main bronchus should be withdrawn by 2 inches to lie within distal trachea; left lower lobe atelectasis; otherwise normal." What additional step should the radiologist take?**

   He or she should phone the physician or nurse treating the patient and include this in the final report. The American College of Radiology's Practice Guidelines advise that the radiologist should directly communicate a report to the physician (or other responsible personnel) or the patient (or responsible legal guardian) in the following situations:

   - Discrepancy between the preliminary and final reads, which could affect management
   - Conditions for which immediate treatment is required (e.g., pneumothorax or a misplaced support line)
   - Significant unexpected findings (e.g., cancer)

22. **A radiologist renders a report on a posteroanterior chest x-ray of a 60-year-old man with dyspnea that reads, "Infiltrate in the right lower lobe, likely pneumonia, clinical correlation is advised." Is this report adequate?**

   No. Even though the infiltrate in the right lower lobe may indeed represent pneumonia, malignancy should be considered either as a differential diagnosis or as an etiologic factor of the pneumonia, and the recommendation for follow-up films to ensure diagnostic resolution should be made clear.

   Failure to include a differential diagnosis may lead to an error in judgment. Failure to suggest the next appropriate step is a recognized area for malpractice.

23. **A radiologist renders a report on a barium enema that reads, "Filling defect in the splenic flexure with abrupt shelflike margins, cannot rule out malignancy; colonoscopy may be of help if clinically indicated." What is wrong with this report?**

When a radiologist suspects a malignancy (or any other significant finding), there is no merit in being ambiguous when reporting the findings. The report should use more assertive language (e.g., "Filling defect in the splenic flexure with abrupt shelflike margins, findings are highly suggestive of colonic cancer and should be confirmed with colonoscopy and biopsy. Findings were conveyed to . . .)." Ambiguous reporting can lead to a lawsuit.

24. **A patient develops anaphylactic shock from iodinated contrast material for excretory urography performed to rule out renal calculi. This older examination (rather than the current standard—a noncontrast helical computed tomography [CT] scan) was performed at the insistence of the referring urologist. Who is to blame: the radiologist or urologist?**

The blame lies with the radiologist. Certain risk management principles should be obvious. The radiologist must follow the principle of *"primum non nocere"*—first, do no harm. Try to avoid a hazardous procedure if a safer alternative is available. Even though anaphylaxis is a recognized complication of iodinated contrast, the physician is considered negligent for not using an examination that is safer than an excretory urogram and is at least as equally diagnostic.

It is important for radiologists to keep referring physicians up-to-date with progress in radiology. In this example, the accepted method of diagnosing renal calculi is no longer with excretory urography but with a noncontrast CT scan.

The ultimate responsibility for the performance of a radiographic procedure is the radiologist's, not the referring physician's. This is important to appreciate since it is radiologists who decide which patients should or should not receive iodinated contrast.

25. **A radiologist reports that a trauma lateral cervical spine is "normal except for straightening which could be positional." Later the patient has weakness in the legs and a CT scan shows "fracture-dislocation" at C7/T1—an area not covered by the lateral film. How was the original reading substandard?**

The report did not mention specifically that the C7/T1 junction was not visualized. It is the radiologist's duty to comment on the adequacy (or its absence) of a radiographic examination and to suggest repeat or alternative radiographs. This must be done as a matter of routine, and it must not be assumed that other clinicians will naturally realize the inadequacy of a study.

26. **A radiologist reports an upper gastrointestinal study as follows: "Findings are highly suggestive of a scirrhous carcinoma of the stomach, endoscopy with biopsy is advised." Biopsy results are negative. What should the radiologist do next?**

The radiologist must advise the physician to repeat the biopsy or assume the diagnosis without further pathologic findings. There are a few situations in imaging in which the findings of malignancy are so strong that negative biopsy results do not exclude the diagnosis. Radiologists should be aware of these situations. Conversely, there are situations in which the findings are so typically benign that it would be negligent to advise a biopsy.

27. **Failure to diagnose breast cancer is the number one cause for litigation in radiology. How may one practice safe mammography?**
   - Communicate with the patients about their examination and the need for follow-up. Communicate with referring physicians.
   - Correlate and follow up on pathologic findings.
   - Compare findings with those of old radiographs, not just the most recent ones but even the more remote films.

- Participate in continuing medical education—breast imaging (and most of radiology) is expanding at an alarming pace.
- Comply with the Practice Guidelines of the American College of Radiology.
- Use computer-aided detection (still experimental).

28. **Only 2% of medical negligence injuries result in claims, and only 17% of claims appear to involve negligent injuries. About 60 cents of every malpractice dollar is taken by administrative and legal costs. Clearly the current tort system is inefficient. What are some reforms that have been suggested?**
    - Creating a "no-fault" system, such as worker's compensation; in this case patients would be compensated for all adverse events that are avoidable, even if the event may not be negligent
    - Capping of noneconomic damages (e.g., for pain and suffering)
    - Eliminating the collateral rule, which prohibits jurors from knowing about payments the plaintiffs have already received from other sources
    - Eliminating joint and several liability
    - Eliminating the doctrine of *res ipsa loquitur*
    - Relocating responsibility from a personal to an institutional level (enterprise liability)

BIBLIOGRAPHY

1. American College of Radiology: ACR Standard for Communication: Diagnostic Radiology. In: Standards 2000–01, ACR, Reston, VA, 2001.
2. Berlin L: Malpractice Issues in Radiology, 2nd ed. American Roentgen Ray Society, Leesburg, VA, 2003.
3. Forster H, Schwartz J, DeRenzo E: Reducing legal risk by practicing patient centered medicine. Arch Intern Med 162:1217–1219, 2002.
4. Friedenberg RM: Malpractice reform. Radiology 231:3–6, 2004.
5. Mohr JC: American medical malpractice litigation in historical perspective. JAMA 283:1731–1737, 2000.
6. Muhm JR, Miller WE, Fontana RS, et al: Lung cancer detected during a screening program using four-month chest radiographs. Radiology 148:609–615, 1983.
7. Robinson PJ: Radiology's Achilles' heel: Error and variation in the interpretation of the roentgen image. Br J Radiol 70:1085–1098, 1997.
8. Studdert S: Medical malpractice. N Engl J Med 350:283–292, 2004.

CHAPTER 74

RADIOLOGY ORGANIZATIONS

E. Scott Pretorius, MD

1. **What is the Radiological Society of North America (RSNA)?**
   The mission of the RSNA, founded 1915, is "to promote and develop the highest standards of radiology and related sciences through education and research." The RSNA is the world's largest organization of its kind. The RSNA publishes the "gray journal," *Radiology*. The RSNA's annual meeting is in Chicago during the last week of November or first week of December.

2. **What is the American Roentgen Ray Society (ARRS)?**
   The ARRS was founded in 1900, shortly after Wilhelm Roentgen's discovery of the x-ray, with the stated goal of "advancement of medicine through the science of radiology and its allied sciences." The ARRS publishes the "yellow journal," the *American Journal of Roentgenology,* which has officially shortened its name to *AJR.* The ARRS meets annually in April or May at varying sites throughout the United States and Canada.

3. **What is the Association of University Radiologists (AUR)?**
   The AUR is the organization of academic radiologists. Subgroups of the AUR include the Society of Chairmen of Academic Radiology Departments, the Association of Program Directors in Radiology, and the American Association of Academic Chief Residents in Radiology. The AUR and its constituent organizations meet annually at varying sites throughout the United States and Canada. It publishes the journal *Academic Radiology.*

4. **What is the American Board of Radiology?**
   The American Board of Radiology, based in Tucson, Arizona, is the organization that administers the written and oral examinations in radiology. The diagnostic radiology written examination is given each September at sites throughout the United States and Canada. The diagnostic radiology oral examination is given annually in early June in Louisville, Kentucky.

5. **What is the American College of Radiology (ACR)?**
   The ACR performs several important functions. It accredits sites that perform mammography, ultrasound, nuclear medicine, and magnetic resonance imaging to maintain appropriate quality standards. Through its American College of Radiology Imaging Network (ACRIN), the ACR conducts multicenter studies in diagnostic radiology. Educational CD-ROMS in all subspecialties of radiology are produced by the ACR. Finally, the ACR has an important role in advocacy for the interests of radiologists, medical physicists, and their patients through work with Congress, the Food and Drug Administration, and state and local governments.

6. **What is the American Council of Graduate Medical Education (ACGME)?**
   The ACGME is the body that accredits American residency training programs, both in radiology and all other fields of graduate medical education. The ACGME develops both requirements and guidelines for residency training programs in all fields. Among its most noted recent actions are the limiting of the resident work week to 80 hours and the requirement that diagnostic radiology residencies include 3 months of training in breast imaging.

7. What are the major subspecialty societies in radiology?

There are many subspecialty societies, and most of them have discounted memberships available for medical students and/or residents (Table 74-1).

TABLE 74-1. RADIOLOGY ORGANIZATIONS AND SELECT NATIONAL SOCIETIES

Society	Abbreviation	Journal	Web Site
Radiological Society of North America	RSNA	*Radiology* and *Radiographics*	www.rsna.org
American Roentgen Ray Society	ARRS	*American Journal of Roentgenology (AJR)*	www.arrs.org
American Board of Radiology	ABR	None	www.theabr.org
American College of Radiology	ACR	*Journal of the American College of Radiology (JACR)*	www.acr.org
Society of Nuclear Medicine	SNM	*Journal of Nuclear Medicine (JNM)*	www.snm.org
International Society of Magnetic Resonance in Medicine	ISMRM	*Journal of Magnetic Resonance Imaging (JMRI)* and *Magnetic Resonance in Medicine*	www.ismrm.org
Association of University Radiologists	AUR	*Academic Radiology*	www.aur.org
Society of Interventional Radiology	SIR	*Journal of Vascular and Interventional Radiology (JVIR)*	www.sirweb.org
American Society of Neuroradiology	ASNR	*American Journal of Neuroradiology (AJNR)*	www.asnr.org
Society for Pediatric Radiology	SPR	*Pediatric Radiology*	www.pedrad.org
Society of Breast Imaging	SBI	None	www.sbi-online.org
Society for Computer Applications in Radiology	SCAR	*Journal of Thoracic Imaging*	www.scarnet.org
Society of Thoracic Radiology	STR	*Thoracic Radiology*	www.thoracicrad.org
Society of Skeletal Radiology	SSR	*Skeletal Radiology*	www.skeletalrad.org

Continued

TABLE 74-1.	RADIOLOGY ORGANIZATIONS AND SELECT NATIONAL SOCIETIES—(CONT'D)		
Society	**Abbreviation**	**Journal**	**Website**
American Institute of Ultrasound in Medicine	AIUM	*Journal of Ultrasound in Medicine (JUM)*	www.aium.org
British Institute of Radiology	BIR	*British Journal of Radiology*	www.bir.org.uk
Canadian Association of Radiologists	CAR	*Canadian Association of Radiologists Journal*	www.car.ca
European Association of Radiology	EAR	*European Radiology*	www.eurorad.org
Royal Australian and New Zealand College of Radiologists	RANZCR	*Australasian Radiology*	www.ranzcr.edu.au
Radiological Society of South Africa	RSSA	*South African Journal of Radiology*	www.rssa.co.za

8. **What are the leading academic journals within diagnostic radiology?**
Radiology, the journal of the RSNA, and the *American Journal of Roentgenology*, the journal of the American Roentgen Ray Society, are the two leading general-purpose radiology journals. There are number of important subspecialty journals, including the *Journal of Interventional Radiology, Journal of the American Journal of Neuroradiology (AJNR)*, *Journal of Pediatric Radiology, Magnetic Resonance in Medicine, Journal of Magnetic Resonance Imaging, Abdominal Imaging*, and *Journal of Nuclear Medicine* (*see* Table 74-1).

9. **What is the NIBIB?**
The National Institute of Biomedical Imaging and Bioengineering is the newest research institute within the National Institutes of Health. Its stated mission is to "improve health by promoting fundamental discoveries, design and development, and translation and assessment of technological capabilities." It has become an important source of funding for hypothesis-driven research in the imaging sciences (http://www.nibib.nih.gov).

KEY POINTS: RADIOLOGY ORGANIZATIONS

1. In the United States, the RSNA and ARRS are the two most important general-interest organizations for radiologists and have broad missions in terms of radiology education and research.

2. The American Board of Radiology administers the written and oral examinations that allow candidates to become board-certified in radiology.

3. The ACR accredits sites that perform diagnostic imaging studies and maintains quality standards.

INDEX

Page numbers in **boldface type** indicate complete chapters.

Artery of Adamkiewicz, 383
Arthritis, **300–304**. *See also* Osteoarthritis;
    Rheumatoid arthritis
  bone scans of, 413
  degenerative. *See* Osteoarthritis
  enteropathic, 302
  inflammatory, 300–301
  psoriatic, 301, 302, 303
  Reiter's syndrome-related, 302
  septic, 307, 308–310
    in children, 310
  tuberculous, 311
Asbestos exposure, 542, 543, 544
Asbestosis, 523
Ascites, intraperitoneal metastases-related, 126, 127
Aspergillosis, invasive pulmonary, 508, 509
Aspiration, of foreign bodies, 463–464
Aspirin
  as erosive gastritis cause, 110
  as osteoid osteoma-related pain treatment, 318
Asplenia, 148, 463, 469
Association of University Radiologists (AUR), 604
Astrocytoma
  calcified, 359
  giant cell, 489
  in infants, 490
  pilocytic, 490
  as primary brain tumor, 358
  spinal, 386
Atelectasis, lung cancer-related, 511–512, 514
Atherosclerosis
  as renovascular hypertension cause, 578
  as stroke cause, 367
Atresia
  biliary, differentiated from neonatal hepatitis, 445
  congenital bronchial, 515
  duodenal, intestinal malrotation-related, 469
  esophageal, 472
  urethral, 569
Atria, cardiac
  borders of, 60
  left, enlargement of, 59–60
  septal defects of, 61, 65, 461
    as right-to-left shunts, 424
  thrombus of, 60, 62
Auerbach's plexus, 471
"Aunt Minnie" approach, to radiographic film
  interpretation, 600
Automatic implantable cardioverter defibrillator
  (AICD), 553–554
Autosomal dominant polycystic kidney disease
  (ADPCKD), 18, 188, 481, 482, 589
Autosomal recessive polycystic kidney disease
  (ARPCKD), 18, 188, 481, 482
Axial plane view, 19
  in the knee, 340
Axillary veins, 549
Azathioprine, 190
Azotemia, renovascular hypertension-related, 579

B
Baastrup's disease, 377, 378
"Babygram," 499
"Bamboo spine," 302
"Banana sign," 570–571
Bankart deformity, 321
Barium allergy, 136
Barium enema, 13, **119–136**
  antibiotic prophylaxis prior to, 123
  of colon cancer, 124–126
  of colonic haustra, 119, 120
  of colonic polyps, 123, 124, 125
  complications of, 123
  contraindications to, 122, 136
  double-contrast (air-contrast), 120–122
    of aphthoid ulcers, 128
    for colon cancer screening, 124
    of colonic involvement in endometriosis,
      134
    comparison with virtual colonoscopy, 134
    of diverticulitis, 131, 133
    of ileocecal valve polypoid carcinoma, 125
    of ischemic colitis, 129, 130
    of rectal adenocarcinoma, 125
    of rectal strictures, 130
    of ulcerative colitis, 128, 129
  of Hirschsprung's disease, 471, 472
  hospital's preparation for, 122
  of intussusception, 466, 467
  left side down decubitus view in, 119, 120
  patient positioning during, 120
  single-contrast, 121, 122
    of diverticula, 132
  technique of, 120–136
Barium impaction, 123
Barium studies, 101-109. *See also* Esophagography
  of common variable immunodeficiency, 117
  of duodenal bulb ulcers, 112, 113
  of reflux esophagitis, 107, 108
  small bowel follow-through, 105–106, 114
  of small bowel obstruction, 95
Barium sulfate, 13, 100–101
Barlow maneuver, 494
Behçet's syndrome, 382
"Bell clapper" deformity, 221
Benzodiazepines, 228
Berylliosis, 519, 521
Biceps tendon, 324
  rupture of, 326–327
  tears or dislocations of, 321
Bile ducts
  anatomy of, 262
  biopsy of, 265
  common
    calculi of, 261
    low obstruction of, 264–265
    measurement of, 586
  as "isolated ducts," 264–265
  obstruction of, 261–262